AF866529

TEXTBOOK OF ANESTHESIA

VOLUME 1
FUNDAMENTALS AND CLINICAL FOUNDATIONS

Dr Krunal Bhatt

ALLIED HEALTH PRESS

Textbook of Anesthesia

Volume 1: Fundamentals and Clinical Foundations

Author: **Dr Krunal Bhatt**

Allied Health Press
4164 Lakeshore Road
Burlington ON L7L 1A4
Canada
www.alliedhealthpress.com
Email: orders@arclereducation.com

ISBN: 978-1-77956-785-7

ABOUT THE AUTHOR

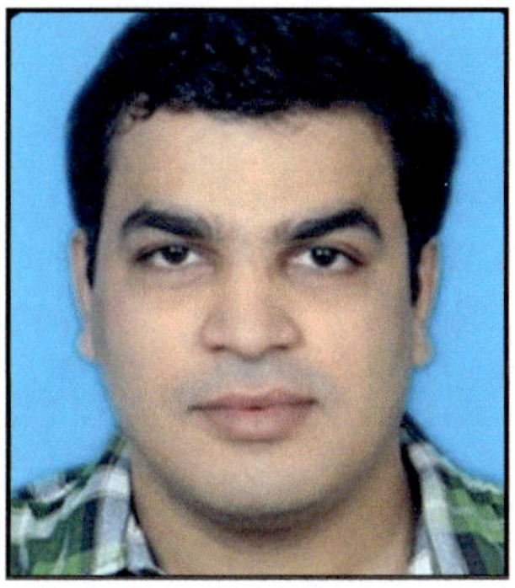

Dr Krunal Bhatt (1982) is presently working at Zydus hospital, Vadodara as a chief clinical intensivist and Anaesthesiologist for one year. He did his MBBS from Baroda Medical College. He has worked as a Medical Officer at various corporate hospitals in Vadodara (2006-2009). He joined Indian armed forces and posted to various locations during his tenure (2009-2018). He has served at Pune, Lucknow, Jodhpur, Jammu and Kashmir. He also has obtained Counter Insurgency ops medal and High Altitude serving medals for his serving tenure at line of control in Kashmir. He did his post-graduation in Anaesthesiology from AFMC, Pune, India in 2018. He is life member of Indian Medical Association, Indian Society of Anesthesiology, Indian Society of Critical Care Medicine, ad European Society of Anaesthesia.

Brief Table of Contents

Chapter Openers

A list of Chapter Outline is presented providing a brief Introduction to what will be covered in the chapter.

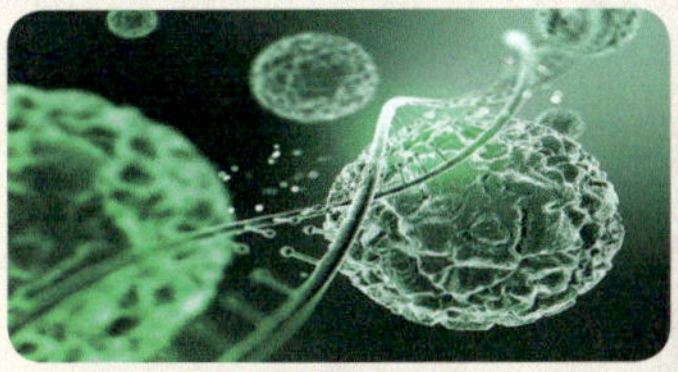

Introduction

Often referred to as the science of life, biology is a broad field of study aimed at comprehending the several kinds of life on Earth, from tiny creatures to sophisticated multicellular entities. Comprising several subfields, including molecular biology, ecology, and evolutionary biology, each of which advances our knowledge of living systems, this field clarifies the mechanisms controlling life events, including development, reproduction, and interaction with the surroundings, which is the central goal of biology. Moreover, biology fills in the void between the natural sciences and medicine by offering a necessary understanding of health, illness, and the interactions between organisms and their environments. Dealing with urgent global issues such as climate change, biodiversity loss, and new diseases depends on an awareness of these complex biological interactions, therefore highlighting the critical part biology plays in modern civilization. Fundamentally, biology explores and tests ideas about the living world using the scientific method. Through methodical observation and experimentation,

LEARNING OBJECTIVES

After studying this chapter, you will be able to:

1. Discuss the scientific method in biology;
2. Explain the cell theory;
3. Discuss the genetics and heredity;
4. Evolution and natural selection;
5. Focus on ecology and ecosystems;
6. Learn about human biology;
7. Evaluate the plant biology;
8. Explain the microbiology;
9. Focus on current trends in biology.

1.1. The Scientific Method in Biology

Learning Outcome

1. Describe the steps of the scientific method;
2. Focus on hypothesis formation;
3. Learn about experimental design.

Learning Outcomes

The beginning of each section of every chapter contains a set of Learning Outcomes that inform students of concepts they should understand. These outcomes help students understand what they should be able to do if they have mastered the material in that section.

Test Your Knowledge

Throughout each chapter, Test Your Knowledge cues you to note which topics have been covered and to self-test your understanding of the material presented.

Test Your Knowledge

1. Explain why correlation does not imply causation in scientific experiments.
2. How does the scientific method help reduce the influence of personal opinions in research?

Chapter Summary

The Summary Section appear at the end of each chapter and summarize main concepts covered throughout the chapter. These points provide key concepts in an engaging and meaningful way.

Summary

The investigation of biological principles highlights the importance of a comprehensive view of life by reflecting the intricate interactions that occur within living systems. The complexity of biology goes beyond individual species or systems, as this essay highlights; it also includes the interactions that mold ecosystems and affect biodiversity. Researchers can conduct in-depth analyses of metabolomic data using sophisticated technologies like MetaboAnalyst, which offer insights into the molecular mechanisms underlying these interactions. As demonstrated by the developments in MetaboAnalyst, for example, the integration of diverse omics data promotes a thorough understanding of metabolic pathways and helps identify important biological markers necessary for research on development and disease (Chong et al., 2018). Additionally, the phenomenon of ecological invasions is a key component of biological research and a vital field of study. The introduction of non-native species into unfamiliar habitats has significant ramifications and calls for multidisciplinary management strategies. Examining the origins and effects of these biological incursions, invasion science has become a crucial field that highlights the need to comprehend ecological dynamics and community interactions. As interest in biological invasions increases, new findings are emerging that put conventional ecological theories and practices to the test. The importance of incorporating various scientific viewpoints is shown by this developing discipline, which also highlights how invasive species shape ecosystems and advances our knowledge of ecological resilience (David et al., 2013). When taken as a whole, these discoveries from invasion science and metabolomics highlight the value of multidisciplinary biology research. Fostering cross-disciplinary collaboration and utilizing technological breakthroughs to improve our comprehension of intricate biological interactions are crucial as we look to the future of biological research. In addition to deepening our understanding of the complexities of life, this method lays the groundwork for tackling urgent environmental issues. Future studies can ensure the continued relevance of biology in a world that is constantly changing by acknowledging the interconnection of biological systems and opening the door to creative solutions that support sustainability and biodiversity conservation. We might imagine a thorough comprehension of life that serves both academia and society at large through ongoing investigation and integration of scientific knowledge.

Knowledge Assessment

The chapter includes material designed to review and reinforce each content. It includes Critical Thinking Questions to help test of your understanding of information presented in the chapter and Short answer Questions to review your understanding of the key concepts presented in the chapter.

Critical Thinking Questions

1. **Who is known as the "Father of Modern Biology"?**
   a. Aristotle
   b. Charles Darwin
   c. Gregor Mendel
   d. Louis Pasteur
2. **What is the basic unit of life?**
   a. Atom
   b. Molecule
   c. Cell
   d. Organism
3. **Which branch of biology studies the interaction of organisms with their environment?**
   a. Genetics
   b. Ecology
   c. Physiology
   d. Botany
4. **Which macromolecule is the main source of energy for living organisms?**
   a. Proteins
   b. Lipids
   c. Carbohydrates
   d. Nucleic acids
5. **DNA is primarily responsible for which function in living organisms?**
   a. Energy production
   b. Protein synthesis
   c. Storing genetic information
   d. Regulating body temperature

Short Answer Questions

1. What is biology, and why is it important to study biology?
2. What are the three main domains of life, and how are they different from one another?
3. Define homeostasis and give an example of how it works in living organisms.
4. What is the cell theory, and why is it fundamental to biology?
5. How do autotrophs and heterotrophs differ in the way they obtain energy?
6. What is the scientific method, and how is it applied in biological research?
7. Discuss how biology helps address global challenges such as climate change, disease, and food security.
8. Explain the levels of biological organization from the smallest unit to the largest. Provide examples at each level.
9. Describe the relationship between structure and function in biology, giving specific examples from cells or organs.
10. How has the discovery of genetics shaped our understanding of inheritance and variation among organisms?

Supplementary Materials

Key Terms: A list of key terms is given for quick reference

KEY TERMS FROM THIS CHAPTER

Annotation enrichment analysis	Biological structure	Cell
Cell theory	Cellular structure	Ecology
Ecosystems	Genetics	Human biology
Microbiology	Natural selection	Organism
Plant biology		

Further Resources: Recommendations for additional readings, websites, and multimedia resources.

References

1. Argelaguet, R., Velten, B., Arnol, D., Dietrich, S., Zenz, T., Marioni, J. C., Buettner, F., et al. (2018). Multi-omics factor analysis—A framework for unsupervised integration of multi-omics data sets. *Molecular Systems Biology, 14*. https://doi.org/10.15252/msb.20178124.
2. Bacher, S., Blackburn, T. M., Essl, F., & Genovesi, P. (2017). *Socio-Economic Impact Classification of Alien Taxa (SEICAT)*. https://core.ac.uk/download/286567949.pdf (accessed on 8th March 2025).
3. Barnett, R., Brace, S., Cucchi, T., & Dobney, K. (2013). *Divergent Evolutionary Processes Associated with Colonization of Offshore Islands*. https://core.ac.uk/download/20664364.pdf (accessed on 8th March 2025).

Detailed Table of Contents

CHAPTER 3

Pharmacology in Anesthesia 69

CHAPTER 4

Preoperative Assessment and Optimization 105

CHAPTER 5

Airway Management in Anesthesia 139

CHAPTER 6

Techniques of Anesthesia 173

CHAPTER 7

Monitoring in Anesthesia 207

CHAPTER 12

Principles of Post-Anesthesia Care 381

Index 413

LIST OF FIGURES

PREFACE

Anesthesia is one of the most significant pillars of modern medicine, revolutionizing the conduct of surgical and diagnostic procedures by offering ways to control pain, alter consciousness, and maintain physiological stability in a humane and safe manner. From its early days using ether and chloroform to advancements in regional, general, and monitored anesthesia care, the specialty has evolved alongside concurrent progress in pharmacology, technology, and clinical practice. The position of anesthesiologist today goes far beyond the operating room, requiring a profound knowledge of systemic physiology, pharmacodynamics, perioperative medicine, and emergency interventions.

As a clinical discipline, anesthesia needs the integration of basic sciences and pragmatic knowledge. Safe administration of anesthesia involves extensive evaluation of the patient, proper selection of technique according to the specific needs of the individual patient, and ongoing monitoring throughout the perioperative course. Anesthetic care, in addition to intraoperative management, involves preoperative assessment, postoperative recovery, and control of acute or chronic pain. For trainees, students, and even practicing clinicians, an organized, comprehensive resource becomes essential for building and honing clinical judgment and decision-making.

Textbook of Anesthesia – Volume 1 has been created to meet this need, with a unifying, practice-oriented introduction to the fundamentals of anesthesia. Guiding readers through basic principles and practices, Volume 1 seeks clarity, clinical relevance, and scientific underpinning. Material has been organized to trace the sequence of anesthetic care chronologically—from introductory principles to practice and technical detail—thereby aiding learning and referral.

Chapter 1 sets forth the history, terminology, and general scope of anesthesia, as well as the specialty's evolution and the many roles of anesthesiologists today. Chapter 2 addresses anatomy and physiology as related to anesthetic care, with special consideration of the systems most salient to anesthetic safety, i.e., the cardiovascular, respiratory, and central nervous systems. Chapter 3 gives the pharmacologic background of anesthesia, which consists of commonly used agents, modes of action, and clinical importance. This includes discussions on induction agents, neuromuscular blocking agents, local anesthetics, and newer adjuvants.

Chapter 4 discusses the preoperative evaluation and optimization process, outlining systematic approaches to risk assessment, management of comorbid conditions, and preparation for surgery. Chapter 5 covers airway management in depth, with detailed discussions of anatomical considerations, devices to assess the airway, and techniques such as endotracheal intubation, supraglottic airway devices, and complex airway algorithms. Chapter 6 introduces the different methods of anesthesia—general, regional, local, and monitored anesthesia care—with emphasis on indications, procedures, and contraindications.

Chapter 7 emphasizes intraoperative monitoring, such as ECG, capnography, blood pressure, oxygen saturation, and depth of anesthesia. It also briefly discusses data interpretation and the use of advanced modalities such as bispectral index and invasive monitoring. Chapter 8 discusses fluid, electrolyte, and blood administration, covering volume resuscitation, maintenance fluids, transfusion practices, and the physiologic effects of fluid shifts during surgery.

Chapter 9 discusses basic pain management, acute pain physiology, assessment, and fundamentals of pharmacologic and non-pharmacologic care. Chapter 10 deals with postpartum pain and recovery with a focus on obstetric complications, labor and cesarean delivery analgesia regimens, and strategies for enhanced maternal recovery. Chapter 11 describes anesthesia complications and emergencies, including airway obstruction, cardiovascular instability, anaphylaxis, and malignant hyperthermia, with step-by-step response algorithms.

Chapter 12 concludes the book with post-anesthesia care principles, including recovery room policies, common postoperative issues, and discharge requirements. The chapter discusses the importance of close observation during recovery and management of common postoperative challenges like nausea, pain, hypoxia, and delirium.

The book is of great help to postgraduate and undergraduate medical students, anesthesia residents, and allied health professionals involved in perioperative care. It is also a handy reference for early-career anesthesiologists who wish to stay up to date.

INTRODUCTION TO ANESTHESIA

1

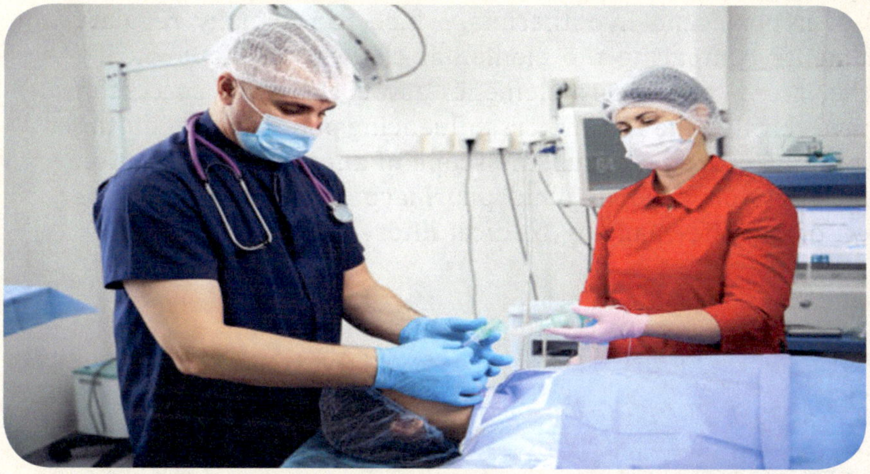

Introduction

Anesthesia is essentially a medical treatment that creates a condition of insensitivity to pain, mainly for the purpose of making surgery and clinical interventions possible. Not only does this sophisticated practice seek to eradicate pain in the course of surgery, but it also creates a temporary loss of consciousness or feeling, depending on the needs of the procedure. The definition is heterogeneous in methods, including general anesthesia, causing reversible loss of consciousness, and regional or local anesthesia acting on a specific segment of the body. The intricacies of such a definition highlight how the practice of anesthesia has developed into a sophisticated science, with advances leading to better patient outcomes. As the profession has evolved, safety and efficacy of anesthetic care have become the burning question, highlighting the need for continuous innovation in techniques and protocols to minimize risks associated with anesthesia (Argo et al., 2019). Anesthetic practice is not problem-free and free of issues, namely issues of morbidity and mortality in patients. With

LEARNING OBJECTIVES

After studying this chapter, you will be able to:

1. Discuss the history of anesthesia
2. Describe the mechanisms of action
3. Discuss the classes of anesthetic agents
4. Know anesthesia administration
5. Highlight risks and complications
6. Understand the advancements in anesthesia

increasing complexities in surgery and patients increasingly older and medically ill, the need for precise definitions in the death cases of anesthesia is a fact. The distinction between "operative deaths" and "anesthetic deaths" gets vague, giving rise to ongoing controversy in the medical community. Whereas preventable deaths have gone down in total, factors such as the patient's pre-existing conditions and intraoperative complications continue to play their part. Addressing these complex problems requires a firm understanding of the consequences and responsibilities involved in anesthetic practice. Clarification of such definitions is thus crucial in informing professional accountability and promoting improvement in anesthesia safety and patient care (Argo et al., 2019). Secondly, anesthesia has been extensively scientifically validated, leading to innovative techniques and technologies. For instance, the induction of artificial hypobiosis is a significant advancement in anesthesia, aimed at regulating physiological conditions to enhance surgical outcomes. This technique relies on the development of hypoxia and hypothermia, which can actually regulate metabolic activity in the body. Experiments comparing the elemental changes in blood during such induced states have identified the micro- and macro-elements associated with successful anesthetic outcomes. Multiple studies have clarified the parameters influencing patient safety during anesthesia, with direct implications for clinical practice. Thus, the scope of anesthesia's definition extends beyond pain relief to include critical physiological and pharmacological considerations required for the proper implementation of this life-changing medical intervention (Figure 1.1).

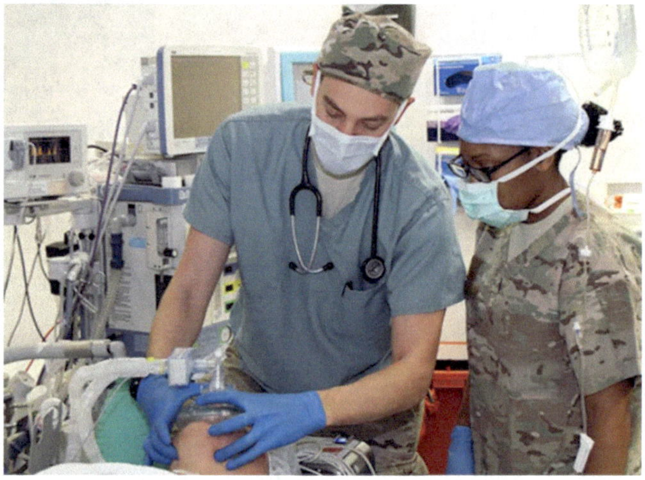

Figure 1.1. Anesthesia is fundamentally defined as a medical intervention.

Source: https://cdn.britannica.com/53/197253-004-630C8542.jpg.

Explanation of Anesthesia and Its Purpose

Anesthesia is a critical part of modern medicine, enabling patients to receive diagnostic and surgical interventions with minimized pain and distress. Anesthesia refers to the administration of drugs that induce temporary loss of consciousness or sensation. Surgeons can now undertake complicated procedures without exposing patients to agony, as anesthesia tends to suppress the body's response to painful stimuli. The primary objective of anesthesia is to render surgical operations painless, but it also aims to maintain essential bodily functions and to maintain physiological balance during surgery. As the world sees advances in pharmacology and technology, anesthetic techniques have advanced, enabling medical professionals to tailor anesthesia to individual patient needs and the nature of the surgery. An interesting feature of anesthesia is the management of neuromuscular block (NMB), which is required for procedures that involve muscle relaxation. Different agents are used in NMB, and the choice of such agents can significantly affect clinical outcomes and healthcare costs. For example, a clinic and cost study of new approaches combining sugammadex and rocuronium showed substantial cost savings in management and improved patient recovery times. In fact, this approach reduced the average cost of NMB management by 36%. It facilitated faster discharge from recovery rooms, demonstrating the twofold nature of anesthesia: enhancing patient comfort and optimizing hospital resource utilization (Baratto et al., 2016). In addition, anesthesia monitoring of levels of consciousness has been further made sophisticated by the introduction of modern technologies. Indices such as qCON and qNOX, based on the electroencephalogram, have been designed to more precisely assess anesthesia depth and sensitivity to stimulation. These provide vital information to anesthesiologists for monitoring to determine whether patients are adequately anesthetized and when they are near recovery. The variable performance of these indices during recovery and induction underscores the nuances of anesthesia administration and underscores the need for continuous monitoring during the procedure (Agustí et al., 2016). Ultimately, the delicate balance among effective anesthesia, patient safety, and cost-effectiveness underscores its relevance in today's surgeries, making it an important area of study and practice in the health sector.

Types of Anesthesia: General, Regional, and Local

The landscape of anesthesia is variegated, comprising three broad categories: general, regional, and local anesthesia. General anesthesia creates a reversible loss of pain perception and sensation throughout the body, and patients are completely unaware during surgeries. General anesthesia is usually applied to major surgeries such as open-heart surgery or massive orthopedic surgery, where maximum immobilization and loss of sensation of pain are essential. Through general anesthesia, the anesthesiologist sustains the desired level by a mix of intravenous agents and inhaled anesthetics. Besides, advances in anesthetic techniques and monitoring have significantly enhanced patient safety during general anesthesia, making it a safe option for complex surgeries. Regional anesthesia, on the other hand, blocks groups of nerves to prevent sensation in a particular region of the body while maintaining consciousness. It is widely employed in procedures such as cesarean section, joint replacement, and certain vascular surgeries. Spinal anesthesia and peripheral nerve block are some examples, offering analgesia with greater control of postoperative pain and fewer systemic effects than general anesthesia. Recent studies indicate that regional anesthesia not only decreases opioid requirements but also potentially leads to lower recovery times and lengths of hospital stay for patients, as regional anesthesia minimizes opioid side effects (Eric et al., 2020). The growing focus on the benefits of regional anesthesia is in line with trends towards opioid-sparing strategies in surgery, which reflect a desire for patient-centered care and enhanced recovery pathways (Eric et al., 2020). Local anesthesia is the most restrictive type of anesthesia, affecting only a local area to numb the patient, leaving the patient completely awake and conscious. It is most often used in minor surgeries, dentistry, and diagnostic procedures. Local anesthetics, including lidocaine and procaine, may be applied with injections or topical treatment, successfully numbing the immediate area around the surgical site. The simplicity and effectiveness of local anesthesia make it a better choice for outpatient surgery, where a quick recovery is desirable. As the focus increases on less use of opioids and subsequent complications in the postoperative period, local anesthesia is a valuable component of multimodal analgesia strategies, allowing effective pain management with less dependence on systemic opioid medications (Marcus, 2015) (Figure 1.2).

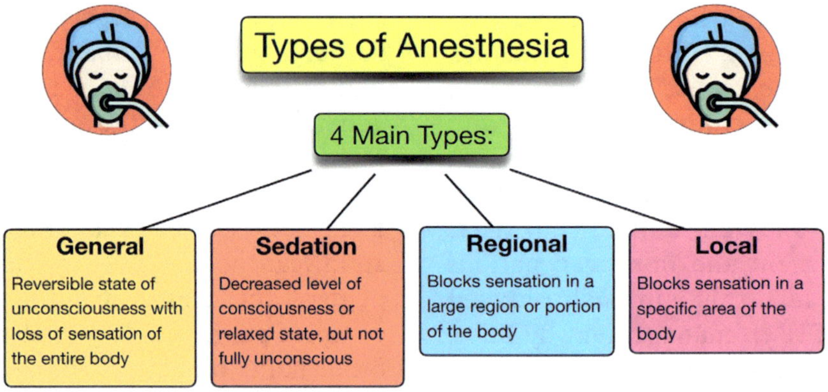

Figure 1.2. Types of anesthesia: general, regional, and local.

Source: https://images.squarespace-cdn.com/content/v1/5e48489da899cd09424943db/e2049b8d-97b2-40ff-881b-baa59042c50a/anesthesia-types-general-sedation-local-regional.jpeg.

Importance of Anesthesia in Modern Medicine

The role of anesthesia in modern medicine cannot be overstated, as it is at the heart of enhancing the surgical experience for both the patient and the physician. Anesthesia provides access to a broad range of operations, enabling safe procedure completion that would otherwise be deemed too dangerous. The ability to manage pain adequately during and after surgery enhances the patient experience and leads to better clinical outcomes. For instance, advances in anesthesia and medication have increased patient comfort, reduced hospital stays, and minimized complications. Due to regional anesthesia and sedation, the extent and safety of surgery have expanded, facilitating outpatient surgeries that were unthinkable in previous decades. These developments illustrate the central position anesthesia holds in the story of surgical medicine and patient care. Further, anesthesia practice extends beyond the operating room, influencing specialties such as obstetrics, chronic pain, and emergency medicine. Regional anesthesia, for example, like epidurals in obstetrics, significantly improves the experience of delivery by reducing pain without the administration of systemic drugs that could damage the mother or fetus. Furthermore, anesthetics remain a fundamental component of the management of acute and chronic pain syndromes, demonstrating their adaptability within the healthcare model. It has been shown that effective pain control with anesthesia leads to faster recovery, lower rates of postoperative complications, and greater patient satisfaction (Cornell University, 1999). This varied application demonstrates how anesthesia not only enhances the success of surgery but also improves well-being and health across numerous medical conditions. Evolution in anesthesia methods has also been a significant factor in increasing patient safety protocols in modern medicine. Continuous research in monitoring technology and anesthetic agents has reduced the incidence of adverse effects from anesthesia to an extent that complex procedures are being performed with minimal risk. Further, the development of specialized programs for anesthesiologists ensures that experts are well-equipped to address routine and unexpected issues during surgical procedures. With ongoing advancements in the healthcare industry, the role of anesthesia specialists will likely expand, encompassing new techniques and technologies to meet the needs of diverse patient groups. Anesthesiology's professionalization, supported by extensive research and clinical practice guidelines, once again highlights the specialty's significance in improving general surgical safety and effectiveness (Cornell University, 1999). The development of anesthesia ultimately continues to be a pillar in contemporary medicine, summarizing its crucial position as a game-changer in patient care.

1.1. History of Anesthesia

Learning Outcome

1. Early methods of pain relief in ancient civilizations
2. Development of anesthesia in the 19th century
3. Key figures in the history of anesthesia

The evolution of anesthesia through history marks a milestone in the course of surgical procedures and patient treatments. Surgical procedures before the middle of the 19th century were typically brutal and traumatic and carried out without any form of alleviating pain experienced by patients. Practices such as alcohol consumption and opiates were employed to anesthetize feelings, but these were predominantly ineffective and unpredictable. The big breakthrough, however, came in 1846, when American dentist William Morton demonstrated the anesthetic properties of ether in a surgical procedure at the Massachusetts General Hospital. This was the dawn of modern anesthesia, as it opened up the possibility of performing surgery without pain that had long become de rigueur for patients. Following Morton's trailblazing demonstration, the field of anesthesia expanded greatly with many agents and techniques being discovered. In subsequent decades, nitrous oxide and chloroform became ubiquitous as inhalational anesthetics, and a range of surgical operations could be performed with greater ease and efficiency. Joseph Clover, in particular, pioneered the use of a hissing vapor inhaler in 1868, a major step forward in the administration of anesthesia.

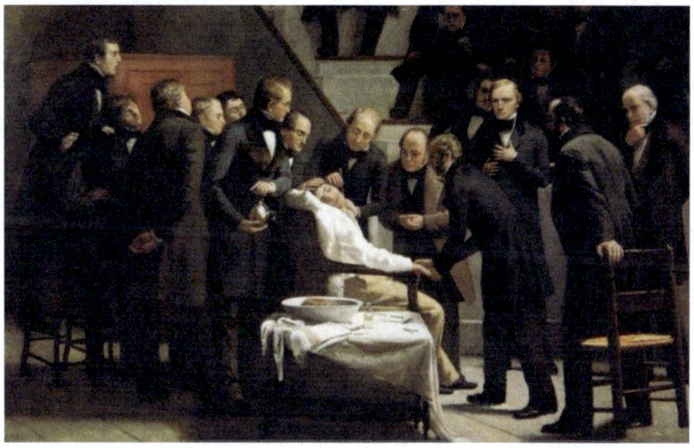

Figure 1.3. The historical evolution of anesthesia marks a pivotal shift in surgical practices and patient care.

Source: https://wfsahq.org/wp-content/uploads/First-Operation-Under-Ether-painting-1-e1588345193673.jpg.

The experience gained through early practice enabled anesthesiologists to standardize dosage and delivery methods, particularly to improve patient safety. Problems associated with the safety of anesthetic drugs were not eventually addressed at once; complication reports began appearing, and more research into the pharmacologic profiles of anesthetic drugs and their physiologic effects on patients had to be performed. Safety remains a central concern in anesthesia administration today. This is especially so in patient groups with specific medical conditions, such as preeclampsia, where careful monitoring is important to the health of both the mother and the fetus. There has been reported variability in pre-neuraxial coagulation testing, and variability in determining safe hemostatic conditions has been reported to compound these complexities further (Butwick et al., 2013). Furthermore, understanding about anatomical and physiological characteristics of patients has significantly advanced since the earliest years of anesthesia and thus more accurate diagnostic tools are now available for assessing procedure readiness (Rycke et al., 2008). As the history of anesthesia illustrates, continuous innovation and strict adherence to safety protocols are crucial to the evolution of anesthetic methods, with the realization that patient safety remains the highest priority in anesthesia delivery today (Figure 1.3).

1.1.1. Early Methods of Pain Relief in Ancient Civilizations

The quest for ancient pain-relief methods across societies reveals a long history of methods before modern anesthesia. Ancient Egyptian communities employed herbal remedies and natural substances such as opium for their analgesic properties. These practices were also intertwined with religious ideologies, suggesting that pain relief was physically as well as spiritually an issue. Furthermore, application of acupuncture within ancient China demonstrates the early incorporation of physical methods, with a focus on correcting the body's energy balance in an effort to avoid pain. Not only does this holistic practice demonstrate the advanced knowledge of the human body, but it also highlights the cultural importance of pain control as a starting point for medical knowledge that continues today in one form or another. In addition to physical and herbal resources, music as a therapeutic agent in ancient societies is also important. From historical accounts, music was used in most societies, e.g., the Greeks and Romans, to minimize pain and enhance emotional well-being. Music's ability to alter physiological responses earned it a place in rituals and healing ceremonies as an agent of relaxation and pain relief. The therapeutic potential of music is in accord with more contemporary findings confirming the efficacy of its use in non-pharmacological treatments, and indicates that ancient therapy, in many ways, was a step ahead of its time. This integrated method of pain relief not only reveals the ingenuity of past societies but also presents a model that is still being explored by medicine today, particularly in the context of expanding non-surgical options for patient treatment. Further, religious and spiritual rituals played an important role in pain alleviation in ancient societies, making pain relief processes more complicated to explain. Diseases were seen as manifestations of spiritual disarray or divine wrath by most cultures, which rendered rituals, prayers, and sacrifices a form of seeking relief. These short treatments were normally complemented by more tangible strategies like herbalism, yielding a rich tapestry of pain relief strategies. These blends reveal the extent of health and wellbeing in ancient times, a sign that pain relief was not merely a bodily activity but a pervasive strategy encompassing the emotional, spiritual, and intellectual realms. By tracing these ancient methods, modern practitioners can appreciate the legacy of earlier wisdom in their search for effective pain management.

1.1.2. Development of Anesthesia in the 19th Century

The 19th century was an era of revolution in medicine, particularly through the development of anesthesia, which transformed the landscape of surgical practice. Before this advancement, surgery was characterized by agonizing pain, often resulting in patient shock or death. With the introduction of ether and chloroform as anesthetics, surgery became more humane and complex. This innovation was successful not only for science, but also a consequence of a profound change in the social attitudes to surgery as such. Increased popular trust in surgeons might be regarded as the anesthetic demonstrated itself to eradicate pain, thus resulting in improved surgical results (Nebiolo et al., 2017). As surgeons practiced the art of surgery, they also gained a better reputation, as physicians increasingly developed a consciousness of their professional standing as medical doctors, not just butchers. Anesthesia's use was an extension not just of innovations in technique but also of close relation to other broader trends in medical technology and training throughout the 19th century. The development of special surgical training and the creation of hospitals with surgery departments further illustrated the utilization of anesthesia as an accepted surgical procedure.

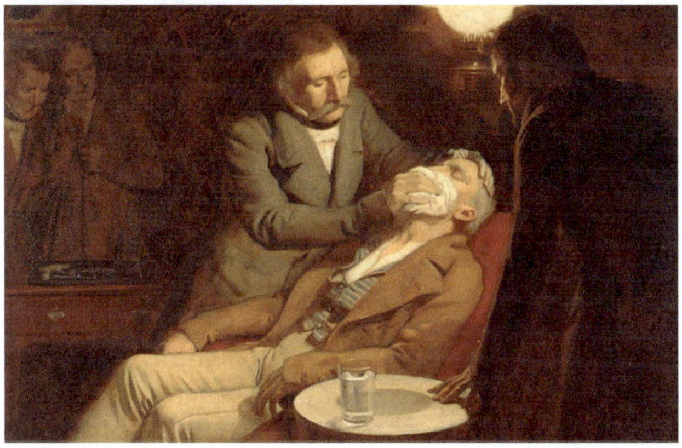

Figure 1.4. The 19th century marked a transformational era in the field of medicine.

Source: https://daily.jstor.org/wp-content/uploads/2018/02/ether_dental_surgery_1050x700.jpg.

The unveiling of scalpels and syringes, which were excavated by archaeological searches, shows the increased development and refinement of medical technology at this period (Veit et al., 2013). The emphasis on surgical practice, with the successful use of anesthetics, enabled more complex surgeries, thereby guaranteeing a standard of care that rested on patient comfort. This reciprocal development of technology and knowledge brought surgery to a position of respect and respectability as a medical technique. Anesthesia not only benefited patients' bodies but also drove a broader cultural change in the medical profession. That the public gained a perception of surgical operations as a viable option rather than solely as a last resort reflects a change in medical practice. It became popularized through the popularization of anesthesia as a component of skillfully executed surgical procedures that gained broader acceptance through successful public demonstrations in addition to patient reports testifying to the advantage through these innovations. The 19th century thus witnessed not just technological breakthroughs that allowed anesthesia to thrive but also a paradigm shift in society's perception of surgical medicine. Both of them opened up a society willing to accept medical innovations that improved the human way of life and removed the centuries-long fear associated with surgery (Figure 1.4).

1.1.3. Key Figures in the History of Anesthesia

The history of anesthesia in modern medicine is the result of the efforts of many pioneers who laid the foundation for its safe and effective administration. Among the most significant figures in the history of anesthetics is Dr. William Morton, a 19th-century dental surgeon. Morton is typically credited with the first public demonstration of ether anesthesia in 1846, which he conducted at Massachusetts General Hospital. This demonstration fundamentally changed the landscape of surgical procedures, allowing operations to be performed without causing patients pain. Morton's work not only put anesthesia at the center of medical practice but also stimulated extensive interest and experimentation, leading to anesthetic techniques and substances becoming more sophisticated. Another important historical figure in anesthesia is Dr. James Simpson, who introduced chloroform into the practice in the 1840s. His extensive testing and evaluation settled chloroform's value as a surgical anesthetic, and thus it became a common replacement for ether. The work of Simpson extended beyond purely practical applications; he also sought to promote the social acceptance of anesthesia, emphasizing its humanitarian potential. His research represented a tremendous advance for obstetric anesthesia, specifically in childbirth, easing the suffering of labor. Simpson's advocacy and creativity contributed to the group's knowledge of anesthesia, furthering the investigation of numerous anesthetic agents that would follow. Continuing into the 20th century, Dr. John Snow became a prominent figure in the development of anesthetic practice, especially the creation of inhalational anesthetics. His cautious exploration of the effects of different agents, particularly ether and chloroform, revolutionized the practice of inhalation anesthesia. Snow's research was characterized by attention to detail and scientific method, and he is thus a pioneer in the field of anesthetic safety. He also valued the importance of watching patients under anesthesia, the cornerstone of modern anesthetic practice. The results derived from Snow's work proved to be paramount in guiding anesthetic practice, ensuring patient safety, and minimizing surgical complications, a cornerstone milestone in anesthetic history.

Test Your Knowledge

1. What were the major milestones in the development of anesthesia, and how did they transform surgical practice?
2. Who are the key pioneers in the history of anesthesia, and what were their significant contributions?

1.2. Mechanisms of Action

Learning Outcome

1. How anesthetics affect the nervous system
2. The role of neurotransmitters in anesthesia
3. Differences in mechanisms between various types of anesthetics

An understanding of the mechanisms of action of anesthetic drugs is core to understanding how anesthesia effectively achieves a reversible state of unconsciousness or loss of sensation. General anesthesia is characterized by amnesia, muscle relaxation, and insensitivity to pain in the entire body. This is achieved by various drugs that can be classified as volatile and intravenous agents, both of which affect in different ways at the molecular level. These medications regulate neurotransmitter systems and neuronal excitability, so the patient is unaware or in pain throughout the surgeries. The significance of this mechanism justifies advances in anesthesia techniques so that clinicians can modulate anesthetic depth to optimal levels and enhance patient outcomes, thereby highlighting the relationship between molecular pharmacology and clinical practice in anesthesia, as underlined in Calvieri et al. (2014). Local anesthetics represent another interesting aspect of the mechanisms of action relevant to anesthesia. Unlike general anesthetics, local anesthetics are designed specifically to interfere with nerve impulse conduction, leading to reversible blockade of sensation in targeted areas of the body. The agents mainly act by inhibiting sodium influx through voltage-gated sodium channels in neuronal membranes, stabilizing the membrane and preventing the generation of action potentials. This nerve conduction block anesthetizes the site to be operated on effectively, making it painless. Notably, local anesthetics include lidocaine and prilocaine, which are available in various formulations such as creams and gels. By being aware of the precise mechanism of action of local anesthetics, medical professionals can better predict their efficacy and treat side effects through surgery, as explained by Calvieri et al. (2014).

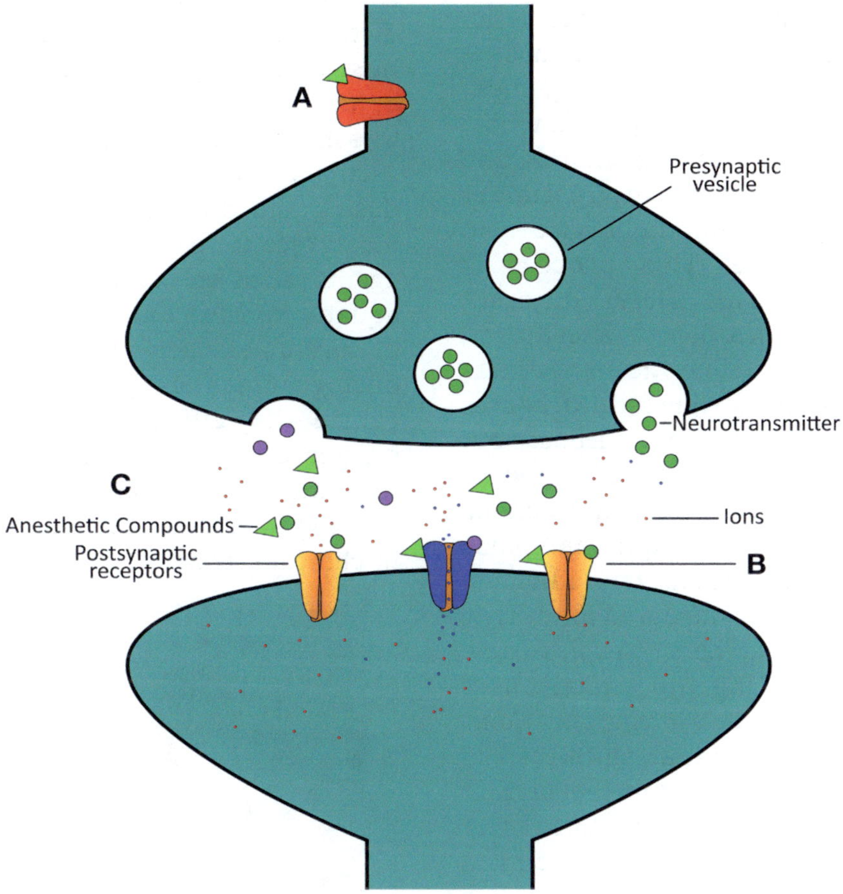

Figure 1.5. Mechanisms of anesthetic action.

Source: https://www.frontiersin.org/files/Articles/313717/fphys-08-01138-HTML/image_m/fphys-08-01138-g001.jpg.

New technologies in anesthesia, such as the proposed Receptor-centered Magnetic Resonance anesthesia, illustrate ongoing improvements in our understanding of anesthetic action. This emerging technique postulates the creation of a flawless anesthetic based on electromagnetic principles. It induces anesthesia without the common side effects that arise with drug metabolism. With high-resolution magnetic resonance technology, this method is likely to target specific receptors in a patient's body, reducing unwanted side effects. This discovery underscores the need for further study of the mechanism of action of anesthetic agents to improve safety and efficacy. As anesthesia practice evolves, embracing new models of drug action could revolutionize how anesthetics are administered and monitored, as discussed in Figure 1.5.

1.2.1. How Anesthetics Affect the Nervous System

The activity of anesthetics within the nervous system is a central focus in understanding how they function during surgery. Anesthetics primarily exert their effects on neuronal receptors, an action that has consequences for neurotransmission and synaptic function. Anesthetics can prevent pain transmission and induce sedation by modulating neurotransmitter activity, such as gamma-aminobutyric acid (GABA) and glutamate. This process is multifaceted, as it varies across different mechanisms of anesthetics. General anesthetics, for example, create a reversible unconsciousness condition that makes it possible for procedures to be performed without patient awareness but ultimately with both analgesia and amnesia. It is worth understanding these interactions to best utilize anesthetic techniques, minimize side effects, and plan methods for individual patient needs. In addition, improved anesthetic technology has led researchers to explore new strategies for maximizing the effectiveness of anesthesia with the fewest complications. Research suggests a potential shift toward electromagnetic theories of anesthesia that interact with selective neuronal receptors rather than relying solely on traditional chemical substances. Theoretical ideal-anesthetic concepts introduced in recent studies include using high-resolution magnetic resonance techniques to establish precise electromagnetic models for anesthesia administration. By avoiding the need for massive amounts of drugs, these technologies have the potential to minimize side effects related to absorption and distribution within the body, thereby safeguarding neurological integrity during procedures (Golyanishchev et al., 2016). Investigations of these emerging modalities can offer valuable insights into how anesthetics might be employed more efficiently and safely, transforming the art of surgical anesthesia. In addition to procedural applications, the influence of anesthetics on the nervous system can vary from extremely agent-dependent to extremely situation-dependent. For instance, certain anesthetics have direct and potent sedative effects. In contrast, others may cause persistent cognitive disturbance following anesthesia, particularly in susceptible populations such as the elderly or those with underlying neurological illness. One must understand the pharmacodynamics of each anesthetic agent in the design of optimal dosing and the reduction of side effects. The most recent research on various anesthetic agents, such as metomidate and clove oil, in aquatic species underscores the importance of careful, species-specific consideration and dosing guidelines (Watson et al., 2015). By considering efficacy and safety, researchers can more effectively ensure positive outcomes for patients undergoing anesthesia, ultimately refining anesthetic administration techniques in clinical settings (Figure 1.6).

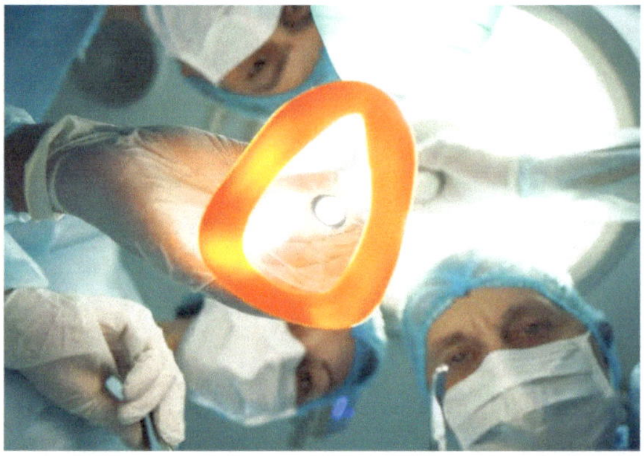

Figure 1.6. Surgeons are preparing to administer anesthesia before surgery.

Source: https://media.post.rvohealth.io/wp-content/uploads/sites/3/2020/02/320564_2200-732x549.jpg.

1.2.2. The Role of Neurotransmitters in Anesthesia

Neurotransmitters play a key role in the mechanism of anesthesia, primarily through central modulation of neuronal and synaptic transmission in the central nervous system. Their action is at the hub of the process of generating the desired anesthetic state, such as unconsciousness, analgesia, and muscle relaxation. Most anesthetic agents work by modulating the release, uptake, and receptor binding of some neurotransmitters, such as GABA and glutamate. For instance, the majority of inhalational anesthetics exert their action through an augmentation of GABAergic neurotransmission, potentiating inhibitory neurotransmission. The potency of this enhancement leads to lower neuronal excitability and is responsible for the anesthetic effect.

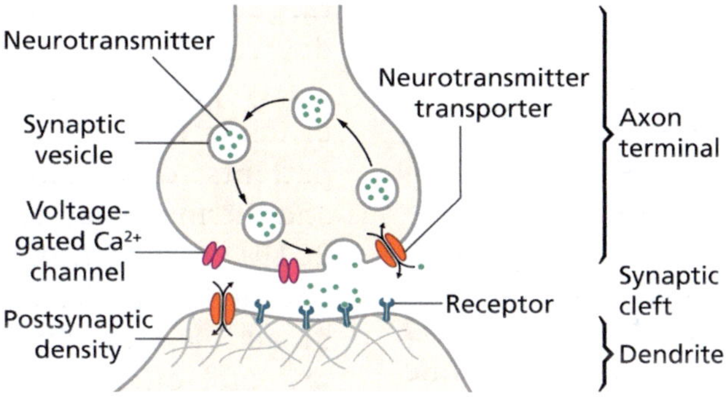

Figure 1.7. The role of neurotransmitters in anesthesia.

Source: https://ars.els-cdn.com/content/image/3-s2.0-B978012802381500004X-f04-02-9780128023815.jpg.

These neurotransmitter-anesthetic interactions depict a deep interplay that is pivotal to clinical anesthetic practice, underscoring the importance of understanding neurotransmitter dynamics for the provision of effective and safe anesthesia. Besides, recent research highlights the contribution of neurotransmitter systems to anesthetics' pharmacodynamics. Anesthetics have been found by research to alter neurotransmitter profiles and associated signaling pathways to induce phenomenal alterations in consciousness and pain perception. General anesthetics, for instance, have been found to alter neuronal membrane function, affecting neurotransmitter release and receptor activation. The study of these events clarifies how anesthetics influence synaptic transmission and lead to physiological changes, such as decreased heat capacity and altered relaxation times, in biological membranes (Antonov et al., 2007). This information informs the design of more selective anesthetic drugs with fewer side effects and improved therapeutic effects. This line of inquiry into anesthetic-neurotransmitter interaction is a model of the ongoing evolution of anesthetic science. Eventually, the interaction between neurotransmitter dynamics and consciousness holds deep practical implications for anesthesiology and neurology. Emerging theories suggest a connection between quantum-mechanical processes and neuronal functioning, speculating that consciousness may be a product of the interaction between nuclear spin ensembles in neurons (Hu et al., 2002). Such perspectives lead anesthesiologists to examine the roles of neurotransmitters not only in sedation and analgesia but also in overall modulation of consciousness. As further research is conducted, clarifying how anesthetics act on neurotransmitter systems can dictate future advances in anesthesia techniques and postoperative care. Therefore, the study of neurotransmitters and anesthesia is a crucial intersection of pharmacology, neurology, and consciousness studies, with the potential to advance clinical practice and provide theoretical insights into the nature of consciousness (Figure 1.7).

1.2.3. Differences in Mechanisms Between Various Types of Anesthetics

The mechanisms of action of various anesthetics are highly diverse and manifest distinct profiles in clinical practice. General anesthetics such as sevoflurane and desflurane act through different mechanisms to produce loss of consciousness and analgesia. Sevoflurane is a volatile anesthetic with a rapid induction and emergence profile owing to its low blood solubility, leading to rapid equilibration between brain tissue and blood. Conversely, desflurane also has a rapid onset due to its low blood-gas partition coefficient. Still, it is typically characterized as having less hypotensive effect, which is advantageous for intraoperative hemodynamic control. Both drugs are capable of reducing cognitive function temporarily following surgery. Yet the degree of impairment observed and the duration of its recovery vary widely, thereby influencing postoperative outcomes, especially in susceptible groups such as the elderly (Allard et al., 2014). The differences in anesthetic mechanisms are also more than just differences in clinician effectiveness, as they dictate their physiological actions and side-effect profile. Opioid anesthetics, like fentanyl, exert their analgesic effect primarily through mu-opioid receptor activation in the central nervous system, producing intense analgesia but also initiating threats of respiratory depression. In contrast, local anesthetics like lidocaine exert their effect through sodium channel blockade, thereby preventing nerve impulse transmission at the site of administration without affecting consciousness. This discrimination is critical in regional anesthesia interventions or in situations where general anesthesia is not suitable. The specific neuronal pathway targeted by these anesthetics primarily determines their therapeutic effects and safety profiles, underscoring the importance of tailored anesthetic strategies for individual patients, depending on the type of surgery and intrinsic medical conditions (Burish et al., 2019). In addition, the pharmacokinetics of anesthetics underlie their varied mechanisms of action and clinical course. Agents like propofol offer rapid onset and recovery due to their unique metabolism in the liver and other tissues, with a context-sensitive half-life that is much shorter than that of many intravenous anesthetics. Agents like thiopental offer longer-lasting action in proportion to their redistribution and elimination characteristics. These differences call for careful deliberation by anesthesiologists in the selection of drugs for the maintenance and induction of anesthesia. Understanding the interaction between the drug's pharmacodynamic profile, the needs of the procedure, and patient considerations remains crucial, particularly in preventing postoperative cognitive dysfunction with age and anesthetic exposure (Allard et al., 2014).

Test Your Knowledge

1. Explain the role of forensic pathologists.
2. Write a short note on post-mortem computed tomographic angiography (PMCTA).
3. What is exhumation?

1.3. Types of Anesthetic Agents

Learning Outcome

1. Inhalational anesthetics and their uses
2. Intravenous anesthetics and their applications
3. Local anesthetics and their specific functions

Anesthetic medications have an important role in medicine, primarily by inducing an anesthetic condition that is used for painless operations. General and local anesthetics are two significant categories of anesthetics. General anesthetics such as propofol and isoflurane induce a reversible loss of consciousness to enable comprehensive operation while keeping the patient comfortable. Local anesthetics, including lidocaine or bupivacaine, block nerve impulses in localized areas of the body to allow minor operations without disrupting general consciousness. Medical professionals must understand the differences between these two classes of anesthetics, each with specific indications, contraindications, and potential side effects that impact patient outcomes during and after surgery.

Administration of anesthetic drugs also plays an important role in managing acute postoperative pain. Acute postoperative pain is intricately related to patient satisfaction and can impact recovery paths considerably. Opioids, often administered in conjunction with anesthetic drugs, have been linked to several adverse events that pose substantial risks, the most important of which is the potential for transitioning from acute to chronic pain. In response to these challenges, anesthesiologists are increasingly mandated to develop comprehensive analgesic plans from preoperative assessment through discharge. Employing multimodal analgesia consisting of the administration of general and local anesthetics, clinicians aim to minimize opioid dependence and total pain relief, ultimately amounting to enhanced surgical results and patient satisfaction as required in the perioperative surgical home model concept (Baratta et al., 2016).

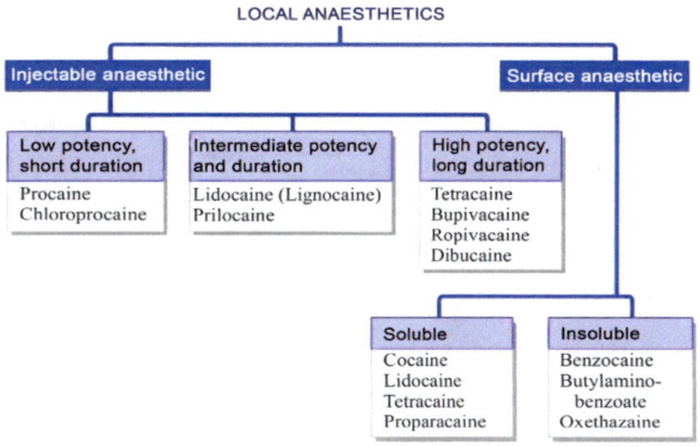

Figure 1.8. Anesthetic agents serve a crucial role in the field of medicine.

Source: https://pharmacyfreak.com/wp-content/uploads/2023/10/Local-anaesthetic-drugs.webp.

Moreover, the mechanisms by which anesthetic drugs exert their effects are of significant scientific interest, particularly with respect to cognitive processes. Studies on the effects of general anesthetics, such as propofol, on brain activity have provided insights into how they disrupt cognitive processing. The unbinding paradigm of cognition posits that general anesthesia impairs the integration of cognitive information, as evidenced by altered brain wave patterns measured by electroencephalography (EEG). Research indicates that the induction of propofol anesthesia leads to a significant reduction in information integration at the gamma frequency band of EEG, as predicted by theories of consciousness and anesthetic action (Choi et al., 2008). Having these processes in mind not only highlights the sophisticated nature of anesthetic agents but also the need for continuous research to optimize their use in favor of greater safety and efficacy in surgery (Figure 1.8).

1.3.1. Inhalational Anesthetics and Their Uses

Inhalational anesthetics constitute a core component of modern-day anesthesia practice, the method of which is to induce and maintain general anesthesia quickly. Agents given in vapor form have both anesthetic and analgesic effects, allowing smooth continuation of the surgery without compromising patient safety and comfort. General inhalation anesthetics, such as sevoflurane, desflurane, and isoflurane, have varying pharmacokinetic properties that influence their onset, potency, and recovery characteristics. The selection of a specific inhalational agent is based on the type of surgery, patient status, and the anesthesiologist's preference, underscoring the need for individualized anesthesia administration. For instance, sevoflurane, which possesses induction qualities and minimal side effects, has become increasingly popular for use on an outpatient basis, demonstrating the evolving world of how inhalational anesthetics are used. Utilization of inhalational anesthetics is not without challenges, particularly in controlling potential complications associated with their use. Postoperative ailments such as residual neuromuscular blockade are hazardous, particularly in elderly patients, who are at higher risk of both morbidity and mortality as a result of anesthesia. How much more vital is meticulous monitoring and reversal of neuromuscular blockade in these patients, which cannot be overstated, since airway obstruction and respiratory collapse occur more frequently in elderly patients. While traditional acetylcholinesterase inhibitors reverse neuromuscular blockade, newer drugs such as sugammadex offer a potentially superior option. However, the pharmacokinetics of such agents may be disrupted in elderly patients, which necessitates careful understanding of their impact within the broader scheme of inhalational anesthetics (Bertoncello et al., 2017). In addition, the evolution of inhalational anesthetics has been accompanied by scientific advancements indicative of both innovation and function within the discipline. Research evaluating anesthetic medications over the last three decades indicates that sevoflurane, for instance, not only achieved a high popularity score but also a significant expectation score, indicating its significant place in contemporary anesthesia practice. Inhalational anesthetics, too, have adapted to different patient populations, both high-risk and outpatient surgery. Additionally, while some older agents in the armamentarium of anesthetics have shown longevity, newer agents like sugammadex herald a shift towards optimizing patient outcomes and enhancing safety protocols in anesthetic use (Kissin et al., 2015). This ongoing development underlines the significance of inhalational anesthetics as critical agents in the anesthetic arsenal, facilitating improved surgical technique and patient recovery (Figure 1.9).

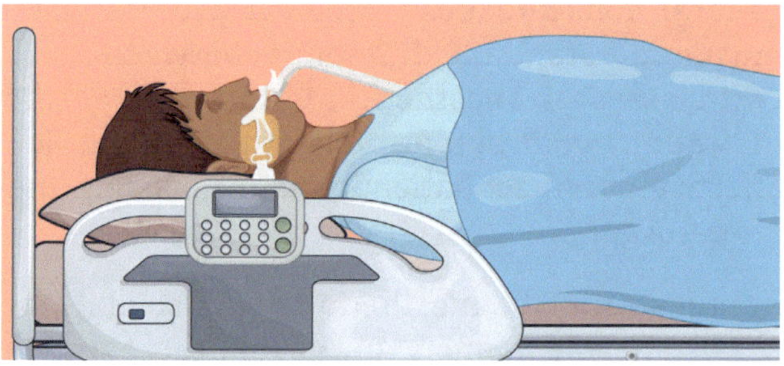

Figure 1.9. Inhalational anesthetics play a pivotal role in modern anesthesia practice.

Source: https://www.jove.com/files/media/science-education/science-education-thumbs/15191.jpg.

1.3.2. Intravenous Anesthetics and Their Applications

Intravenous anesthetics represent a significant advancement in anesthesia, with rapid onset of sedation and analgesia for the majority of surgical procedures. Intravenous drugs are administered primarily through a peripheral or central venous catheter, facilitating rapid delivery into the bloodstream and enabling almost immediate effects on the central nervous system. Their rapid onset is particularly valuable in emergency departments, where immediate sedation can be critical. Intravenous anesthetics are versatile in their applications, ranging from short outpatient procedures, such as dental surgery, to longer and more invasive interventions, in which they are combined with other types of anesthesia, such as inhaled agents, to enhance effectiveness and patient comfort during the perioperative period. The pharmacological profiles of the drugs make them ideal agents for both the induction and maintenance of anesthesia, thereby making anesthesia delivery easier (Calvieri et al., 2014). Propofol, etomidate, and thiopental are intravenous anesthetics currently used in routine clinical settings, each with distinct pharmacokinetic and pharmacodynamic properties. Propofol, due to its high metabolism rate and short recovery time, is the drug of preference for the majority of outpatient surgeries, both inducing sedation and antiemetic effects. Etomidate is favored on the grounds of hemodynamic stability, and it's an excellent option in cardiovascular-compromised patients because it minimizes fluctuations of blood pressure.

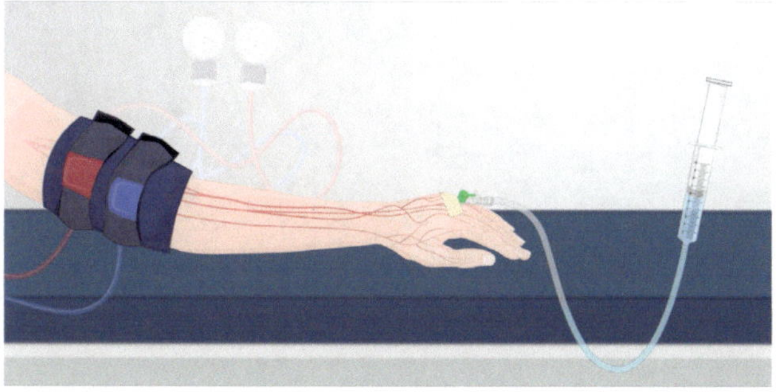

Figure 1.10. Intravenous anesthetics represent a significant advancement in the field of anesthesia.

Source: https://www.jove.com/files/media/science-education/science-education-thumbs/14749.jpg.

Thiopental, although less frequently used in practice nowadays, laid the groundwork for newer agents with faster recovery and fewer side effects. Individual characteristics of each agent determine the anesthesiologist's choice to provide individualized patient care to address unique clinical needs (Brown et al., 2018). Intravenous anesthetics have a role beyond surgery and are utilized in pain management and sedation in intensive care unit conditions. Intravenous anesthetics can be used to sedate mechanically ventilated patients, allowing comfort while permitting necessary medical procedures. Moreover, intravenous anesthetics have been used in procedural sedation, where short-acting agents enable rapid recovery, particularly for outpatient procedures or diagnostic testing that require patient cooperation. The ability to administer drugs safely allows health care providers to optimize patient experience and outcome, underscoring the importance of sufficient monitoring and dosing strategies. Ongoing research into new intravenous agents reveals the potential for even greater safety and efficacy in anesthetic practice to guide the future direction of perioperative care (Calvieri et al., 2014) (Figure 1.10).

1.3.3. Local Anesthetics and Their Specific Functions

The use of local anesthetics is a bulwark of modern analgesic therapy, providing localized pain relief for a vast range of medical interventions. The medications act by preventing the entry of sodium ions into neurons through voltage-gated sodium channels responsible for action potential generation and conduction. With these channels blocked, nerve impulses are effectively deterred, resulting in the reversible abolition of sensation in the region of application. Thus, local anesthetics are invaluable in surgical and minor non-surgical procedures, from dental operations to minor dermatological procedures. Their ability to produce pain relief with minimal or no systemic effects renders them unique in anesthetic practice. Thus, the use and mechanism of action of local anesthetics are crucial for achieving maximum patient benefit during treatment. Local anesthetics are also classified into two broad classes: amino esters and amino amides with distinct pharmacological properties and clinical applications. Amino esters, such as benzocaine, have a rapid onset of action and a short duration and are thus ideal for surface procedures of the skin. Amino amides such as lidocaine and prilocaine are more commonly used owing to their prolonged action and fewer allergic reactions. This differentiation not only guides critical care selection based on specific procedural needs but also influences product development used within clinics. For instance, lidocaine is typically used in topical formulations, such as gels and creams, to provide regional analgesia in dermatological treatments (Abelho et al., 2006). Choice among them is imperative, as it influences both the efficiency and safety of the anesthesia used. Also, the action of local anesthetics can be influenced by inflammatory conditions and variations in local tissue pH. Inflammatory conditions can alter physiological status, and the decreased effectiveness of these agents results from the fact that the acid environment usually present in inflammation can inhibit anesthetic penetration into tissue, and the agents lose their effectiveness as blockers of nerve conduction. The Meyer-Overton hypothesis of anesthetic potency varying with lipid solubility also draws attention to the thermodynamic intricacies involved in local anesthetic action (Abelho et al., 2006). Awareness of these factors is essential for clinicians to anticipate challenges in achieving the desired analgesia and adjust dosages and techniques accordingly. Lastly, a thorough understanding of local anesthetics and their functions ensures optimal pain control in accordance with the patient's requirements.

Test Your Knowledge

1. How do general anesthetics affect the central nervous system to produce unconsciousness, analgesia, and muscle relaxation?
2. What are the cellular and molecular mechanisms by which local anesthetics block nerve impulse transmission?

1.4. Anesthesia Administration

Learning Outcome

1. Preoperative assessment and patient evaluation
2. Techniques for administering anesthesia
3. Monitoring during anesthesia administration

Administration of anesthesia is a core feature of modern surgical practice, evolving in complexity with advances in medical technology. Anesthetics are used to induce states of controlled unconsciousness and analgesia, rendering patients' pain-free as well as insensible to surgical incisions. Careful attention to the patient's medical history, including prior conditions that complicate anesthesia care, is necessary for this procedure. Practitioners should also consider potential risks associated with anesthesia agents, thereby possessing a balanced understanding of pharmacology and patient-specific factors. Furthermore, anesthetic planning involves team discussions between surgical teams to ensure that all aspects of patient care are covered during anesthesia, surgery, and postoperatively. In intensive care unit (ICU) settings, the demands on anesthesia administration rise as patients must be monitored continuously and urgent changes in clinical status must be addressed. Recent research has demonstrated that drug administration, patient observation, and communication are typical activities performed simultaneously with the control of alarm systems used to monitor patients' vital signs and responses to anesthesia (Edworthy et al., 2013). The cognitive workload placed on anesthesiologists working in such settings is substantial as it must be maintained to preserve distraction-free sustained attention and alarm distraction control in high-stakes procedures. Additionally, performance is diminished under simultaneous alarm exposure, underscoring the importance of sound system design and communication as strategies to promote anesthesiology practice under stress. Furthermore, with the continued increase in demand for anesthetic services, especially in areas with scarce resources, there's a pressing need to increase the number of trained anesthesia personnel. In Japan, for instance, the shortage of practicing anesthesiologists has spurred innovative initiatives, such as developing training programs for non-physician anesthesia personnel, including nurse practitioners and perianesthesia nurses (Henker et al., 2021). These training programs aim to create a standardized curriculum that can refine the quality of care delivered across various operating environments.

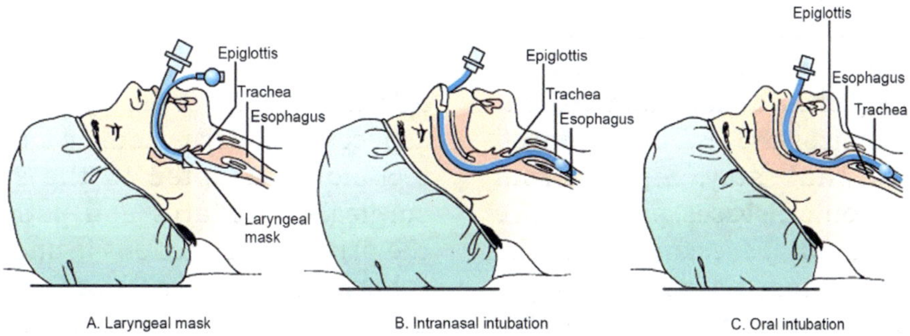

Figure 1.11. Methods of anesthesia administration.

Source: https://img.brainkart.com/article/article-Methods-of-Anesthesi-ONB.jpg.

By implementing robust training models, including simulation and didactic instruction, organizations can train a broader range of health professionals to administer anesthesia effectively. Such innovations in training can make a significant difference in patient safety and outcomes, and they reflect the growing appreciation of the important contributions that non-physician providers make to the practice of anesthesiology (Figure 1.11).

1.4.1. Preoperative Assessment and Patient Evaluation

Preoperative assessment and patient evaluation are critical components of the anesthetic management, serving as the foundation for safe surgical care. This is a step that involves a thorough assessment of the medical history of the patient, the patient's general health status, and possible risk factors potentially contributing to complications during surgery and anesthesia. For instance, patients with such chronic illnesses as diabetes mellitus can have some complications if they are not adequately assessed. Studies reveal that preoperative referral to a clinic for elevated glycosylated hemoglobin (HbA1c) has been found to significantly reduce adverse outcomes in patients treated with total joint arthroplasty. When preoperative HbA1c is managed, postoperative complications decline substantially, and therefore meticulous preoperative evaluation is necessary to establish optimal patient health (Breakwell et al., 2015). This method not only ensures maximum patient safety but also minimizes the risk of prolonged postoperative hospital stay. Apart from evaluation of the chronic diseases, preoperative assessment focuses on assessment of the patient's pain management needs, an integral component of the anesthetic plan. Adequate relief of acute postoperative pain helps reduce perioperative morbidity and enhance patient satisfaction. But opioid use, though common, carries a risk for adverse events and makes postoperative recovery difficult, especially among opioid-tolerant patients. The resulting risk of increasing dose to allow pain control underscores the need for multimodal pain management interventions from preoperative times. Anesthesiologists are in a unique position to design coordinated analgesic plans that address pain management correctly while minimizing the risk of complications due to opioid use (Baratta et al., 2016). This coordinated approach makes pain management not merely reactive but proactive and patient-centered. Finally, the significance of thorough preoperative evaluation and assessment of patients is evident in the impact on surgery outcomes. By establishing potential risks and implementing appropriate management techniques, patient satisfaction and safety can be enhanced through the perioperative cycle. Using pain control and medical history assessments, a comprehensive evaluation of the patient's health is conducted, enabling informed decisions regarding surgery and anesthesia. With the evolving terrain of surgical care, rigorous preoperative assessments will become priceless, highlighting the priority of these tests to achieving optimal surgical results. Details obtained at the time are a precious asset for anesthesiologists, allowing for tailored anesthesia regimens and the ability to predict potential complications ahead of time, ultimately resulting in improved patient outcomes.

1.4.2. Techniques for Administering Anesthesia

Administration of an anesthetic is a critical aspect of modern medicine that encompasses techniques adapted to the specific needs of surgical procedures and patient care. One of the primary distinctions in anesthetic technique is between general and local anesthesia. General anesthetic, which are commonly used for major surgeries, induces a reversible state of unconsciousness that is crucial for inpatient immobility and pain relief. It uses a combination of intravenous and volatile agents that alter consciousness, cause amnesia, and induce muscle relaxation to the entire body. Alternatively, local anesthesia selectively anesthetizes limited areas, leaving patients conscious while pain in those areas is alleviated. Local anesthetic agents, which are primarily aminoesters and aminoamides, act by inhibiting sodium ion influx into nerve membranes, thereby blocking pain signal transmission (Calvieri et al., 2014). Among modern approaches to anesthesia administration, regional anesthesia stands out for its safety and effectiveness. Techniques such as the fascia iliaca block are only a few examples of innovations in regional anesthesia, whose impact is significant pain relief without the need for inordinate systemic medication. The procedure involves infiltration of local anesthetics into the fascia iliaca plane to anesthetize nerves innervating the lower limbs. In 2016, a study comparing fascia iliaca block guided by ultrasound with spinal morphine reported that, although the block was less effective for pain relief during the first 24 hours of surgery, it did not significantly increase side effects compared to spinal morphine (Anderson et al., 2016). These results show continued research into anesthetic modality development to achieve maximum comfort and outcomes for the patient while using varying principles of anesthesia. Besides, anesthesia delivery methods also continue to evolve due to advancements in technology and pharmacology. Ultrasound-guided regional block procedures have revolutionized the precision with which anesthetics are administered, dramatically reducing the frequency of complications. By allowing physicians to visualize anatomical structures in real time using imaging technologies, needle placements are more accurate, and anesthetic success rates are less variable. Additionally, the development of newer local anesthetics with enhanced pharmacokinetic characteristics offers more prolonged analgesia with reduced toxicity, ideal for outpatient procedures and early recovery strategies. Investigational studies and clinical trials continue to refine such procedures, with a focus on achieving effective pain relief while respecting patient comfort and safety across a variety of surgical environments, reflecting dynamic change in anesthetic practice under modern medicine (Figure 1.12).

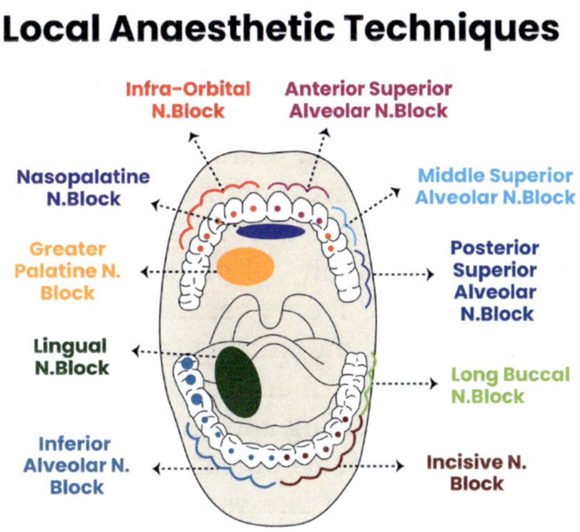

Figure 1.12. Techniques for administering anesthesia.

Source: https://www.instagram.com/p/DCbuJvVsK9Q/.

1.4.3. Monitoring During Anesthesia Administration

Effective monitoring during the administration of anesthesia is essential to ensure patient safety and the best results. The anesthetic process consists of an ambiguous balance of the sedatives, analgesics, and muscle relaxants, and thus needs constant monitoring of the patient's physiological status. Monitors measure vital parameters such as heart rate, blood pressure, and oxygen saturation, which provide real-time information on hemodynamic stability. Sophisticated monitoring technology, including electrocardiography (ECG) and capnography, broadens the ability to detect complications early. Anesthetists must be attentive, adjusting anesthetic protocols based on real-time data from such machines. This adaptability is critical during procedures, as patient status can shift rapidly, necessitating accurate and ongoing monitoring to mitigate anesthesia-related risks. The addition of processed electroencephalogram (EEG) measurements to anesthesia monitoring has shown promise for improving patient safety, with particular relevance for older patients. Research reveals that using EEG indices to assess sedation depth can provide the potential for the prediction of unfavorable cognitive outcomes, which are common among older patients undergoing anesthesia. Despite its promise, the variability of patient response to various anesthetic agents has limited the use of EEG as a standard monitoring technique in the clinical setting. New methods of analysis, such as 1/f frequency scaling and multiscale entropy, show potential to identify small effects of altered brain activity during anesthesia delivery. With these new EEG assessments, anesthesiologists can better understand loss of consciousness and provide a more personalized anesthetic strategy to meet patient needs, ultimately improving safety and efficiency in geriatric anesthesia (Caitlin et al., 2018). Monitoring practices have also evolved from traditional methods to include the latest advancements in the behavior of EEG responses to inhalation anesthetics. Studies in equine models have shown the complex effects of anesthetic drugs such as isoflurane and halothane on cerebral function, as reflected in subject-to-subject variation in EEG activity. This underscores the challenge of interpreting EEG patterns, especially in the presence of anesthesia-related complications. These findings encourage clinicians to maintain a state of alertness regarding the potential EEG effects of various anesthetic drugs. As the practice evolves, integrating advanced monitoring strategies, such as in-depth EEG analysis, can enhance anesthesiologists' ability to detect subtleties in patients' reactions, thereby promoting safer anesthetic practice (Aleman et al., 2015). In the end, nuanced monitoring under anesthesia is evidence of the devotion to ongoing optimization of patient care and outcomes.

Test Your Knowledge

1. What are the common routes and techniques used for administering anesthesia, and how do they influence the onset and duration of anesthetic effects?
2. What factors must be considered when selecting an appropriate method of anesthesia administration for a patient?

1.5. Risks and Complications

Learning Outcome

1. Common side effects of anesthesia
2. Serious complications and their management
3. Factors influencing anesthesia risk

In anesthesia, understanding the risks and complications associated with its administration is of utmost significance to both surgical success and patient safety. The indispensable tool in surgery pain management, anesthesia is riddled with intrinsic risks that are likely to trigger varying complications according to the technique applied. For instance, epidural analgesia (EDA) is very difficult to utilize; aside from its benefit in providing relief from postoperative pain, it has serious risks, including infection, hematoma formation, and neurologic injury. These complications underscore the importance of diligent screening and surveillance of the patients, and this is more important in high-risk populations, such as those with concomitant medical illnesses or those undergoing complex procedures like pancreatoduodenectomy, wherein histological analysis has been able to detect alterations in postoperative complications after anesthetic methods (Ceppa et al., 2019).

Furthermore, the consequences of anesthetic choices may extend beyond immediate surgical risk. Long-term complications of anesthesia can include cognitive dysfunction, particularly in the elderly, and psychological effects on recovery. Differences in anesthetic practice, such as the relative effectiveness of EDA compared to general anesthesia on outcomes in patients, should be considered.

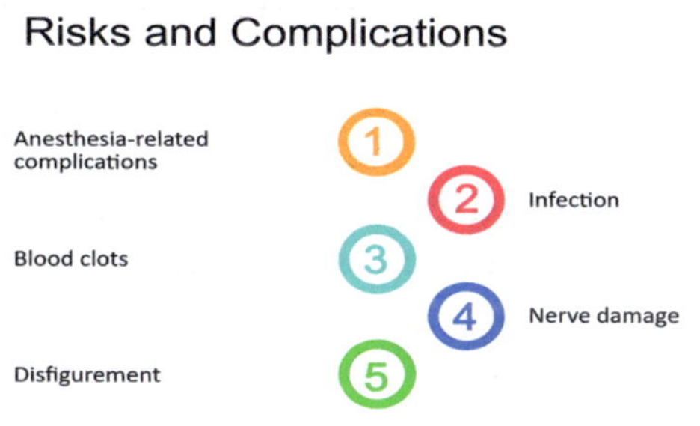

Figure 1.13. Risks and complications.

Source: https://fastercapital.co/i/Cosmetic-Enhancements--How-Windowdressing-Masks-Reality--Risks-and-Complications.webp.

The data reveal that EDA can have the potential to abolish some of the risks, such as unplanned intubation and pulmonary embolism, while lowering pain scores after surgery at the same time (Ceppa et al., 2019). Anesthesiologists should recognize these correlations when designing personalized plans to meet the needs of the individual patient, ensuring maximum safety and efficiency. Apart from being responsible for immediate anesthesia-specific complications, systemic effects should also be considered. These include complications that may arise from the surgical procedure itself, such as infection, thrombosis, and mechanical ventilation for over 48 hours, which may be exacerbated by anesthesia. For instance, mechanical ventilation for over 48 hours and septic shock have been associated with critical relationships to anesthetic practices employed in the operating room (Ceppa et al., 2019). Therefore, an overall risk assessment and interprofessional planning between surgical and anesthetic teams are essential in avoiding such risks. Emphasizing the importance of a thorough evaluation of the patient's history, medical history, and indications for surgery can also be useful in managing potential complications and optimizing patient outcomes during and after anesthetic procedures (Figure 1.13).

1.5.1. Common Side Effects of Anesthesia

The anesthetic injection, as required to ensure patient comfort and protection throughout surgery, is often accompanied by a range of everyday side effects. The most common are postoperative nausea and vomiting (PONV), and these can have a considerable impact on a patient's recovery process. PONV occurs in a large proportion of patients undergoing general anesthesia, and despite widespread prophylactic care, some patients continue to experience this unpleasant symptom. The effects of PONV do not stop at mere discomfort; they can lead to prolonged hospital stays, increased healthcare costs, and further complications that can extend the recovery process of a patient. Notably enough, the use of some medication, such as Promethazine, remains common despite associated side effects, further indicating the need for ongoing research into more effective alternatives for the management of PONV in clinical environments (Britton et al., 2022). Apart from PONV, other anesthetic side effects include dizziness, sleepiness, and alterations in mental status that can be of protracted duration postoperatively. These are particularly worrisome in elderly patients, who may be more susceptible to the neuropsychological action of anesthetic agents. On top of this, patients also complain of sore throat and hoarseness, particularly after intubation, and muscle soreness due to the anesthetics' relaxing action. While these side effects are generally transient, their occurrence makes patients feel uneasy and uncomfortable, which affects their satisfaction with the surgical intervention. Having these potential effects enables healthcare providers to adequately prepare patients in advance so they are aware of what to expect in the healing process (Aleman et al., 2015). Anesthesia specialists are now placing greater emphasis on individualizing care to minimize such side effects while optimizing operative outcomes. Patient individualization can involve selecting specific anesthetic agents with favorable side-effect profiles, closely monitoring patient responses intraoperatively, and prudent postoperative care strategies. Second-line drugs such as Amisulpride have been identified to be effective in the management of PONV in case of failure of first-line agents. Data indicate that Amisulpride offers a safer profile than conventional antiemetics such as Promethazine, which is associated with significant side effects (Britton et al., 2022). By enhancing anesthesia practitioners' knowledge of these medications and their associated side-effect profiles, practitioners are better positioned to individualize anesthetic plans to maximize patient outcomes and reduce the incidence of adverse postoperative experiences (Figure 1.14).

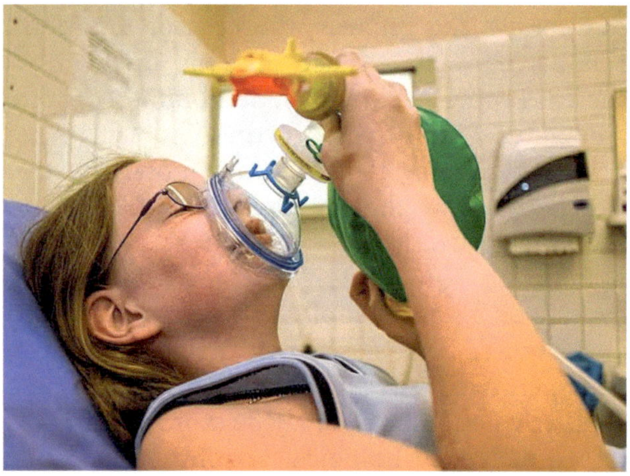

Figure 1.14. Common side effects of anesthesia.

Source: https://media.post.rvohealth.io/wp-content/uploads/2020/09/young_girl_nitrous_oxide-732x549-thumbnail-732x549.jpg.

1.5.2. Serious Complications and Their Management

Evolution in anesthesia has significantly enhanced patient safety in the operating room, but the risk of serious complications remains an important problem in anesthesiology. The most problematic problem is probably perioperative mortality risk that, at times, can be a consequence of preventable causes. Improvements in monitoring and anesthetic technology have made surgery safer, but the complexity of the patient population—older patients have more comorbidities—has introduced new hazards. Significantly, forensic pathology anesthetic-related deaths remain a challenging area as it involves the detection of unnatural deaths and surgery and anesthesia-related complications from natural health decline (Murphy et al., 2019). The requirement for high-quality control practices cannot be overstressed, as the methods have strong risk-reducing features and improved patient outcomes (Argo et al., 2019). Epidural anesthesia is a common technique for controlling pain during labor and postoperative pain, but it is not without risk. One of the risks is the formation of an epidural abscess, although this is rare. Infection is a consideration when epidural catheters are placed, necessitating careful monitoring and care. The clinical presentation of an epidural abscess typically includes fever and back pain, usually appearing several days post-procedure. Treatment is effective with early diagnosis and management, usually with the requirement of intravenous antibiotics to prevent possible severe morbidity. The favorable outcomes in such patients emphasize the importance of vigilance and early medical intervention to prevent epidural anesthesia complications (Liu et al., 2010). Prevention and control of anesthesia complications must prioritize evidence-based as well as personalized measures, according to patients' needs. Implementing regular screening of risky patients and applying high-technology monitoring equipment can significantly reduce the risk of life-threatening adverse events during anesthesia. Continuous education and training for anesthesiologists and perioperative professionals are also vital to keeping them informed of the latest guidelines and standards. Coordination between surgical teams and anesthesiologists is also necessary, as this provides a forum in which every patient's individual risks are thoroughly assessed. By highlighting the need for proactive action and emphasizing the implementation of strict risk management practices, health systems are better positioned to improve patient safety and outcomes in anesthesia (Argo et al., 2019).

1.5.3. Factors Influencing Anesthesia Risk

In anesthesia, knowledge of the myriad factors that influence anesthesia risk is important for patient safety and optimal outcomes. Patient characteristics, including age, comorbid conditions, and body mass index, greatly influence how patients respond to anesthetic drugs. Older patients, for instance, may exhibit altered pharmacokinetics and pharmacodynamics, so the selection and dosing of anesthetic medications need to be prudent. In addition, comorbid patients such as those with cardiovascular disease or respiratory disease can also be at increased risk under surgery, as these diseases compromise their physiological reserve. Proper preoperative assessment of the patient is necessary to identify such vulnerabilities and, accordingly, adjust the anesthesia plan to reduce the risk of anesthesia-related complications. Another crucial factor concerning anesthesia risk is the experience and skill of the anesthesiologists. Studies have also shown that more experienced professionals achieve better results because they handle unforeseen complications more effectively. For example, the stress levels of specialized fields, such as cardiac anesthesiology, can lead to higher burnout among anesthesiologists (Arcadipane et al., 2018). Burnout not only impacts the health of the individual but can also result in reduced decision-making and procedural skills during stress. Therefore, fostering a conducive work environment and wellness programs in anesthetic departments can mitigate these risks, thereby enhancing patient care and safety during anesthesia. Finally, the method of anesthesia administered also determines risk factors. Various techniques, such as general anesthesia, regional anesthesia, or monitored anesthesia care, have varying risk profiles and recovery implications. For example, intrathecal anesthesia is advantageous due to reduced opioid requirement, but it will disturb the post-operative course if not managed with proper care. Intrathecal opioid injection during cesarean section was reported to on the initiation of breastfeeding, but it affected the gain of infant weight, which warrants further research on its implications (Anbarafshan et al., 2016). Recognizing the subtleties of various anesthetic modalities enables practitioners to balance benefits and risks appropriately, thus maximizing patient outcomes within the context of anesthesia.

Test Your Knowledge

1. What are the common risks and complications associated with anesthesia, and how can they be prevented or managed?
2. How do patient-related factors influence the likelihood of anesthetic complications?

1.6. Advances in Anesthesia

Learning Outcome

1. Technological innovations in anesthesia delivery
2. Research on anesthetic agents and safety
3. Future trends in anesthesia practice

The latest advances in anesthesia have revolutionized surgical procedures, enhancing patient safety and postoperative recovery. Some important advances include the development of anesthetic drugs with faster onset and offset times and fewer side effects. The newer inhalation agents, such as sevoflurane and desflurane, have emerged as alternatives to traditional agents, offering more convenient anesthetic depth control and faster recovery following surgery. This pharmacokinetic enhancement is significant for outpatient procedures, when rapid recovery is the key to patient satisfaction and workflow optimization. Moreover, the integration of simulation technology into clinical education has radically changed the way anesthesia is taught, making it possible to train anesthesiologists in a way that effectively addresses complications. Thus, beyond improving the pragmatic aspects of anesthesia, such innovations also underpin the growing emphasis on patient-centered care in the operating room. With the global healthcare context evolving, so is the development of anesthesia, especially with respect to accessibility and equity. There is an urgent need for low- and middle-income countries (LMIC), where surgical disease burden remains disproportionately heavy. In a recent review, the disparity in access to functional neurosurgery methods in these countries was pointed out, citing that even though there's a growing prevalence of conditions such as epilepsy, patients are not treated accordingly because of systemic hindrances. Initiatives to collaborate between HICs and LMICs can facilitate learning from each other and the allocation of resources, resulting in better implementation of these cutting-edge procedures. Increasing awareness of surgical inequalities across the globe can drive initiatives towards enhancing access to surgical care and hence making a contribution toward overall ends in the field of public health, as well as outcomes of anesthetic practice in different contexts (Fezeu et al., 2018).

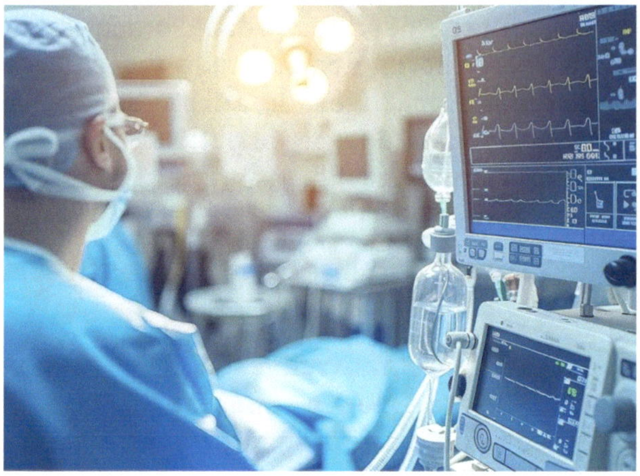

Figure 1.15. Recent advancements in anesthesia have significantly transformed surgical practices.

Source: https://stloralsurgery.com/wp-content/uploads/advances-in-anesthesia-1200x900.jpg.

Another significant factor in fostering anesthesia is overcoming the psychological aspects of surgical care. Literature reviews indicate that preoperative anxiety remains a substantial problem for the majority of patients, while treatment of anxiety has not been equally advanced in terms of practice. Three dominant themes related to preoperative anxiety were identified using a comprehensive review of the literature: causes, clinical concerns, and effective management. Psychological preparation of the patient requires more emphasis despite progress in anesthetic techniques and postoperative care. By integrating anxiety management protocols into the anesthesia process, healthcare professionals enhance the overall patient experience, leading to better surgical outcomes. Research in the future ought to be focused on determining standardized interventions that address preoperative anxiety in the frame of modern anesthesia practice (Mitchell et al., 2003). Addressing both the physiological and psychological components of anesthesia offers a more holistic approach to patient care (Figure 1.15).

1.6.1. Technological Innovations in Anesthesia Delivery

The practice of anesthesia has witnessed tremendous changes in recent years mainly due to technological progress that enhances the safety and efficacy of anesthesia delivery. Advances in automated systems capable of monitoring and regulating anesthesia levels have made closed-loop anesthesia delivery feasible. Such computerized systems employ advanced algorithms combined with real-time monitoring to adjust anesthetic agents minute by minute based on an individual patient's response. As discussed, the evolution of these closed-loop systems involves sophisticated control methods and patient modeling, which can potentially offer better clinical outcomes while maintaining patient safety. By reducing variability from manual administration, these technologies not only promote a higher degree of patient comfort but also contribute to more efficient practice in the operating room, eventually transforming surgical care (Copot et al., 2020). Moreover, the integration of artificial intelligence (AI) in anesthesia practice is a paradigm shift in how anesthesia is practiced. With the capacity to analyze large volumes of data from many different sources, AI can predict oncoming complications or shifts in a patient's physiological status in real time. This predictive capacity not only enhances the anesthesiologist's capability to make evidence-based decisions but also facilitates the overall objectives of precision medicine. By tailoring anesthesia delivery to each patient's unique properties, healthcare practitioners can achieve improved safety and efficacy. The drug-delivery system and automated monitoring research continues to demonstrate compliance with closing present technological gaps and implementation barriers while opening new avenues in clinical settings (Copot et al., 2020). Beyond automation and AI, emerging technologies such as telemedicine and sophisticated monitoring equipment have paved the way for anesthesia delivery, opening new avenues in patient management. Technologies for remote monitoring make it possible for anesthesiologists to observe patients undergoing surgery from a remote location, thereby maximizing the utilization of resources and delivering expert care even in underdeveloped parts of the world. Moreover, advancements in monitoring devices have made it easier to identify intraoperative awareness, an uncommon but essential element of general anesthesia, which has remarkable effects on patient experiences. By designing devices that not only sedate but also neutralize the minimal aspects of patient awareness, medical professionals can better safeguard against adverse consequences as a result of surgical awareness. They collectively depict a promising future for anesthesia delivery as technology continues to evolve and adapt to changing landscapes.

1.6.2. Research on Anesthetic Agents and Safety

The landscape of anesthesia has undergone a significant transformation in recent decades, particularly in the areas of safety and efficacy of anesthetic agents. Scientific studies have repeatedly highlighted the imperative to delineate the mechanisms and side effects of various anesthetics. At the heart of this is the requirement for categorization and investigation of perioperative mortality, which remains a cause of concern despite advances in practice. Research into these adverse events makes evident a high percentage of deaths related to anesthesia that are within the purview of preventable, intermingling the borders of anesthetic science with surgical proficiency. As noted, persistent issues are complications from airway and circulatory homeostasis maintenance, as well as side effects from drugs that result in iatrogenic death. Thus, the critical evaluation of anesthetic drugs puts a high value on training and procedural rigor to preclude risk (Argo et al., 2019). Further research into some anesthetic drugs, such as ropivacaine and tetracaine, reveals their relevance to contemporary clinical practice. Studies have demonstrated that these local anesthetics provide effective analgesia during procedures such as intravitreal injections, which are crucial for managing conditions such as diabetic macular edema. In one comparative study of the long-term effectiveness and safety of ropivacaine versus tetracaine 0.5%, patients reported very little pain during procedure, further solidifying the place of these medications in patient comfort. The findings inform the broader narrative that topical anesthesia is safe and effective for targeted interventions and that the appropriate anesthetic is key to achieving optimal clinical outcomes (Collini et al., 2015). This study demonstrates the convergence of theory and practice in anesthesia, leading to improved patient safety and satisfaction. Incorporating findings from extensive research into anesthetic practice is pivotal to enhancing patient safety in the perioperative environment. As anesthesia care continues to advance to address the complexities of modern medicine, the evolving patient population of older, multiple-comorbid patients increases the need for ongoing monitoring and assessment. The inclusion of current research not only plots the various complications with general and spinal anesthesia but also provides much-needed guidelines for the development of quality control techniques. Through the emphasis on the epidemiology of anesthetic-related mortality and complications, clinicians are able to understand the causal relationships at fault for such a situation. Ultimately, an overarching strategy that integrates ongoing research findings into the practice of clinical anesthesiology will be most crucial for reducing risk and promoting safety throughout anesthesia (Argo et al., 2019) (Figure 1.16).

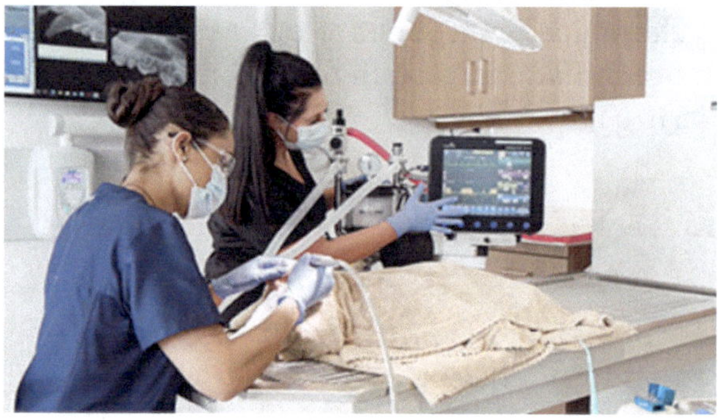

Figure 1.16. Research on anesthetic agents and safety.

Source: https://www.midmark.com/images/default-source/animal-health/spark-picture-2.png?sfvrsn=c8230f8e_1.

1.6.3. Future Trends in Anesthesia Practice

Technological advancements and the growing emphasis on patient-centered care are poised to transform anesthesia practice in a dramatic way. One recent trend is the widespread adoption of multimodal analgesia protocols aimed at minimizing opioid use. These protocols not only reduce the risk of opioid addiction, which is currently a significant public health problem, but also enhance patient recovery outcomes. Furthermore, the coordination of regional anesthesia techniques allows anesthesiologists to better tailor pain management. With the increasing prevalence of these technologies, anesthesiologists can play a significant role in developing standards that prioritize personalized patient care, particularly for patients at higher risk of developing chronic postoperative pain (Pozek et al., 2018). By embracing these evolving practices, anesthesia providers can significantly influence overall surgical outcomes, driving both clinical excellence and patient satisfaction. Anesthesia practice's integration of data analytics and artificial intelligence (AI) is also a revolutionary trend. These technologies have the potential to enhance decision-making, particularly in predicting patient response to anesthetics and anticipating complications. Through advanced algorithms and real-time monitoring, anesthesiologists can tap into significant volumes of data to inform their decisions, calibrating anesthetic protocols to a patient's individual physiology and medical history. Furthermore, anesthesia information management systems can facilitate enhanced communication among providers, keeping patient records up-to-date and at their fingertips throughout procedures (Beckerman, 2025). As healthcare increasingly moves toward a more data-centric model, the implementation of such technologies will not only enhance individual patient care but also enable larger initiatives that optimize clinical workflows and resource utilization. Interdisciplinary collaboration involving anesthesiologists, surgeons, and other health care providers is key to unlocking the potential of these emerging trends. Through a multidisciplinary approach, medical teams can optimize perioperative care, with particular focus on improving patient experiences and outcomes through integrated efforts. For example, anesthesiologists are positioned in the perioperative surgical home model to have a substantial impact on multiple dimensions of patient management, ranging from preoperative evaluation to postoperative pain control measures. Such collaboration can result in tailored analgesic regimens that result in considerably improved recovery times and reduce the need for opioids (Pozek et al., 2018). In an increasingly complex health environment, developing a culture of teamwork and communication will position the anesthesia practice to adapt fluidly, so that innovations serve the ultimate mission of delivering effective and safe patient care.

Test Your Knowledge

1. What recent technological and pharmacological advances have improved the safety and effectiveness of anesthesia?
2. How have modern monitoring systems and minimally invasive techniques transformed anesthetic practice?

SUMMARY

The intricate specialty of anesthesia is a cornerstone of modern medicine, significantly transforming the surgical and patient management landscape. Understanding anesthetic concepts not only optimizes the perioperative course but also maximizes patient safety and comfort. As highlighted in the descriptions within this chapter, advances in anesthetic medications and methods have dramatically improved clinical outcomes, enabling health professionals to manage diverse patient populations effectively. The increasing use of technology and personalized approaches in anesthesia will likely continue to optimize anesthesia, reducing surgical risk and complications. This trend underscores the critical need for ongoing education and refresher courses in anesthesia to ensure professionals remain adept with new methods and standards of care. In addition, the requirement of intensive training in the application of anesthesia cannot be overstated. As highlighted in current veterinary practice, the need for skilled practitioners proficient in anesthesia management outweighs that in human medicine. For instance, the role of veterinary students in surgery clinics, focusing on rabbits, illustrates how practical training can lead to improved clinical success and well-being of the animals. Effective administration of anesthetic protocols in this case emphasizes the need for experienced knowledge and hands-on ability. Thus, involving such hands-on training in academic programs will not only enhance the skills of future professionals but also ensure improved standards of care in all aspects of healthcare provision, including veterinary practice. In summary, the specialty of anesthesia is dynamic and crucial, with implications that extend beyond human medicine to veterinary medicine. With the growing need for proficient anesthetic care, training programs must be prioritized to equip healthcare professionals with the skills and knowledge they need to address this multifaceted field. Concerns such as keeping pace with technological advancements and addressing individual patients' needs become priorities for future professional development. Emphasis on theoretical and practical education in anesthetic techniques will enable us to cultivate a new generation of practitioners who are best positioned to deliver safe, effective anesthetic care and, hopefully, improved outcomes for all patients. Commitment to sustained improvement and adaptation within the field will be crucial in addressing new challenges as they arise and optimizing overall provision of anesthesia care.

One of the main concepts in anesthesia research is the development of anesthetic techniques and their clinical practice. New approaches introduced to enhance patient care have played a central role in reducing anesthesia-related risks. An illustration is the proposal to design the ideal anesthetic using a receptor-focused magnetic resonance technique, which presents a revolutionary alternative to traditional pharmacologic agents. This new technique relies on creating an electromagnetic model to minimize the potential side effects traditionally associated with anesthetics. This technique addresses the electromagnetic nature of drug interactions at the receptor level and has the potential to offer greater safety and efficacy in anesthesia practice by keeping pace with current technology development and individualized medicine (Golyanishchev et al., 2016). The use of intra-abdominal pressure management in laparoscopic interventions also underscores the critical relationship between surgical and anesthetic techniques. A recent study examined the physiological effects of differential intra-abdominal pressures on hemodynamic stability and how these pressures affected various intra-procedural factors. Findings from the survey revealed that despite large excursions in mean arterial pressure (MAP) and blood gas parameters, these remained within the target range, indicating the resiliency of patients under effective care regimens. These realities are required to guide anesthesiologists in their practice, particularly in understanding the physiological responses elicited by different surgical techniques and the accompanying anesthesia principles (Afonso et al., 2011). This is a reflection of the dynamic character of anesthesia, where the anesthetic techniques must adapt to the operating conditions and the patients' physiological responses. Furthermore, the ongoing debate regarding the details of anesthesia is coupled with an understanding of pharmacodynamics and the need for innovation. As ongoing studies seek safer anesthesia methods, the potential for 3D modeling of receptor interactions is increasingly relevant. By building an extensive database of receptor locations and corresponding pharmacologic effects, physicians may tailor anesthetic approaches to patient profiles to optimize therapeutic effects. This shift to individualized anesthesia not only maximizes patient safety but also increases overall satisfaction with anesthetic care. As technology in this field continues to advance, practitioners must stay abreast of these developments so that gains in anesthetic technology are transformed into productive uses for improved patient care (Golyanishchev et al., 2016).

KEY TERMS FROM THIS CHAPTER

- Anesthesiologists
- Archaeological
- Hypothermia
- Neuromuscular block (NMB)
- Regional anesthesia
- Sensation
- Anesthetic techniques
- Clinical interventions
- Hypoxia
- Patient demographic
- Safe hemostatic
- Sophisticated science

CRITICAL THINKING QUESTIONS

1. **Who is known as the "Father of Modern Anesthesia"?**
   a. William T. G. Morton
   b. John Snow
   c. Crawford Long
   d. Joseph Lister
2. **Which of the following is NOT a goal of anesthesia?**
   a. Analgesia
   b. Amnesia
   c. Paralysis
   d. Infection control
3. **General anesthesia typically affects which of the following systems?**
   a. Nervous system
   b. Endocrine system
   c. Skeletal system
   d. Immune system
4. **The "triad of anesthesia" includes all EXCEPT:**
   a. Hypnosis
   b. Analgesia
   c. Muscle relaxation
   d. Antibiotics
5. **Which of the following agents is used for induction of general anesthesia?**
   a. Atropine
   b. Propofol
   c. Succinylcholine
   d. Epinephrine

Short Answer Questions

1. What is the primary goal of general anesthesia?
2. What is the difference between local and regional anesthesia?
3. How does local anesthesia block pain?
4. What is the purpose of muscle relaxants in anesthesia?
5. What is the difference between an anesthetist and an anesthesiologist?

Answer to Critical Thinking Questions

1. (a); 2. (d); 3. (a); 4. (d); 5. (b)

REFERENCES

1. Heimburg, T., & Jackson, A. D. (2007). The thermodynamics of general anesthesia. *Biophysical Journal*, *92*(9), 3159–3165. https://doi.org/10.1529/biophysj.106.099754Afonso, C. C. G. M., Marigliani, B., Gama, F. A. B., Azevedo, G. C., Miguel, G. P. S., Azevedo, J. L., José, et al. (2011). Invasive monitoring of the clinical effects of high intra-abdominal pressure for insertion of the first trocar. https://core.ac.uk/download/pdf/290403.pdf (accessed on 28th June 2025).
2. Agustí, M., Fontanet, J., Gabarrón, E., Gambus, P., et al. (2016). Comparison of the qCON and qNOX indices for the assessment of unconsciousness level and noxious stimulation response during surgery. https://core.ac.uk/download/81578685.pdf (accessed on 28th June 2025).
3. Aleman, M. R., Brosnan, R. J., Fletcher, D. J., Holliday, E., et al. (2015). Electroencephalogram of healthy horses during inhaled anesthesia. https://core.ac.uk/download/323071267.pdf (accessed on 28th June 2025).
4. Aleman, M., Brosnan, R. J., Fletcher, D. J., Holliday, E., et al. (2015). Qualitative and quantitative characteristics of the electroencephalogram in normal horses during administration of inhaled anesthesia. https://core.ac.uk/download/323068610.pdf (accessed on 28th June 2025).
5. Allard, M., Anderson, D., Applegate, R. L., Azer, J., et al. (2014). Cognitive dysfunction following desflurane versus sevoflurane general anesthesia in elderly patients: A randomized controlled trial. https://core.ac.uk/download/323070409.pdf (accessed on 28th June 2025).
6. Anbarafshan, M., Davari-Tanha, F., Kaveh, M., Khashayar, P., et al. (2016). Effects of intrathecal opioids use in cesarean section on breastfeeding and newborns' weight gaining. https://core.ac.uk/download/287941006.pdf (accessed on 28th June 2025).
7. Anderson, K., Grant, A., Harrison, P., Kearns, C., et al. (2016). A randomized, controlled, double-blind, non-inferiority trial of ultrasound-guided fascia iliaca block vs. spinal morphine for analgesia after primary hip arthroplasty. https://core.ac.uk/download/74232536.pdf (accessed on 28th June 2025).
8. Antonov, V. F., Antonov, V. F., Blume, A., Bovill, J. G., Brown, D. A., Böckmann, R. A., Böttner, M., et al. (2007). The influence of anesthetics, neurotransmitters and antibiotics on the relaxation processes in lipid membranes. https://core.ac.uk/download/44173701.pdf (accessed on 28th June 2025).
9. Arcadipane, A., Bignami, E., Blangetti, I., Cattaneo, S., et al. (2018). Burnout in cardiac anesthesiologists: Results from a national survey in Italy. https://core.ac.uk/download/188829816.pdf (accessed on 28th June 2025).
10. Argo, A., Buscemi, R., Karch, S. B., Lanzarone, A., Roccuzzo, R., & Zerbo, S. (2019). Perioperative and anesthetic deaths: Toxicological and medico-legal aspects. https://core.ac.uk/download/224993621.pdf (accessed on 28th June 2025).
11. Baratta, J. L., Schwenk, E. S., Viscusi, E. R., Wenzel, K., et al. (2016). Managing opioid-tolerant patients in the perioperative surgical home. https://core.ac.uk/download/46975930.pdf (accessed on 28th June 2025).
12. Baratto, F., Carron, M., Ori, C., Zarantonello, F., et al. (2016). Sugammadex for reversal of neuromuscular blockade: A retrospective analysis of clinical outcomes and cost-effectiveness in a single center. https://core.ac.uk/download/53528510.pdf (accessed on 28th June 2025).

13. Beckerman, C. (2025). The patient as a construction and a non-participant member of a change-process. https://core.ac.uk/download/pdf/6643568.pdf (accessed on 28th June 2025).

14. Bertoncello, F., Carron, M., & Ieppariello, G. (2017). Profile of sugammadex for reversal of neuromuscular blockade in the elderly: Current perspectives. https://core.ac.uk/download/158825140.pdf (accessed on 28th June 2025).

15. Blugerman, G., D'Angelo, J. A., Habbema, L., Lisborg, M., et al. (2011). Application of the liposuction techniques and principles in specific body areas and pathologies. https://core.ac.uk/download/17179833.pdf (accessed on 28th June 2025).

16. Breakwell, S., Kallio, P. J., Nolan, J., Olsen, M., et al. (2015). Anesthesia preoperative clinic referral for elevated HbA1c reduces complication rate in diabetic patients undergoing total joint arthroplasty. https://core.ac.uk/download/213081699.pdf (accessed on 28th June 2025).

17. Britton, S., Campbell, Y., & Chan, C. (2022). The utilization of amisulpride as a rescue drug for postop patients compared to promethazine for the treatment of postoperative nausea and vomiting: An educational module. https://core.ac.uk/download/552575912.pdf (accessed on 28th June 2025).

18. Brown, L. E., Dai, J. B., Daigle, R., Forman, S. A., et al. (2018). High-throughput screening in larval zebrafish identifies novel potent sedative-hypnotics. https://open.bu.edu/bitstream/2144/32909/3/ALN-D-17-01664_R2_manuscript.pdf (accessed on 28th June 2025).

19. Burish, M. J., Ganguly, K., Gulati, T., Hishinuma, A., et al. (2019). Large-scale changes in cortical dynamics triggered by repetitive somatosensory electrical stimulation. https://core.ac.uk/download/323072309.pdf (accessed on 28th June 2025).

20. Burokiene, V. Y. (2023). On the intraoperative awareness general anesthesia. https://core.ac.uk/download/591386666.pdf (accessed on 28th June 2025).

21. Butwick, A., & Sultan, P. (2013). Platelet counts and coagulation tests prior to neuraxial anesthesia in patients with preeclampsia: A retrospective analysis. https://core.ac.uk/download/29416263.pdf (accessed on 28th June 2025).

22. Calvieri, S., Cantisani, C., D'Andrea, V., Frascani, F., et al. (2014). New patents on topical anesthetics. https://core.ac.uk/download/54511696.pdf (accessed on 28th June 2025).

23. Ceppa, E. P., Colgate, C. L., Fennerty, M. L., House, M. G., et al. (2019). Post-pancreatoduodenectomy outcomes and epidural analgesia: A 5-year single institution experience. https://core.ac.uk/download/187423802.pdf (accessed on 28th June 2025).

24. Choi, B. M., Mashour, G. A., Noh, G. J., Kim, S., & Lee, U. (2008). Propofol induction reduces the capacity for neural information integration: Implications for the mechanism of consciousness and general anesthesia. https://core.ac.uk/download/pdf/288135.pdf (accessed on 28th June 2025).

25. Clough, A. V., Cummens, B., Densmore, J. C., Jacobs, R. F., et al. (2013). *Rattus* model utilizing selective pulmonary ischemia induces bronchiolitis obliterans organizing pneumonia. https://core.ac.uk/download/213078972.pdf (accessed on 28th June 2025).

26. Collini, S., Pacella, E., Pacella, F., Salducci, M., et al. (2015). Ropivacaine vs tetracaine in topical anesthesia for intravitreal injection. https://core.ac.uk/download/54527194.pdf (accessed on 28th June 2025).

27. Copot, D., Ghita, M., Muresan, C., Neckebroek, M., et al. (2020). Closed-loop control of anesthesia: Survey on actual trends, challenges and perspectives. https://core.ac.uk/download/368712192.pdf (accessed on 28th June 2025).

28. Cornell University. (1999). *College of Veterinary Medicine*. https://ecommons.cornell.edu/bitstream/handle/1813/38459/COS_v90_1998_99_16.pdf?sequence=1&isAllowed=y (accessed on 28th June 2025).

29. De Rycke, L., Gielen, I., Hermans, K., van Bree, H., et al. (2008). Diagnosis of dental problems in pet rabbits (*Oryctolagus cuniculus*). https://core.ac.uk/download/55795678.pdf (accessed on 28th June 2025).

30. Drover, C. M., Drover, D. R., Vaughn, D. A., MacIver, M. B., Cohen, M. S., et al. (2018). Do complexity measures of frontal EEG distinguish loss of consciousness in geriatric patients under anesthesia? https://core.ac.uk/download/323076544.pdf (accessed on 28th June 2025).

31. Edworthy, J., Hellier, E., Meredith, C., Rose, M., et al. (2013). Learning medical alarms whilst performing other tasks. https://core.ac.uk/download/29818949.pdf (accessed on 28th June 2025).

32. Fezeu, F., Henderson, F., Larson, P. S., Melmer, T., et al. (2018). Challenges and solutions for functional neurosurgery in developing countries. https://core.ac.uk/download/323062978.pdf (accessed on 28th June 2025).

33. Golyanishchev, M. (2016). Hypothesis of Rfmra development–the receptor-focused magnetic and resonant anesthesia. https://core.ac.uk/download/301580510.pdf (accessed on 28th June 2025).

34. Henker, R., O'Donnell, J. M., Sakai, T., Tamura, T., et al. (2021). Certified registered nurse anesthetist and anesthesiologist assistant education programs in the United States. https://core.ac.uk/download/636419491.pdf (accessed on 28th June 2025).

35. Hu, H., & Wu, M. (2002). Spin-mediated consciousness theory: An approach based on pan-protopsychism. https://core.ac.uk/download/pdf/85302.pdf (accessed on 28th June 2025).

36. Huang, J., Lv, Y., Rubinsky, B., Wang, Y., et al. (2019). A study on nonthermal irreversible electroporation of the thyroid. https://core.ac.uk/download/323081132.pdf (accessed on 28th June 2025).

37. Jones, B. (2021). Increased access (knowledge) of health promotion & preventative care reduces chronic disease within African American communities. https://core.ac.uk/download/520100766.pdf (accessed on 28th June 2025).

38. Kalachnyuk, L., Melnichuk, D., & Umanska, A. (2018). Indicators of the element range of rat's blood in term artificial hypotyposis. https://media.neliti.com/media/publications/297432-indicators-of-the-element-range-of-rats-59679f83.pdf (accessed on 28th June 2025).

39. Kissin, I., & Vlassakov, K. V. (2015). Scient metrics of anesthetic drugs and their techniques of administration, 1984–2013. https://core.ac.uk/download/28952631.pdf (accessed on 28th June 2025).

40. Liu, H., & Tumber, S. S. (2010). Epidural abscess after multiple lumbar punctures for labor epidural catheter placement. https://core.ac.uk/download/323071341.pdf (accessed on 28th June 2025).

41. Mitchell, M. J. (2003). Patient anxiety and modern elective surgery: A literature review. https://core.ac.uk/download/104290.pdf (accessed on 28th June 2025).

42. N/A. (2012). A costly dental destination: Hospital care means states pay dearly. https://core.ac.uk/download/71357939.pdf (accessed on 28th June 2025).

43. N/A. (2022). Music in health and diseases. https://core.ac.uk/download/534904022.pdf (accessed on 28th June 2025).

44. Nebiolo, M. (2017). Surgery as a science: The intellectual and practical evolution of European surgery from the 16th to the 18th century. https://core.ac.uk/download/80463099.pdf (accessed on 28th June 2025).

45. Pozek, J. P. J., Schwenk, E. S., & Viscusi, E. R. (2018). Managing prolonged pain after surgery: Examining the role of opioids. https://core.ac.uk/download/213444274.pdf (accessed on 28th June 2025).

46. Raichle, M. E. (2015). The brain's default mode network. *Annual Review of Neuroscience, 38*, 433–447. https://doi.org/10.1146/annurev-neuro-071013-014030 (accessed on 28th June 2025).

47. Siu, E. Y., & Moon, T. S. (2020). Opioid-free and opioid-sparing anesthesia. *International Anesthesiology Clinics, 58*, 34–41. https://doi.org/10.1097/aia.0000000000000270 (accessed on 28th June 2025).

48. Veit, R. (2013). A ray of sunshine in the sickroom: Archaeological insights into late 19th- and early 20th-century medicine and anesthesia. https://core.ac.uk/download/215547654.pdf (accessed on 28th June 2025).

49. Watson, M. T. (2015). The use of tricaine methane sulfonate, clove oil, metomidate, and 2-phenoxyethanol for anesthesia induction in alewives (*Alosa pseudoharengus*). https://core.ac.uk/download/215521192.pdf (accessed on 28th June 2025).

ANATOMY AND PHYSIOLOGY RELEVANT TO ANESTHESIA

2

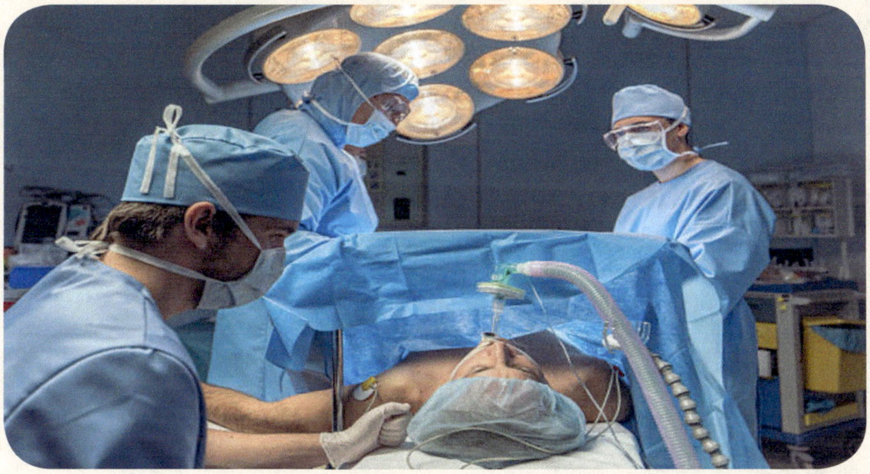

LEARNING OBJECTIVES

After studying this chapter, you will be able to:

1. Basic anatomy relevant to anesthesia
2. The nervous system and anesthesia
3. Cardiovascular physiology in anesthesia
4. Respiratory physiology and anesthesia
5. Pharmacology of anesthetic agents
6. Patient considerations in anesthesia

Introduction

A comprehensive understanding of human anatomy and physiology largely drives the art of anesthesia. This basic knowledge is helpful to anesthesiologists when dealing with complex physiological responses to anesthetic agents, ensuring safe patient care and efficient pain relief. For instance, the addition of regional anesthesia techniques, such as the surface anatomy-guided clavipectoral fascia plane block, underscores the significance of anatomical landmarks in achieving positive anesthetic effects. This technique, first applied in 2017, demonstrates how well a block reduces the risk of more invasive techniques such as the Interscalene Block, particularly for clavicle surgery. Thus, understanding anatomical structures and variations is crucial for optimizing patient outcomes in surgical interventions (Purnomo et al., 2025). Also, the evolution of image-guided techniques, such as ultrasonography, in combination with traditional ones, enhances the precision of anesthesia administration. In older adults, physiological changes associated with age can pose a complicating element in the already challenging task of successful spinal anesthesia. Evidence shows that visualization of neuraxial anatomy using ultrasonography to injecting spinal anesthesia significantly increases the likelihood that the first attempt is successful and decreases complications such as needle redirections during repetition. This development is not only most important in the provision of adequate anesthesia but also in alleviating pain and potential trauma to the patient, which could be particularly damaging in older adults (Arda Işıker et al., 2023). As this industry continues to advance, combining novel imaging techniques with conventional anatomical knowledge highlights the importance of this dualistic approach in enhancing anesthetic methods. The dynamic interaction between physiology and anatomy in anesthesia extends beyond procedural considerations to include anesthetic drug pharmacodynamics and pharmacokinetics. Understanding the body systems—e.g., circulatory, respiratory, and nervous systems—enables anesthesiologists to predict patients' reactions to various drugs. Drug metabolism and action can be significantly affected by factors such as body weight, age, and underlying medical disease, and hence anesthetic plans need to be tailored to individual patients. This personalized method not only ensures maximum safety in procedures but also enables optimal postoperative recovery. Therefore, the importance of complete anatomical and physiological data is paramount in anesthesia practice, affecting both the technological and clinical aspects of the anesthetic procedure (Purnomo et al., 2025; Arda et al., 2023) (Figure 2.1).

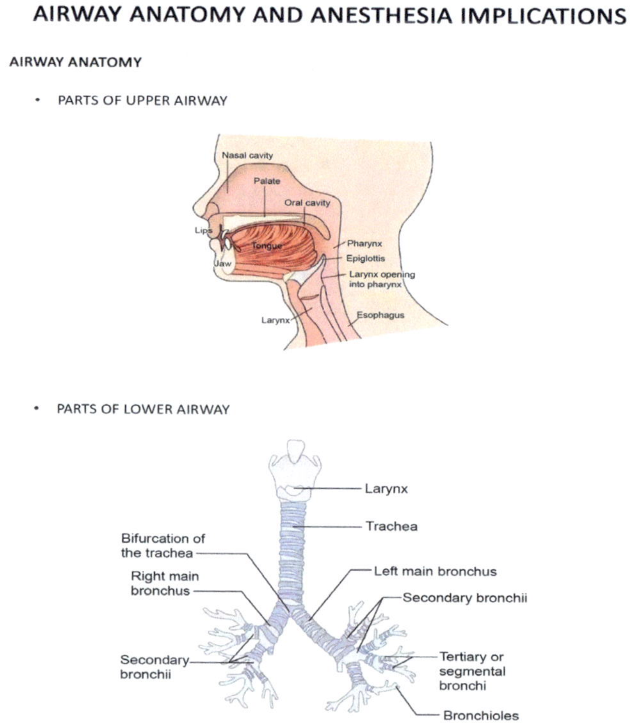

Figure 2.1. The field of anesthesia relies heavily on a comprehensive understanding of human anatomy and physiology.

Source: https://conceptualanesthesia.com/wp-content/uploads/2024/02/1.-Airway-anatomy-and-physiology-and-Anesthesia-Implications_page-0001-min.webp.

Definition of Anesthesia

Anesthesia, as part of modern medicine, can be defined as a condition in which there is a loss of sensation, coupled with or without loss of consciousness. The motive is to enable surgical and diagnostic procedures by ensuring patients experience no pain or distress. This is achieved with various anesthetic agents and techniques, which are further divided into general anesthesia, in which the patient is made unconscious, and regional or local anesthesia, in which a specific body part is targeted. The mode of anesthesia matters and depends on several issues, such as the nature of the surgical procedure, the patient's medical history, and the dangers associated with the application of different anesthetic procedures. The combined interaction between physiology and anatomy is instrumental in the administration of anesthesia. Anesthesiological landmarks and their identification during regional anesthesia are instrumental in facilitating effective analgesia through procedures such as nerve blocks or epidural anesthesia, where precise placement of needles is essential. Moreover, the body's physiological responses to anesthetic agents are complex; anesthetic mechanisms interact with neural activity, receptor sites, and systemic processes. For instance, the local anesthetic effect on sodium channels in nerve fibers suppresses pain impulse conduction, underscoring the importance of understanding both the structure and function of the nervous system in anesthesia practice (Hilton et al., 1989). Such information ultimately assists anesthetists in tailoring anesthetic plans for patients. Additionally, the history of anesthetic practice itself has evolved over time from primitive to more sophisticated methods that exploit technological and pharmacologic advancements. Newer anesthetics have not only made anesthesia safer and more efficient but also more versatile in application in numerous facets of medicine. In addition, research continues to examine the physiological consequences of anesthesia across diverse patient groups, in this case, whether factors such as obesity or age will influence the pharmacokinetic and pharmacodynamic characteristics of anesthetic drugs (Breckenridge et al., 1972). And although progress is continually being made, it remains vital for practitioners to remain vigilant for such developments so that the relationship between anatomy and physiology is factored into decisions to optimize patient care during anesthesia.

Importance of Anatomy and Physiology in Anesthesia

The value of anatomy and physiology in the practice of anesthesiology cannot be overstated, as a thorough understanding of these subjects is the basis for safe, effective anesthetic practice. Anesthesiologists must have detailed knowledge of human body structure and function to administer anesthesia. For instance, the anatomy and physiology of the central nervous system and its channels are significant in the selection of anesthetic drugs and techniques. Additionally, understanding airway anatomy allows providers to anticipate and manage potential complications during anesthetic induction. Such foundational knowledge empowers practitioners to make more informed decisions based on patient characteristics, further enhancing patient safety and clinical outcomes. Additionally, patient anatomical differences, such as obesity, present difficulty for anesthetic management. Research indicates that body mass index influences sensory regression times with spinal anesthesia. In a study comparing levels of sensory blocks produced by hyperbaric 0.75% bupivacaine, it was found that the hypothesis, which indicated differences in sensory regression times between obese and non-obese patients, was not validated. The absence of statistically significant differences reiterates the need for the anesthesiologist to modify their strategy based on individual anatomical considerations and physiological response, reinforcing the need for an individualized practice in anesthesia. Appreciations of such correlations are essential to developing strategies to minimize risks associated with anomalous anatomies. Lastly, the interplay between anatomy, physiology, and pharmacology confirms the importance of these disciplines in anesthesia. , Complete knowledge of drug metabolism, receptor interactions, and physiological effects is essential for maximizing anesthetic techniques. Some anesthetic agents have differential potency based on differences in patient anatomy and health status, illustrating the close connection between anatomical variation and drug action. The re-tuning of drug dosages and the optimal selection of drugs most appropriate to the patient's unique anatomy and physiology constitute one of the most critical elements of anesthesia practice. Thus, the integration of these disciplines not only renders anesthetic administration safer and more efficient but also equips caregivers with the ability to deal with complex clinical scenarios in terms of providing the best outcomes for patients undergoing surgical procedures.

2.1. Basic Anatomy Relevant to Anesthesia

Learning Outcome

1. Overview of the human body systems
2. Key anatomical structures involved in anesthesia
3. Variations in anatomy among patients

Understanding the anatomy of the human airway is critical in anesthesia because it directly affects how airway management should be conducted. The airway has two broad divisions: the upper and lower airways. The upper airway is made up of anatomical structures such as the nasal cavity, pharynx, and larynx, while the lower airway is made up of the trachea and bronchi. Knowledge of these anatomical regions is essential for successfully intubating a patient and securing an adequate airway during anesthesia. For instance, anatomical variations such as irregular jaw development or enlarged tonsils may make visualization and passage to the vocal cords more difficult, so it is essential to be prepared to use alternative methods or devices to ensure patient safety during anesthesia administration. As important is respect for the cardiovascular system and its implications for anesthesiology practice. The heart, major vessels, and overall circulatory dynamics become focal points on the operating room table during surgery, particularly in monitoring and managing blood pressure and cardiac output. Anesthetics can alter hemodynamics; thus, practitioners need to assess individual cardiovascular anatomy in preparation for reactions to anesthetic agents. For example, variations in coronary artery anatomy can substantially impact anesthesia management, especially in patients with underlying cardiovascular disease. Profound knowledge of these factors allows anesthetists to tailor their practice, ensuring hemodynamic stability and minimizing the risk of induction and maintenance of anesthesia complications, once more putting forward the significance of anatomy in medical practice. MeSH terms: Anatomy/physiology, Anesthesia/administration and dosage, Anesthetics/administration and dosage. In addition, the anatomy of the neuromuscular system has a significant impact on the anesthetic process management. Anesthesia has a profound impact on muscle function, and knowledge about the anatomical organization of nerve and muscle is pivotal for the administration of neuromuscular blocking agents. Information regarding the pattern of nerve innervations and muscle groups facilitates anesthetists in anticipating the onset and duration of blockades during surgery. In addition, anatomical variations of pathways of the brachial or lumbosacral plexus can be critical determinants in regional anesthesia techniques. Anatomical variation in landmarks, for instance, requires accurate localization for effective peripheral nerve blocks to optimize surgical conditions while minimizing patient discomfort and risk. This interdependence between the anatomic structure and anesthesia supports the basic integration of anatomy in developing competent anesthesia practice, as cited in relevant scholarly literature (Cornell University, 1996; Florencia et al., 2005).

2.1.1. Overview of the Human Body Systems

The human body is made up of a multifaceted array of systems that work cohesively towards the function of homeostasis and the maintenance of life processes. Each system, from the circulatory to the nervous, has its own function in overall health and well-being. The circulatory system, for instance, is tasked with the dissemination of oxygen and nutrition through the bloodstream, facilitated by the heart's rhythmic contractions.

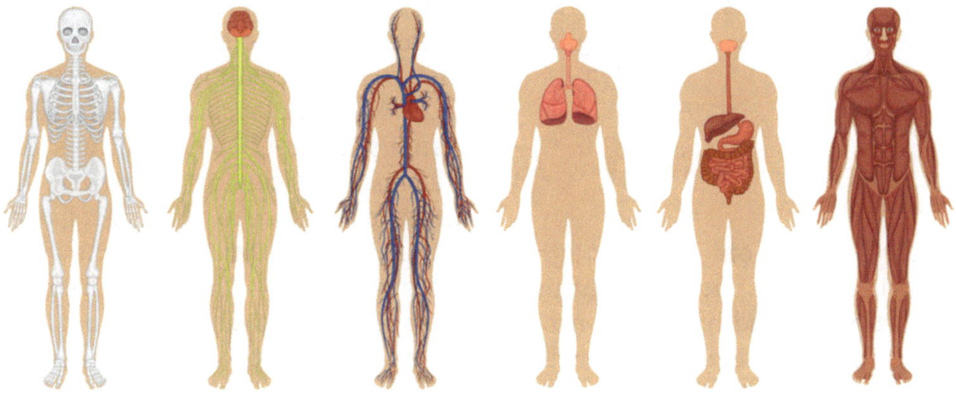

Figure 2.2. Overview of the human body systems.

Source: https://libapps-au.s3-ap-southeast-2.amazonaws.com/accounts/10951/images/humanbodysystems.jpg.

The smooth functioning of this system is paramount in anesthesia, as cardiovascular status must be monitored during surgery. The manner in which these systems interact points to the necessity of an overall approach to patient care in the context of anesthesia, in which any form of imbalance can lead to serious complications, necessitating thorough knowledge of human anatomy and physiology to minimize risks to a bare minimum. The respiratory system is also essential, especially when anesthetized with agents that can disrupt normal respiratory processes. Gas exchange—oxygen and carbon dioxide exchange—happens in the alveoli, relying on the proper functioning of the respiratory system. During anesthesia, the providers must stay vigilant regarding airway management and also ventilation, as well as the patient's respiratory status throughout the operation. Changes in the respiratory gas balance can lead to hypoxemia or hypercapnia, and these must be treated promptly. The necessity of a thorough understanding of the mechanics of respiration and the accompanying physiological responses ensures that anesthesia personnel can predict and prevent anticipated complications and provide the interrelationships among systems necessary to deliver a safe anesthetic. A secondary necessity in anesthesiology is the interaction between the nervous and endocrine systems. The nervous system, responsible for the control of body function and responses, corresponds with the endocrine system in regulating metabolic activity through the secretion of hormones. This is especially relevant when discussing how anesthetic agents act in the body, as most act on both nerve conduction and hormonal balance, thereby modifying patients' responses to anesthesia. Anesthesia can suppress the autonomic nervous system, which manages involuntary body functions, and thus enhances the demand for anesthesiologists to monitor and manage such responses with caution. Lastly, knowledge of the functions and interaction of these body systems allows informed decision-making during anesthesia, facilitating safe patient outcomes and enhanced performance in operating rooms (University of Vermont, 1948; Metzinger et al., 2001) (Figure 2.2).

2.1.2. Key Anatomical Structures Involved in Anesthesia

Anesthesia relies heavily on a thorough understanding of critical anatomical structures that govern both action and administration of anesthetic agents. Of the structures, the central nervous system, more specifically the brain and spinal cord, plays an indispensable role. Brain regions, notably the thalamus, cortex, and brainstem, play a pivotal role in governing awareness and sensory perception during anesthesia. The spinal cord is also significant because it transmits signals from peripheral nerves to the brain, and therefore it is a target for most types of regional anesthesia, such as epidurals and spinal blocks. Consolidated knowledge of these anatomical structures assists anesthesiologists in effectively managing patient sedation and pain relief, achieving a balance between adequate anesthesia and patient safety—a matter of utmost importance in operating rooms, given the directive against inducing awareness and pain during procedures (Ruholl et al., 2021). Peripheral nerves are also a vital anatomical component in anesthesia. These nerves that travel between the spinal cord and other regions of the body are generally the focus of regional anesthesia techniques that target anesthetizing the feeling in specific locations. Peripheral nerves, such as the femoral, sciatic, and brachial plexus, serve specific regions and must be precisely localized to enable successful administration of the anesthetic. Understanding the anatomical course and variations of these nerves enables the development of optimal anesthetic protocols, reducing the risk of complications such as nerve damage or inadequate pain relief. With the use of advanced imaging techniques such as ultrasound guidance, the accuracy of nerve blocks has increased, allowing anesthesiologists to visualize these structures in real time and optimize the effectiveness and safety of regional anesthesia procedures (Bartsch et al., 2010). Apart from the peripheral and central nervous systems, anatomical conditions of the airway are most critical for anesthetic management. Anesthesia, due to its effects on respiratory function, requires thorough knowledge of airway anatomy for smooth intubation and ventilation management. Anatomical landmarks such as the pharynx, larynx, and trachea must be adequately assessed before anesthesia induction to prevent complications such as difficult intubation or airway obstruction. Moreover, variations in anatomy caused by conditions such as obesity or congenital abnormalities can also pose extra problems. Airway management in a successful context not only ensures efficient delivery of anesthetics but also safeguards the well-being of the patient during the surgery process. Therefore, awareness of the complexities of airway anatomy is an important part of the preparation and application of safe and effective anesthetics (Ruholl et al., 2021).

2.1.3. Variations in Anatomy Among Patients

Anatomical variations among patients are a significant concern in anesthesia practice, influencing the efficacy and safety of anesthetic interventions. Anatomical variations may result from genetic causes, developmental abnormalities, or acquired diseases, necessitating specialized anesthetic management. For instance, patients with conditions such as achondroplasia exhibit apparent physiologic characteristics, including short stature and potential skeletal deformities, that may make procedures challenging and require precise anatomical knowledge. Such distinctions not only can affect the approach to accessing the nerve block and airway management but also the nature of the equipment utilized and the dosage of the anesthetic agents. Anesthesiologists must be aware of such differences since ignorance of anatomical differences could lead to adverse outcomes or failed anesthesia, suggesting the need for rigorous preoperative assessments. Anatomical variation extends beyond physical patient attributes; it also includes medical histories that predispose patients to anesthesia-related complications. For example, those patients with skeletal abnormalities have associated cardiovascular abnormalities as well, as noted by studies that found that individuals with achondroplasia have increased cardiovascular disease. Anesthesia providers need to consider these variables, as variations in awareness of current anatomical and physiological conditions may significantly influence patient outcomes. A thorough understanding of the impact of variations on the principles of anesthesiology is necessary to minimize dangers and enhance the level of care. Therefore, maximizing anesthetic outcomes necessitates readjusting anesthesia procedures and protocols to account for patient-specific anatomical deviations. Furthermore, the recognition of anatomical variations in conjunction with patient demographics, such as age, sex, and comorbidities, adds to the intricacies of anesthetic practice. For instance, studies have shown that specific populations, e.g., those with special care needs or healthcare disparities, have higher surgical condition rates. The midlevel dental provider paper discusses the growing need to address healthcare access for underserved populations, emphasizing the importance of specialized anesthesia practice across various clinical settings. For this reason, anesthesiologists must receive ongoing education and training to be aware of the anatomical presentations they may encounter. Ongoing learning is central to advancing the safety and efficiency of anesthesia care, ultimately leading to enhanced patient outcomes across anatomical environments, which are required for the development of effective anesthesia practice.

Test Your Knowledge

1. Which anatomical structures are most important for airway management, and why is their understanding critical during anesthesia?
2. How does knowledge of spinal and peripheral nerve anatomy guide the safe administration of regional and local anesthesia?

2.2. The Nervous System and Anesthesia

Learning Outcome

1. Central nervous system functions
2. Peripheral nervous system and pain pathways
3. Impact of anesthesia on nervous system activity

The interface of anesthesia with the nervous system is a complex relationship that is integral to the field of anesthesiology. Anesthesia affects the central nervous system (CNS) for analgesia, sedation, and muscle relaxation primarily. Understanding the anatomical structures and physiological functions of the nervous system is a prerequisite for anesthesiologists for appropriate perioperative care. For instance, regional anesthesia techniques rely on a full appreciation of nerve pathways and their related anatomical landmarks.

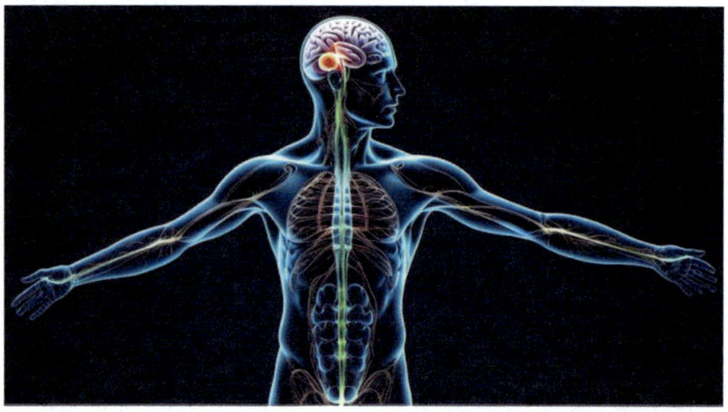

Figure 2.3. The nervous system and anesthesia.

Source: https://t3.ftcdn.net/jpg/07/40/60/02/360_F_740600281_ob14aimawHd4VFTfyK0JJFu3ypJzKzoH.jpg.

This not only allows practitioners to minimize patient pain but also optimizes therapeutic effect through targeted intervention. Furthermore, an understanding of the selective actions of various anesthetic drugs on neurophysiological mechanisms can guide the selection of drugs appropriate to individual patient needs. Monitoring anesthesia's effect on the nervous system is central to ensuring patient safety and successful surgical outcomes. Intraoperative neurophysiological monitoring, as with endoscopic and endonasal surgery, provides real-time feedback on the functional integrity of vulnerable neural structures during surgery. Employing advanced modalities like electroencephalography and somatosensory evoked potentials allows Anesthesiologists to quantify the efficacy of anesthesia without causing potential neurological damage (Doan et al., 2016). This multimodality approach offers a safer environment by providing mechanisms to detect changes indicating imminent neural damage, enabling corrective actions to be taken in the blink of an eye. All these technologies aim at emphasizing close inter-association of anesthesia and neurophysiological health, and they call for competent monitoring. Additionally, pain pathway and sensory processing knowledge are necessary in tailoring anesthesia to specific patients. For instance, the activity of the auditory nerve during sensory processing reveals the effects of anesthetic drugs on specific nerve pathways (Clark et al., 2025). Patterns of single-fiber discharge in the auditory nerve are essential sources of information regarding sensory perception under anesthesia. Mapping these pathways assists in optimizing anesthetic techniques to not only relieve surgical pain but also postoperative pain effectively. This integrated strategy not only enhances patient comfort but also significantly influences recovery times and overall success of surgery, emphasizing the importance of applying anatomical and physiological knowledge to anesthesia practice (Figure 2.3).

2.2.1. Central Nervous System Functions

The central nervous system (CNS) is central to facilitating homeostasis in the body, influencing a broad array of physiological processes. The brain and spinal cord coordinate the body's responses to stimuli both within and outside the body, enabling adaptation to varying environments. Sensory processing is one of the principal functions of the CNS, where peripheral sensory inputs are conveyed through ascending pathways to the brain for interpretation. This is of crucial significance when working with anesthesia, since anesthetic agents must effectively modulate sensory pathways to produce pain relief and maintain homeostasis during surgery. Understanding these mechanisms directs anesthetic regimens and predicts how different patients will respond to other anesthetic agents, which is crucial in optimizing patient outcomes under anesthesia. In addition to sensory processing, CNS is also responsible for more complicated cognitive processes, including memory, consciousness, and attention, with significant concerns in the area of anesthetics. Mechanisms of consciousness are involved with intricate networks that are predominantly dependent on the engagement of the thalamus and cortex, which provide reportable and qualitative conscious experience. This difference between conscious and unconscious conditions is crucial when anesthetized, where it is frequently aimed at controlling levels of consciousness for surgical interventions. Research indicates that some anesthetic drugs might selectively affect specific neural networks to cause desired amounts of sedation or unconsciousness, thereby reducing side effects. The interaction between anesthetic techniques and their impact on cognitive function underscores the importance of understanding CNS mechanisms in detail to ensure optimal safety and efficacy of anesthesia across different operating environments (Bernard, 2012). Exposure to radiation has been determined to profoundly influence the CNS integrity and functionality that might lead to cognitive disorders, and so is the case with anesthetic issues. For instance, it has been demonstrated that radiation is never suitable for neurogenesis in critical brain areas, such as the hippocampus, and modulates cognitive recovery after anesthesia. The implication is immense because it underscores the importance of accounting for neurological interactions in giving anesthetic drugs, particularly among patients with a history of CNS impairment following radiation or other treatment. important critical anesthetic management may then involve modified approaches to address the varying degrees of neuroplasticity and radiosensitivity in patients' brains. By identifying anesthetic strategies that account for such CNS functions, clinicians are better able to achieve recovery and cognitive preservation, underscoring the intimate interconnectedness between CNS anatomy and physiology and anesthetic practice (Azami et al., 2012).

2.2.2. Peripheral Nervous System and Pain Pathways

The peripheral nervous system (PNS) plays a significant role in transmitting pain information from peripheral tissues to the central nervous system, and it is a fundamental concept of learning pain management in anesthesia. The PNS includes sensory, motor, and autonomic fibers that convey detection and response to noxious stimuli through well-defined pain pathways. Nociceptors, which are specialized sensory receptors located throughout the body, activate the pain pathway in response to potentially harmful stimuli such as mechanical tension or thermal extremes. When stimulated, these nociceptors transmit electrical impulses through afferent neurons to the spinal cord, where synaptic transmission occurs. Pain pathways subsequently ascend through the spinothalamic tract to the thalamus, ultimately to the cortex, where pain perception is achieved. Understanding these pathways allows anesthesiologists to guide their interventions appropriately, whether regional or via systemic agents, to modulate pain perception and improve patient outcomes. Knowledge of pain pathways is not only vital for conventional treatment methods but also for more contemporary interventions, such as occipital nerve stimulation (ONS). Originally applied to occipital neuralgia, ONS has been used to treat other headache conditions, such as migraine and cluster headache. New research identifies patient phenotyping as a framework for individualized treatment based on the most probable responders to ONS.

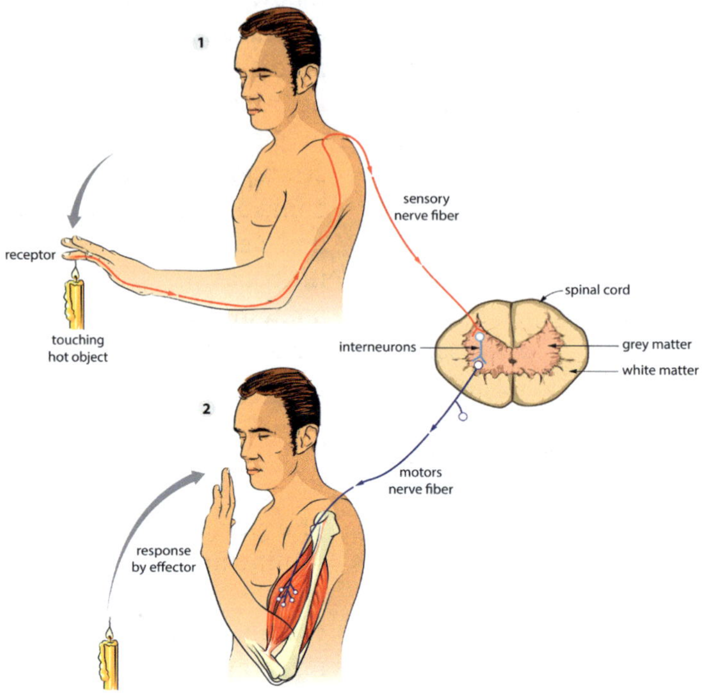

Figure 2.4. Peripheral nervous system and pain pathways.

Source: https://www.acquiredbraininjury-education.scot.nhs.uk/wp-content/uploads/360969659-Reflex.jpg.

This sophisticated assessment, as recorded, has the potential to improve patient outcomes through personalized treatment regimens. The incorporation of such approaches into pain management regimens reflects a broader respect for the role of the PNSs in processes of pain and the complexity of actually diminishing chronic conditions of pain (Bartsch et al., 2010). Anesthesia procedures that incorporate these considerations are a means of guaranteeing the quality of care for patients suffering debilitating pain. In addition, pain pathway anatomy also meaningfully overlaps with the physiology that governs anesthetic intervention. Understanding how peripheral nerves are linked to central pain-processing components clarifies how anesthetics interfere with pain-signal transmission. Local anesthetics, for instance, act by blocking sodium channels in nerve fibers, which prevents the ability to conduct action potentials and permits subsequent pain signal transmission to the central nervous system. These pharmacologic maneuvers enhance the effectiveness of surgical procedures by reducing intraoperative and postoperative pain. In the context of ongoing research into new therapeutic approaches, the growth of knowledge concerning PNS dynamics has profound clinical consequences for anesthesia, particularly in respect of tailoring methods to the patient and optimizing the therapeutic efficacy of anesthetic medication (Freed et al., 1951). This ongoing advancement underscores the necessity for anesthesiologists to remain as up to date as possible on the evolving science of anatomy and physiology in pain management (Figure 2.4).

2.2.3. Impact of Anesthesia on Nervous System Activity

Anesthesia exerts a profound influence on the nervous system, primarily through its effects on neurotransmission and synaptic plasticity. Anesthetic induction alters the dynamics of neural circuits, leading to a homogenization of brain activity with extensive cortical silence and reduced thalamocortical communication. Disruption is not only selective for sensory processing but also for cognition, as anesthetics affect the release and reuptake of neurotransmitters such as gamma-aminobutyric acid (GABA) and glutamate. In addition, the control of such neurotransmitters results in the analgesic and sedative effects of most anesthetic drugs. Studies have revealed that by amplifying GABAergic inhibition, anesthetics abolish conscious awareness and alter pain perception, which is important in operating rooms to avoid patient discomfort and movement during potentially painful procedures. Further, enhanced imaging technologies have enabled more advanced studies of the effects of anesthesia on nervous system activity. For instance, two-photon microscopy has revolutionized scientists' ability to visualize neuronal activity in living tissue, providing insight into how anesthetics affect neuronal activity at the cellular level. This nonlinear imaging technique enables researchers to monitor calcium dynamics and blood flow within the brain at various depths, hence illuminating anesthesia's impact on neural connectivity and function. The possible implications of such research are enormous, as they not only advance our understanding of anesthesia's momentary effects during surgical procedures but also provide insight into longer-term repercussions for neuronal health and plasticity, particularly in vulnerable groups such as the elderly. With the association of anesthesia with neural function, understanding of the resulting anatomical and physiological mechanisms is of utmost importance. Ramon y Cajal's early work established the premises for neuron-to-neuron interactions and the structural details of nerve cells and their axonal interconnects. The anesthetic drug compromises these interconnects, although specific pathways and points of interference vary significantly by anesthetic. For example, inhaled anesthetics may have effects on different brain regions than intravenous drugs, and other effects on recovery and cognition after surgery. With ongoing revelations of specific mechanisms, applying the latest imaging and analytical techniques will further elucidate how anesthesia reorganizes nervous system activity, thereby informing best practices in anesthesia delivery and patient care (Georgiev et al., 2010; Giovanni et al., 2011).

Test Your Knowledge

1. How does anesthesia affect the central and peripheral nervous systems to produce analgesia, sedation, and loss of consciousness?
2. Why is an understanding of neurophysiology essential for the safe and effective administration of anesthetic agents?

2.3. Cardiovascular Physiology in Anesthesia

Learning Outcome

1. Heart function and blood circulation
2. Effects of anesthesia on blood pressure and heart rate
3. Monitoring cardiovascular status during anesthesia

An understanding of cardiovascular physiology is relevant to anesthesiologists because it directs them through the complexities of anesthesia administration. The cardiovascular system plays a significant role in maintaining homeostasis during surgery because it provides tissues with oxygen and nutrients and removes metabolic waste products. An understanding of hemodynamics, i.e., blood pressure, cardiac output, and systemic vascular resistance, is critical during anesthesia. Anesthetics can induce changes in these parameters that lead to hemodynamic instability. With an adequate understanding of these concepts, practitioners can anticipate and respond to possible complications, ensuring the patient's safety throughout the operation. Monitoring cardiovascular status is at the foundation of anesthetic practice, allowing real-time dynamic modulation of anesthetic drugs to maintain optimal physiological conditions. The cardiovascular effects of anesthetic medications must also be studied; different drugs exert different effects on heart rate, contractility, and vascular tone. Volatile anesthetics, for instance, may lead to vasodilation with a reduction in systemic vascular resistance and potentially result in hypotension. Other agents, such as etomidate, may provide hemodynamic stability and are therefore preferred in patients with pre-existing cardiovascular compromise. Anesthesiologists must evaluate the patient's baseline cardiovascular condition, including hypertension or congestive heart failure. Information provided through this helps individualize anesthesia protocols, minimizing undesirable cardiovascular responses. Additionally, the intricate relationship between anesthesia and autonomic nervous regulation necessitates understanding how various agents interact with sympathetic and parasympathetic activity to influence cardiovascular dynamics during surgery.

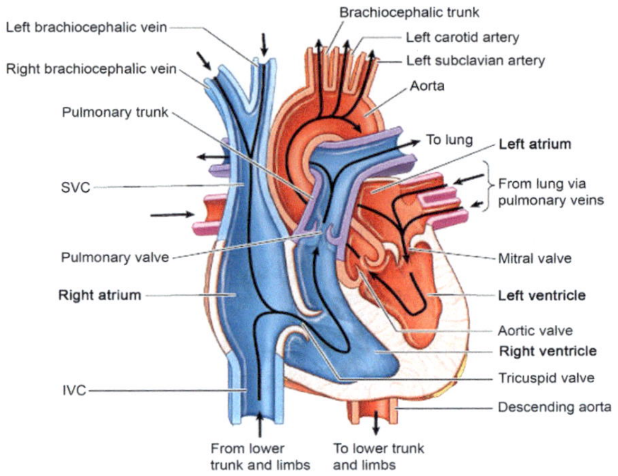

Figure 2.5. The cardiovascular physiology in anesthesia.

Source: https://aneskey.com/wp-content/uploads/2016/06/image00859.jpeg.

Preanesthetic evaluation is an important step towards optimizing cardiovascular well-being before anesthesia. Estimation of cardiac reserve and risk stratification are a few procedures, which allow the anesthesiologist to customize perioperative management protocols in advance. Methods such as echocardiography or non-invasive cardiac output monitoring can provide data on a patient's functional status and guide anesthetic selection. In addition, preoperative optimization of comorbidities—such as blood pressure control or diabetes management—can have a tremendous impact on perioperative outcomes. These maneuvers must be instituted because underlying cardiovascular disease can have a critical impact on patients' ability to tolerate the physiological insults related to surgery and anesthesia. Lastly, an all-encompassing integration of cardiovascular physiology into anesthetic management not only optimizes the procedure's safety and efficacy but also continues to further the general objective of enhancing patient outcomes in the operating room, as reiterated in the literature (University of Vermont, 1948; University of Vermont, 1950) (Figure 2.5).

2.3.1. Heart Function and Blood Circulation

The heart is the central pump of the circulatory system, channeling blood throughout the body. Its rhythmic contractions are necessary to maintain hemodynamic stability, distribute oxygenated blood to tissues, and eliminate metabolic end products. An understanding of heart function is most crucial to anesthesiologists since alterations in cardiac output and systemic vascular resistance can have a tremendous influence on a patient's responsiveness to anesthetics. Techniques such as echocardiography and invasive monitoring support assessing cardiac performance, especially during surgery. Studies in cardiac remodeling and repair, such as the use of scaffolds for myocardial infarction, are encouraging developments.

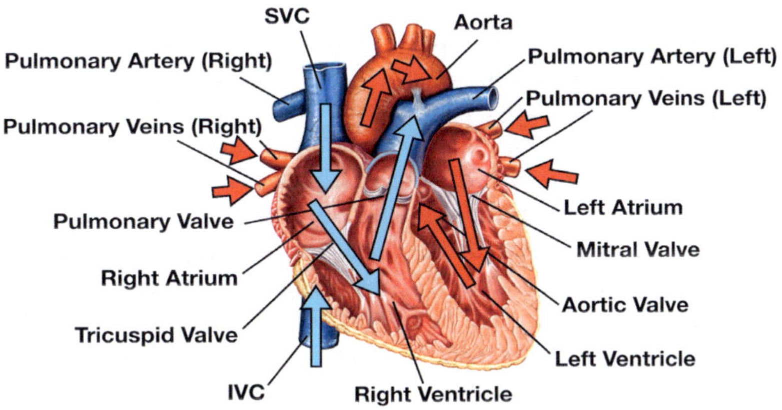

Figure 2.6. Heart function and blood circulation.

Source: https://images.squarespace-cdn.com/content/v1/5e48489da899cd09424943db/1615050389310-5OV8SZNDSHXC32M5Y079/austin+kosier+heart+anatomy+diagram+cardiac+blood+flow+circulation+pathway+steps.

For instance, studies have shown that poly-l-lactide scaffolds functionalized with granulocyte colony-stimulating factor increase cellular colonization and neovascularization, ultimately improving cardiac function and potentially affecting anesthesia-related factors in high-risk cardiac procedures (Chello et al., 2017). Circulation of the blood is a complex mechanism with not only the heart but a network of vessels—e.g., arteries, veins, and capillaries—that facilitates the exchange of gases and nutrients. The difference between the systemic and pulmonary circulations is critical to understanding how these systems achieve homeostasis. The systemic circulation delivers oxygenated blood from the left side of the heart to peripheral tissues, whereas the pulmonary circulation returns deoxygenated blood from the right side of the heart to the lungs for oxygenation. For patients with cardiovascular abnormalities such as single-ventricle physiology, the balance between pulmonary and systemic blood flow becomes increasingly important. Experimental sheep models have shown that interventions, such as pharmacologic agents, affect blood flow dynamics in congenital heart disease. Such a nuanced understanding aids anesthesiologists in predicting hemodynamic responses to surgery and thereby directs anesthesia management approaches (Chang et al., 1996). Further, integration of physiological principles with anesthetic practice can enhance outcomes in patients. Under anesthesia, a thorough awareness of cardiac performance and blood flow dynamics is critical, particularly in respect to the influence of anesthetics on myocardial contractility and vascular resistance. Anesthetic management can affect heart rate, preload, and afterload, thereby impacting cardiac output. Each anesthetic agent has unique characteristics that can alter vascular tone and myocardial oxygen demand, so titration should be performed carefully. For example, vasodilator agents can reduce systemic vascular resistance, leading to hemodynamic changes that anesthesiologists must manage. The dynamic interaction between cardiac function, circulatory perfusion, and the action of anesthetic drugs underscores the significance of being skillful in anatomy and physiology prior to practicing anesthesia in patients with variable cardiovascular profiles (Figure 2.6).

2.3.2. Effects of Anesthesia on Blood Pressure and Heart Rate

The administration of an anesthetic has profound effects on hemodynamic variables like blood pressure and heart rate. The variations are crucial as changes can have significant impact on the outcome of the patient during surgeries. Most anesthetic drugs, in most situations, lower blood pressure due to the vasodilatory effects, reducing systemic vascular resistance. This can result in an increase in heart rate as a compensatory response, allowing the body to maintain cardiac output and perfusion pressure. This interaction between these two very significant signs indicates that constant monitoring under anesthesia is required, as any abnormality will indicate suboptimal tissue perfusion or evolving complications. For example, research shows that anesthesia's hemodynamic actions are differential according to the agent and route of administration and necessitate an individualized plan of anesthetic care according to the physiology of the patient and the surgery. Further, different types of anesthesia have varying effects on cardiovascular stability. General anesthesia with the inhalational or intravenous agents will typically cause significant falls in both diastolic and systolic blood pressure secondary to drug effects upon vascular tone. Regional anesthesia techniques generally preserve hemodynamics to a greater extent but carry some risk of hypotension, particularly when local anesthetic volume is widespread. Also, the patient's posture during surgery and the development of comorbid conditions like hypertension or heart disease can complicate anesthesia-cardiovascular relationships. Therefore, anesthesiologists must be vigilant in monitoring and managing these changes during the surgical period to prevent adverse effects and ensure patient safety. Important data regarding the cardiovascular impact of anesthesia are available from advanced imaging modalities, which provide improved insights into microcirculatory behavior and blood flow. For instance, new instruments such as two-photon microscopy have significantly enhanced visualization of blood vessels and measurement of blood flow at the tissue level in intact systems. This level of resolution permits investigation into how varying anesthetic conditions affect blood pressure and heart rate at the microcirculatory levels, revealing mechanisms for the described cardiovascular changes. Studies reveal that anesthetized conditions can significantly alter patterns of blood flow due to differences in wall shear stress, indicating hemodynamic variation between anesthetized and active states. With these advanced imaging techniques, researchers can uncover mild cardiovascular physiologic effects of anesthetics and design more efficient controls to minimize the risks of anesthetic delivery, thereby maximizing outcomes in diverse clinical settings (Giovanni et al., 2011; Meyer et al., 2016) (Figure 2.7).

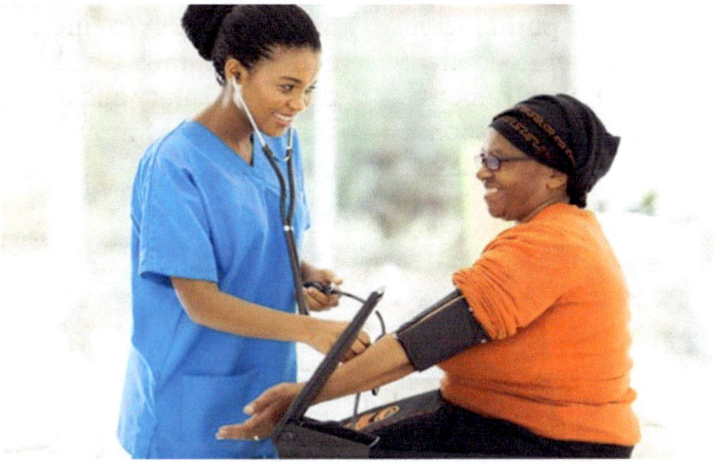

Figure 2.7. Effects of anesthesia on blood pressure and heart rate.

Source: https://www.hopkinsmedicine.org/-/media/images/health/1_-conditions/high-blood-pressure/seniorpatientnurse64044.jpg?h=358&iar=0&mh=360&mw=520&w=520&hash=52E5C59CCCB10AC74F156A56DA22DFDF.

2.3.3. Monitoring Cardiovascular Status During Anesthesia

Cardiovascular status monitoring during anesthesia is a critical component of perioperative care to ensure patient safety and optimal management of physiological responses. Anesthesia profoundly affects hemodynamic parameters, including heart rate, blood pressure, and cardiac output. For instance, anesthetic drugs cause vasodilation and reduced myocardial contractility, which can lead to considerable alterations in cardiac performance. Close observation and accurate monitoring of cardiovascular status are essential to the prompt detection and correction of any ensuing complications, e.g., hypotension or arrhythmias. The integration of state-of-the-art monitoring devices, i.e., invasive arterial catheters and non-invasive monitors, can provide real-time information on a patient's cardiovascular status, enabling anesthesiologists to make informed decisions throughout the surgical process. Anatomy and physiology of cardiovascular function have significant implications for the heart and vasculature's response to anesthesia. The intricate organ of the heart, including the myocardium, the valvular apparatus, and conduction systems, is susceptible to the action of various anesthetic agents, which may affect its rhythm and mechanical adequacy. Of special relevance are illnesses such as ischemic heart disease or metabolic syndrome, which may exacerbate the cardiovascular effects of anesthesia. For instance, dysregulation of calcium-handling mechanisms in coronary smooth muscle, which is prevalent in some patients with metabolic syndrome, can complicate anesthetic management, particularly the hemodynamic response. The recognition of such anatomical and pathological facts is the foundation for optimizing cardiovascular monitoring under anesthesia to prevent adverse effects during surgical interventions (Badin et al., 2018). Moreover, the need for vigilant monitoring is underscored by the risk of an acute cardiovascular event developing intraoperatively due to a pre-existing condition like coronary artery disease. Monitoring cardiovascular status effectively involves not only routine parameters but also evaluating the effectiveness of perioperative therapies. It is important for anesthesiologists to appreciate the physiological impact of cardiac pathologies, i.e., myocardial infarction, in order to deliver patient care appropriate to their requirements. For example, understanding the heart's response to stressors during anesthesia can maximize the results in patients suffering from underlying cardiovascular disease, thus emphasizing the importance of employing integrative monitoring approaches. The development of new models and methods to monitoring cardiovascular status becomes a valuable asset in enhancing operative safety and encouraging individualized care strategies in anesthetic practice (Amodeo et al., 2013).

Test Your Knowledge

1. How do anesthetic agents influence heart rate, blood pressure, and cardiac output during surgery?
2. Why is continuous cardiovascular monitoring essential during anesthesia, and how does it help prevent complications?

2.4. Respiratory Physiology and Anesthesia

Learning Outcome

1. Anatomy of the respiratory system
2. Gas exchange and anesthesia implications
3. Management of the airway during anesthesia

Respiratory physiology should be known in the practice of anesthesia, as it provides the foundation for effective airway management during surgery. The primary function of the respiratory system is to facilitate gas exchange, in which oxygen enters the bloodstream and carbon dioxide is excreted.

Pulmonary functioning, including lung volume, airway resistance, and gas diffusion, should be assessed by anesthesiologists. Such parameters are particularly relevant when general anesthesia is given, since it may depress respiratory drive and alter normal physiological responses. Airway obstruction and hypoventilation can readily become more serious issues under anesthesia, particularly in patients with preexisting respiratory illness. Therefore, adequate airway management techniques and technology, including intubation and ventilatory support, are essential for maintaining optimal oxygenation and preventing the consequences of suboptimal respiratory function. The association between respiratory physiology and anesthetic pharmacology is also a crucial part of perioperative care.

Anesthetics can precipitate varying degrees of respiratory depression that must be titrated cautiously according to the patient's response and type. Agents can manipulate lung compliance, airway reactivity, and ventilation mechanics, as well as the effectiveness of gas exchange. Furthermore, the anesthesiologist must take precautions against postoperative respiratory morbidity, i.e., atelectasis or pneumonia, particularly in risk factor-positive patients such as those with obesity or a history of smoking. Furthermore, regional anesthesia, i.e., neuraxial blocks, has different effects on the respiratory system compared to general anesthesia, thus requiring a dexterous understanding of both respiratory and anesthetic grades to ensure patient safety and recovery outcomes. The importance of diligent patient assessment prior to anesthesia cannot be overestimated, as it is a key indicator of future respiratory complications that could arise during the surgical process.

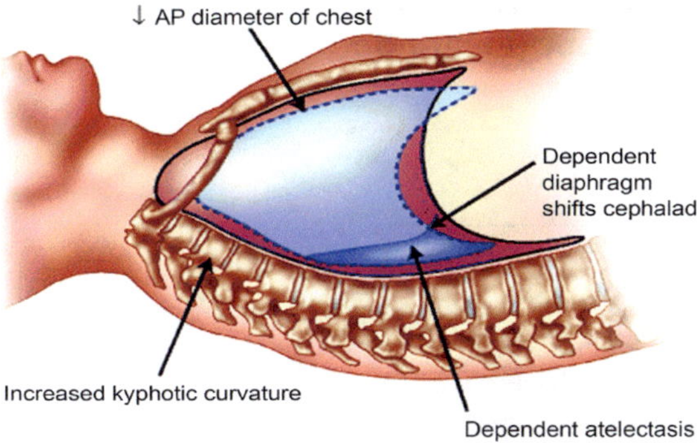

Figure 2.8. Understanding respiratory physiology is essential in anesthesia.

Source: https://media.springernature.com/lw685/springer-static/image/chp%3A10.1007%2F978-0-387-88493-6_4/MediaObjects/159338_1_En_4_Fig1_HTML.gif.

A Full Complete assessment in the guise of a comprehensive medical history and pulmonary function tests can reveal underlying respiratory illness, which can add complexity to anesthetic risks. Those with underlying conditions like obstructive sleep apnea or chronic obstructive pulmonary disease need careful consideration and may potentially be treated with tailored anesthetic strategies or postoperative care plans to ensure safe results.

Additionally, the cartography of airway and lung tissue anatomy can guide interventions and inform anesthetic strategies. Incorrect assessments can introduce inefficient management during procedures and could result in life-threatening complications, making it absolutely crucial for anesthesiologists to remain well-informed about respiratory physiology and the impact of their interventions on patients' general health (Bălălău et al., 2018; N/A, 2018) (Figure 2.8).

2.4.1. Anatomy of the Respiratory System

The anatomy of the respiratory system is key to understanding the physiology of anesthesia. The system consists of the upper and lower airways, each of which transports air during respiration. The upper airway comprises structures such as the nasal cavity, pharynx, and larynx, which significantly contribute to air filtration, moisture addition, and warming of inhaled air. They also play protective roles by preventing foreign material from entering the lower airway, thereby ensuring lung function. The larynx, more familiarly referred to as the voice box, contains the vocal cords and serves as a guard to the trachea, ensuring that food and fluid pass to the esophagus. This difference is important in highlighting the significance of the upper airway in maintaining respiratory mechanics, particularly in anesthetic management, where airway management is paramount for patient safety. Proceeding to the lower respiratory system, we see that it includes the trachea, bronchi, bronchioles, and alveoli, and all the structures play a crucial role in gas exchange and respiration. The trachea bifurcates into the bronchial tree to give rise to the right and left main bronchi, which segment again into smaller bronchi and bronchioles. This process increases surface area for gas exchange while facilitating oxygen delivery to the alveoli as well. The alveoli, which are small air sacs containing a dense network of capillaries, are the sites of the critical exchange of oxygen and carbon dioxide. Anesthetic medications can directly affect gas exchange, and hence it is critical that anesthetists are familiar with this anatomy so that effective ventilation is maintained and surgical complications are avoided. The respiratory apparatus is also intimately related to vascular structures, as pulmonary arteries transport deoxygenated blood from the heart to the lungs for oxygenation. The relationship between the respiratory and cardiovascular systems underscores the importance of respecting both systems when administering anesthesia. Interference with the structural integrity and function of the respiratory system can lead to severe impairment during anesthesia control. Anesthetics influence respiratory drive and tone of the airways, and thus there is always a need for monitoring and control. Thus, thorough awareness of respiratory anatomy and its physiological expressions not only enhances the practice of anesthesia but also yields the best outcomes for patients undergoing surgery requiring anesthesia management (Figure 2.9).

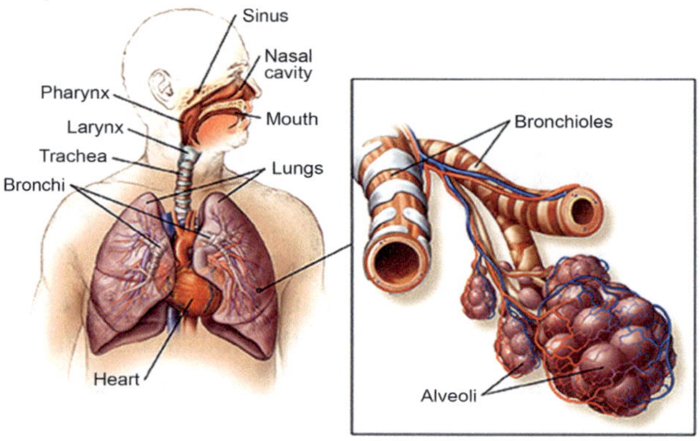

Figure 2.9. The anatomy of the respiratory system plays a pivotal role in understanding the physiology relevant to anesthesia.

Source: https://api.kramesstaywell.com/Content/ea71e7eb-cb87-49b4-826a-a5b60118a08f/medical-illustrations/Images/P01300_1.

2.4.2. Gas Exchange and Anesthesia Implications

The process of gas exchange is vital to the delivery of adequate oxygen to tissues and the elimination of carbon dioxide from the body. This occurs in the respiratory system, particularly in the alveoli, where carbon dioxide is released, and oxygen diffuses into the blood. Anesthesia is of great significance to gas exchange, as many agents affect respiratory status and the effectiveness of gas exchange. For instance, volatile anesthetics can cause alterations in lung mechanics, lessening the capacity for adequate ventilation and leading to intraoperative hypoxia. Thus, anesthesia management would entail diligent monitoring of gas-exchange parameters to ensure adequate tissue oxygenation during anesthesia, particularly in patients with pre-existing respiratory disease or comorbidities. Besides, the use of non-invasive ventilatory support techniques, such as high-flow nasal therapy (HFNT), has been increasing in the clinical setting, primarily in patients with respiratory failure. HFNT makes it possible to deliver humidified and heated gas in a high flow rate, leading to significantly elevated oxygen supply and assistance in maintaining normative gas exchange. Used as a component of an anesthetic regimen, HFNT can be very beneficial to patients whose lung function is impaired, particularly in perioperative conditions. By optimizing inspired oxygen fractions, HFNT is sufficient to avoid desaturation and overall enhance patient outcomes when applied under anesthesia. With researchers continuing to examine the interaction between respiratory interventions and anesthetic strategies, the incorporation of HFNT into standard care protocols may significantly affect patient management at risk for impaired gas exchange, and reinforces the significance of cutting-edge techniques in anesthesia. Physiological features of gas exchange are most pronounced in patients with congenital heart disease or those with right ventricular outflow tract obstruction (RVOTO). Techniques such as percutaneous pulmonary valve implantation (PPVI) have demonstrated significant improvement in hemodynamic indices, confirming the critical role of efficient gas exchange in overall cardiovascular function under anesthesia. More importantly, studies have shown that alleviation of RVOTO can reduce right ventricular pressure and improve exercise tolerance after the procedure, with more serious implications for the anesthetic management of patients with chronic RVOTO. Anesthesiologists must be careful when assessing and managing both circulatory and respiratory dynamics during anesthesia in patients with such complex profiles. By understanding the intricate link between gas exchange and implications of anesthesia, healthcare practitioners can better tailor their interventions to optimize patient safety and procedural success in even more challenging clinical environments (Cortegiani et al., 2019; Bonhoeffer et al., 2006) (Figure 2.10).

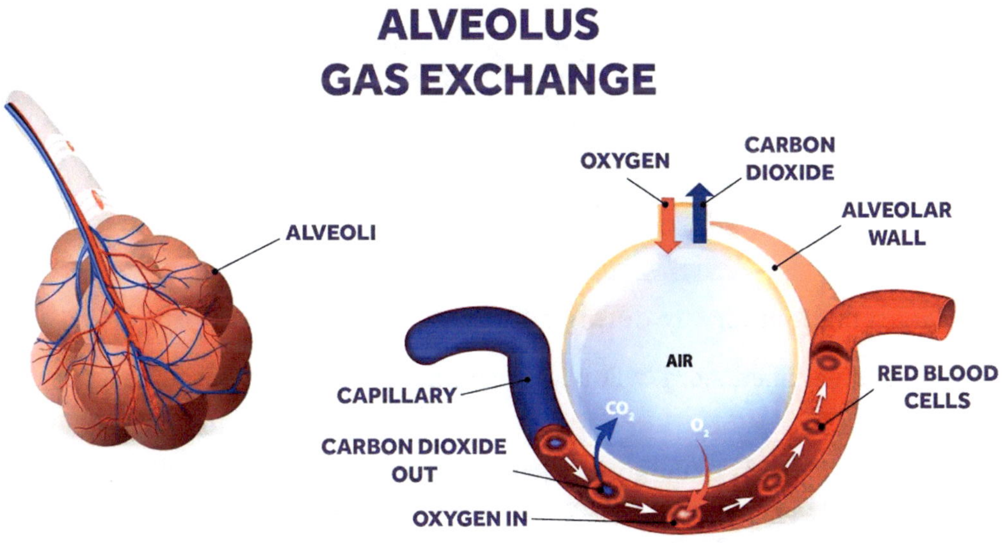

Figure 2.10. Gas exchange and anesthesia implications.

Source: https://www.eakinrespiratory.com/wp-content/uploads/2023/11/Alveolus-gas-exchange-final.webp.

2.4.3. Management of Airway During Anesthesia

Effective management of the airway during anesthesia is crucial to patient safety and effective surgical outcomes. Knowledge of the anatomy of the airway and the breathing structures involved, and of their physiological behavior, enables the anesthesiologist to perform appropriate ventilation and intubation techniques. Relaxation of the pharyngeal muscles, induced by anesthesia, increases the risk of airway obstruction. Thus, there needs to be a vigilant preoperative assessment to identify potential challenges, such as anatomical variations or known airway pathologies. Preemptive measures, such as the use of airway aids, such as oropharyngeal and nasopharyngeal airways, may maintain patency during induction. Besides, accurate knowledge of anatomical landmarks will allow clinicians to perform laryngoscopy properly and aid successful intubation without causing trauma to neighboring tissues, thereby making the process more complicated and interfering with patient recovery. The complications arising from faulty airway management can be dire and encompass respiratory distress and aspiration pneumonia. As highlighted in the literature, deep neck infections, including retropharyngeal and peritonsillar abscesses, may obstruct the airway and pose significant problems during anesthesia. Such conditions often require a multidisciplinary approach due to complications, such as mediastinitis and septic shock, that can develop from these infections (Bălălău et al., 2018). Surgical care may involve drainage of abscesses and management of airway obstruction, both important for patient safety but demanding close liaison between surgical and anesthetic teams.

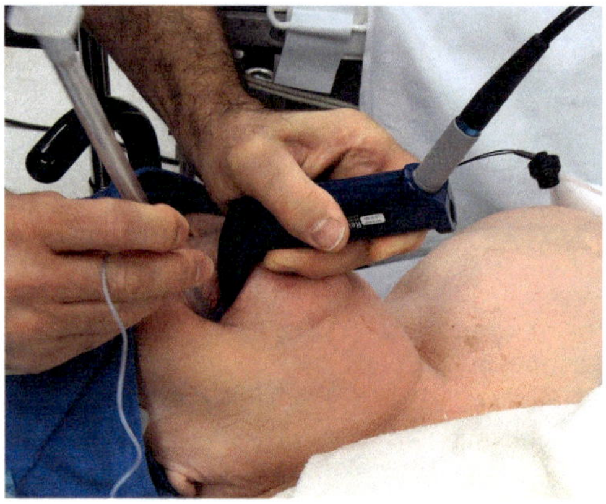

Figure 2.11. Management of airway during anesthesia.

Source: https://upload.wikimedia.org/wikipedia/commons/thumb/3/36/Glidescope_02.JPG/960px-Glidescope_02.JPG.

Psychological impact on patients undergoing such invasive procedures should also be considered, with particular emphasis on ensuring informed consent and open discussion of potential outcomes and complications. Development in airway management continues to improve outcomes in challenging situations. Studies have also examined the use of small animal models to refine such airway techniques, particularly in rodents, where routine intubation is extremely challenging (Molthen et al., 2006). Such innovations not only expand the understanding of airway structures but also improve anesthetic techniques in various species. The development of specialized laryngoscopes can enable easier visualization and tracheal access, ultimately leading to higher rates of successful intubations and improved ventilation control. With advancing research, these findings need to be adopted by practitioners, and airway management guidelines should be updated and modified regularly to reflect different patient populations and surgical conditions. Through repeated education and modification, risks can be minimized, and patient outcomes can be improved when on anesthesia (Figure 2.11).

Test Your Knowledge

1. How do anesthetic agents affect respiratory rate, tidal volume, and gas exchange?
2. Why is careful monitoring of ventilation and oxygenation critical during anesthesia?

2.5. Pharmacology of Anesthetic Agents

Learning Outcome

1. Types of anesthetic agents
2. Mechanisms of action of anesthetics
3. Pharmacokinetics and pharmacodynamics in anesthesia

Pharmacology of anesthetic agents is central to understanding the mechanisms by which they exert their effects on the body during surgery. Anesthetic agents, classified as general and local, have distinct mechanisms of action that shape patient management in anesthesia to a large extent. General anesthetics induce loss of consciousness and are administered by inhalation or intravenous administration and act on neurotransmitter systems, notably the GABA system, that reduce neuronal excitability. Conversely, bupivacaine and the other local anesthetics inhibit the transmission of nerve impulses within a localized area, providing analgesia while preserving complete consciousness.

Anesthesiologists can tailor anesthetic care to the individual's physiological and anatomical characteristics by understanding these pharmacological principles, improving surgery success, and limiting side effects. Within the clinical context, the choice of an anesthetic drug can be a response to pharmacokinetic and pharmacodynamic factors, but also to patient-specific information such as body mass index (BMI) and comorbidities. Research into the impact of obesity on the sensory regression time of spinal anesthesia highlights the need for individual patient characteristics to be taken into account in anesthesia care. A study that compared sensory regression time with hyperbaric 0.75% bupivacaine revealed that the' variability of sensory blockade in non-obese patients and obese patients was not statistically different, which means that the pharmacodynamic characteristics of anesthetics can be consistent despite body composition diversity. This information is valuable because practitioners make modifications to anesthesia plans, obtaining efficacy and safety in diverse groups, which can significantly influence post-operative outcome and patient satisfaction (Hilton et al., 1989).

Furthermore, biochemical processes influenced by anesthetic medications extend beyond basic sedation or analgesia and affect an extensive array of physiological systems. This complexity necessitates a thorough grasp of both the underlying anatomy and the pharmacologic effects of anesthetics. Anesthetists must be adept at detecting potential interactions between anesthetics and other drugs, including their effects on cardiovascular, respiratory, and neurological functions. The use of adjuncts like opioids and sedatives tends to make the pharmacology of the drugs more complicated, thereby requiring close attention during administration of anesthetics. With advances in the field, education in the pharmacology of anesthetic agents continues to be important so that practitioners are prepared to handle the intricacies of anesthesia across various patient populations (University C, 1996) (Figure 2.12).

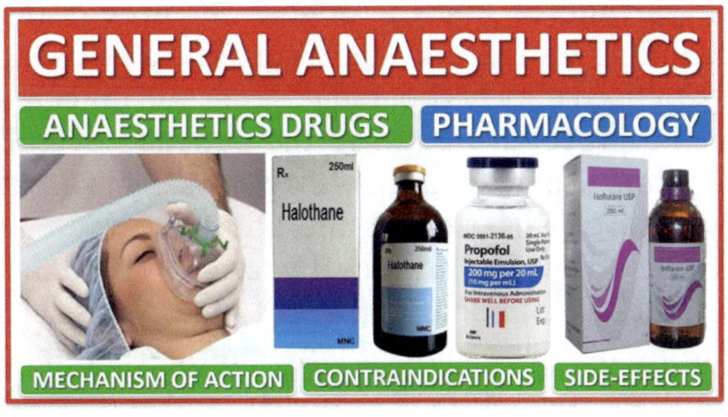

Figure 2.12. The pharmacology of anesthetic agents.

Source: https://i.ytimg.com/vi/1Z6mxIaFsqI/maxresdefault.jpg.

2.5.1. Types of Anesthetic Agents

The anesthetic drug environment is rich and critical to medical and surgical practice, and it is a multifaceted situation between their physiological activity and their clinical application. In general terms, anesthetic drugs are divided into two large categories: general and local anesthetics. General anesthetics induce unconsciousness and a lack of sensation of pain in the entire body and are usually administered by inhalation or intravenous injection. Conversely, local anesthetics are used to provide pain relief at a localized site by inhibiting nerve conduction in that area, and hence are best suited for minor surgery. Local anesthesia classification not only helps one choose the best drug for a particular medical procedure but also assists anesthesiologists in understanding the physiological mechanism involved with each anesthetic's action, thereby impacting patient safety and efficacy. The mechanisms of action of anesthetic agents are key to understanding their actions on the central nervous system and other physiological processes. General anesthetics primarily target neurotransmitter receptors, such as GABA and N-methyl-D-aspartate (NMDA) receptors, which are key to blocking neuronal activity. Inhibition results in a general state of unconsciousness and insensitivity to pain. In contrast, local anesthetics block sodium channels of peripheral nerves, effectively preventing action potentials and sensation. The anesthetic agent used dictates not only the desired outcome of the procedure but also the patient's overall physiological response. As emphasized in recent literature, variation in the administration of anesthetics can profoundly affect outcomes of studies conducted on small animal models, calling for specialized anesthetic regimens tailored to address specific physiological requirements (Cicone et al., 2017). Clinical application of anesthetic agents requires careful balance of specific patient factors along with the physiological actions of each administered drug. For instance, administration of anesthetics can greatly influence cardiac performance because some of them can induce dose-dependent depression of the cardiovascular system. In studies on the interaction between anesthetics and neural dynamics, physiological values have been found to relate to anesthetic effects, with significant influences on electrocortical activity and overall brain function established. This knowledge allows anesthesiologists to anticipate potential complications from surgery and anesthesia. Further, advancements in anesthetic techniques and technology also necessitate ongoing evaluation of the physiological effects of these drugs to enhance patient safety and optimal outcomes (Bojak et al., 2010). Thus, the selection and monitoring of the anesthetic agent become paramount in improving effective anesthesia practice (Figure 2.13).

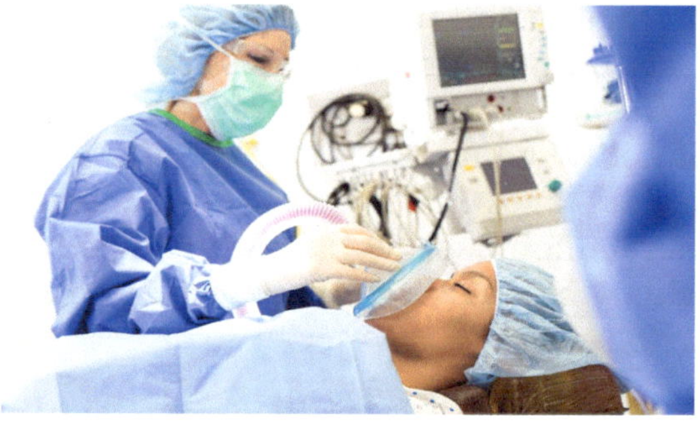

Figure 2.13. Types of anesthetic agents.

Source: https://www.unasourcesurgery.com/wp-content/uploads/2022/02/AAS-Types-of-Anesthesia-487195922-1024x683.jpg.

2.5.2. Mechanisms of Action of Anesthetics

The mechanisms of action through which anesthetics exert their effects are intricate and closely linked with the physiological characteristics of neuronal membranes. Anesthetics have been shown to interact with lipid bilayers, altering membrane fluidity and permeability. This ability to disrupt neuronal membrane integrity is central to their action. By causing fundamental changes in the operation of neurons in response to electrochemical input, anesthetics can inhibit synaptic transmission, leading to diminished neuronal excitability. These changes can decrease the neurons' capacity to generate action potentials, which is another way the total analgesic effect occurs. This corresponds with findings by Ramon y Cajal, the discoverer of the neuron doctrine, who identified the importance of single neurons in the conveyance of nervous impulses and described the requirement for axonal signaling in anesthesia (Georgiev et al., 2010). Anesthetics are also known to influence neurotransmitter receptors, particularly those of GABA and NMDA. GABAergic receptors are responsible for inhibitory neurotransmission within the central nervous system, and anesthetic agents most commonly augment GABA activity, thereby increasing inhibitory action. This leads to potent inhibition of synaptic neurotransmission and can cause anesthesia by increasing sedation. Conversely, NMDA receptors are crucial to excitatory neurotransmission, and certain anesthetics block these receptors, contributing to the blunting of pain perception and consciousness. Fluid dynamics in neuronal membranes are directly responsible for anesthetic potency, as indicated by research on free energy differences between neuronal membranes in the presence of anesthetics, which show measurable changes in excitability with varying anesthetic concentrations (Heimburg et al., 2018). The different effects of anesthetics on neuronal excitability and membrane properties are indicative of their sophistication. Various anesthetic agents possess differential physicochemical properties that determine their mode and intensity of action. Lipid-soluble anesthetics, for instance, produce decreases in phase transition temperature of the neuronal membranes and thus have a depressant effect on the central nervous system. This impact is crucial in demonstrating how anesthetics lower the threshold for action potentials and impair everyday synaptic interaction. The mechanisms of these processes reveal how profoundly anesthetics affect the entire neural structure, and hence prove effective in clinical applications. Understanding the relationship between anesthetic action and neuronal physiology finally enhances the safe and effective administration of anesthesia in clinical practice and maximizes patient outcomes (Heimburg et al., 2018) (Figure 2.14).

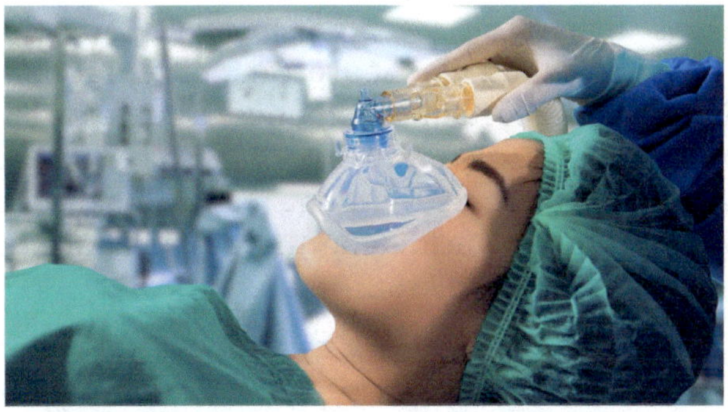

Figure 2.14. The mechanisms through which anesthetics.

Source: https://cdn.britannica.com/78/240878-138-E9CB8517/How-Does-Anesthesia-Work.jpg.

2.5.3. Pharmacokinetics and Pharmacodynamics in Anesthesia

There is a need to understand the basic principles of pharmacokinetics and pharmacodynamics to effectively administer anesthetic medications, which influence both patient outcomes and safety profiles. Pharmacokinetics deals with how drugs are absorbed, distributed, metabolized, and excreted by the body, and this is of serious interest when administering anesthesia because it significantly affects drug concentrations in tissue spaces and overall effectiveness. For instance, the absorption rates of anesthetics can vary significantly by route of administration, e.g., intravenous, inhalational, or regional. Further, intrinsic patient-related factors such as age, weight, and comorbidities, as well as anatomical features of the vascular and pulmonary systems, will modify drug kinetics and require individually tailored dosing regimens to produce optimal anesthetic depth with fewer adverse effects. Pharmacodynamics, on the other hand, refers to drug-site of action relationships in the body, with an emphasis on the mode of action and the resulting physiological effects. This is a vital consideration in anesthesia because it describes how an anesthetic drug's desired effects, such as sedation, pain relief, or muscle relaxation, are achieved. The efficacy and safety of anesthetic drugs depend on receptor specificity and the ability to modulate neurotransmitter action. For instance, certain anesthetics can selectively block excitatory processes and enhance inhibitory processes in the central nervous system, thereby achieving the best balance of sedation and analgesia.

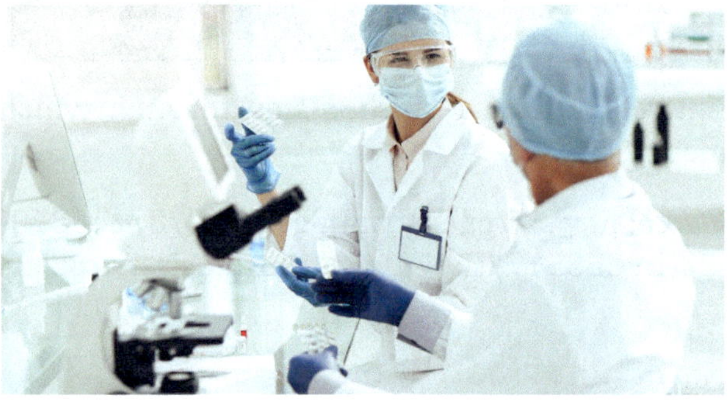

Figure 2.15. The principles of pharmacokinetics and pharmacodynamics is essential for the effective administration of anesthetic agents.

Source: https://www.nebiolab.com/wp-content/uploads/2020/01/shutterstock_new_1859542000.webp.

An understanding of these interactions forms the foundation for anesthesiologists to predict patients' responses to varied agents and to reduce risks from drug interactions and patient variability, testifying to the significance of a thorough knowledge of both pharmacokinetics and pharmacodynamics. The mutual interaction between pharmacokinetics and pharmacodynamics is further illustrated by studies on some nonsteroidal anti-inflammatory drugs (NSAIDs) used in specialized settings, such as veterinary anesthesia.

A pharmacokinetic and clinical efficacy study of firocoxib demonstrated that, although it effectively inhibited cyclooxygenase enzymes, analgesic responses in Asian elephants were limited by the dosing schedule employed. Similarly, analgesic investigations following dehorning in cattle concluded that pharmacokinetic profiles influenced the overall efficacy of pain management regimens, with emphasis on multimodal regimens to optimize analgesia.

These findings demonstrate that the careful application of pharmacokinetic and pharmacodynamic theory in veterinary and human anesthesia not only permits optimal pain relief but also enhances patient comfort during surgical procedures, thereby improving anesthetic practice across disciplines (Figure 2.15).

Test Your Knowledge

1. How do the pharmacokinetic and pharmacodynamic properties of anesthetic agents influence their clinical use?
2. What factors affect the absorption, distribution, metabolism, and elimination of anesthetic drugs?

2.6. Patient Considerations in Anesthesia

Learning Outcome

1. Preoperative assessment and history
2. Special populations and anesthesia considerations
3. Postoperative recovery and monitoring

Awareness of the patient's concerns during anesthesia is crucial to achieving safe and efficient surgical outcomes. Patients' unique physiological and anatomical features have the potential to influence how they respond to anesthetic agents to a significant degree. For instance, patients with some skeletal disorders, e.g., those with achondroplastic conditions, demonstrate increased cardiovascular risks, leading to a greater requirement for comprehensive preoperative assessments. Studies indicate that such patients have co-existing conditions, such as scoliosis and kyphosis, that pose positioning and intraoperative airway management challenges (Choi et al., 2020). Understanding these patient-specific anatomical variations allows anesthesiologists to tailor their techniques, optimize drug dosing, and select optimal monitoring strategies considering unparalleled anatomical challenges. In addition to anatomical considerations, the physiologic well-being of a patient also plays a clear role in contributing to the anesthetic strategy. For instance, comorbid patients, such as those with coronary artery disease or recent myocardial infarction, present particular challenges to perioperative cardiovascular stability. Case series indicate that a high percentage of achondroplasia patients undergo cardiac procedures, thus keeping anesthesiologists vigilant during preoperative evaluation and intraoperative management (Choi et al., 2020). The presence of these diseases often necessitates modifications to anesthetic plans to ensure hemodynamic stability intraoperatively, underscoring anesthesia providers' responsibility to apply their physiologic and pathophysiologic knowledge to effectively counter threats. Furthermore, advances in intraoperative monitoring techniques have improved the outcome of complicated operations. For example, multimodal neurophysiological monitoring during endoscopic and endonasal procedures allows anesthesiologists to assess the functional integrity of critical nervous structures in real time. The technique is fundamental in patients with anatomical variations that could affect surgical access and carry a high risk of neurological complications. By integrating improved monitoring modalities, anesthesia delivery can enhance patient safety and enable more aggressive intervention when necessary. Eventually, understanding and responding to the diverse patient considerations in anesthesia not only enhances surgical efficiency but also significantly improves patient satisfaction and recovery rates.

2.6.1. Preoperative Assessment and History

Preoperative history and evaluation constitute the cornerstones of the discipline of anesthesia, used to assess both the patient's readiness for surgery and the intricate interplay among anatomy, physiology, and anesthetic management. The evaluation begins with a comprehensive review of the patient's medical history, including chronic illnesses, history of prior surgery, and any response to anesthesia, all of which may affect the anesthesiologist's plan. Furthermore, a thorough physical examination is essential for detecting anatomical variations and unexpected complications that may arise during surgery. These tests identify risk factors such as obesity or airway difficulty, which are essential for planning an anesthetic based on the patient's anatomical and physiological features. Early identification of these factors not only ensures patient safety but also enhances the success of surgery, making preoperative assessment an important component of perioperative care. Evaluation of physiological parameters, particularly those that may affect anesthetic drug metabolism and response, is equally important. Cardiovascular, respiratory, and renal function tests fall under this category, as they help determine how the body will respond to anesthetic drugs. For instance, it is critical to understand the cardiac condition of a patient to select appropriate medications and doses, especially in patients with preexisting ailments like hypertension or heart failure.

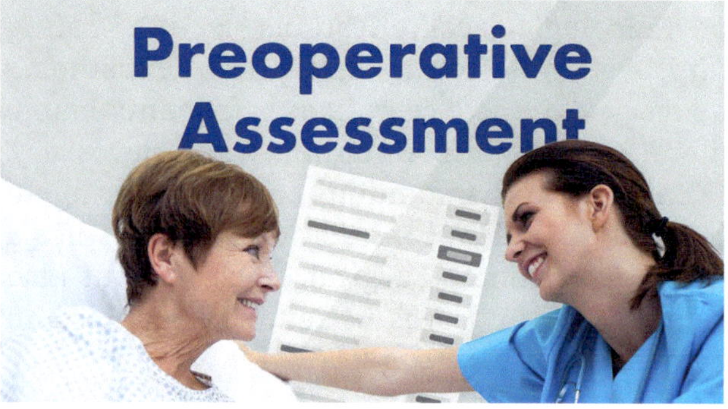

Figure 2.16. The preoperative assessment and history.

Source: https://ausmed-images.s3-ap-southeast-2.amazonaws.com/ausmed.com/ausmed-course/COURSE122_01v2.0.jpg.

Respiratory evaluations also play a crucial role in patients with chronic obstructive pulmonary disease or sleep apnea, since conditions of the latter affect airway management significantly with induction. These kinds of physiological assessments have a one-to-one correlation with the anatomical and physiological principles applicable to anesthesia, allowing practitioners to create a comprehensive anesthetic administration plan with patient safety as a top priority, in addition to compliance with the clinical standards of care. The use of advanced monitoring techniques also adds a pivotal role during the perioperative process, particularly with regard to neurophysiological assessments. With the advent of multimodality nerve monitoring modalities, anesthesiologists can monitor in real time the nervous system structure's functional integrity during surgery. This is especially important during complicated operations, where anatomy is complex and the risk of neurological compromise is increased. Evidence from the literature indicates that these modalities, including electroencephalography and somatosensory evoked potentials, enhance procedure safety by providing immediate feedback on neural function (Doan et al., 2016). In effect, the scope of preoperative testing not only reflects the preeminence of anatomy and physiology in anesthesiology but also emphasizes the necessity for an individualized, patient-centered model of surgical care (Figure 2.16).

2.6.2. Special Populations and Anesthesia Considerations

Anesthesia management differs markedly across special populations due to anatomical and physiological variations that necessitate tailored approaches. Pediatric patients represent one of the most vulnerable populations due to their distinctive pharmacokinetics and metabolic rates that deviate significantly from those of adults. Their immature organ systems, for instance, may metabolize anesthetic drugs more quickly, creating different pain management needs and recovery durations. Additionally, airway anatomy factors are just as significant; pediatric airways are approximately smaller, therefore more likely to be obstructed during anesthesia. Such added susceptibilities require pediatric anesthesiologists to use specialized methods and equipment; hence the need for a customized approach to ensure both effectiveness and safety in these children, informed by findings on age-related differences in pharmacology (University C, 1998). The elderly patient population also presents unique anesthetic challenges, mainly due to physiological changes associated with aging and comorbid illness, which complicate anesthetic management. This patient population typically exhibits alterations in drug metabolism, increased sensitivity to anesthetic medications, and an increased risk of cardiovascular and respiratory complications. These factors must be closely monitored and dosing adjusted to preclude the hazards of general anesthesia, such as excessive sedation or postoperative delirium. Moreover, pre-existing co-morbid conditions might pose added challenges, often requiring multidisciplinary perioperative management and treatment.

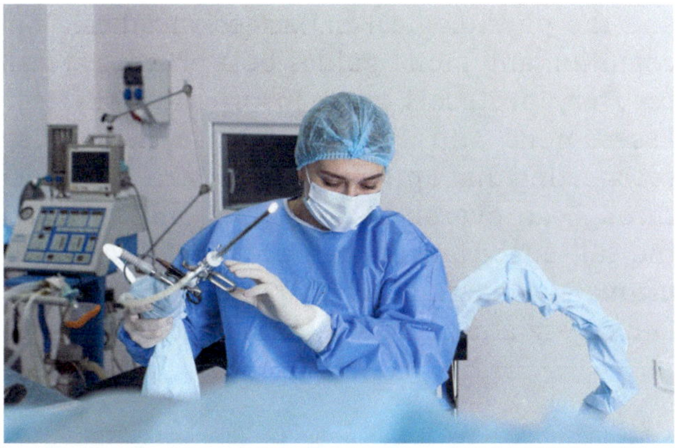

Figure 2.17. Special populations and anesthesia considerations.

Source: https://radiusanesthesia.com/wp-content/uploads/2022/04/anesthesiahysteroscopy.jpg.

As such, knowledge of the specific anatomical and physiologic idiosyncrasies in the elderly emphasizes the need for tailored anesthesia strategies to reduce the risk for complications and optimize outcomes in this vulnerable group (Cornell University, 1999). Obese patients are another critical special population whose anatomical idiosyncrasies may differentially affect anesthesia considerations. The altered body fat distribution can affect the pharmacodynamics and distribution of anesthetic agents, making conventional dosage calculations less precise. Also, the increased vulnerability to airway complications, such as obstructive sleep apnea, demands more sophisticated airway management maneuvers during the induction and maintenance phases of anesthesia. Furthermore, the physiological stress imposed on various organ systems in obese patients can make perioperative management challenging; e.g., cardiovascular stress can be heightened during induction. Careful preoperative assessment, including imaging and functional tests, plays a crucial role in planning for such patients. Lastly, integration of anatomical and physiological data into customized anesthetic plans is critical to account for the intricacies that are involved in anesthetizing obese populations (Figure 2.17).

2.6.3. Postoperative Recovery and Monitoring

The postoperative recovery phase is a crucial part of obtaining good outcomes following surgical procedures. It is inherently related to the principles of anatomy and physiology in anesthesiology. During the recovery phase, the physiological response of the patient to anesthesia and surgical trauma is monitored closely in order to avoid any complications. Routine checks are performed on various parameters, including heart rate, blood pressure, and oxygen saturation. Understanding the intricate association between the autonomic nervous system and these physiological markers enables medical practitioners to accurately assess recovery status. This constant monitoring not only allows for timely intervention when unexpected changes occur, but it also improves a more favorable healing climate. Clinicians must be vigilant, as unexpected postoperative course abnormalities such as prolonged sedation or respiratory arrest may be signs of underlying anatomical problems secondary to surgical trauma, highlighting the significance of balanced recovery pathways. Effective postoperative monitoring also entails ensuring the integrity of neurological function, particularly in operations involving critical areas such as the skull base. Multimodal monitoring methods provide a holistic dimension to such an analysis, in which various neurological activities are assessed in real time using methodologies such as somatosensory evoked potentials and electromyography. Such monitoring is imperative in procedures where nearby neural structures are at risk in order to guarantee the following: any compromised evidence can be immediately rectified. These technologies are used by clinicians to assess the functional integrity of critical pathways within the central nervous system, thereby minimizing the risk of permanent damage. Anatomical understanding of nerve tracts informs anesthesia delivery and recovery parameters, enabling patients to regain full function as expeditiously and safely as possible, thereby highlighting the synergy among anatomy, physiology, and monitoring practice in the postoperative setting (Doan et al., 2016). Postoperative recuperation is not simply reacting to physical parameters; it must involve psychological aspects that may result after surgical interventions. Patients will often experience all kinds of emotional responses, including anxiety and confusion, particularly during the recovery time from anesthesia to full consciousness. It is essential to note the interplay of physiological recuperation and psychological welfare. Healthcare practitioners are encouraged to employ practices that foster a facilitating environment, with effective communication and reassurance during the recuperation period. This understanding of the anatomy of the brain's cognitive pathways and the physiological impact of anesthesia on cognition and mood guides best practice. Total recovery protocols must incorporate physical assessment and emotional care measures, recognizing that optimal outcomes are achieved through an overall strategy that encompasses the full spectrum of the recovery experience, ultimately culminating in patient satisfaction and safety after surgery (Kumar et al., 2012).

Test Your Knowledge

1. How do the pharmacokinetic and pharmacodynamic properties of anesthetic agents influence their clinical use?
2. What factors affect the absorption, distribution, metabolism, and elimination of anesthetic drugs?

SUMMARY

The outcome of an investigation into anatomy and physiology related to anesthesia underscores the fundamental relationship between physiological knowledge and anesthetic practice. Anesthesia is not a technical procedure; it entails an appreciation of the intricate physiology involved in maintaining homeostasis during surgical procedures. With detailed knowledge of anatomical structures, their roles, and physiological responses, anesthesiologists are better positioned to anticipate complications and modify anesthetic procedures to meet individual patient requirements. This is even more important when considering differences in presenting patients, e.g., those recognized in different species, such as cats with kidney disease, where perfusion dynamics are integral to anesthetic management (Daminet et al., 2017). Further, the implications of neurological events, i.e., cerebrovascular accidents, highlight the importance of thorough familiarity with the anatomy and physiology of the central nervous system. In cats where acute presentation is indicative of CVAs, prompt intervention takes a predominant role. Understanding the value of patient history and the impact of systemic disease on neurological outcome can enhance anesthetic planning, thereby ensuring that risks are kept to a minimum. This is particularly so in the veterinary field, where systemic disease and anesthesia crossover might affect patient prognosis in general (Beltran et al., 2017). Last but not least, it must be said that the application of anatomical and physiological principles to anesthetic practice cannot be stressed enough. Enhanced comprehension guarantees improved clinical outcomes, indicating that anesthesiologists must remain on their toes in either branch. The nuances of vascular physiology in chronic disease and the intricacies of acute neurologic events inform not only immediate anesthetic decision-making but also long-term patient management strategies. As the practice of anesthesia expands, greater recognition of these interdependencies will eventually translate into more productive, safer anesthetic care in both human and veterinary medicine.

An understanding of the relationship between anatomy and physiology is at the core of the work of anesthetists in the anesthetic field. The intricate human body anatomy and its physiological processes are the foundation of effective anesthetic practice. Knowledge of the cardiovascular system, for instance, is pivotal because anesthesia significantly affects heart function. Anesthesiologists must also know how agents influence myocardial oxygen demand and systemic vascular resistance, which are key factors to ensuring hemodynamic stability during surgical procedures. In fact, cardiac disorders such as myocardial infarction (MI) must be tackled by a specially tailored anesthetic approach to manage risk and ensure patient safety. By examination of the heart's anatomy and understanding of physiological responses to standardized anesthetic drugs, experts can maximize patient outcomes as well as minimize complications (Amodeo et al., 2013). The anatomy of the respiratory system, in turn, plays a vital role in anesthesia administration. A thorough understanding of the interactions among airway structures, pulmonary mechanics, and gas exchange is essential for controlling airway complications. Choice of anesthetic agents can influence respiratory drive, airway patency, and lung function, and thus overall anesthesia management. Anesthesiologists should be well versed in intubation, anatomical landmarks, and the physiology of ventilation to maximally assist optimal oxygenation during surgery. A thorough knowledge of these factors is needed not only for preoperative assessments but also in the prediction and management of intraoperative complications that may arise (Breckenridge et al., 1972). Additionally, the sophisticated anatomy and physiology of the nervous system play a significant role in determining the pharmacodynamics of anesthetic drugs. Understanding the anatomy of the central and peripheral nervous systems aids in selecting appropriate regional anesthesia techniques. Physiological principles of block efficacy and nerve conduction guide anesthesiologists' dosing and techniques. Differences in patients' anatomy can also create diverse effects from anesthetic drugs, so a tailored approach is tailored to anatomy. By integrating anatomical and physiological information, anesthesiologists can enhance their practice, providing every patient with safe and effective anesthetic care that is appropriate to their physiological makeup (Amodeo et al., 2013).

KEY TERMS FROM THIS CHAPTER

- Achondroplasia
- Anesthesia administration
- Clavicle surgery
- Gamma-aminobutyric acid (GABA)
- Immature organ systems
- Nervous system
- Obesity
- Pharmacodynamics
- Analgesia
- Cardiovascular anatomy
- Drug metabolism
- Human anatomy
- Modern medicine
- N-methyl-D-aspartate (NMDA)
- Pain management
- Pharmacology

CRITICAL THINKING QUESTIONS

1. **Which of the following nerves must be anesthetized for an effective axillary block?**
   a. Median nerve
   b. Ulnar nerve
   c. Radial nerve
   d. All of the above
2. **The primary site of action for inhalational anesthetics is:**
   a. Neuromuscular junction
   b. Cerebral cortex
   c. Reticular activating system
   d. Spinal cord
3. **What is the primary buffer system in the blood relevant to acid-base balance during anesthesia?**
   a. Phosphate buffer
   b. Protein buffer
   c. Bicarbonate buffer
   d. Hemoglobin buffer
4. **Which organ is primarily responsible for the metabolism of most intravenous anesthetic agents?**
   a. Heart
   b. Liver
   c. Kidneys
   d. Lungs
5. **The epidural space is located between:**
   a. Dura mater and arachnoid mater
   b. Dura mater and the vertebral periosteum
   c. Arachnoid mater and pia mater
   d. Pia mater and spinal cord

Short Answer Questions

1. Discuss the anatomy of the respiratory system and its significance in the administration of anesthesia.
2. Explain the physiological principles of oxygen transport in the body and how anesthesia can affect it.
3. Describe the anatomy of the cardiovascular system and its relevance during anesthesia.
4. How does the nervous system's anatomy influence the administration of regional anesthesia?
5. What is the role of the liver in drug metabolism, and why is its function critical in anesthesia?

Answer to Critical Thinking Questions

1. (d); 2. (c); 3. (c); 4. (b); 5. (b)

REFERENCES

1. Biondi-Zoccai, G., De Falco, E., Peruzzi, M., Cavarretta, E., Mancone, M., Leoni, O., Caristo, M. E., Lotrionte, M., Marullo, A. G. M., Amodeo, A., Pacini, L., Calogero, A., Petrozza, V., Chimenti, I., D'Ascenzo, F., & Frati, G. (2013). A novel Closed-Chest porcine model of chronic ischemic heart failure suitable for experimental research in cardiovascular disease. *BioMed Research International, 2013*, 1–8. https://doi.org/10.1155/2013/410631Azami, N. S., Jahanshahi, M., & Khoshbin Khoshnazar, A. R. (2012). Gamma radiation-induced impairment of hippocampal neurogenesis, comparison of single and fractionated dose regimens. https://core.ac.uk/download/84432196.pdf (accessed on 28th June 2025).
2. Baars, B. J. (2012). The biological cost of consciousness. https://core.ac.uk/download/pdf/290570.pdf (accessed on 28th June 2025).
3. Badin, J. K., Bruning, R. S., & Sturek, M. (2018). Effect of metabolic syndrome and aging on Ca2+ dysfunction in coronary smooth muscle and coronary artery disease severity in Ossabaw miniature swine. https://core.ac.uk/download/228066171.pdf (accessed on 28th June 2025).
4. Bălălău, C., Domuța, M., Egor, S., Sargarovschi, M., Mărginean, G., et al. (2018). Management of deep space infections of the neck. https://core.ac.uk/download/216808113.pdf (accessed on 28th June 2025).
5. Bartsch, T., & Paemeleire, K. (2010). Occipital nerve stimulation for headache disorders. https://core.ac.uk/download/55758140.pdf (accessed on 28th June 2025).
6. Beltran, E., Drees, R., & Wittaker, D. E. (2017). MRI and clinical characteristics of suspected cerebrovascular accident in nine cats. https://core.ac.uk/download/160499853.pdf (accessed on 28th June 2025).
7. Blugerman, G., D'Angelo, J. A., Habbema, L., Lisborg, M., et al. (2011). Application of the liposuction techniques and principles in specific body areas and pathologies. https://core.ac.uk/download/17179833.pdf (accessed on 28th June 2025).
8. Bojak, I., Frascoli, F., Liley, D. T. J., van Veen, L., et al. (2010). Meta bifurcation analysis of a mean field model of the cortex. http://arxiv.org/abs/1008.4043 (accessed on 28th June 2025).
9. Bonhoeffer, P., Coats, L., Deanfield, J. E., Derrick, G., et al. (2006). Physiological and clinical consequences of relief of right ventricular outflow tract obstruction late after repair of congenital heart defects. https://core.ac.uk/download/1675374.pdf (accessed on 28th June 2025).
10. Breckenridge, R., Cunius, K. M., Dembert, M., et al. (1972). *Ariel–Volume 5 Number 2*. https://core.ac.uk/download/213440701.pdf (accessed on 28th June 2025).
11. Chang, R., Fineman, J. R., Hanley, F. L., Klein, J. R., et al. (1996). Hemodynamic effects of epinephrine, bicarbonate and calcium in the early postnatal period in a lamb model of single-ventricle physiology created in utero. https://core.ac.uk/download/pdf/82026830.pdf (accessed on 28th June 2025).
12. Chello, M., Crescenzi, A., De Marco, F., Gambardella, C., et al. (2017). Implantation of a poly-L-lactide GCSF-functionalized scaffold in a model of chronic myocardial infarction. https://core.ac.uk/download/74230989.pdf (accessed on 28th June 2025).
13. Choi, J. H., Gordon, J. S., Maynes, E. J., O'Malley, T., et al. (2020). Cardiac interventions in patients with achondroplasia: A systematic review. https://core.ac.uk/download/322850156.

pdf (accessed on 28th June 2025).

14. Cicone, F., Denoël, T., Gnesin, S., Prior, J. O., et al. (2017). Cardiac radionuclide imaging in rodents: A review of methods, results, and factors at play. https://core.ac.uk/download/84058455.pdf (accessed on 28th June 2025).
15. Clark, L. F., Kiang, N. Y. S., & Takeshi, T. E. C. (2025). Discharge patterns of single fibers in the cat's auditory nerve. https://core.ac.uk/download/pdf/85249703.pdf (accessed on 28th June 2025).
16. Cornell University. (1999). *College of Veterinary Medicine*. https://ecommons.cornell.edu/bitstream/handle/1813/38459/COS_v90_1998_99_16.pdf?sequence=1&isAllowed=y (accessed on 28th June 2025).
17. Cortegiani, A., Gregoretti, C., & Spoletini, G. (2019). Physio pathological rationale of using high-flow nasal therapy in the acute and chronic setting: A narrative review. https://core.ac.uk/download/224993362.pdf (accessed on 28th June 2025).
18. De Meyer, G., De Wilde, D., Segers, P., Trachet, B., et al. (2016). The influence of anesthesia and fluid-structure interaction on simulated shear stress patterns in the carotid bifurcation of mice. https://core.ac.uk/download/55742526.pdf (accessed on 28th June 2025).
19. Di Giovanni, G., Muscat, R., Pierucci, M., Valentino, M., et al. (2011). Two-photon microscopy: Sequential imaging studies *in vivo*. https://core.ac.uk/download/46602303.pdf (accessed on 28th June 2025).
20. Doan, A. T., Evans, J. J., Kenning, T. J., Lober, R. M., et al. (2016). Intraoperative neurophysiological monitoring for endoscopic endonasal approaches to the skull base: A technical guide. https://core.ac.uk/download/83050037.pdf (accessed on 28th June 2025).
21. Edelstein, B. L. (2010). *Training New Dental Health Providers in the U.S. (Full Report)*. https://core.ac.uk/download/71355422.pdf (accessed on 28th June 2025).
22. Freed, M. (1951). The phantom limb. https://open.bu.edu/bitstream/2144/26009/1/Freed_Murray_1951_web.pdf (accessed on 28th June 2025).
23. Georgiev, D. D., & Glazebrook, J. F. (2010). SNARE proteins as molecular masters of intraneuronal communication. https://core.ac.uk/download/pdf/9637295.pdf (accessed on 28th June 2025).
24. Heimburg, T., Jackson, A. D., Music, T., Wang, X., et al. (2018). The free energy of bio membrane and nerve excitation and the role of anesthetics. http://arxiv.org/abs/1801.10455 (accessed on 28th June 2025).
25. Hilton, G. L. (1989). Sensory regression time from subarachnoid block with hyperbaric 0.75% bupivacaine in the obese patient. https://core.ac.uk/download/130355392.pdf (accessed on 28th June 2025).
26. Işıker, A., Onay, M., Akcan, A., Akkemik, Ü., & Güleç, M. (2023). Evaluating the role of vertebral anatomy examination by ultrasonography before administering spinal anesthesia in geriatric patients: A prospective randomized trial. *Turkish Journal of Geriatrics*. https://www.semanticscholar.org/paper/4c52c991e7a64a483ff75a1823413c172e841065 (accessed on 28th June 2025).
27. Kottwitz, J. R. (2019). Determination of safe and effective dosing regimens for nonsteroidal anti-inflammatory drugs in African and Asian elephants. https://core.ac.uk/download/650412371.pdf (accessed on 28th June 2025).

28. Kumar, S., Ramamoorthy, M., & Thiagarajan, B. (2012). Endoscopic tympan mastoid exploration [Functional endoscopic ear surgery–FEES]. https://core.ac.uk/download/pdf/9634108.pdf (accessed on 28th June 2025).
29. Metzinger, T. (2001). "Consciousness": Selected bibliography 1970–2001. https://core.ac.uk/download/pdf/12236278.pdf (accessed on 28th June 2025).
30. Molthen, R. C. (2006). A simple, inexpensive, and effective light-carrying laryngoscope blade for orotracheal intubation of rats. https://core.ac.uk/download/213083259.pdf (accessed on 28th June 2025).
31. N/A. (2018). Download entire issue: *Gibbon Surgical Review, 1*(1), 2018. https://core.ac.uk/download/155271707.pdf (accessed on 28th June 2025).
32. Páez, F., Casarin, M., & Irastorza, R. (2005). Pelvic examinations under anesthesia: An important teaching tool. https://core.ac.uk/download/56355378.pdf (accessed on 28th June 2025).
33. Purnomo, H. D., & Witjaksana, R. (2025). Surface anatomy-based clavipectoral fascia plane block for clavicle surgery. *Indonesian Journal of Anesthesiology and Reanimation*. https://www.semanticscholar.org/paper/ef32abd0569b0d1fad3347c7c312f52ed84f3741 (accessed on 28th June 2025).
34. Ruholl, H., & Smith, K. (2021). Virtual cadaver dissection prior to clinical experiences in nurse anesthesia. https://core.ac.uk/download/428365734.pdf (accessed on 28th June 2025).
35. Stock, M. L. (2015). Comparison of oral non-steroidal anti-inflammatory drugs in cautery dehorned calves. https://core.ac.uk/download/38939766.pdf (accessed on 28th June 2025).

PHARMACOLOGY IN ANESTHESIA

3

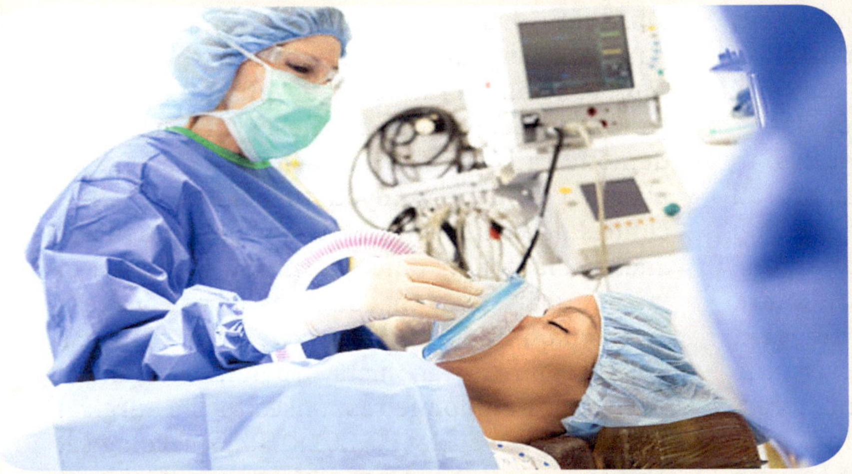

LEARNING OBJECTIVES

After studying this chapter, you will be able to:

1. Discuss the types of anesthetic agents
2. Focus on mechanisms of action
3. Learn about administration routes
4. Know monitoring and safety
5. Understand special considerations
6. Explain the advances in anesthetic pharmacology

Introduction

The field of anesthesia involves the multifaceted use of pharmacological agents that bring about a reversible state of unconsciousness to enable surgical procedures and other interventions without pain-related distress. An understanding of the pharmacology of such drugs is invaluable to anesthesiologists in effectively managing patients. Anesthetics can be classified as general and local agents, each with distinct mechanisms of action and specific applications. General anesthetics generally have an action on the central nervous system and produce loss of consciousness, while local anesthetics block sensation in a regional area and therefore provide relief from pain without upsetting the general consciousness of the patient. This aspect makes it all the more necessary to possess a deep understanding of the pharmacodynamics and pharmacokinetics of these drugs because their incorrect application can lead to serious complications or inadequacy of analgesia during and after the treatment. In the anesthesia discipline, management of chronic pain is a problem of paramount importance that converges with the pharmacological answer. Chronic pain, as typically defined, persisting beyond the normal healing time, affects a considerable proportion of the population, as contextualized by statistics showing that more than 14% of adults experience it [4]. The ramifications of inadequate pain control are more than physical; they extend into the psychological and social domains, harming the patient's quality of life. Given this, the anesthesiologist must be concerned not only with the short-term consequences of anesthetic agents but also with the long-term management of pain. This dual responsibility calls for general information of not only the anesthetic drugs but also the adjunct drugs, such as opioids and non-opioid analgesics, to reverse pain and enhance patient status overall (Dowell et al., 2016). Moreover, the overlap of consciousness and drug interactions among anesthetic drugs is a challenging field of study. Patient consciousness levels should be assessed when under anesthesia, as they determine corresponding drug doses to be administered. New advances involve the realization of a theory-based consciousness index that measures brain reaction to stimuli across varying consciousness states, including anesthesia (Adenauer et al., 2013). This empirical approach provides a more advanced means of measuring anesthetic depth and enables practitioners to tailor anesthetic plans more accurately to meet patient requirements. Because knowledge of the action of anesthetic agents and the resulting neurological response becomes more sophisticated through research, the application of pharmacology within anesthesia continues to improve, making treatment safer and more effective for patients.

Definition of Pharmacology

The word pharmacology comes from the intricate study of drugs and their interactions with biological systems. Pharmacology is a discipline that encompasses all aspects of drug synthesis and manufacture, the mechanisms of action of drugs, their therapeutic effects, and their side effects. It is fundamental to medical practice, particularly in anesthesiology, where precision in drug use significantly affects patient outcomes. Anesthetics are a group of pharmacologic agents used to induce temporary unconsciousness, analgesia, and muscle relaxation required for surgery. As noted by Brown et al. in their study on multimodal general anesthesia, close familiarity with the pharmacodynamics and pharmacokinetics of anesthetic drugs is essential for achieving peak patient safety and treatment during surgical interventions (Talmage et al., 2018). The general dynamics of anesthesia pharmacology demonstrate the way in which a variety of agents can be employed to achieve desired clinical outcomes effectively and safely. General anesthesia, for instance, formerly consisted of inhalational agents that suppress consciousness and immobility, with adjunctive agents such as opioids and α-2 agonists providing enhanced control of autonomic responses to the surgical stimulus (Talmage et al., 2018). Pharmacological principles underlying drug interactions highlight the value of taking a multimodal approach to anesthesia. By employing a combination of drugs that act through different mechanisms, anesthetists can achieve more effective analgesia and sedation with less potential for side effects from elevated doses of individual drugs, thereby paving the way for safer patients and better recovery. In addition, the ongoing development in the field of pharmacology continually educates anesthetic practice, pushing the limits of safer and more effective therapy. With the opioid epidemic raising concerns about dependency and abuse, anesthesiologists increasingly are considering diverse pharmacologic regimes to deal with such problems while delivering effective anesthesia. The formation of recommendations and guidelines, as outlined by applicable clinical trials and professional agreements, reflects the flexible nature of pharmacology in addressing evolving challenges. Lastly, the definition of pharmacology, at least in the context of anesthesia, outlines a multifaceted discipline that balances efficacy and safety through advanced knowledge of drug activity and interactions (Figure 3.1).

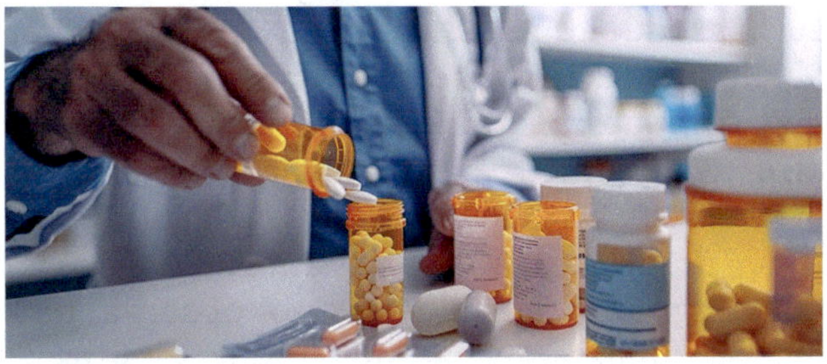

Figure 3.1. The definition of pharmacology.

Source: https://www.diginerve.com/blogs/wp-content/uploads/2025/04/Top-30-Important-Drugs-You-Must-Remember-for-NEET-PG-2025-1.webp.

Importance of Pharmacology in Anesthesia

Pharmacology in anesthesia cannot be exaggerated, as it is the basis for the establishment of good anesthetic practice. Anesthesiologists use a wide range of pharmacologic agents to induce and maintain anesthesia in operating patients. These extend not only to incorporate anesthetics but also ancillary drugs like analgesics, muscle relaxants, and antiemetics, all complementing each other to offer patient comfort and protection. It is critical to understand pharmacokinetics and pharmacodynamics, as they govern how drugs are metabolized, eliminated, distributed, and absorbed in the body. Proper knowledge enables anesthesiologists to tailor anesthetic regimens to individual patient needs, considering factors such as age, comorbidities, weight, and drug interactions. As a result, pharmacology is a primary driver of maximizing therapeutic outcomes and minimizing side effects during anesthesia (Chen et al., 2020). Also, pharmacological innovation has led to the development of novel anesthetic medications that enhance surgical practice by providing better patient safety and recovery profiles. In particular, the development of short-acting anesthetics enables faster recovery from anesthesia, facilitating faster post-anesthesia care and fewer complications. Also, the use of target-controlled infusion devices reflects the integration of pharmacological concepts with technology, enabling more precise delivery of anesthetic medication. Ongoing research in the area has led to agents with better safety profiles, lowering the risk of postoperative nausea and vomiting, which is a frequent complication of anesthesia.

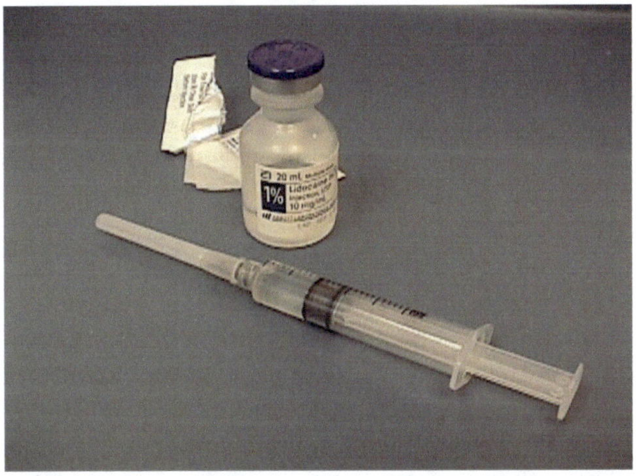

Figure 3.2. Importance of pharmacology in anesthesia.

Source: https://www.operationalmedicine.org/Powerpoint/Lectures/Lidocaine.jpg.

The influence of pharmacology is not limited to the operating room, as perioperative care is affected by methods like enhanced recovery after surgery (ERAS) protocols, whose objective is to maximize preoperative and postoperative patient experiences (Stout et al., 2018). The pharmacology's role in anesthesia also encompasses patient education and informed consent. An understanding of drugs used in anesthetic practice equips anesthesiologists to discuss the concerns, benefits, and risks with patients. Being able to explain how each agent acts, what action is anticipated, and what side effects may occur helps boost confidence in the anesthesia care team and enhance the quality of the patient experience. Apart from that, pharmacology aids in the identification and management of potential complications, such as post-anesthetic or anaphylactic shock. Consequently, pharmacology not only guides anesthesia practice in clinical settings but also serves as a nexus for beneficial interactions between patients and healthcare workers, ultimately resulting in better surgical outcomes and patient satisfaction (Chen et al., 2020) (Figure 3.2).

Overview of Anesthetic Agents

The context of anesthetic drugs has been markedly altered by advances in pharmacology and technology, rendering anesthetic practice safer and more efficient. Anesthetic drugs are broadly classified into two categories: general and local anesthetics. General anesthetics induce a reversible loss of consciousness, effectively blunting pain, awareness, and reflexes. Local anesthetics, however, target a given location, inhibiting sensation in a defined area without rendering the patient unconscious. The choice of anesthetic agent depends on various aspects, including the type of surgery to be performed, the patient's medical history, and the desired effect of analgesia. Recent advances in technology for the delivery of anesthesia have improved precision and patient outcomes, and the practice has become more responsive to individual physiological needs (Thomas et al., 2024). In recent years, the development of agents like ketamine has transformed anesthetic practice into a more versatile use of anesthetics in both surgical and non-surgical contexts. Ketamine is a member of the dissociative anesthetics, which are defined by their unique pharmacological profile that not only causes anesthesia but also analgesia. The usage is also not restricted to traditional perioperative contexts, showing immense potential in acute and chronic pain diseases. Ketamine has also emerged as an adjuvant to general anesthesia, assisting with reduced opioid consumption and enhanced patient recovery times, particularly in enhanced recovery after surgery (ERAS) protocols. This all-purpose drug is increasingly being used for procedural sedation, especially in low-resource settings, due to its efficacy and safety (Afify et al., 2023). Further, the development of robotic and computerized anesthetic technology has also transformed the administration of such medicines. These innovations enable real-time, accurate titration of anesthetic drugs, allowing anesthesiologists to observe and respond to patients' physiological responses to interventions. Artificial intelligence in anesthetic practice introduces another level of safety and effectiveness, enhancing communication and decision-making in high-risk operating rooms. As the role of technology grows stronger in the field, anesthetic agents are no longer evaluated solely on pharmacologic profiles but also on their compatibility with advanced mechanical devices that enhance patient care (Thomas et al., 2024). As research progresses and technology develops further, the future of anesthetic agents will continue to expand and improve considerably in clinical settings.

3.1. Types of Anesthetic Agents

Learning Outcome

1. General anesthetics
2. Local anesthetics
3. Adjunctive medications

The pharmacological identification of anesthetic drugs is integral to the practice of anesthesia, where drugs are most fundamentally divided into two categories: general and local anesthetics. General anesthetics induce reversible loss of consciousness and are typically used in major surgery, while local anesthetics produce localized anesthetic effects without affecting consciousness. However, the pharmacology of these drugs is very different. General anesthetics, such as the volatile anesthetics and intravenous agents like propofol, exert their effects through effects on a variety of receptors, enhancing inhibitory neurotransmission primarily through gamma-aminobutyric acid type A receptor (GABA(A)R) mechanisms and are responsible for their sedation (Li et al., 2010). Local anesthetics such as lidocaine and bupivacaine inhibit sodium channels on nerve fibers, thereby blocking impulse transmission in localized areas. Anesthesiologists must understand these distinctions to choose patient-specific anesthesia plans that are optimal for safety and efficacy. Intravenous anesthetic agents represent a significant category of general anesthetics, with drugs like propofol, etomidate, and thiopental of very short onset and duration of action. Propofol is particularly utilized due to its excellent induction and recovery profile, offering fast sedation with minimal postoperative nausea. Its effect mainly augments the function of GABA(A)R, thereby augmenting inhibitory neurotransmission in the central nervous system (Li et al., 2010). In contrast, etomidate is characterized by minimal cardiovascular effects and is thus the drug of choice in patients with compromised hemodynamics. It does not, however, provide analgesia, and thus concomitant administration with other analgesic agents is required. Furthermore, thiopental, although currently less frequently used, is still used reference-wise historically, and is a milestone in the barbiturate family, indicating ongoing progress in anesthetic choice and use according to patient profile and surgical needs. Volatile anesthetics, administered by inhalation, constitute the other vital component of general anesthesia, with agents including sevoflurane, isoflurane, and desflurane. These agents are characterized by their ability to induce immobility and unconsciousness through modulation of multiple neurotransmitter systems, with a significant effect on GABA(A) R-mediated inhibitory transmission (Li et al., 2010). The demands of the delivery system, i.e., the need for precision vaporization, distinguish inhalation agents, with close observation during administration necessary to confirm adequate depth of anesthesia. Each of the volatile anesthetic agents possesses special pharmacokinetic properties that impact such factors as the time of onset and recovery, as well as the effect on hemodynamics. Desfluranes' properties of quick induction and recovery, for instance, render it suitable for outpatient procedures, while isoflurane's' cardiovascular stabilizing effects require careful consideration in high-risk situations. With the development of an anesthetic practice, an understanding and perception of these drugs increasingly enhances the art and science of surgical anesthesia (Figure 3.3).

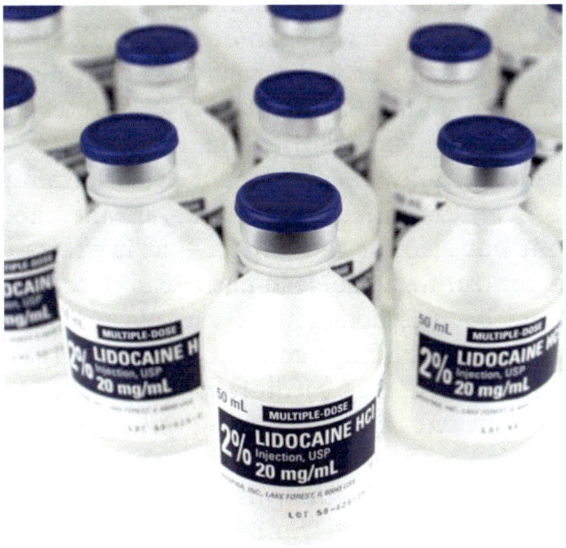

Figure 3.3. The classification of anesthetic agents plays a crucial role in the practice of anesthesia.

Source: https://www.mountainside-medical.com/cdn/shop/products/Hospira_Lidocaine_2_for_Injection_50mL_25Pk_8cf77a60-12a2-4fe5-8ee7-ef69bf68d17a_500x500.jpg?v=1722512740.

3.1.1. General Anesthetics

The quest for general anesthetics has undergone a revolution over the past 150 years, driven by developments that reflect the complex dynamics of pharmacologic agents and their interactions at the molecular level. It remains to be understood how the agents induce anesthesia, particularly as they induce unconsciousness by altering brain function. Current theories suggest general anesthetics primarily disrupt communication among and within cortical regions of the brain, impeding neural network function critical to consciousness. The implications of these findings are broad, as they can foreshadow an integrated conceptualization of anesthesia that links clinical practice and theoretical neuroscience, with consequential insights into the nature of unconsciousness and the mechanisms of neurophysiological communication under general anesthesia (Logan et al., 2019). Of the many selections of general anesthetics available, ketamine alone has its own characteristic pharmacological profile and mechanisms of action. Initially used in the 1960s, ketamine has been identified not only as an anesthetic agent but also for the impact that it exerts on the central nervous system. It exerts complex effects by interacting with various molecular targets, producing considerable analgesia without disrupting cardiorespiratory stability. The current understanding tilts towards ketamine's ability to disrupt corticocortical transfer of information, primarily in the top-down direction from frontal to parietal regions, thus leading to the induction of the anesthetic state (Li et al., 2016). This understanding not only supports the promotion of an experience for the application of ketamine in anesthesiology, but it also comes with the promise of potential applications in the treatment of refractory depression as well as PTSD. With the evolution of anesthesiology, knowledge of general anesthetic pharmacokinetics and pharmacodynamics remains a very high priority. Pharmacologic advances in drug formulation and drug delivery systems highlight the transition towards tailored anesthetic approaches based on the patient's requirements and the needs of a specific surgical condition. The advent of newer agents added to the anesthetic arsenal to offer optimized sedation regimens that avoid risks traditionally presented by anesthetic therapy. Ongoing future investigation is necessary to further elucidate the nuances of these agents' effects and refine the overall safety and efficacy of anesthetic care. Taken together, these developments argue that anesthetic pharmacology not only enhances surgery but also contributes to broader medical paradigms of patient health and mental well-being, reaffirming the continued importance of general anesthetics in contemporary clinical practice.

3.1.2. Local Anesthetics

Local anesthetics form the foundation of modern-day anesthesia, rendering regional analgesia that causes very little pain during surgical and diagnostic interventions. Local anesthetics block sodium channels in the neuron's membrane reversibly, resulting in a failure of action potential generation and conduction. Through specifically compromising the transmission of nerve impulses, local anesthetics allow practitioners to perform surgery without inducing general anesthesia. Local anesthetic flexibility encompasses several techniques, including infiltrative, regional, and topical, each useful in distinct clinical situations. Furthermore, the local anesthetic selected—e.g., lidocaine, bupivacaine, or ropivacaine—is based on the duration of action required and the demands of the operation, underscoring the necessity of pharmacologic knowledge in anesthesia practice. Advances in imaging technology, particularly ultrasound, have transformed the use of local anesthetics. Ultrasound guidance has become essential in achieving precise placement of local anesthetic agents, enhancing the efficacy and safety of nerve blocks. Evidence indicates that the use of ultrasound significantly reduces complications such as vascular damage and local anesthetic systemic toxicity, and enables the generation of new and improved nerve blocks. Ultrasound integration not only improves visualization of anatomical structures but also improves general local anesthetic pharmacology knowledge and its influence on patient outcomes.

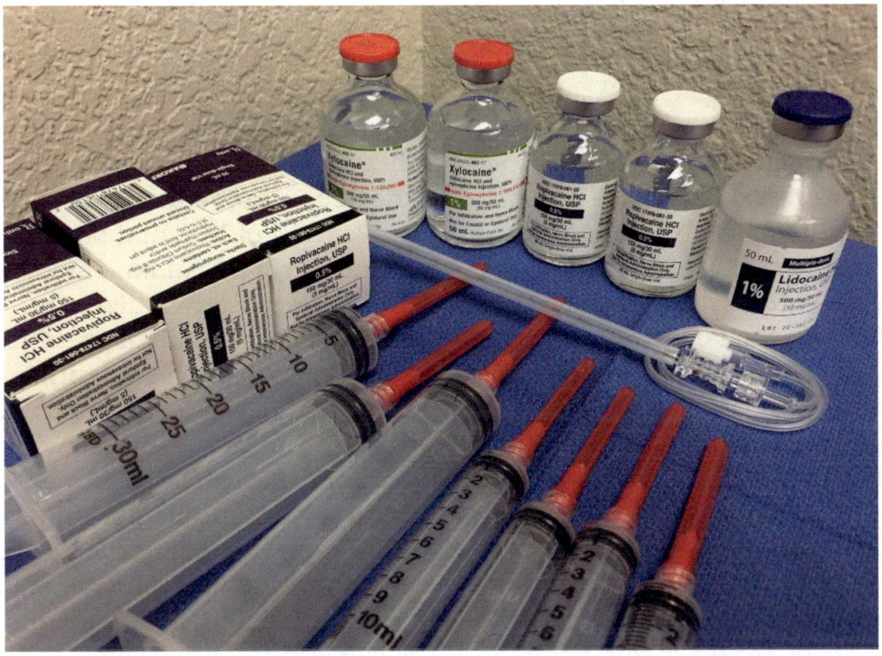

Figure 3.4. Local anesthetics play a fundamental role in modern anesthesia.

Source: https://images.squarespace-cdn.com/content/v1/55ccc7c0e4b0b3e97680f13b/1518629255728-BQWI98Z33VLF5OQ9INT1/Local+Anesthetics.

With the evolution of the field, practitioners must stay up to date on the use of this technology to optimize anesthesia practice, thereby underscoring the need for continual education and training in local anesthetics (Michael et al., 2018). In pediatric anesthesia practice, the pharmacology of local anesthetics has unique considerations that demand high-level expertise and techniques. While the pain relief offered by local anesthetics is effective in children undergoing surgery, vigilant consideration of pharmacokinetics, dosing, and side effects must be made for this group of patients. Literature identifies a need for practical guidelines to address the complexities of ultrasound-guided regional anesthesia in children, with safe and effective outcomes (N/A, 2015). Anesthesiologists may reduce local anesthetic risks and achieve optimal therapeutic outcomes by being mindful of anatomical variability and the development of physiology in children. As pediatric local anesthesia knowledge continues to grow, remain updated on optimal practices, thus promoting a safety and effectiveness culture in anesthesia practice among children (Figure 3.4).

3.1.3. Adjunctive Medications

The use of adjunctive drugs during anesthesia is a significant aspect of modern perioperative care, enhancing patient outcomes without sacrificing or exaggerating analgesia and minimizing the potential deleterious effects of the surgical procedure. Drugs utilized as adjuncts include non-opioid analgesics, anxiolytics, and neuromuscular blockers, each contributing to the anesthetic regimen in specific ways. Non-opioid pain relievers such as acetaminophen and nonsteroidal anti-inflammatory drugs (NSAIDs) can commonly be utilized to alleviate pain and decrease opioid usage, which has significant risks in terms of respiratory depression and dependency. Having a multimodal approach to analgesia that incorporates these adjunct therapies allows anesthesiologists to provide a more comprehensive pain management protocol that addresses immediate and postoperative pain successfully. Anxiolytics constitute another important class of adjunctive medications, especially employed for anxious patients concerning surgical procedures. The use of medications such as midazolam results in smoother induction and recovery phases during anesthesia. In addition to decreasing preoperative anxiety, anxiolytics also enhance patient satisfaction as a whole by creating a more serene atmosphere during the process of surgery. The anxiolytic effects of these medications can also be used to decrease the amount of general anesthetic required, potentially with a reduction in postoperative complications and recovery time. Current literature increasingly supports that the management of anxiety with adjunctive medications can lead to improved recovery outcomes and decreased hospital stay, illustrating their role in contemporary anesthetic practice. Additionally, adjunctive therapy can play a critical role in achieving the safety and efficacy of venous thromboembolism (VTE) prophylaxis in surgical patients. The application of pharmacologic treatment agents, such as low molecular weight heparin or direct oral anticoagulants, assists in managing the controversial trade-off between the prevention of VTE and bleeding complications, especially in trauma patients. The Western Trauma Association algorithm emphasizes the importance of patient-specific pharmacologic prophylaxis to ensure optimal patient safety and outcomes and posits that risk management during surgery is best achieved through a prudent, judicious application of medication therapy (Eric et al., 2020). Also, the inclusion of non-pharmacologic adjunct methods, like immersive virtual reality for pain relief, presents an additional opportunity for enhancing the anesthetic experience while potentially reducing opioid use (Firoozabadi et al., 2020). This evolution in multimodal anesthetic techniques underscores ongoing research and practice to address patients' needs more effectively.

Test Your Knowledge

1. What are adjunctive medications, and how do they enhance the safety and effectiveness of anesthesia?
2. Explain the roles of sedatives, analgesics, muscle relaxants, and antiemetics as adjuncts in anesthetic practice.

3.2. Mechanisms of Action

Learning Outcome

1. Pharmacokinetics of anesthetic agents
2. Pharmacodynamics in anesthesia
3. Interaction with neurotransmitter systems

Understanding the mechanisms of action of anesthetic drugs is at the core of anesthesiology, as it informs both drug selection and patient safety. Anesthetic drugs primarily exert their effects by modulating neurotransmitter receptors in the central nervous system. Specifically, most anesthetics have sites of action at transmembrane receptors, such as N-methyl-D-aspartate (NMDA) and GABAA receptors. Studies have established that certain hydrocarbons are capable of potentiating GABAA receptor current but inhibiting NMDA receptor function, and thereby causing the desired sedation and analgesic action; fascinatingly, modulation of NMDA receptor function has been determined to be characterized by a water solubility threshold of 1.1 mM, suggesting a complex interdependence of the chemical composition of anesthetics and their pharmacologic effect (Brosnan et al., 2014). Further, the pharmacodynamics of anesthetic agents also include their effects on cardiovascular stability during surgical procedures. Anesthesia-induced cardiac arrest is a serious issue, particularly in children. In studies, it has been proven that the risk is significantly increased in the induction and maintenance of anesthesia through states of bradycardia, hypotension, and abnormal oxygenation. These states often precede cardiac arrest, and the monitoring of vital signs under continuous observation becomes a requirement. Understanding the mechanisms underlying such cardiovascular changes will be useful to anesthesiologists in the prevention of such changes, with a view to ensuring optimal patient outcomes (Prabakti et al., 2005). Beyond the effects of novel receptors, the pharmacological characteristics of anesthetics can vary depending on their molecular complexity and solubility. For instance, it has been observed that hydrocarbons with novel functional groups can vary in their interactions with receptor types. These variations not only impact the potency of the anesthetics but also their safety profiles. The differential modulation observed for GABAA and NMDA receptors suggests that anesthetic side effects may be avoided if insight into the specific mechanisms at play is gained. Consequently, increased research into these interactions will result in an encyclopedic knowledge base that will allow anesthesiologists to tailor their interventions to individual patient needs and conditions, thereby enhancing the entire anesthesia care practice (Brosnan et al., 2014).

3.2.1. Pharmacokinetics of Anesthetic Agents

Pharmacokinetics of anesthetic drugs involves understanding the process of absorption, distribution, metabolism, and excretion of the drugs in the body. This is required for optimal doses and improving patient management under anesthesia. Anesthetic drugs may vary widely in pharmacokinetics, dictating the onset, duration of action, and overall effectiveness. For instance, drugs such as propofol have a rapid onset and brief effect duration due to their beneficial distribution attributes, like rapid elimination and recovery. Conversely, the pharmacokinetics of drugs such as remimazolam characterize its unique ultrashort-acting profile, with the potential to be metabolized rapidly by tissue esterases. This feature can minimize postoperative complications related to sedation. Awareness of these differences is important for clinicians to modify anesthetic technique according to individual patient requirements and procedural demands. Secondly, even the pediatric population presents inherent difficulties with the pharmacokinetics of the anesthetic drug. Preterm and term infants exhibit different metabolic trends and developmental characteristics that govern drug processing in the body. Accordingly, the majority of anesthetics administered to this vulnerable population are off-label, often based on adult data due to the lack of specific clinical trials. This extrapolation may lead to dosing errors and increased risks of adverse effects in neonates. Considering these challenges, there is an urgent need to study more extensively the pharmacokinetics of anesthetic drugs in neonates. This is required for the development of evidence-based guidelines that ensure efficacy and safety in their use for anesthesia and analgesia for surgical and procedural procedures (Tesoro et al., 2020). The pharmacokinetics of anesthetic medications also must consider age, body composition, and comorbidities, which could have a significant influence on drug metabolism and excretion. For example, older patients might experience altered pharmacokinetic response due to physiological changes in the aging process, resulting in prolonged action of certain anesthetics. Additionally, patients with renal or hepatic dysfunction may exhibit altered pharmacokinetics that necessitate dose adjustments. The importance of these differences is significant because they illustrate the necessity of customized anesthetic regimens crafted to address each patient's individual profile. Clinicians must be vigilant and aware of the variable pharmacokinetic characteristics of anesthetics to prevent complications and maintain a secure overall practice of anesthesia. With advancing science, increased awareness of variables will enable improved clinical outcomes for patients in diverse populations.

3.2.2. Pharmacodynamics in Anesthesia

The concept of pharmacodynamics is especially relevant in anesthesia, where anesthetic drugs produce their effects on the body. Drug-receptor interactions play a crucial role in achieving the desired effects, such as unconsciousness, analgesia, and muscle relaxation. As stated in current literature, anesthesia could require a multimodal approach because it involves the application of a range of drugs with differing mechanisms to maximize effect while limiting side effects. Brown et al discuss enhancing past methodology by what they call multimodal general anesthesia and emphasize the interaction of neuroanatomical circuits and neurophysiological mechanisms to strengthen the efficacy of anesthetic agents during surgery (Talmage et al., 2018). This approach not only surpasses the limitations of single-agent anesthetics but also aims to maximize patient outcome through drug synergy. Among the many classes of anesthetics, the pharmacodynamics of agents like ketamine are of utmost significance. Ketamine, with its defining dissociative effect, affects several neurotransmitter systems, including N-methyl-D-aspartate (NMDA) receptors, and is a critical element in anesthetic and analgesic regimens. Their metabolites, (S)- and (R)-ketamine, also play a role in the drug's clinical activity, which is responsible for its analgesic and anti-inflammatory properties (Zanos et al., 2018). The ability of ketamine to interact with numerous receptor systems not only demonstrates the complexities of anesthetic drug interactions but also its potential as a multi-purpose drug in multimodal anesthesia approaches." The pharmacodynamic profile highlights ketamine's efficacy in perioperative pain management with a favorable safety profile compared with usual opioids and as a valuable addition to modern anesthetic practice. Pharmacodynamics is not only the examination of individual drugs but also the overall regulation of anesthesia. The MAC principle provides a basis for quantifying the potency of inhalational anesthetics and their interactions when administered in combination with adjunct agents (Talmage et al., 2018). MAC has essential clinical implications, as it informs dosing and anesthetic drug titration to achieve desired surgical conditions without inducing hemodynamic perturbations. Moreover, the understanding that multiple drugs are capable of modifying the concentration-effect profiles of parent anesthetics enlarges the anesthesiologist's scope for personalization of anesthetic regimens to individual patient requirements. Ultimately, this personalization can translate into improved patient outcomes and safety, underscoring the central role of pharmacodynamics in the anesthetic profession and the ongoing evolution of practice (Figure 3.5).

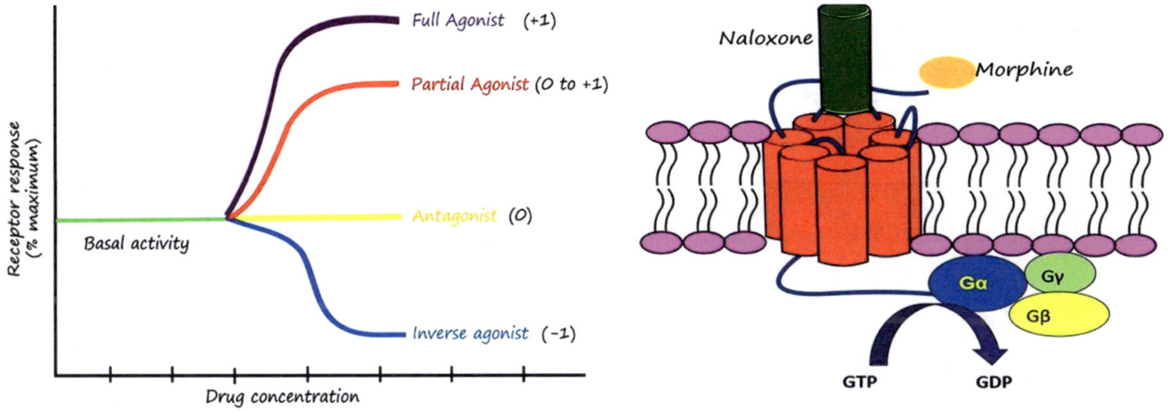

Figure 3.5. The concept of pharmacodynamics plays a crucial role in anesthesia.

Source: https://i.ytimg.com/vi/3k7iVixdYrU/maxresdefault.jpg.

3.2.3. Interaction with Neurotransmitter Systems

The action of anesthetic agents on neurotransmitter systems is at the heart of the understanding of their pharmacological effects under conditions of surgery. General anesthetics primarily act on GABA and glutamate receptors and modulate the central nervous system's balance between inhibition and excitation. Anesthetics, for instance, stimulate GABA receptors, leading to a sedative effect that permits unconsciousness and amnesia. This action is further augmented by inhibition of excitatory glutamate transmission, specifically NMDA receptors, which diminishes synaptic transmission and contributes to an anesthetic-induced state of unresponsiveness. These interactions underlie the complex pharmacodynamics of anesthetics and provide a basis for explaining potential neurotoxic effects observed in certain groups, notably pediatric and geriatric patients. Therefore, knowledge of mechanisms is critical to optimize anesthetic use and reduce risk of anesthesia-induced cognitive deficits (Perouansky et al., 2009). The modulation of mental processes by neurotransmitter systems extends beyond GABA and glutamate to other essential pathways that anesthetics may influence. For example, gamma hydroxybutyric acid (GHB) is in the spotlight for its two faces as both a neurotransmitter and a drug with applications in the treatment of narcolepsy and as an anesthetic adjunct. GHB is an agonist at some GHB receptors and GABAB receptors, whose actions are sedation and anesthesia. The GHB modulation of neurotransmitter release can create anxiolytic and hypnotic effects, demonstrating the diversity of neurotransmitter systems that can be controlled under anesthesia. The understanding of these interactions not only makes optimal use of anesthetics feasible but also indicates the relevance for drug abuse, since the recreational potential of GHB means that its safety and abuse liability are issues (Castelli, 2008). The actions of anesthetics and neurotransmitter systems are more in focus nowadays, with novel evidence of their long-term effects on cognitive ability. Experiments have shown that exposure to general anesthetics can cause neurotoxic changes, particularly in susceptible individuals, and there is also the postoperative cognitive dysfunction issue. These actions may be mediated by specific neurotransmitter systems, as alterations in brain-derived neurotrophic factor and calcium signaling pathways have been observed following anesthetic administration. The clinical implications of these findings warrant further investigation of the mechanisms of neurodegeneration and cognitive impairment. By extensive investigation of these neurotransmitter interactions, clinical practitioners can better assess the dangers of anesthetic-induced neurocognitive changes, ultimately leading to improved patient outcomes and more reflective anesthetic practice (Perouansky et al., 2009).

Test Your Knowledge

1. How do anesthetic drugs produce their effects at the cellular and receptor levels?
2. Why is an understanding of dose–response relationships important in the safe administration of anesthesia?

3.3. Administration Routes

Learning Outcome

1. Inhalational anesthetics
2. Intravenous anesthetics
3. Regional anesthesia techniques

The administration route of anesthetic agents plays a central role in determining their efficacy, onset, and margin of safety in clinical practice. Various routes, including intravenous, intramuscular, intranasal, and oral, are suited to different patient requirements and clinical scenarios. Intravenous administration is generally preferred for its rapidity and controllability and is therefore best suited to procedures requiring instant sedation. Conversely, intramuscular routes are valuable when intravenous access is not readily available. Oral and intranasal routes have also gained popularity due to ease of administration, most commonly with pediatric patients or perioperative control of anxiety. All routes share distinctive pharmacokinetic properties that influence drug absorption and bioavailability, underscoring the importance of administering the correct route to achieve maximum anesthetic effect. The versatility of drugs like ketamine most clearly demonstrates the significance of routes of administration in pharmacologic application in anesthesia. Ketamine is a dissociative anesthetic drug that can be delivered by a variety of routes to allow the practitioner to tailor his or her modality according to patient-specific concerns and procedural requirements. Such versatility optimizes its utility throughout the spectrum of clinical contexts, including the management of acute and chronic pain, particularly when standard analgesics may prove inadequate. Intramuscular and intravenous ketamine provide rapid analgesia, while oral and nasal formulations are particularly beneficial in patient acceptance and comfort. Thus, familiarity with the pharmacological profile and potential for use of ketamine in each route of administration is essential for effective pain and sedation control in different patient populations (Zoroufchi et al., 2020). Although the heterogeneity of administration routes enhances the adaptability of anesthetic drugs, clinicians must also exercise caution with side effects from these routes. For instance, although esketamine has been shown to have significant analgesic effects with minimal impact on respiratory function, clinicians must proceed carefully in clinical settings. Pharmacological profile, including rapid metabolism and extensive use in pediatric and emergency settings, contributes to the complexity of the decision to use it (Zhang et al., 2022). Aftercare strategies must accommodate varied responses to the drug depending on the route of administration. Anesthesia practitioners assist in informed decision-making by understanding the pharmacodynamics of these drugs and delivering patient safety and optimal results throughout the continuum of care. Finally, a sophisticated understanding of administration pathways allows clinicians to utilize anesthetics' pharmacologic characteristics to their advantage while minimizing risks associated with anesthesia practice.

3.3.1. Inhalational Anesthetics

The use of inhalational anesthetics has revolutionized anesthesia practice by offering a unique pharmacologic approach to effectively controlling pain and consciousness in surgery. The agents, such as halothane, isoflurane, and desflurane, are administered via the respiratory system and are characterized by their induction and recovery profiles. The pharmacokinetics of volatile anesthetics are influenced extensively by several physiological factors, including cardiac output, ventilation-perfusion ratios, and the solubility of anesthetics in blood and tissues. In addition, the manner in which the drugs exert their effects on the central nervous system is still being developed, illustrating the character of action, which also comprises modulation of neurotransmitter systems and neuronal excitability. The selection of an appropriate inhalational anesthetic is not only a matter of personal choice. Still, it is a more subtle process including patient-related issues, surgical requirements, and drug pharmacologic properties. With the increasing population of elderly patients, there are good reasons to be worried about the dangers of employing inhalational anesthesia, especially its heightened sensitivity to postoperative morbidity and mortality, such as respiratory failure and neurologic dysfunction in the elderly patient. Close monitoring is essential to avoid potential adverse effects, particularly in patients with comorbidities.

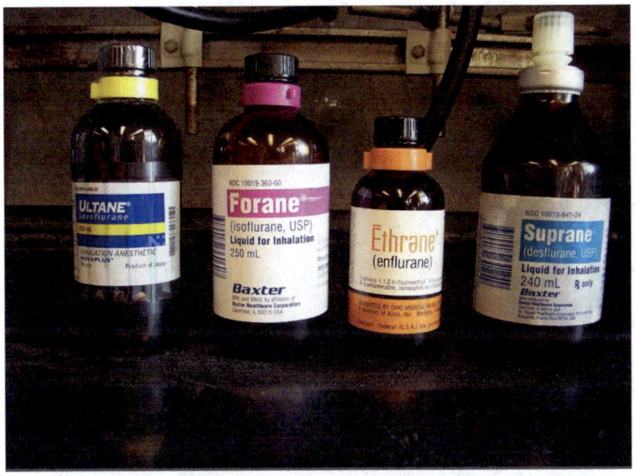

Figure 3.6. The use of inhalational anesthetics has revolutionized the practice of anesthesia.

Source: https://upload.wikimedia.org/wikipedia/commons/1/18/Fluranebottles.jpg.

These considerations necessitate anesthesiologists keeping pace with evolving drug information, particularly as novel drugs and delivery methods emerge that can enhance the safety and efficacy of inhalational anesthetics (Bertoncello et al., 2017). New research has drawn attention to the potential effects of inhalational anesthetics beyond their anesthetic characteristics, and more specifically, how they may act on cancer biology. Recent research suggests that bupivacaine, an agent traditionally relegated to regional anesthesia classification, possesses features that affect cancer cell biology, perhaps as regards affecting cancer recidivism following surgery. Although this discovery does not have a direct application to inhalational anesthetics, it underscores the importance of understanding how anesthetic agents act in multifarious ways to influence patient outcomes.

This is what emphasizes the need for more studies into the way inhalational anesthetics, and other means of anesthesia, might affect not just control of pain but also wider post-surgical effects on patients, thus justifying the development of personalized anesthetic regimens in today's medical practice (Chen et al., 2016) (Figure 3.6).

3.3.2. Intravenous Anesthetics

Intravenous anesthetics are a mainstay of modern anesthetic practice, offering rapid onset and simplicity of administration. Intravenous agents are breathed directly into the circulation, allowing precise control over the level and length of anesthesia.

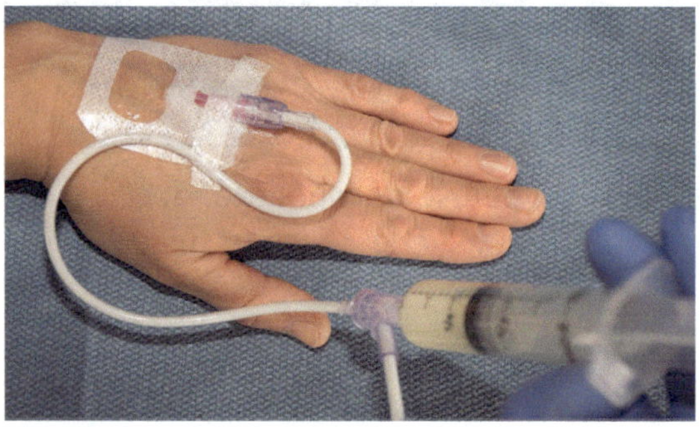

Figure 3.7. Intravenous anesthetics.

Source: https://chblob.icloudhospital.com/images/6-8b8cd2fb-109b-4d6d-9a2c-5fec3bb55bf2.jpg.

Propofol, etomidate, and thiopental are standard agents with unique pharmacodynamic properties that guide their applications in clinical practice. Propofol, for instance, is favored for its antiemetic properties and rapid recovery, making it suitable for outpatient procedures. Its speedy onset of action makes it an acceptable option both as an induction agent and for maintaining anesthesia, making it a useful tool in contemporary anesthesia practice. Such characteristics make intravenous anesthetics an essential addition to the anesthetic repertoire, making patient management easier and improving overall surgical results. The pharmacokinetics of intravenous anesthetics strongly influence their clinical safety and efficacy profiles. Drugs are typically characterized by rapid redistribution from the central nervous system to peripheral tissues, which accounts for their rapid onset of action. Their lipid solubility allows their quick passage through the blood-brain barrier. Understanding the pharmacodynamic interactions of these agents is crucial, as they have varying effects on cardiovascular stability and respiratory function.

For instance, while propofol may cause hypotension in some patients, etomidate tends to be hemodynamically stable and therefore is an ideal choice for patients with compromised cardiovascular functions. These differences necessitate careful examination of the agent selected based on individual patient profiles and surgical requirements, further validating the use of customized medication approaches in anesthesia. Further, the application of intravenous anesthetics clinically must also consider potential issues and side effects. Adverse effects can be mild or severe and can affect patients' recovery and overall safety. For instance, propofol's sedative effects can induce respiratory depression if not monitored, especially in patients who are prone to it, such as the geriatric or patients with pre-existing respiratory conditions. Intravenous anesthetics also tend to cause postoperative nausea and vomiting, against which adjunctive antiemetic therapies are needed to neutralize discomfort. As observed in the European Society for Pediatric Anesthesiology guidelines, the use of anesthesia in children introduces additional complexities in the choice of agents and monitoring methods (Adamek et al., 2018). It is thus crucial to have a thorough understanding of the pharmacological properties and patient choice factors in the best use of intravenous anesthetics with optimal patient outcomes in procedural and surgical settings (Calvieri et al., 2014) (Figure 3.7).

3.3.3. Regional Anesthesia Techniques

The topography of regional anesthesia techniques has been significantly altered, most notably with the advent of ultrasound guidance. Not only is the use of ultrasound more precise in localizing the nerves, but it also provides higher patient safety by reducing complications such as vascular trauma and local anesthetic systemic toxicity. There is evidence to indicate that ultrasound-guided techniques are superior to earlier techniques, and they decrease adverse effects like pneumothorax and phrenic nerve block (Michael et al., 2018). Moreover, with earlier nerve stimulation, tactile feedback could occasionally lead to misplaced local anesthetics, whereas with ultrasound, one can visualize anatomical structures in real time. This shift to imaging technology reflects how the practice of pharmacy is changing, and, in doing so, anesthetic surroundings are being reshaped, reducing the risk of complications and generally enhancing the quality of treatment provided to patients undergoing surgery. In addition to evolving technology, the choice of anesthetic medications is critical to the effectiveness and safety of regional anesthesia. Levobupivacaine, now an alternative to bupivacaine as a new agent, is noted for its pharmacokinetic advantages. As the S (-)-enantiomer of pure bupivacaine, levobupivacaine has a reduced incidence of adverse drug reaction when administered appropriately, making it a desirable option for physicians (Bajwa et al., 2013). Clinical research indicates levobupivacaine to be an equally potent substitute for bupivacaine without the possibility of inducing the latter's potential harms, such as cardiac toxicity. This favorable profile makes levobupivacaine the leading edge of modern anesthetic regimens, where patient safety is given top priority. The use of these new agents underscores the benefits of research and development in anesthetic pharmacology, particularly in terms of patient safety. In addition, regional anesthesia encompasses various techniques tailored to surgical requirements, thereby reinforcing the importance of patient-specific treatment. Techniques such as nerve blocks and spinal anesthesia are tailored to treat localized pain and can effectively reduce postoperative pain and shorten recovery times. Each technique requires exhaustive knowledge of anatomy, pharmacology, and patient-related factors to deliver the maximum benefit. The evolution of methods, such as novel blocks facilitated by ultrasound, not only enhanced existing techniques but also created new horizons for regional anesthesia (Michael et al., 2018). As practitioners become more competent in employing these technologies, the balance between providing adequate analgesia and minimizing potential risks remains the hallmark of the intersection between pharmacology and anesthesia practice. Generally, regional anesthesia techniques exhibit an interactive relationship among emerging practices, fostering safety and efficiency in patient care.

Test Your Knowledge

1. What are the different routes of administering anesthetic agents, and how do they affect the onset, duration, and intensity of anesthesia?
2. What factors influence the choice of administration route for anesthetic drugs in clinical practice?

3.4. Monitoring and Safety

Learning Outcome

1. Importance of patient monitoring
2. Adverse effects of anesthetic agents
3. Strategies for minimizing risks

In the complex world of anesthesia pharmacology, monitoring and safety are the top priorities. Within this context lies the implementation of rigorous guidelines to avert issues such as venous thromboembolism (VTE), something that patients undergoing anesthesia are highly concerned about. Evidence-based practice emphasizes initiating pharmacologic prophylaxis within 24 hours of trauma to maximize outcomes. For example, the Western Trauma Association (WTA) recommends an algorithm that sets categorical parameters for risk assessment, while pointing out that early intervention can significantly reduce the incidence of VTE in high-risk individuals, particularly trauma patients. This policy emphasizes individualization based on patient profiles, balancing safety and appropriate anesthetic care across diverse clinical environments, which can impact postoperative recovery and long-term health outcomes (Eric et al., 2020). Of related interest, neuromuscular blockade monitoring, especially among elderly patients, is a critical safety procedure in anesthesiology. Aging affects neuromuscular transmission, which results in an increased likelihood of residual blockade, potentially being the etiology of severe postoperative outcomes, including respiratory failure and extensive recovery. Acetylcholinesterase inhibitors such as neostigmine are commonly used to reverse neuromuscular blockade but is not without disadvantage. The new agent sugammadex has been found to reverse neuromuscular effects effectively, particularly with rocuronium. But its pharmacokinetics are age-dependent, necessitating strict monitoring when administered to elderly patients. Thus, stringent monitoring should be combined with the use of such pharmacologic tools to ensure their safety and effectiveness in vulnerable populations, underscoring that patient-centered monitoring remains the basic tenet of anesthetic practice (Carron et al., 2017). Moreover, the interconnection between patient monitoring and pharmacologic intervention extends far beyond the realm of anesthesia administration itself. Periodic observation of a patient's physiological condition, including hemodynamic and neuromuscular function, must be in keeping with the timing and dose of administered anesthetics and adjuvants. Advances in technology for monitoring devices, such as state-of-the-art hemodynamic and neuromuscular transmission monitoring devices, can enhance the clinician's ability to detect and respond early to adverse effects. Taking a proactive role in monitoring not only ensures timely intervention but also develops the culture of safety in the operating room. As anesthesiologists work through the details of pharmacology, the synergy of diligent monitoring and safety protocols remains essential in delivering quality anesthesia care, ultimately leading to improved patient outcomes and reduced complication rates (Eric et al., 2020) (Figure 3.8).

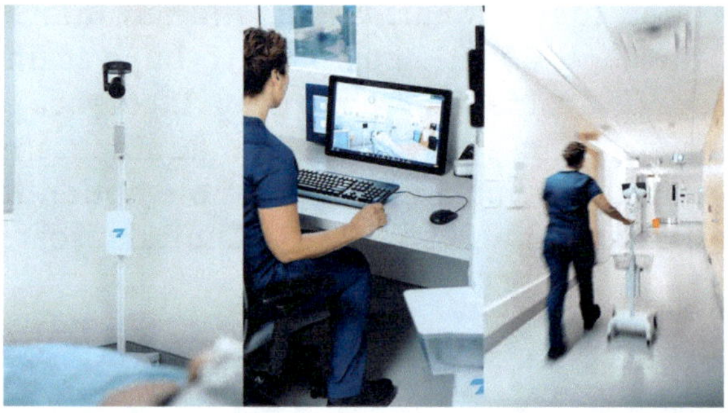

Figure 3.8. The complex field of pharmacology in anesthesia, monitoring and safety emerge as paramount considerations.

Source: https://www.capsahealthcare.com/wp-content/uploads/2024/07/Patient-Observation-1200x680-1.png-1024x580-1.webp.

3.4.1. Importance of Patient Monitoring

Patient monitoring is a primary component in the practice of anesthesia and is an important safeguard for incidents of ill effect during surgery. Adequate monitoring allows anesthesiologists to monitor patients' vital signs, including heart rate, blood pressure, oxygen saturation, and ventilation parameters. Monitoring is continuous and permits any variations from normal expectations to be identified and addressed in a prompt manner. Failure to monitor patients adequately during the process of induction and maintenance of anesthesia can lead to severe complications, which can worsen to become life-threatening. Hence, the integration of newer monitoring technologies has revolutionized anesthesia practice, allowing clinicians to make decisions in real time with confidence and appropriate judgment regarding patient safety and drug administration strategies.

Thus, emphasis cannot be overemphasized on the need for careful patient monitoring as it is the pillar of quality and safety in operative anesthesia practice, establishing pharmacology's role in ensuring maximum patient care in anesthesia. Moreover, the value of monitoring patients extends to anesthetic pharmacology management, particularly in titrating anesthetic agents. Accurate monitoring not only facilitates the identification of appropriate dosages but also helps in establishing the patients' physiological responses to various anesthetics. Each individual will respond variably to anesthetic agents due to variations in age, comorbidities, and genetic variations in drug-metabolizing pathways. Real-time monitoring gives anesthesiologists the data to dynamically adjust drug doses so as not to underdose or overdose. Additionally, monitoring is particularly valuable in special populations—such as pediatrics or geriatrics—where physiological responses may differ markedly from those in the general adult population. The drug-patient monitoring synergy finally offers a greater safety margin for anesthetized patients, allowing care to be tailored to individual needs during surgery.

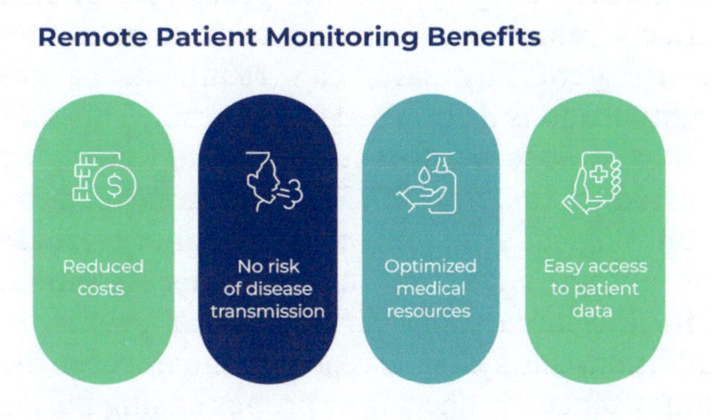

Figure 3.9. Importance of patient monitoring.

Source: https://www.scalefocus.com/wp-content/uploads/2022/08/SCF_Remote_patient_monitoring_image1-1.jpg.

Finally, patient monitoring also plays an important part in post-anesthesia care, directly affecting recovery and reducing postoperative complications. Continuous monitoring enables caregivers to identify any adverse response to anesthetic agents such as hypotension, respiratory depression, or emergence delirium. Early identification of complications may enable rapid interventions and avoid bad clinical outcomes. Furthermore, effective monitoring during the recovery phase can affect discharge timing decisions in the postoperative environment, with patients being discharged only if they have met predetermined criteria for recovery prior to discharge from the healthcare environment. Alongside the evolving global healthcare landscape, the importance of effective patient monitoring as a component of anesthesia practice is likely to grow. Adoption of fresh monitoring technologies and protocols can make recovery processes more rational and enhance patient safety, thus reaffirming the pivotal role that pharmacology plays in anesthesia and surgical care (Iorio et al., 2020; Calkins et al., 2017) (Figure 3.9).

3.4.2. Adverse Effects of Anesthetic Agents

The use of anesthetic medication is a crucial part of modern surgery; yet, the possibility of side effects remains a problem. Local anesthetics, while generally safe, can result in severe complications if absorbed systemically. This self-inflicted absorption results in local anesthetic systemic toxicity (LAST), characterized by neurological symptoms in the form of seizures or arrhythmias that may further manifest into life-threatening cardiovascular events. In addition, this systemic reaction underscores the importance of adhering to proper dosing norms to minimize risks. The pharmacological profile of local anesthetic drugs necessitates a thorough understanding of their mechanisms and potential side effects to enhance patient safety during procedures (Dontukurthy et al., 2021). Thus, monitoring techniques and prophylactic procedures become essential in reducing the occurrence of LAST and rendering the benefits of local anesthesia larger than potential hazards. Injection anesthetics like barbiturates and newer agents like propofol also possess unique risks, though more so for veterinary use, but applicable in human contexts as well. Despite barbiturates being established over many years as potent anesthetic and anticonvulsant agents, they produce protracted recoveries and respiratory depression. Propofol, with its anesthetic onset of just a few minutes, has resulted in hypotension and possible apnea and necessitates careful cardiovascular monitoring on administration. These effects require clinicians to remain alert and adjust their anesthetic plans based on each agent's properties and risks (Stephanie, 2015). Similarly, dissociative agents induce a state of altered awareness that yields unpredictable pharmacokinetic effects, rendering it challenging for clinicians to hold patients stable during surgery. Its side effects are essential to understand to optimize outcomes in anesthesiology practice. Considering these multifaceted adverse effects, pharmacologic regulation of anesthesia should entail rigorous safety precautions and strategies to minimize risk. Clinicians must incorporate practices such as ultrasound-guided regional anesthesia, which have been shown to reduce complication rates of local anesthetic systemic absorption. Anesthetic selection must also be tailored to the individual patient based on their clinical status, comorbidities, and potential drug interactions. Continuing education and implementation of evidence-based guidelines could go a long way in reducing the incidence of anesthetic drug-related adverse effects. With the advancement in the field of anesthesiology, safety of patients versus successful anesthesia continues to be a prime concern, setting the path for pharmacology in anesthetic practice (Stephanie, 2015; Dontukurthy et al., 2021) (Figure 3.10).

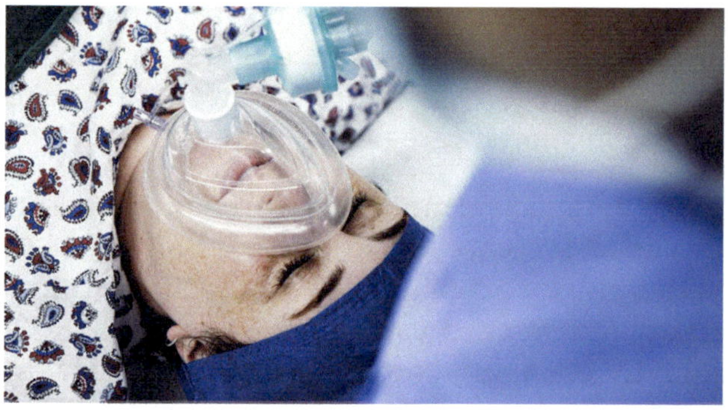

Figure 3.10. Adverse effects of anesthetic agents.

Source: https://post.medicalnewstoday.com/wp-content/uploads/sites/3/2021/11/general_anesthesia_GettyImages910493382_Header-1024x575.jpg.

3.4.3. Strategies for Minimizing Risks

The administration of anesthetics involves inherent risk; therefore, the use of thorough strategies to reduce possible adverse effects is necessary. One important technique is the careful selection and dosing of pharmacologic agents based on individual patient considerations such as comorbidities, age, and body weight. Using principles of pharmacokinetics and pharmacodynamics, anesthesiologists can individualize drug selection and dosage to optimize safety. This becomes particularly critical in the context of patients requiring extracorporeal membrane oxygenation (ECMO) because alterations in drug metabolism can compromise therapeutic efficacy and produce undesirable side effects. As described (Aebi et al., 2017), the changes caused by ECMO can significantly affect the pharmacokinetics of medications, so it is vital to customize dosing regimens to address individualized requirements for enhancing patient safety and therapeutic outcome. Outside of individualized dosing, multimodal analgesia is also quite effective in reducing opioid dependence and, consequently, the accompanying risks of tolerance and addiction. Multimodal analgesia is a regimen whereby a combination of non-opioid analgesics and regional anesthetic modalities is used in a way that produces sufficient pain relief while minimizing opioid exposure. The opioid crisis has aggravated the necessity for such measures, so new alternatives such as stem cell therapy (SCT) and non-opioid anesthetic techniques have come under study. As elaborated in the study (II A et al., 2024), SCT has proved to be beneficial in reducing chronic pain by taking advantage of the body's capacity to heal without the adverse connections associated with opioid drugs. By making a multimodal pain strategy a priority, clinicians not only can best manage pain but also can enhance public health efforts to reduce addiction to opioids. Communication and collaboration among the care team are essential in maximizing patient safety with anesthesia. Standardized preoperative screening protocols can aid in the identification of patients at increased risk for complications and can provide these patients with necessary precautions before the procedure. Regular multidisciplinary meetings and ongoing education of anesthesia professionals on emerging pharmacologic options and recent research can also help ensure these safety precautions. Monitoring the patient in real time during anesthesia allows for instantaneous identification and treatment of any unwanted effects. This proactive approach is essential for minimizing anesthesia risks, as it promotes a culture in which patient safety is paramount and enables anesthesia practices to evolve in line with the latest scientific evidence and clinical practice.

Test Your Knowledge

1. Why is continuous patient monitoring essential during anesthesia, and which vital parameters must be closely observed?
2. How do modern monitoring technologies enhance patient safety and help prevent anesthetic complications?

3.5. Special Considerations

Learning Outcome

1. Pediatric anesthesia
2. Geriatric anesthesia
3. Anesthesia in patients with comorbidities

Relevant to the field of anesthesia, the patient population, comorbidities, and the nature of surgery significantly influence pharmacologic regimens. Age, weight, and comorbidities significantly influence the metabolism and excretion of anesthetic drugs. For instance, elderly patients have altered pharmacokinetics due to physiological changes, thereby increasing the risk of complications. Further, patients with chronic conditions such as diabetes or cardiovascular disease may require personalized anesthetic regimens to prevent complications. By considering these factors, anesthesiologists can customize their approach, enabling the selected agents to provide maximum efficacy while minimizing risk. Personalization requires close familiarity with the individual patient's profile, thereby guiding surgical success and recovery directly. Such customized practices are made possible by ongoing research aimed at improving anesthetic protocols centered on patient care. The use of technology, especially artificial intelligence (AI), also has a crucial contribution towards enhancing the effectiveness of anesthetic methods and monitoring. An AI's ability to handle large sets of data enables clinicians to forecast outcomes according to patient-specific characteristics, hence enabling improved real-time decision-making. The development of machine learning models that identify risk factors and suggest appropriate pharmacological interventions is a trend in precision medicine in anesthesia. Even though there are potential benefits, integrating these AI systems is not without challenges, including ethical concerns about data procurement and validation. Although the future of AI in anesthesia keeps unfolding, it is imperative that the principles of AI are embraced by practitioners so that technology doesn't replace but complements clinical intelligence. The integration of such knowledge with artificial intelligence can revolutionize anesthetic management but remains a persistent challenge due to poor adoption, which underscores the need for further studies in the area (Singh et al., 2022). Postoperative side effects, such as PONV, exemplify the critical need for global pharmacological management in anesthesia. Given the fact that PONV can occur in a high rate of patients undergoing surgery like craniotomies, it is necessary to employ multimodal prevention and treatment of this side effect. The administration of more than one drug with differing mechanisms of action can markedly reduce the incidence of PONV and increase patient satisfaction. A survey of new clinical trials demonstrated the efficacy of the combination of ondansetron and dexamethasone in this context, highlighting the importance of an active approach to symptom management. Knowledge of the multifactorial etiology of PONV will enable anesthesiologists to better individualize their interventions to address this common complication, ultimately improving patient care and the surgical experience (Uribe et al., 2019).

3.5.1. Pediatric Anesthesia

The subtleties of pediatric anesthesia present a unique challenge that demands a rigorous understanding of pharmacological principles applicable to this special group. Unlike adults, children exhibit broad pharmacologic variability in pharmacokinetics and pharmacodynamics, primarily due to variation in body composition, organ maturity, and developmental stage. All these demands careful consideration in selecting anesthetic agents because their metabolism and drug response may markedly deviate from adult standards. Thus, anesthetists must familiarize themselves with evidence-based practice and guidelines that ensure safe and effective medication administration in children. Recent advances in neuroscience and pharmacology have begun to elucidate the complexities inherent in the administration of anesthetics in children, emphasizing the need to adapt clinical practice to the changing nature of knowledge in these sciences (Sepúlveda et al., 2021). Further, susceptibility to postoperative complications such as vomiting and nausea is a matter of great concern in pediatric anesthesia. Pediatric patients are most vulnerable to postoperative nausea and vomiting (PONV), and the latter can significantly influence their course of recovery and outcomes. Prophylactic intervention is emphasized in the literature as very important for effectively preventing these unwanted reactions, and it is predicated on the patient's individual risk factors. The development of detailed guidelines meant to manage PONV, alongside recommendations for pharmacologic treatment, underscores the interface among clinical insight and robust evidence in enhancing pediatric care. By implementing multimodal approaches with newer agents, clinicians can create anesthetic protocols that reduce the incidence of PONV, thereby improving the postoperative experience for pediatric patients (Tong et al., 2020). In general, the altered dynamics in pediatric anesthesia underscore the importance of ongoing education and research in pharmacology. With an increased awareness among clinicians regarding the neurodevelopmental implications of anesthetic drugs in children, clinicians are optimally positioned to implement measures that safeguard the health of their young patients. Pivoting towards the synergy of clinical acumen and advanced scientific expertise will enable a more precise approach to pediatric anesthesia, ultimately enhancing efficacy and safety in operating rooms. The new knowledge of pharmacologic interactions and neurodevelopmental consequences requires an adaptive approach to clinical practice, so that anesthetists are always at the forefront of children's care while minimizing the harmful effects of anesthesia in the vulnerable population (Sepúlveda et al., 2021) (Figure 3.11).

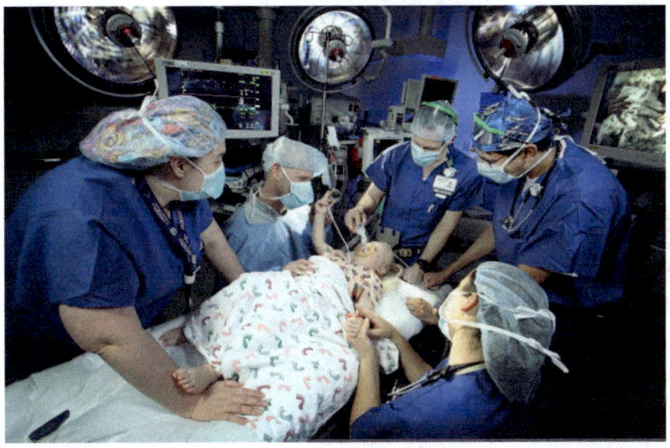

Figure 3.11. The intricacies of pediatric anesthesia pose unique challenges.

Source: https://anesthesiology.hopkinsmedicine.org/wp-content/uploads/2022/04/Pediatric-Anesthesiology-Fellowship.jpg.

3.5.2. Geriatric Anesthesia

As the population ages, anesthesia practice must advance with the unique physiological and pharmacological challenges of the aging patient. The elderly patient has altered sensitivities to anesthetics due to altered pharmacokinetic and pharmacodynamic interactions. Altered body composition, reduced hepatic and renal function, and variations in protein binding all contribute significantly to drug metabolism and action in the elderly. Specifically, the tolerance to an anesthetic is lost; hence, a conservative approach to dosage and administration is to be followed. Titration of anesthetics, i.e., adjusting their dosage to balance them, is not only essential for achieving successful surgical outcomes but also for preventing untoward effects, such as postoperative states common in the elderly, e.g., delirium and cognitive dysfunction (Reuben et al., 2024). The presence of polypharmacy in elderly patients also poses additional challenges in anesthetic management. Ager patients may be prescribed more than one medication, and this can lead to drug interactions and medication-related side effects. The anesthetic agents will interact with the co-prescribed drugs and exacerbate side effects or lessen the intended therapeutic effect. Anesthesiologists must thus conduct a comprehensive reconciliation of medicines, both prescription and nonprescription, to tailor anesthetic protocols accordingly. These are crucial not just for the patient's safety but also for optimizing the overall success of the operation and avoiding the risk of prolonged hospitalization, which is generally associated with elderly patients (Reuben et al., 2024).

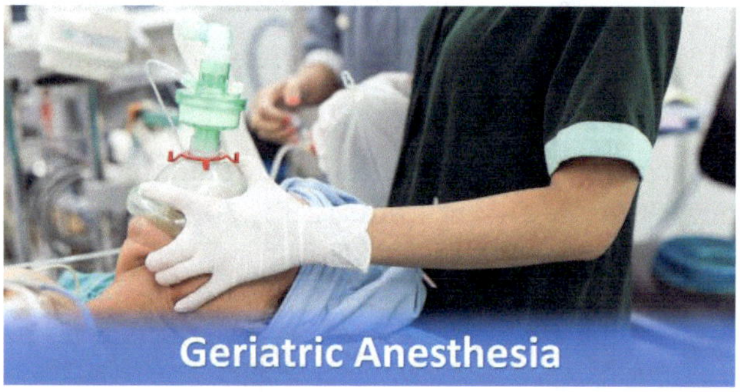

Figure 3.12. Geriatric anesthesia.

Source: https://cdn.docplexus.com/117/7/4/954083c2-1749-44e8-962a-2907042a0908_t.jpg.

The recognition and management of perioperative neurocognitive disorders (NCDs) in the elderly also contribute to the challenge of geriatric anesthesia. NCDs can present in several forms, such as preoperative delirium, delayed cognitive recovery, and postoperative NCD, which require prompt identification and management. The pathophysiology of these conditions is multifactorial and comprises predisposing and precipitating events amenable to both pharmacologic and nonpharmacologic approaches. Nonpharmacologic interventions such as geriatric assessment and cognitive prehabilitation should be the initial approach, with pharmacologic interventions such as dexmedetomidine and nonsteroidal anti-inflammatory drugs as adjunct therapy in agitated patients. If the anesthesiologist implements these practices, they can enhance care for agitated patients and minimize adverse outcomes, demonstrating the importance of individualized treatment in geriatric anesthesia (Figure 3.12).

3.5.3. Anesthesia in Patients with Comorbidities

The management of anesthesia in comorbid patients is a significant challenge that calls for a firm understanding of the pharmacology principles. Comorbid patients are typically those with underlying chronic medical conditions such as obesity, diabetes, or cardiovascular disease, not just complicating the administration of anesthesia but also influencing the choice of anesthetic drugs. Anesthesiologists should be aware of how these comorbidities will influence drug metabolism and excretion when they choose anesthetic technique and dosing. For instance, in patients with renal impairment, the elimination of some anesthetics will be slowed, indicating the need for cautious dosing. Also, special caution should be taken to avoid drug interactions that may occur as a result of the numerous drugs that patients are being administered, which may add to postoperative complications and prolonged recovery time. Innovations in anesthetic techniques have made anesthetic regimens more tailored to the needs of patients with comorbidities. Regional anesthesia, for instance, can minimize systemic effects and provide localized pain relief, and is therefore a candidate of choice for obese or respiratory-compromised patients. By focusing on a multi-modal approach, the use of adjunctive drugs that optimize analgesia and reduce opioid requirements, anesthesiologists can significantly minimize risks associated with anesthesia in such high-risk populations. Additionally, by including patient-specified factors like body mass index (BMI) and cardiac function in preoperative assessments, an individualized anesthesia protocol becomes possible. These personalized plans ultimately aim to optimize patient outcomes and prevent perioperative adverse events. Moreover, the presence of comorbidities necessitates close postoperative monitoring since such patients are at greater risk for postoperative complications like DVT and PE. There is evidence that indicates that specific populations, including patients with obesity, may carry higher risks for postoperative complications. However, real-world studies yield conflicting evidence for the impact of obesity on DVT and PE outcomes alone. Anesthesiologists and surgical services must be careful to implement pharmacologic interventions, including anticoagulation, based on each patient's individual risk profile to avoid such complications. This approach can include the use of low-molecular-weight heparins or adjustment of anticoagulant dosage based on an individual's medical history and status. Awareness of the complexities of anesthesia in patients with comorbidities will ultimately translate to improved patient safety and enhanced surgical recovery (Sloan et al., 2019; Rohan et al., 2020).

Test Your Knowledge

1. What anatomical and physiological differences in children must be considered when administering anesthesia?
2. What are the key safety considerations and challenges unique to pediatric anesthesia practice?

3.6. Advances in Anesthetic Pharmacology

Learning Outcome

1. Development of new anesthetic agents
2. Role of technology in anesthesia
3. Future trends in anesthetic pharmacology

Advances in anesthetic pharmacology over the past several years have significantly enhanced clinical outcomes and patient safety during perioperative care. The quest for better and more secure anesthetic agents has influenced research into natural products, a process that has previously yielded a rich supply of medicinal leads. By leveraging the diversity of global biodiversity, researchers are identifying new anesthetic agents of plant origin that, in addition to pain relief, have fewer side effects than traditional synthetic agents. Recent progress in high-throughput screening has accelerated this process by enabling rapid identification of bioactive molecules that can be chemically modified for use as anesthetics. Besides, such advancement demands inter-disciplinary research to optimize the novel therapeutic prospects of natural compounds, towards more targeted anesthetic modalities across various surgical environments (Chaachouay et al., 2024). The mechanisms of pain have become clearer to provide novel anesthetic options addressing dental and orofacial pain in itself, being common patient complaints. Modern advances have led to the use of novel pharmacological modalities, including local anesthetics, non-steroidal anti-inflammatory agents, and muscle relaxants, that provide widespread pain control in dental practice. The ongoing evolution of these pharmacologic agents has led to more effective preparations, such as liposome-encapsulated local anesthetics, which release the anesthetic drug over a prolonged period. This new approach, in addition to minimizing patient discomfort, also aims to decrease systemic side effects, thus leading to greater overall satisfaction with dental care. The ongoing development of the specialty will ensure greater understanding of the biochemical mechanisms that produce pain and will further tailor anesthetic interventions to deliver more accurate and effective dental pain control protocols to dentists (Pahade et al., 2023). Emergent technologies in anesthetic delivery systems reflect the convergence of pharmacology and innovation in anesthesia. New techniques, such as microneedles and site-specific drug delivery systems, are being developed to optimize the effectiveness of anesthetic agents and to make administration methods easier. These advances not only enhance the comfort of the delivery process for the patient but also improve the pharmacokinetics of anesthetic drugs, enabling precise delivery and longer action duration. Furthermore, advances in monitoring technology enable anesthesiologists to customize drug delivery based on real-time feedback, thereby allowing more individualized administration of anesthesia. As these technologies continue to advance, they also hold promise for revolutionizing anesthetic practice, with the end goal of optimizing anesthesia safety and effectiveness across various surgical specialties (Chaachouay et al., 2024) (Figure 3.13).

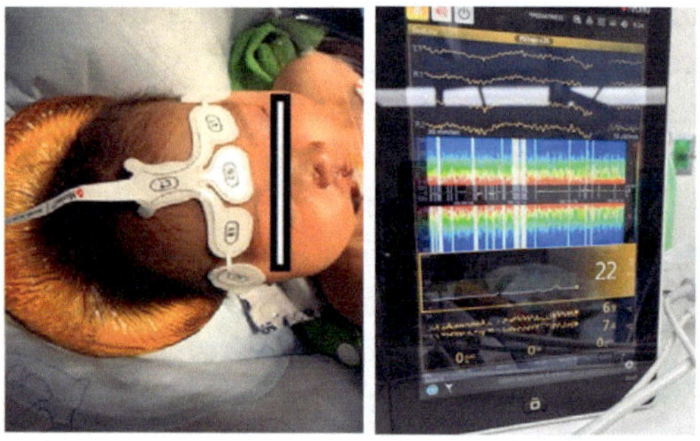

Figure 3.13. Recent developments in anesthetic pharmacology.

Source: https://www.mdpi.com/jcm/jcm-10-02175/article_deploy/html/images/jcm-10-02175-g002.png.

3.6.1. Development of New Anesthetic Agents

The search for new anesthetic medications is driven by demands for increased safety, efficacy, and patient comfort during surgery. The history of inhalation anesthetics has, over time, developed a trend for the use of fluorinated agents, beginning with halothane. The medication revealed significant disadvantages, such as hepatotoxicity, prompting the development of newer medications like enflurane, isoflurane, desflurane, and sevoflurane. With each successive generation of inhalation anesthetics, there was incremental improvement, with attention to removing solubility issues, enhancing the onset time, and altering recovery profiles. Despite their progress, existing agents remain far from perfect, underscoring a strong need for anesthetics with broader safety margins and improved patient outcomes. The identification of ideal inhalation anesthetics remains a multifaceted issue, with structure-activity relationships that need to be clarified to guide the synthesis of candidate compounds that overcome the current deficits of available ones (Wang et al., 2019). Intravenous anesthetics have also progressed significantly, most significantly, ketamine, which was originally synthesized as a fast-acting anesthetic. Its unique pharmacological profile makes it distinct from traditional agents, mainly due to its effects on NMDA receptors, offering both anesthesia and analgesia with fewer effects on respiration. More recent research has extended ketamine's application from perioperative care to chronic pain therapy, as well as, most intriguingly, the treatment of depression. This transformation is driven by a growing awareness of the multiple functions of ketamine in pharmacotherapy, highlighting how it can revolutionize treatment paradigms across various branches of medicine. Through ongoing research into the mechanisms of action and effectiveness of ketamine, anesthesiology can identify new paths and applications for existing compounds and provide evidence for the need to revisit and reassess earlier agents based on current clinical needs (Nader, 2017). Despite the clinical advances in today's anesthetic agents, issues persist in identifying new drugs with optimized pharmacological profiles. Synthesis of fluorinated halocarbons and other novel compounds in the search for better anesthetics has yielded compounds that demonstrate anesthetic potency but have issues with efficacy and safety. The volatility of anesthetic potency with respect to the molecular structure complicates the design process, necessitating detailed experimental evaluations. In addition, the regulatory context for drug approval entails yet another facet of sophistication, typically requiring substantial evidence of safety and efficacy before introducing new anesthetics into practice. With the advancements the field is experiencing, it is still important that scientists embrace their understanding of both pharmacokinetics and pharmacodynamics to enable the development of the next generation of anesthetic drugs and to improve the quality of anesthesia care (Wang et al., 2019) (Figure 3.14).

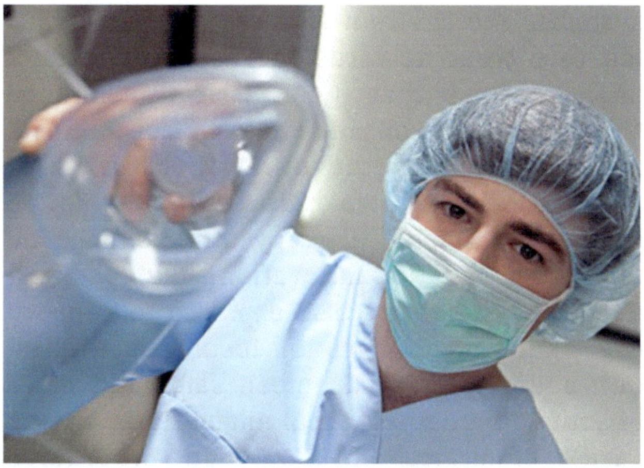

Figure 3.14. Development of new anesthetic agents.

Source: https://www-tc.pbs.org/prod-media/newshour/photos/2013/10/16/154769208_blog_main_horizontal.jpg.

3.6.2. Role of Technology in Anesthesia

The use of technology in anesthesia has been revolutionized with the advent of sophisticated monitoring systems and computer technology. These technologies have improved patient safety and optimized anesthetic outcomes through continuous online monitoring of critical physiological parameters such as heart rate, blood pressure, and oxygen saturation. Automated monitoring equipment can detect a departure from the normal range and provide the anesthesiologist with a timely warning to intervene. In addition, the application of technology in anesthetic delivery has made processes more efficient, eliminating the risk of human error in drug administration. The more complex the surgical procedures, the greater the reliance on such technologies, not just freeing practitioners from drudgery but also ensuring that patient care is prioritized and precision is the rule. Artificial intelligence (AI) is at the forefront of anesthetic technology, transforming how anesthesiologists manage drug delivery and patient monitoring. In particular, machine learning algorithms have the ability to process vast volumes of data and produce predictive models that improve decision-making in anesthesia management. For example, AI systems can detect patterns in individual patients' responses to anesthesia drugs, enabling personalized dosage recommendations that maximize efficacy while reducing adverse effects. These innovations reverse the trend from reactive to proactive anesthesia care, allowing practitioners to anticipate and be ready for potential complications without exception. Furthermore, the integration of tele-anesthesia through remote monitoring technologies erases the logistic challenges of the operating room, so that anesthesiologists can see information anywhere, enhancing outcomes of surgery as well as patient safety (Cascella et al., 2023). Furthermore, the intersection of technology and pharmacology in anesthesia holds considerable potential for advances in clinical practice. Electronic equipment that facilitates the capture and processing of electronic health records helps construct customized anesthetic protocols based on real-world evidence. This evidence-based strategy enables clinicians to consider intrinsic and extrinsic factors that affect drug interactions and pharmacokinetics across patient populations. By using digital biomarkers gathered from wearables, anesthesiologists can track the impact of medications on a patient's health in real time and adjust treatment during procedures as needed. While these developments carry the potential to move forward clinical outcomes, they also raise critical ethical considerations toward data privacy, informed consent, and the inherent bias surrounding algorithmic-driven decision-making, and therefore call for ongoing discourse on governance and patient rights on AI usage in anesthesia (Johnson et al., 2023) (Figure 3.15).

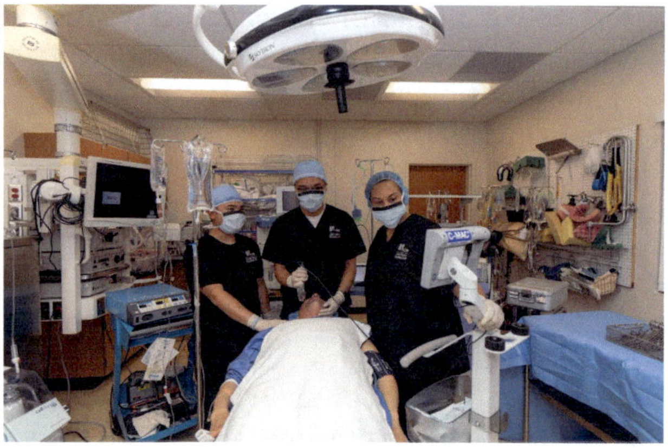

Figure 3.15. The role of technology in anesthesia has undergone significant transformation.

Source: https://skylinecollege.edu/anesthesiatech/images/scene-3.jpg.

3.6.3. Future Trends in Anesthetic Pharmacology

With further advances in anesthetic pharmacology, new techniques are being developed that promise to enhance the safety and efficacy of anesthesia. Among these advancements, low-intensity ultrasound (US) is a revolutionary technique. Ultrasonic neuromodulation has been introduced as a non-invasive, pharmacologically sound method of modulating neural activity. This method capitalizes on mechanical interactions at a cellular scale, and its promise lies in providing clinicians another option for targeted nerve stimulation under anesthesia. The improved spatial localization and depth targeting are specific strengths compared to other existing modalities. With ongoing research validating its safety and effectiveness, US neurostimulation will be able to complement traditional methods of anesthesia in the near future, with better pain control and optimized patient outcomes, thereby revolutionizing the practice of anesthesiology in the future to a great extent (Blackmore et al., 2019). Furthermore, enhancing the drug-like pharmacological properties of local anesthetics is a vital area of study to overcome existing limitations. New local anesthetics are overshadowed by drawbacks, including a short duration of action and dose-dependent side effects on the cardiac and central nervous systems. The reaction to these drawbacks has led to a trend towards the use of adjuvants and additives that synergistically enhance the effects of local anesthetics. The adjuncts not only prolong the duration of sensory-motor block but also reduce the cumulative dose requirements, thereby diminishing side effects. Formulation innovations like liposomal delivery systems are also explored to improve the pharmacokinetics of local anesthetics. Consequently, this can mean safer and more effective regimens of local analgesia in a wide variety of surgical and therapeutic procedures (Swain et al., 2017). Moreover, the direction of future anesthetic pharmacology is increasingly focused on personalized medicine through the application of pharmacogenomics. Knowledge of the genetic determinants of individual variation in response to anesthetic drugs will allow for drug choice and dosing to be tailored to the patient's individual profile. This strategy is intended to maximize efficacy and safety by reducing adverse effects and maximizing anesthesia management. As the genetic basis of drug metabolism and sensitivity comes to be better understood, clinicians will be able to make more rational decisions based on the individual patient's profile. The integration of artificial intelligence and machine learning with pharmacological models will also play an essential role in predicting patient responses and thus matching treatment regimens better to individual needs. In general, personalized anesthetic pharmacology can change patient care and outcomes in anesthesia.

Test Your Knowledge

1. What recent developments in anesthetic drugs have improved their safety, efficacy, and recovery profiles?
2. How have novel anesthetic agents and formulations influenced the management of high-risk patients and complex surgeries?

SUMMARY

The pharmacologic contribution to anesthesia is more than the mere dispensing of anesthetic drugs but rather the overall concept of drug interaction, efficacy, and safety profile. Anesthetics are critical to ensuring patient comfort during surgical procedures, with the prerequisite of a proper balance between sedation and responsiveness. As can be seen from the statistics, up to 50% of ready anesthetic medicine is wasted, amounting to massive wastage that not only translates to unnecessary costs but also affects environmental sustainability. Mitigating such wastage is at the core of ethical medical practice, where the maximization of resource use is the principle. Increasing drug-use efficiency can yield major economic savings for the system while promoting a healthier health system, eventually translating into improved outcomes for patients and health systems (Barbariol et al., 2021). Also, the implications of pharmacology for anesthetic practice are further underscored by new discoveries that improve drug formulations and administration methods. The introduction of new agents, such as direct oral anticoagulants, has changed the landscape of perioperative care, particularly in patients at risk for thromboembolic complications. It is crucial to balance the benefits of these new treatments with the risks, primarily of bleeding complications in at-risk patient groups. The ongoing assessment of clinical practice not only focuses attention on the necessity of tailored pharmacologic treatment but also on continuing education and physician updates. By incorporating recent research into clinical guidelines, the profession of anesthesiology can enhance practices, reducing risks as well as streamline pharmacologic management of patients under anesthesia (Nigel et al., 2019). Finally, the climax of this review calls for a renewed devotion to the principles of pharmacology as a driving force towards better anesthetic outcomes. As anesthesia practice evolves over time, so do drug management and elimination strategies. Faced with drug wastage, as research has found, requires an integrated approach that ensures coordination among anesthesiologists, pharmacists, and medical administrators to devise efficient workflows. Besides, educating patients about medication safety and the associated risks of anesthesia is paramount for informed consent and overall therapeutic efficacy. The quest for excellence in pharmacology within the scope of anesthesia will ensure sustainable practicewith ensuring , while ensuring the highest standards of patient care and safety, heralding future growth in this important area. Anesthesia, being a component of medical and surgical practice, relies heavily on pharmacology to render the patient comfortable and safe. An understanding of how anesthetic agents interact with the central nervous system is crucial for optimizing their use. Cerebral blood flow, for example, must be tightly regulated during anesthetic hours to be able to supply adequately to the brain's metabolic demand. This regulation entails a precise balance between oxygen and nutrient supply and the efficient removal of waste products, underscoring the intrinsic relationship between pharmacology and physiological response (Claassen et al., 2021). As anesthetic agents influence cerebral flow and neurologic function, pharmacological characteristics regulate anesthesia outcomes, impacting both efficacy and safety of patient care during surgery. Moreover, newer editions of classic books in the anesthesiology branch, such as The Basics of Anesthesia, cover significant advances in the subject and identify pharmacological knowledge needs for anesthesiologists to adopt contemporary practice. The seventh edition provides a concise yet comprehensive overview of current anesthetic practice, demonstrating the evolving landscape of anesthesiology. It addresses areas such as anesthetic neurotoxicity and opioid epidemic, emphasizing the importance of learning about pharmacology in emerging complications of clinical practice (Gonzalez et al., 2018). These resources serve not only as study materials but also as a bridge between pharmacologic theory and its application, equipping practitioners to address contemporary challenges in patient care. Furthermore, the evolution of anesthetic practice is reflected in the growing body of pharmacology literature, which recognizes patient heterogeneity in response to anesthetic agents. Advanced age and obesity affect the patient's metabolism of anesthetics and mandate unique strategies for anesthesia management (Gonzalez et al., 2018). Greater controversy in revised material offers clinical correlations better assimilated by the reader into understanding pharmacology's role in anesthesiology. Thus, these books are critical in providing a glimpse into the best practices in the safe delivery of anesthesia and emphasizing the anesthesiologist's critical role as a perioperative physician and a perioperative care leader that ensures outstanding outcomes for diverse groups of patient populations.

KEY TERMS FROM THIS CHAPTER

- Biological systems
- Central nervous system
- Enhanced recovery after surgery (ERAS)
- Neural network
- Nonsteroidal anti-inflammatory drugs (NSAIDs)
- Pediatric patients
- Pharmacokinetics
- Technological innovation
- Cardiovascular
- Chronic pain
- Gamma-aminobutyric acid
- Neurotransmission
- Optimize anesthesia practice
- Pediatric population
- Pharmacological efficacy
- Venous thromboembolism (VTE)

CRITICAL THINKING QUESTIONS

1. **Which of the following is a commonly used inhalational anesthetic?**
   a. Propofol
   b. Isoflurane
   c. Ketamine
   d. Fentanyl
2. **Which intravenous agent is known for its rapid onset and short duration of action?**
   a. Midazolam
   b. Etomidate
   c. Propofol
   d. Thiopental
3. **Which opioid is most commonly used in anesthesia for pain management?**
   a. Morphine
   b. Fentanyl
   c. Codeine
   d. Tramadol
4. **What is the primary mechanism of action of local anesthetics?**
   a. Inhibition of GABA receptors
   b. Blockage of sodium channels
   c. Activation of potassium channels
   d. Inhibition of acetylcholine release
5. **Which of the following drugs is used as a neuromuscular blocking agent?**
   a. Succinylcholine
   b. Sevoflurane
   c. Lidocaine
   d. Propofol

Short Answer Questions

1. Describe the pharmacokinetics and pharmacodynamics of inhalational anesthetic agents.
2. Explain the mechanism of action and clinical use of intravenous anesthetics.
3. What are muscle relaxants, and how are they classified? Discuss their role in anesthesia.
4. Discuss the pharmacological management of postoperative nausea and vomiting (PONV).
5. What is the importance of premedication in anesthesia?
6. How are hypotension and hypertension managed pharmacologically during anesthesia?

Answer to Critical Thinking Questions

1. (b); 2. (c); 3. (b); 4. (b); 5. (a)

REFERENCES

1. Absalom, A. R., De Keyser, R., & Struys, M. M. R. F. (2011). Closed loop anesthesia. *Anesthesia & Analgesia, 112*(3), 516–518. https://doi.org/10.1213/ane.0b013e318203f5adAdamek, D., Akin, A., Al-Zaben, A., Alm, J., Amminnikutty, M., Amoli, K., Anderson, R., et al. (2018). Postoperative pain management in children: Guidance from the pain committee of the European Society for Pediatric Anesthesiology (ESPA Pain Management Ladder Initiative). https://core.ac.uk/download/157582937.pdf (accessed on 28th June 2025).
2. Aebi, M., Shah, A. G., Anderson, K., Arlt, F., Barr, D., Barthelemy, J., Beiderlinden, M., et al. (2017). Medication complications in extracorporeal membrane oxygenation. https://core.ac.uk/download/129191716.pdf (accessed on 28th June 2025).
3. Afify, E. E. S., Mohamed, S., & Khedr, M. B. (2023). Ketamine: Recent evidence and current uses. *Benha Journal of Applied Sciences, 8*, 111–117. https://doi.org/10.21608/bjas.2023.208756.1165 (accessed on 28th June 2025).
4. Anderson II, J., Azi, C. I., Carsrud, N. D. V., Chawla, A., et al. (2024). Exploring the potential of stem cell therapy and non-opioid anesthesia and pain reduction: Reducing the negative impact on the individual and society. https://core.ac.uk/download/621451718.pdf (accessed on 28th June 2025).
5. Bajwa, S. J. S., & Kaur, J. (2013). Clinical profile of levobupivacaine in regional anesthesia: A systematic review. *Journal of Anesthesiology Clinical Pharmacology, 29*, 530–530. https://doi.org/10.4103/0970-9185.119172 (accessed on 28th June 2025).
6. Barbariol, F., Deana, C., Lucchese, F., Cataldi, G., Bassi, F., Bove, T., Vetrugno, L., et al. (2021). Evaluation of drug wastage in the operating rooms and intensive care units of a regional health service. *Anesthesia & Analgesia*. https://doi.org/10.1213/ane.0000000000005457 (accessed on 28th June 2025).
7. Barrington, M. J., & Uda, Y. (2018). Did ultrasound fulfill the promise of safety in regional anesthesia? *Current Opinion in Anesthesiology, 31*, 649–655. https://doi.org/10.1097/aco.0000000000000638 (accessed on 28th June 2025).
8. Berry, S. H. (2015). *Injectable Anesthetics*. https://doi.org/10.1002/9781119421375.ch15 (accessed on 28th June 2025).
9. Bertoncello, F., Carron, M., & Ieppariello, G. (2017). Profile of sugammadex for reversal of neuromuscular blockade in the elderly: Current perspectives. https://core.ac.uk/download/158825140.pdf (accessed on 28th June 2025).
10. Blackmore, J., Shrivastava, S. K., Sallet, J., Butler, C., & Cleveland, R. O. (2019). Ultrasound neuromodulation: A review of results, mechanisms and safety. *Ultrasound in Medicine & Biology, 45*, 1509–1536. https://doi.org/10.1016/j.ultrasmedbio.2018.12.015 (accessed on 28th June 2025).
11. Brosnan, R. J., & Pham, T. L. (2014). Hydrocarbon molar water solubility predicts NMDA vs. GABAA receptor modulation. https://core.ac.uk/download/323068772.pdf (accessed on 28th June 2025).
12. Calkins, H., Hindricks, G., Cappato, R., Kim, Y. H., Saad, E., Aguinaga, L., Akar, J. G., et al. (2017). 2017 HRS/EHRA/ECAS/APHRS/SOLAECE expert consensus statement on catheter and surgical ablation of atrial fibrillation: Executive summary. *Journal of Arrhythmia, 33*, 369–409. https://doi.org/10.1016/j.joa.2017.08.001 (accessed on 28th June 2025).

13. Calvieri, S., Cantisani, C., D'Andrea, V., Frascani, F., et al. (2014). New patents on topical anesthetics. https://core.ac.uk/download/54511696.pdf (accessed on 28th June 2025).

14. Carron, M., Bertoncello, F., & Ieppariello, G. (2017). Profile of sugammadex for reversal of neuromuscular blockade in the elderly: Current perspectives. *Clinical Interventions in Aging, 13*, 13–24. https://doi.org/10.2147/cia.s134108 (accessed on 28th June 2025).

15. Casali, A. G., Gosseries, O., Rosanova, M., Boly, M., Sarasso, S., Casali, K. R., Casarotto, S., et al. (2013). A theoretically based index of consciousness independent of sensory processing and behavior. *Science Translational Medicine, 5*. https://doi.org/10.1126/scitranslmed.3006294 (accessed on 28th June 2025).

16. Cascella, M., Tracey, M., Petrucci, E., & Bignami, E. (2023). Exploring artificial intelligence in anesthesia: A primer on ethics, and clinical applications. *Surgeries, 4*, 264–274. https://doi.org/10.3390/surgeries4020027 (accessed on 28th June 2025).

17. Castelli, M. P. (2008). Multi-faceted aspects of gamma-hydroxybutyric acid: A neurotransmitter, therapeutic agent and drug of abuse. *Mini-Reviews in Medicinal Chemistry, 8*, 1188–1202. https://doi.org/10.2174/138955708786141025 (accessed on 28th June 2025).

18. Chaachouay, N., & Zidane, L. (2024). Plant-derived natural products: A source for drug discovery and development. *Drugs and Drug Candidates, 3*, 184–207. https://doi.org/10.3390/ddc3010011 (accessed on 28th June 2025).

19. Chen, C., Gao, G., Xu, Y., Pu, L., Wang, Q., Wang, L., Wang, W., et al. (2020). SARS-CoV-2–positive sputum and feces after conversion of pharyngeal samples in patients with COVID-19. *Annals of Internal Medicine, 172*, 832–834. https://doi.org/10.7326/m20-0991 (accessed on 28th June 2025).

20. Chen, L., Hankin, J., Ma, D., Xuan, W., et al. (2016). Local anesthetic bupivacaine induced ovarian and prostate cancer apoptotic cell death and underlying mechanisms *in vitro*. https://core.ac.uk/download/77011206.doc (accessed on 28th June 2025).

21. Claassen, J. A. H. R., Thijssen, D. H. J., Panerai, R. B., & Faraci, F. M. (2021). Regulation of cerebral blood flow in humans: Physiology and clinical implications of autoregulation. *Physiological Reviews, 101*, 1487–1559. https://doi.org/10.1152/physrev.00022.2020 (accessed on 28th June 2025).

22. D'Souza, R., & Hsu, G. (2024). *Pharmacology in Geriatric Anesthesia*. BENTHAM SCIENCE PUBLISHERS eBooks. https://doi.org/10.2174/9789815238877124010005 (accessed on 28th June 2025).

23. D'Souza, R., Ashraf, R., Rowe, H., Zipursky, J. S., Clarfield, L., Maxwell, C., Arzola, C., et al. (2020). Pregnancy and COVID-19: Pharmacologic considerations. *Ultrasound in Obstetrics and Gynecology, 57*, 195–203. https://doi.org/10.1002/uog.23116 (accessed on 28th June 2025).

24. Dontukurthy, S., & Tobias, J. D. (2021). Update on local anesthetic toxicity, prevention and treatment during regional anesthesia in infants and children. *The Journal of Pediatric Pharmacology and Therapeutics, 26*, 445–454. https://doi.org/10.5863/1551-6776-26.5.445 (accessed on 28th June 2025).

25. Dowell, D., Haegerich, T. M., & Chou, R. (2016). CDC guideline for prescribing opioids for chronic pain–United States, 2016. *MMWR Recommendations and Reports, 65*, 1–49. https://doi.org/10.15585/mmwr.rr6501e1 (accessed on 28th June 2025).

26. Egan, T. D., & Svensén, C. (2018). Multimodal general anesthesia: A principled approach to producing the drug-induced, reversible coma of anesthesia. *Anesthesia & Analgesia, 127*, 1104–1106. https://doi.org/10.1213/ane.0000000000003743 (accessed on 28th June 2025).

27. Firoozabadi, R., El-Haddad, M. E., Drever, S., Soltani, M., Githens, M., Kleweno, C. P., Sharar, S. R., et al. (2020). Case report: Virtual reality analgesia in an opioid sparing orthopedic outpatient clinic setting: A case study. *Frontiers in Virtual Reality, 1*. https://doi.org/10.3389/frvir.2020.553492 (accessed on 28th June 2025).

28. Gan, T. J., Belani, K. G., Bergese, S. D., Chung, F., Diemunsch, P., Habib, A. S., Jin, Z., et al. (2020). Fourth consensus guidelines for the management of postoperative nausea and vomiting. *Anesthesia & Analgesia, 131*, 411–448. https://doi.org/10.1213/ane.0000000000004833 (accessed on 28th June 2025).

29. Gonzalez, A., & Kimatian, S. J. (2018). The basics of anesthesia, 7th edition. *Anesthesiology, 129*, 1194–1195. https://doi.org/10.1097/aln.0000000000002432 (accessed on 28th June 2025).

30. Hemmerling, T. M., & Jeffries, S. D. (2024). Robotic anesthesia: A vision for 2050. *Anesthesia & Analgesia, 138*, 239–251. https://doi.org/10.1213/ane.0000000000006835 (accessed on 28th June 2025).

31. Iorio-Morin, C., Hodaie, M., Sarica, C., Dea, N., Westwick, H. J., Christie, S., McDonald, P. J., et al. (2020). Letter: The risk of COVID-19 infection during neurosurgical procedures: A review of Severe Acute Respiratory Distress Syndrome Coronavirus 2 (SARS-CoV-2) modes of transmission and proposed neurosurgery-specific measures for mitigation. *Neurosurgery, 87*, E178–E185. https://doi.org/10.1093/neuros/nyaa157 (accessed on 28th June 2025).

32. Johnson, M., Patel, M., Phipps, A., van der Schaar, M., Boulton, D., & Gibbs, M. (2023). The potential and pitfalls of artificial intelligence in clinical pharmacology. *CPT Pharmacometrics & Systems Pharmacology, 12*, 279–284. https://doi.org/10.1002/psp4.12902 (accessed on 28th June 2025).

33. Key, N. S., Khorana, A. A., Kuderer, N. M., Bohlke, K., Lee, A. Y. Y., Arcelus, J. I., Wong, S. L., et al. (2019). Venous thromboembolism prophylaxis and treatment in patients with cancer: ASCO clinical practice guideline update. *Journal of Clinical Oncology, 38*, 496–520. https://doi.org/10.1200/jco.19.01461 (accessed on 28th June 2025).

34. Kong, H., Xu, L. M., & Wang, D. X. (2022). Perioperative neurocognitive disorders: A narrative review focusing on diagnosis, prevention, and treatment. *CNS Neuroscience & Therapeutics, 28*, 1147–1167. https://doi.org/10.1111/cns.13873 (accessed on 28th June 2025).

35. Ley, E. J., Brown, C. V. R., Moore, E. E., Sava, J., Peck, K. A., Ciesla, D. J., Sperry, J. L., et al. (2020). Updated guidelines to reduce venous thromboembolism in trauma patients: A Western Trauma Association critical decisions algorithm. *Journal of Trauma and Acute Care Surgery, 89*, 971–981. https://doi.org/10.1097/ta.0000000000002830 (accessed on 28th June 2025).

36. Li, G., Chiara, D. C., Cohen, J. B., & Olsen, R. W. (2010). Numerous classes of general anesthetics inhibit etomidate binding to γ-aminobutyric acid type A (GABAA) receptors. *Journal of Biological Chemistry, 285*, 8615–8620. https://doi.org/10.1074/jbc.m109.074708 (accessed on 28th June 2025).

37. Li, L., & Vlisides, P. E. (2016). Ketamine: 50 years of modulating the mind. *Frontiers in Human Neuroscience, 10*. https://doi.org/10.3389/fnhum.2016.00612 (accessed on 28th June 2025).

38. Nader, N. D. (2017). Ketamine: An update on cellular and subcellular mechanisms with implications for clinical practice. *Pain Physician, 2*, E285–E301. https://doi.org/10.36076/ppj.2017.e301 (accessed on 28th June 2025).

39. Pahade, A., Bajaj, P., Shirbhate, U., & John, H. (2023). Recent modalities in pain control and local anesthesia in dentistry: A narrative review. *Cureus*. https://doi.org/10.7759/cureus.48428 (accessed on 28th June 2025).

40. Perouansky, M., Hemmings, H. C., & Riou, B. (2009). Neurotoxicity of general anesthetics. *Anesthesiology, 111*, 1365–1371. https://doi.org/10.1097/aln.0b013e3181bf1d61 (accessed on 28th June 2025).

41. Prabakti, Y., Siahaan, E. M. P., Sidhartani, M., et al. (2005). Cardiac arrest in a child during a combined general epidural anesthesia procedure. https://core.ac.uk/download/11702556.pdf (accessed on 28th June 2025).

42. Rosen, R., Vandenplas, Y., Singendonk, M., Cabana, M. D., DiLorenzo, C., Gottrand, F., Gupta, S. K., et al. (2018). Pediatric gastroesophageal reflux clinical practice guidelines. *Journal of Pediatric Gastroenterology and Nutrition, 66*, 516–554. https://doi.org/10.1097/mpg.0000000000001889 (accessed on 28th June 2025).

43. Sepúlveda, P., Epulef, V., & Campos, G. (2021). Why do we use the concepts of adult anesthesia pharmacology in developing brains? Will it have an impact on outcomes? Challenges in neuromonitoring and pharmacology in pediatric anesthesia. *Journal of Clinical Medicine, 10*, 2175–2175. https://doi.org/10.3390/jcm10102175 (accessed on 28th June 2025).

44. Singh, M., & Nath, G. (2022). Artificial intelligence and anesthesia: A narrative review. *Saudi Journal of Anesthesia, 16*, 86–93. https://doi.org/10.4103/sja.sja_669_21 (accessed on 28th June 2025).

45. Sloan, M., Sheth, N. P., & Lee, G. C. (2019). Is obesity associated with increased risk of deep vein thrombosis or pulmonary embolism after hip and knee arthroplasty? A large database study. *Clinical Orthopedics and Related Research, 477*, 523–532. https://doi.org/10.1097/corr.0000000000000615 (accessed on 28th June 2025).

46. Stout, K., Daniels, C. J., Aboulhosn, J., Bozkurt, B., Broberg, C. S., Colman, J. M., Crumb, S. R., et al. (2018). 2018 AHA/ACC guideline for the management of adults with congenital heart disease: A report of the American College of Cardiology/American Heart Association Task Force on Clinical Practice Guidelines. *Circulation, 139*. https://doi.org/10.1161/cir.0000000000000603 (accessed on 28th June 2025).

47. Swain, A., Nag, D. S., Sahu, S., & Samaddar, D. P. (2017). Adjuvants to local anesthetics: Current understanding and future trends. *World Journal of Clinical Cases, 5*, 307–307. https://doi.org/10.12998/wjcc.v5.i8.307 (accessed on 28th June 2025).

48. Tesoro, S., Marchesini, V., Fratini, G., Engelhardt, T., & De Robertis, E. (2020). Drugs for anesthesia and analgesia in the preterm infant. *Minerva Anesthesiologic, 86*. https://doi.org/10.23736/s0375-9393.20.14073-2 (accessed on 28th June 2025).

49. Uribe, A., Stoicea, N., Echeverria-Villalobos, M., Todeschini, A. B., Gutierrez, A. E., Folea, A. R., & Bergese, S. D. (2019). Postoperative nausea and vomiting after craniotomy: An evidence-based review of general considerations, risk factors, and management. *Journal of Neurosurgical Anesthesiology, 33*, 212–220. https://doi.org/10.1097/ana.0000000000000667 (accessed on 28th June 2025).

50. Voss, L. J., García, P. S., Hentschke, H., & Banks, M. I. (2019). Understanding the effects of general anesthetics on cortical network activity using *ex vivo* preparations. *Anesthesiology, 130*, 1049–1063. https://doi.org/10.1097/aln.0000000000002554 (accessed on 28th June 2025).

51. Wang, Y. Z., Ming, X. X., & Zhang, C. P. (2019). Fluorine-containing inhalation anesthetics: Chemistry, properties and pharmacology. *Current Medicinal Chemistry, 27*, 5599–5652. https://doi.org/10.2174/0929867326666191003155703 (accessed on 28th June 2025).

52. Zanos, P., Moaddel, R., Morris, P. J., Riggs, L. M., Highland, J. N., Georgiou, P., Pereira, E. F. R., et al. (2018). Ketamine and ketamine metabolite pharmacology: Insights into therapeutic mechanisms. *Pharmacological Reviews, 70*, 621–660. https://doi.org/10.1124/pr.117.015198 (accessed on 28th June 2025).

53. Zhang, H., Li, H., Zhao, S., & Bao, F. (2024). Remimazolam in general anesthesia: A comprehensive review of its applications and clinical efficacy. *Drug Design Development and Therapy, 18*, 3487–3498. https://doi.org/10.2147/dddt.s474854 (accessed on 28th June 2025).

54. Zhang, X., Zhang, N., Liu, D., Ding, J., Zhang, Y., & Zhu, Z. Q. (2022). Research advances in the clinical application of esketamine. *Ibrain, 8*, 55–67. https://doi.org/10.1002/ibra.12019 (accessed on 28th June 2025).

55. Zoroufchi, B. H., Abdollahpour, A., & Saffarieh, E. (2020). A review on the recent application of ketamine in management of anesthesia, pain, and health care. *Journal of Family Medicine and Primary Care, 9*, 1317–1317. https://doi.org/10.4103/jfmpc.jfmpc_875_19 (accessed on 28th June 2025).

PREOPERATIVE ASSESSMENT AND OPTIMIZATION

4

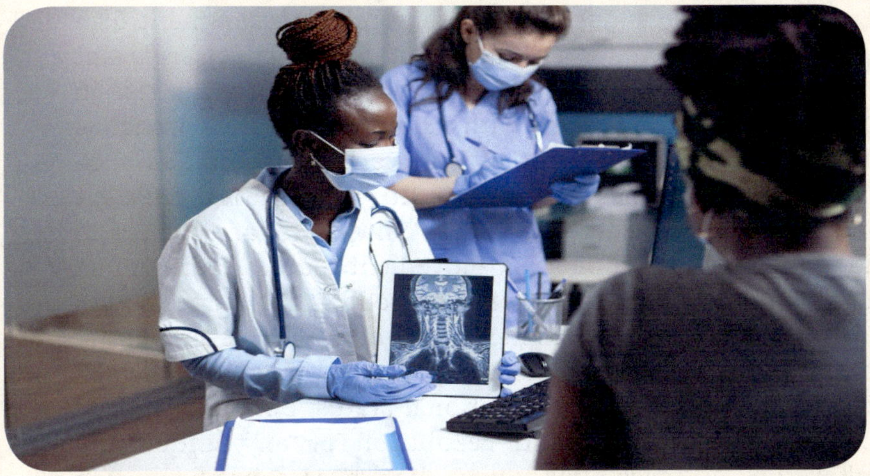

LEARNING OBJECTIVES

After studying this chapter, you will be able to:

1. Discuss the objectives of preoperative assessment
2. Explain the components of preoperative assessment
3. Focus on risk stratification
4. Know optimization strategies
5. Discuss the role of multidisciplinary teams
6. Know challenges in preoperative assessment

Introduction

The importance of preoperative optimization and evaluation cannot be overstated in surgical procedures, as these operations profoundly influence patient outcomes. In recent years, there has been an emphasis on enhanced recovery after surgery (ERAS) protocols, which aim to minimize the surgical stress response and expedite recovery through multidisciplinary interventions. Preoperative optimization is the foundation of such protocols, as it enables the identification and modulation of patient-specific risk factors before entering the operating room. Through a systematic evaluation of physiological, nutritional, and psychological health, providers can tailor anesthetic and surgical strategies to maximize postoperative recovery and reduce complications. Current evidence supports the benefits of implementing systematic preoperative optimization protocols. In a 2019 prospective analysis, the addition of aggressive preoperative rehabilitation and medical optimization programs significantly improved the outcomes associated with radical cystectomy. For instance, patients with bladder cancer who presented to surgery and participated in enhanced prehabilitation programs achieved better preoperative laboratory tests, with indicators of health measures improvement such as nutrition and physical strength. This proactive management of the patient detects not only anemia and malnutrition but also facilitates early interventions, such as iron supplementation and glucose control, designed to improve operative outcomes and reduce hospital stay. The immediate clinical ramifications of these observations form the basis of enhanced recovery after surgery (ERAS) pathway design in surgical practice. Furthermore, the relationship between preoperative optimization and postoperative morbidity underscores the importance of assessing patients' readiness for surgery. While certain variables, such as malnutrition and elevated blood glucose, were found among the cohort of interest, physical strength and muscle mass measures emerged as predictors of postoperative complications. Understanding this relationship enables practitioners to guide preoperative practice towards maximizing physical preparedness in patients. Exploration of these factors is thus essential to paradigms informing surgical practice and underscores the need for successful preoperative assessment within ERAS protocols, ultimately contributing to better patient outcomes and experiences across the surgery continuum (Jalanko et al., 2025).

Definition of Preoperative Assessment

Preoperative assessment is a fundamental instrument in optimizing patient safety and enhancing surgical outcomes. It is a systematic evaluation performed to surgery, the aim of which is to identify hidden dangers and design an individualized strategy to control them. It involves taking the medical history, performing an examination, and conducting investigations, which collectively inform the operating team about the patient's overall condition and specific comorbidities. The occurrence of adverse cardiac events highlights the importance of preoperative evaluation, and the estimates have been as high as 1.4% to 3.9% in the perioperative period for patients undergoing surgery. Having a comprehensive preoperative evaluation enables healthcare providers to identify patients at higher risk, making it easier to intervene appropriately to prevent complications and enhance perioperative care in general (Kelsey et al., 2023). In addition to cardiopulmonary considerations, preoperative assessment also includes evaluation of other aspects relevant to surgical outcomes. For instance, the rise in case volume with rising age demands proactive management of prevalent comorbidities such as diabetes and obesity, which make recovery difficult. The phrase "silver tsunami" refers to the population movement that is leading to an influx of patients presenting for surgery with greater complexity, and thus, there is a necessity for optimum preoperative planning. Through evaluating nutritional status, optimal glycemic control, and resolution of any underlying psychiatric illness, health care providers can tailor interventions to enhance a patient's fitness for surgery. Studies have identified that proactive assessment and optimization measures significantly improve postoperative recovery pathways and lower the risk of surgery-related complications, particularly in high-risk patients (Hedrick, 2023). Furthermore, adopting a multidisciplinary approach enhances the preoperative assessment process by facilitating inter-specialty collaboration to deliver comprehensive patient care. The inclusion of experts from the fields of cardiology, nutrition, and anesthesiology can result in the development of rigorous preoperative testing protocols that address the multidimensional needs of patients. Complete screenings for anemia, malnutrition, and infection risk are some of the most important elements of this approach, potentially supplemented by interventions aimed at smoking abstinence and physical rehabilitation—also referred to as prehabilitation. This combined focus not only enhances physical preparedness for surgery but also assists in aligning patient expectations with varied care and education. Overall, a holistic assessment based on optimization not only ensures patient outcomes but also optimizes the surgical process, thereby contributing to a smooth and effective surgical experience (Hedrick, 2023) (Figure 4.1).

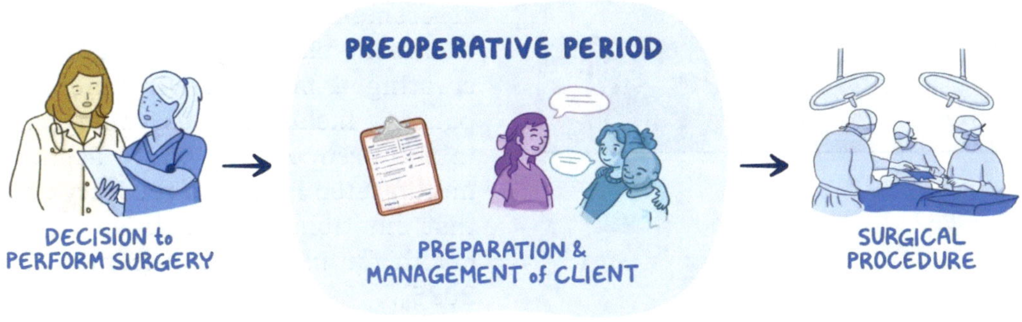

Figure 4.1. Preoperative assessment serves as a critical component in enhancing patient safety and optimizing surgical outcomes.

Source: https://d16qt3wv6xm098.cloudfront.net/cMQjO-Y9Qjy_j6OtmiPkudniTWqqz_z2/_.jpg.

Importance of Preoperative Optimization

Preoperative optimization cannot be exaggerated since it reinforces patients' outcomes and reduces postoperative complications by a great deal. Preoperative optimization involves intensive assessment of patients' health status before surgery, with the goal of identifying risk factors most likely to influence surgical outcomes. For example, intensive evaluations could include determinations of nutrition status, chronic disease, and overall physical fitness. This preoperative evaluation is significant in patients undergoing large operations, such as for colorectal cancer. With an estimated 105,000 new cases of colon cancer in 2020, as per the American Society of Colon and Rectal Surgeons, optimization of such patients preoperatively guarantees that they are optimized to the best possible extent to sustain the stress of surgery, thereby reducing postoperative complications and improving recovery intervals (Jon et al., 2021). Besides, preoperative optimization is needed to correct functional capacity, especially in elderly and comorbid patients. For surgical settings, frail patients are likely to be at risk of complications and extended recovery periods. The current evidence has established that preoperative assessment using detailed geriatric evaluation instruments, such as frailty indexes, is an accurate predictor of postoperative functional status and recovery trajectories. Individuals who present with higher levels of frailty have lower odds of functional recovery post-operatively (Kim et al., 2019). This information puts the need for individualized optimization strategies into perspective, ensuring they increase patients' physical and functional capacity to withstand surgical procedures. Additionally, health optimization among patients prior to surgery may facilitate the initiation of individualized care plans that enhance the surgical process. Preoperative measures can include nutritional optimization, physical rehabilitation, and controlled disease management, all aimed at enhancing patients' resilience during the perioperative period. Multiple studies have consistently shown that these measures can lead to significant short- and long-term outcomes following surgery. Moreover, quality communication and shared decision-making with the clinician can help to establish an appreciation for the value of such optimization strategies.

By ensuring preoperative care and evaluations are top priority, health systems can maximize patient safety and satisfaction and minimize healthcare costs related to complications and more extended hospital stays (Jon et al., 2021).

4.1. Objectives of Preoperative Assessment

Learning Outcome

1. Identifying patient risk factors
2. Establishing baseline health status
3. Planning for perioperative care

The objectives of the preoperative evaluation are crucial to ensure optimal surgical outcomes and patient safety. Of significance, this assessment aims to thoroughly evaluate a patient's medical history, current health status, and any comorbid conditions that may affect the surgery. As examples, diabetes, hypertension, and obesity have massive impacts on surgical risk and recovery trajectories. Such a meticulous examination helps medical practitioners devise personalized strategies for the effective management of these factors. The identification of potential complications through a preoperative assessment is essential as it offers the opportunity to take preventive measures, such as nutritional optimization or special perioperative monitoring protocols. Thus, preoperative assessment not only more confidently guarantees patient safety but also maximizes the likelihood of favorable surgical results, providing a stable basis for the subsequent surgical operation. Besides, another very significant goal of preoperative assessment is to formulate a comprehensive picture of a person's psychological status. Psychological factors, such as anxiety, depression, and emotional status, may notably influence postoperative recovery and satisfaction. Recent studies indicate that surgical patients, particularly those who undergo surgery as a means of big weight loss, can experience heightened stress and emotional tensions that could jeopardize their recovery process. For instance, appropriate management of psychological state during preoperative assessment can lead to more individualized treatment planning and education, ultimately creating a better environment for surgical patients. Inclusion of psychological evaluations in the preoperative phase acknowledges the multifaceted nature of recovery and the reality that emotional health is as vital as physical health for improved outcomes (Galieri et al., 2025).

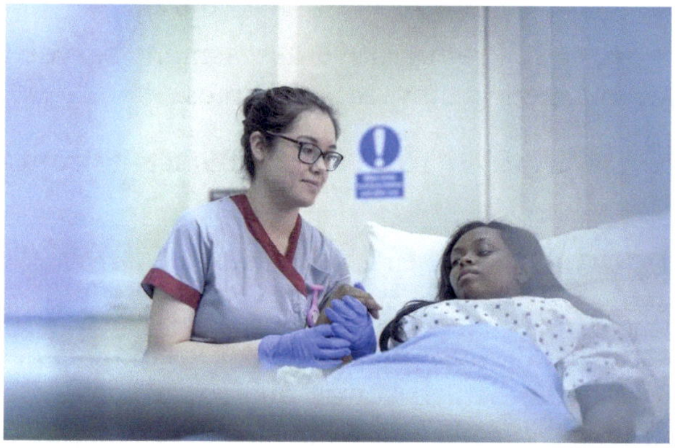

Figure 4.2. The objectives of the preoperative assessment.

Source: https://www.pasadenauc.com/wp-content/uploads/2024/07/pre-operative-assessment.jpg.

Finally, preoperative testing also plays a role in establishing a clear communication line about the surgery and expectations between patients and providers. This goal highlights the value placed on shared decision-making, in which patients are actively engaged in their care process. Informing patients about their surgery, possible risks, and what to expect during recovery can improve their readiness and reduce anxiety about the surgery. For instance, operating room staff must convey individualized information and tailored care plans to individuals undergoing complex surgeries after significant weight loss, as their unique physiological features necessitate special approaches (Giordano et al., 2025). Communication not only helps align patient expectations with clinical realities but also fosters a sense of autonomy and teamwork, ultimately improving satisfaction and adherence to postoperative care practices. Thus, integrating these multifaceted goals into preoperative assessment is crucial for optimizing the surgical experience and outcome (Figure 4.2).

4.1.1. Identifying Patient Risk Factors

Determining patient risk factors is a critical component of preoperative assessment and preparation. As operations themselves place patients at risk, it is imperative to understand each patient's individual profile to minimize complications. One of the most critical components of attention is the assessment of comorbidities, such as chronic diseases like hypertension, diabetes, and obesity. These factors play a significant role in influencing surgeries and postsurgical healing. Further, the timeliness of such an evaluation may impact the physician's ability to perform preoperative interventions in an effort to mitigate risk. The early identification of these risk factors allows health care professionals to optimize patients' health prior to surgery, ultimately yielding improved postoperative outcomes and reduced health care costs. The relationship between aggressive risk assessment and enhanced patient care also reinforces the need for careful preoperative evaluation processes in the operating room. Aside from chronic diseases, some anesthetic and surgical principles must be integrated into risk assessment. One study among Canadian internists highlighted important knowledge gaps in procedure-specific risk estimation, like bleeding and thrombosis complications. This study highlighted that while there is a perceived understanding of the importance of surgical principles by doctors, their ability to accurately estimate the risks is extremely variable. For instance, internists underestimate the risks of bleeding with large operations and overestimate the risks of thrombosis, where greater educational efforts are particularly needed. Closing these knowledge gaps, though, will enable providers to provide better patient counseling regarding their risks and alter preoperative optimization algorithms accordingly. Remediating these knowledge gaps in surgery is critical to minimizing complications and enhancing overall patient safety within the perioperative period, therefore upholding the objective of successful preoperative assessment and optimization. Optimizing modifiable risk factors is also vital for minimizing postoperative complications. According to studies, coordinated preoperative intervention can lead to significant improvements in key health indicators, thereby facilitating improved surgical outcomes. For example, a prospective study of patients undergoing total joint arthroplasty identified that formal preoperative optimization protocols safely improved weight, hemoglobin levels, and glucose control. These improvements were associated with a lower rate of superficial surgical site infection (SSI) compared with usual preoperative management. Both obesity and suboptimal glycemic control are significant determinants of surgical risk, underscoring the importance of active risk management. By implementing evidence-based optimization protocols, health systems can enhance patient readiness for surgery, reduce complication rates, and ultimately offer a safer surgical experience. This endeavor is the quintessence of preoperative assessment and optimization, mirroring patient care strategies aligned with empirical evidence for improved outcomes.

4.1.2. Establishing Baseline Health Status

A comprehensive preoperative assessment is essential in establishing a baseline health status of surgical patients because it enables clinicians to develop any underlying health problems that may influence patient outcomes. Not only does the initial evaluation involve a complete medical history and physical examination, but also laboratory tests and relevant imaging studies. The significance of this process is that it will stratify patients based on risk factors, such as age, underlying medical conditions, and surgical history. For example, elderly individuals or patients with chronic illnesses, such as diabetes and hypertension, can have enhanced surgical risks that need to be optimized before the surgery. With a precise appreciation of a patient's baseline health, clinicians can tailor interventions to maximize preoperative preparation, minimizing complications and maximizing postoperative recovery. This proactive step is highly critical in the modern surgical era, where individualized care must be provided. Furthermore, the ability to ascertain baseline health status enables goal-directed optimization strategies aimed at maximizing patients' overall fitness before surgery. Prehabilitation, a nutrition- and exercise-based practice, has been marketed as a way to enhance patients' preoperative health. The evidence supports that an active role for patients in their own customized exercise programs and dietary modifications improves their tolerance to surgical stress, reduces surgical complications, and shortens hospital stay. One study comparing elderly surgical patients noted that those prehabilitated had fewer adverse outcomes than their non-prehabilitated counterparts. Furthermore, assessing baseline health status provides a basis for comparison in longitudinal assessments of treatment effectiveness, allowing healthcare providers to make informed decisions about care modifications. By targeting effectively modifiable risk factors, healthcare providers maximize patients' global surgical experience, promoting improved outcomes and patient satisfaction. In surgical care, it is also imperative to determine baseline health status by conducting a comprehensive evaluation of psychosocial problems that can affect postoperative recovery. These involve anxiety, depression, and social support, which are critical determinants to be assessed as part of a holistic preoperative evaluation. It was discovered that mental health was a good predictor of recovery, and therefore it is important to tackle these problems to enhance patient outcomes. For instance, anxious patients could benefit from stress management or psychological counseling prior to surgery. Further, understanding patients' social situation, such as living and support arrangements, may help healthcare providers with sufficient information necessary to make proper postoperative arrangements addressing individual needs. By recognizing and addressing both psychosocial and physical health determinants, clinicians can establish an overall baseline health status that enables effective preoperative assessment and optimization, and ultimately results in better surgical outcomes and recovery (Figure 4.3).

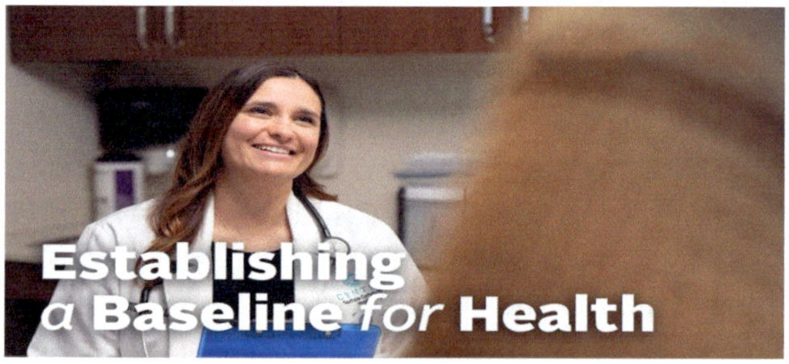

Figure 4.3. A comprehensive preoperative assessment is essential in establishing.

Source: https://i.ytimg.com/vi/AGPeVQmamxY/hq720.jpg?sqp=-oaymwEhCK4FEIIDSFryq4qpAxMIARUAAAAAGAElAADIQj0AgKJD&rs=AOn4CLAszzCi64iuQ9H7784yDloVPT1jJw.

4.1.3. Planning for Perioperative Care

Effective perioperative planning is founded on comprehensive preoperative assessment that strategically identifies and addresses potential patient vulnerabilities. The process begins with meticulous examination of patients' health statuses, considering present conditions, pharmacologic management, and history of surgery. As the European Society of Anesthesiology and Intensive Care Medicine guidelines dictate, these assessments involve a multi-item method that involves clinical evaluation, application of predictive preoperative scores, and biomarkers applied to decision-making (Madison et al., 2024). By diligently acquiring this information, health practitioners can create customized care plans that suit individual patient safety and outcomes while minimizing postoperative complication risk to the lowest levels. At the core of optimizing preoperative care is the implementation of multidisciplinary surgical pause committees (MDSPCs) that foster cross-collaboration among stakeholders in a patient perioperative pathway. The committees are poised to assess and risk-stratify patients based on frailty and other risk factors to provide individualized interventions tailored to each patient's unique needs. The outcomes of recent studies indicate that patients undergoing MDSPC monitoring achieve improved clinical outcomes compared to those without such multidisciplinary attention (Madison et al., 2024). By carefully weighing the risk-benefit ratios of surgical intervention, these committees are very important in determining whether high-risk patients are optimized for surgery or directed away from surgery toward less invasive procedures, thus maximizing surgical success. The worth of preoperative optimization is not merely preparation; it is an entire process of preparing patients for surgery in a holistic approach. It entails both medical and behavioral treatments that facilitate improvement in a patient's overall health before surgery. Efforts such as quitting smoking, maintaining optimal nutritional intake, and managing chronic disease must be included in the preoperative process (Lamperti et al., 2024). In addition, multidisciplinary coordination of care enables optimal implementation of evidence-based guidelines, which have repeatedly proven effective in reducing complications and shortening recovery times. By investing in detailed preoperative planning and coordination, health teams can significantly improve the quality of perioperative care, making patients as well-prepared as possible for the complexities of surgical procedures.

Test Your Knowledge

1. What patient-related factors, such as age, comorbidities, and allergies, increase the risk of complications during anesthesia?
2. How does preoperative assessment of patient risk factors guide anesthetic planning and improve surgical outcomes?

4.2. Components of Preoperative Assessment

Learning Outcome

1. Medical history evaluation
2. Physical examination procedures
3. Laboratory and diagnostic tests

A thorough preoperative assessment is essential to achieve the best surgical outcome and minimize the risk of postoperative complications. The thorough history taking of the patient's medical history is an important component of this assessment and includes identification of coexisting illnesses, previous surgeries, medications, and allergic reactions. These are vital to know, as they can influence anesthesia care and surgical procedures. Also to be assessed are the patient's functional status, including activity levels and physical functioning. For instance, patients with impaired cardiovascular or pulmonary functioning may require specific perioperative arrangements to be made for them to balance risk factors attendant upon surgery and anesthesia. In so doing, caregivers can create well-informed, personalized care plans that are appropriate to each patient's needs, ultimately resulting in improved surgical outcomes and recovery. Another significant area of preoperative evaluation is addressing lifestyle factors, most notably smoking cessation, which has been an important determinant of operative complications. The evidence favors the implementation of smoking-cessation interventions at least four weeks before surgery to prevent postoperative complications, including surgical-site infections. A systematic review noted that several behavioral support sessions together with pharmacotherapy is a significant benefit in achieving successful cessation, hence enhancing patient outcomes (Rachel et al., 2024). This evidence supports the multidisciplinary approach to this issue, whereby anesthesiologists, surgeons, and primary care physicians must collaborate to enhance preoperative smoking-cessation interventions. By placing these interventions first in line, health care professionals will aid patients in achieving better surgical outcomes and overall health improvement, emphasizing the central role of preoperative assessment in delivering maximal surgical care. Moreover, risk evaluation for individual patients goes beyond comprehensive laboratory and diagnostic screening.

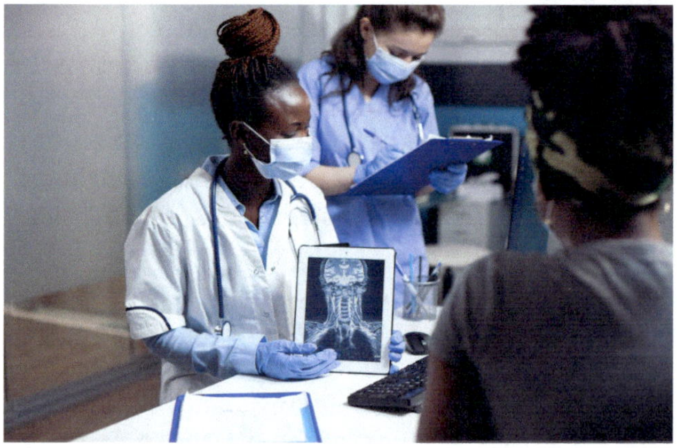

Figure 4.4. A comprehensive preoperative assessment.

Source: https://www.pasadenauc.com/wp-content/uploads/2024/04/medical-clearance-for-surgery.jpeg.

Preoperative testing generally includes routine blood tests, imaging studies, and other studies based on the patient's medical history or the purpose of presentation. For instance, patients undergoing major surgery may require baseline cardiac assessment or pulmonary function tests to ascertain their perioperative risk for complications. Recent developments in precision medicine, exemplified in the management of diseases such as lung cancer, have yielded promising results through personalized treatment strategies. As with biomarker-driven therapies, the integration of genetic and phenotypic information can enhance preoperative planning and postoperative convalescence (Kedar et al., 2025). Hence, by applying a multidisciplinary approach that incorporates state-of-the-art diagnostics along with traditional preoperative assessment, the results of surgery can be optimized and the quality of patient-centered care in surgical practice can be enhanced (Figure 4.4).

4.2.1. Medical History Evaluation

Detailed medical history taking is central to the preoperative assessment process, enabling clinicians to identify potential risks and optimize patient treatment before surgery. Assessment involves careful recording of the patients' previous medical ailments, history of surgery, and family medical history. Special care must also be accorded to comorbidities such as diabetes, hypertension, and cardiovascular disease, which have substantial impacts on surgery outcomes. Through a structured analysis of these variables, healthcare professionals can tailor their practice to meet the specific needs of each patient, thereby enhancing both effectiveness and safety throughout the surgery. This important step not only facilitates predicting the probability of complications but also serves as the foundation for establishing individualized anesthetic and surgical protocols, ultimately leading to improved patient outcomes. In addition to evaluating active medical conditions, a patient's current medications and daily habits are important aspects of the preoperative evaluation. Prescription medications, over-the-counter medications, and nutritional supplements can affect anesthesia and recovery from surgery. As a result, a careful inventory of these items is paramount to anesthesia safety and the prevention of adverse drug events. In addition, lifestyle variables such as alcohol consumption, level of physical activity, and smoking also influence the potential to heal and the potential for postoperative complications in a patient. For example, smoking patients will develop delayed wound healing and increased respiratory complications. Having this knowledge, clinicians can use appropriate optimization strategies, such as smoking cessation therapy, thus physically and psychologically readjusting the patient for surgery. Also, patients with significant weight loss or those being treated with GLP-1 agonists deserve special attention to history and physical examination. These patients may have unique anatomical and physiological derangements that must be identified to optimize surgical outcome. For instance, excessive weight loss may lead to dietary deficiencies that necessitate preoperative vitamin supplementation and dietary counseling to minimize surgical risks. Furthermore, the patients may also undergo significant changes in their comorbidity statuses, with diseases like sleep apnea or metabolic syndrome that must be controlled at all times. As recommended in more recent literature, a proper evaluation of these factors is essential in arriving at an overall surgical plan tailored to the individual patient's requirements (Giordano et al., 2025). The addition of cutting-edge predictive algorithms, such as artificial intelligence-based algorithms, can further improve these evaluations and provide an even more objective foundation for assessing surgical candidacy and postoperative needs (Turan et al., 2025).

4.2.2. Physical Examination Procedures

The physical examination procedures carried out during the preoperative assessment period are part of optimizing patient outcomes and reducing surgical risk. A comprehensive assessment typically begins with a complete medical history assessment including consideration of the patients' current comorbidities, medications, allergies, and surgical history. The health practitioner then carries out a systematic physical assessment, evaluating the vital signs, cardiovascular status, pulmonary status, and neurological status. These assessments not only help to determine if any underlying illnesses would complicate surgery but also provide important information needed for anesthetic planning. Furthermore, as seen in the current literature, bedside assessments have gained value, demonstrating their utility in detecting anatomical complexities that will complicate airway management. Part of preoperative evaluation is also a distinct series of physical examination maneuvers designed to assess respiratory function and risk of complications from underlying cardiopulmonary disease. Certain diseases, such as heart failure and COPD, can significantly elevate perioperative risk and therefore require special testing. Assessment can include auscultation of respiratory sounds and monitoring of oxygen saturation, as these are critical for predicting respiratory complications intraoperatively and postoperatively. The literature suggests that a rigorous preoperative assessment process, including thorough cardiopulmonary evaluations, can accurately identify patients at higher risk of perioperative events. By identifying these risks, medical professionals can use targeted interventions to prepare patients for surgery. In addition, newer advances in technology have enhanced the effectiveness of physical examination protocols in preoperative assessment. Techniques such as, but not restricted to, ultrasound and advanced imaging modalities are now being utilized to provide more comprehensive evaluation of anatomical structures, particularly where more traditional examinations might be found wanting. For instance, during advanced airway examination, techniques such as transnasal endoscopy and virtual endoscopy can provide valuable information about upper airway anatomy. These technologies, apart from assisting in the identification of potential intubation challenges, also help in the formulation of a more sophisticated anesthetic plan and possess more efficient mitigation processes. Thus, bridging traditional physical examinations with technology forms a more robust foundation for optimizing patient outcomes in the perioperative setting (Figure 4.5).

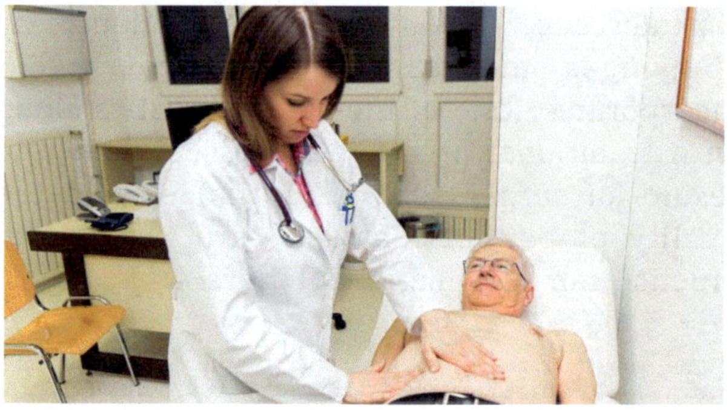

Figure 4.5. The physical examination procedures undertaken during the preoperative assessment phase.

Source: https://soloabadi.com/wp-content/uploads/2024/05/Palpation-Physical-Examination-1024x576.jpg.

4.2.3. Laboratory and Diagnostic Tests

Preoperative assessment largely relies on laboratory and diagnostic testing to adequately prepare patients for the operation. It has several essential functions, including evaluating the patient's physiological status, identifying possible limitations, and providing advice on perioperative care management. Routine tests such as complete blood counts, liver function tests, and metabolic panels are typically part of a comprehensive preoperative evaluation. In colorectal surgery patients, carcinoembryonic antigen (CEA) measurement is particularly significant. It serves as a survival and recurrence marker and is used to measure baseline values for postoperative follow-up. Research indicates that an elevated level of CEA before surgery is correlated with increased mortality among patients with colorectal cancer, rendering it a pivotal component of the diagnostic process (Jon et al., 2021). Imaging studies also play a critical role in the diagnostic pathway leading to surgery. For colorectal carcinoma, abdomen and pelvis CT scans are commonly employed to establish the stage of the disease as well as to look for possible metastases. Oral and intravenous contrast improve visualization of anatomical structures and demarcation of tumors from surrounding tissues, a critical step in preparing surgical plans. Although PET scans are not usually performed for primary staging, they can influence surgical planning in advanced stages (Yau-You et al., 2020). Uniting these imaging techniques with preoperative assessment enables a deep understanding of the patient's condition and supports well-informed decision-making by the surgical team during treatment.

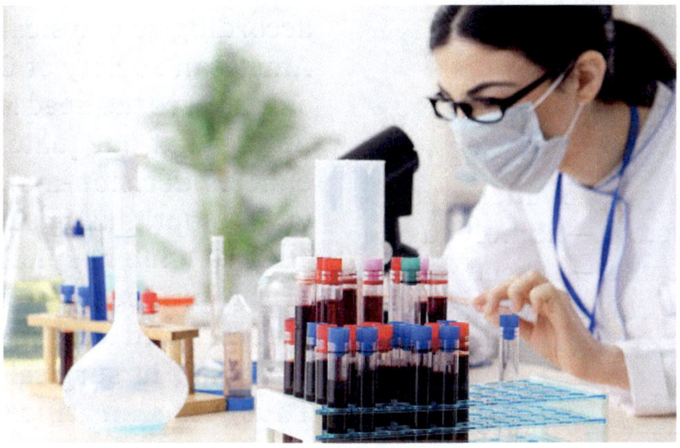

Figure 4.6. Laboratory and diagnostic tests.

Source: https://www.firstlabdiagnostics.com/Heamatology.jpg.

Moreover, performing a histological investigation is critical to confirm the diagnosis of malignancy before any surgery is performed. Through methods such as endoscopic biopsy, professionals are capable of obtaining biopsy specimens for pathological examination, with implications regarding tumor biology and impacting therapeutic decision-making. Complete evaluation of colorectal mucosa is recommended for synchronous lesions detection because even 30% of patients may contain other polyps or cancer. This integrated approach emphasizes the applicability of diagnostic tests not only for staging but also for individualizing treatment protocols (Jon et al., 2021). Lastly, the integration of laboratory and diagnostic tests in preoperative assessments ensures an integral realization of the patient's health, hence optimizing surgical outcomes and recovery avenues (Figure 4.6).

Test Your Knowledge

1. What are the essential components of a preoperative assessment, and how do they help identify potential anesthetic risks?
2. How do medical history, physical examination, and laboratory investigations contribute to planning safe anesthesia care?

4.3. Risk Stratification

Learning Outcome

1. Tools for assessing surgical risk
2. Classification of patients by risk levels
3. Implications of risk stratification on surgical outcomes

Risk stratification is the cornerstone of preoperative evaluation and optimization, particularly for complex surgery. By identifying patients' unique risk factors—namely age, comorbidities, and mental status—surgeons can tailor their preoperative protocol to achieve optimal patient outcomes. Risk stratification involves a meticulous review of physiological and psychological metrics to categorize patients by postoperative risk. For example, a patient with multiple comorbidities may require additional preoperative workup, such as cardiology consultation, while those having a history of mental illness can access combined psychological care services. This varied approach enables health professionals to allocate intervention priority to prevent complications that are reduced with interventions prescribed based on the needs of each individual (Yau-You et al., 2020). The integration of mental health into risk stratification makes it more significant in preoperative assessment protocols. Research indicates that patients who have pre-existing mental health illnesses such as depression and anxiety are much more likely to develop complications following surgery and stay longer in the hospital (Anghela et al., 2020). It calls for a dual focus on physical and mental health factors during preoperative assessment. The inclusion of standardized measures of mental well-being during routine evaluations allows clinicians to screen vulnerable patients earlier in their surgical journey. Treating mental health as a fundamental aspect of health helps surgical teams develop more holistic care plans. These approaches not only enhance patient safety but also provide emotional and psychological support to achieve optimal recovery. Lastly, effective risk stratification is a foundation for optimizing surgical performance in preoperative assessment and preparation. The process enables the creation of evidence-based guidelines that can be adapted to various patient groups according to physical and mental factors. The American Society of Colon and Rectal Surgeons emphasizes the need for evidence-based practice, noting that adequate preoperative assessment enables decision-making in the clinic, which is vital to optimizing surgical care (Yau-You et al., 2020). While hospitals adopt risk stratification in the preoperative process, the emphasis on personalized care manifests in a continuous reduction in surgical morbidity and mortality. Thus, risk stratification not only enhances clinical outcomes but also signifies a paradigm shift toward patient-centric surgical practice.

4.3.1. Tools for Assessing Surgical Risk

Comprehensive preoperative assessment is valuable in determining operative risk, particularly in risky candidates. The Society of Thoracic Surgeons (STS) risk calculator and the European Heart Surgery Risk Assessment System, EuroSCORE II, are used in most cases to estimate postoperative complications and risk of death. The two calculators consider patient-specific data such as comorbidities, age, and surgical procedure type and deliver an assessable risk score that guides clinicians' decision-making. These objective assessments allow for individualized preoperative optimization regimens aimed at minimizing identified risks. Therefore, by applying such tools in routine practice, healthcare providers can maximize patient safety and postoperative outcomes, thereby necessitating a complete assessment in the preoperative setting (Michael et al., 2024). The incorporation of robust risk assessment tools into the preoperative process not only improves surgical outcomes but also fosters a culture of shared decision-making between clinicians and patients. Informing patients about their risk profiles promotes collaborative care, which is paramount when exploring potential interventions or alternatives to surgery. A multidisciplinary team can use information from risk assessments to tailor perioperative care plans that prioritize patient safety and early recovery.

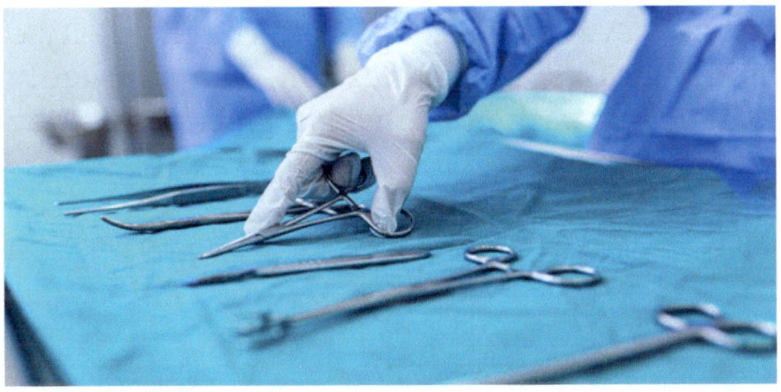

Figure 4.7. Tools for assessing surgical risk.

Source: https://aci.health.nsw.gov.au/__data/assets/image/0004/942673/Perioperative-Toolkit-digital-thumbnail.jpg.

In addition, prehabilitation programs focusing on physical conditioning and nutritional optimization are imperative during the preoperative period. Surgery programs that aim to improve patients' fitness levels can decrease surgical risks considerably and improve recovery times, which are in the principles stated in enhanced recovery after surgery (ERAS) programs that recognize value-based care (Carli et al., 2021). The inclusion of digital health technologies also strengthens the preoperative evaluation of surgical risk by facilitating round-the-clock monitoring of patient data and communication. Wearable devices and smartphone applications measuring vital signs, activity, and patient reports of symptoms enable interactive risk stratification. The devices could report to clinicians in real time and adapt preoperative plans as necessary. Furthermore, the use of systematic postoperative follow-ups through such electronic platforms encourages patient engagement and adherence to preoperative regimens. By presenting patients with educational materials and behavioral cues, health care providers can facilitate adherence to lifestyle changes needed to minimize surgical risks. Hence, the use of both traditional risk-stratification tools and new digital solutions is an inclusive framework that can significantly optimize preoperative assessment modalities and guarantee optimal patient outcomes (Michael et al., 2024) (Figure 4.7).

4.3.2. Classification of Patients by Risk Levels

Risk classification of the patient is a key part of preoperative optimization and evaluation, particularly among surgical candidates with health status varying from normal to severe. It traditionally considers a wide range of parameters, such as medical history, active comorbidities, age, and surgery type. For instance, chronic cardiovascular patients can be categorized as high-risk due to related complications during surgery. The standards offered by the American Society of Colon and Rectal Surgeons (ASCRS) emphasize a comprehensive evaluation to determine the patient's specific risk for surgical procedures. Effective risk stratification allows physicians to efficiently tailor preoperative practices to ensure patients receive the most appropriate care based on their risk factors, thereby minimizing postoperative complications and improving outcomes overall (Stefan et al., 2021). Moreover, the application of systems of risk classification facilitates enhanced patient education and informed consent. By expressing surgical risks and advantages within the framework of each patient's classification, practitioners can communicate the uncertainties of surgery and postoperative recovery in greater detail. This process favors the collaborative model of decision-making, enabling patients to participate more actively in their care plan. ASCRS guidelines recommend the use of formal risk assessment tools to identify patients who require additional preoperative optimization, such as lifestyle modification or medical therapy, before surgery (Yau-You et al., 2020). This advanced planning eventually helps achieve the target of maximizing surgical outcomes and minimizing the incidence of complications related to surgery and underlying health conditions. Furthermore, risk categorization is the most critical factor in developing multidisciplinary approaches for optimal patient care preoperatively. The inclusion of a broad range of experts—such as anesthesiologists, dietitians, and physiotherapists—appears to significantly enhance preoperative care for high-risk patients. The multidisciplinary team collaboration ensures that all conceivable risk factors are addressed holistically, potentially including nutritional supplementation to malnourished patients, best comorbidity management, and prehabilitation programs for maximizing physical condition before surgery. These procedures not only support the patient's well-being but also align with clinical practice guidelines, which ensure evidence-based practice and high-quality care follow-up (Stefan et al., 2021). Thus, systematic classification and interdisciplinary collaboration together promote an active patient safety environment and enhanced surgical success.

4.3.3. Implications of Risk Stratification on Surgical Outcomes

Risk stratification is a critical part of preoperative optimization and surgical outcome assessment. By evaluating an individual patient's risk factors—such as age, comorbidities, and history of surgery—health care professionals can tailor treatment to prevent complications during surgery. With proper utilization, risk stratification can identify high-risk patients who may benefit from increased observation or additional preoperative treatment. Here, studies indicate that extensive preoperative cardiac and pulmonary assessment can significantly enhance patient safety, with a reduced rate of surgical complications (Poldermans et al., 2009). In such a manner, integrating risk stratification into practice not only maximizes surgical outcomes but also enhances the use of resources in healthcare settings. The importance of risk stratification extends beyond simply identifying possible complications; it also guides decision-making regarding surgical intervention. Preoperative optimization based on risk evaluations, either through lifestyle modifications or medication, can markedly enhance a patient's physiological status for surgery.

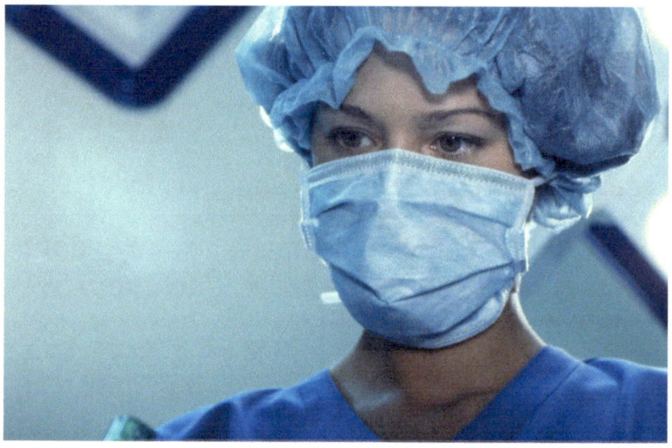

Figure 4.8. Risk stratification is a vital component of preoperative assessment and optimization of surgical outcomes.

Source: https://www.verywellhealth.com/thmb/H1uTjfpZja1zGu0OQmC4GiRv8hU=/1500x0/filters:no_upscale():max_bytes(150000):strip_icc()/91803648-56a9125a3df78cf772a35d41.JPG.

This period of preparation is crucial, as it can prevent complications related to anesthesia and the operation itself. Literature shows that patients who undergo sufficient preoperative optimization and assessment have lower postoperative mortality and morbidity (Englesbe et al., 2015). Thus, the implementation of systematic risk stratification in the preoperative protocol essentially entails anticipatory practices that can improve outcomes, directly addressing the call for comprehensive patient care in the surgical setting. Risk stratification also promotes a culture of shared decision-making between patients and healthcare providers. Clear articulation of risk factors provides patients with the necessary information to understand their health risks and take an active role in their operative decisions. Not only does it empower the patients, but it also encourages adherence to preoperative suggested intervention, which enhances their overall health and readiness for surgery. The practice application of risk-stratification tools also facilitates a more tailored approach to surgical care, in which the unique conditions of each patient are addressed and respected. In total, this patient-focused style of management, placed in the forefront by risk assessment and optimization, is crucial to optimizing surgical outcomes and developing a safer surgical environment for each patient (Figure 4.8).

Test Your Knowledge

1. What systems or criteria are commonly used to classify patients by anesthetic risk, and what factors determine a patient's risk level?
2. How does knowing a patient's risk classification influence the choice of anesthetic technique and perioperative management?

4.4. Optimization Strategies

Learning Outcome

1. Preoperative lifestyle modifications
2. Management of comorbid conditions
3. Nutritional assessment and intervention

In pursuit of successful surgical results, preoperative optimization methods are paramount. A thorough examination of a patient's medical history, comorbidities, and lifestyle is necessary to identify potential risks and implement individualized interventions. For instance, patients scheduled for bariatric surgery or who have experienced significant weight loss are likely to need particular nutritional counseling and evaluation of their unique physiological conditions. A sensitive investigation of comorbidities such as diabetes and hypertension allows practitioners to design optimized plans to facilitate recovery and avoid complications in the postoperative period. Additionally, gaining insight into a patient's weight trend is crucial, particularly for patients who use medication aids, as it can guide appropriate dietary planning and supplemental needs, ultimately optimizing surgery preparedness and outcomes (Giordano et al., 2025). Implementation of evidence-based practices during the preoperative phase can successfully reduce postoperative pulmonary complications (PPCs), a common disease that leads to prolonged hospitalization. Systematic reviews underscore the importance of identifying crucial preoperative determinants, such as older age, reduced preoperative oxygen saturation, and preexisting chronic obstructive pulmonary disease (COPD), as risk factors for developing PPCs. To mitigate such risks, optimization tactics must include vigilant pulmonary assessments and application of lung-protective ventilation techniques during surgery. Intraoperative factors must also be taken into account, as previous studies have linked excessive fluid administration and poor reversal of neuromuscular blockade to increased PPC risk. By actively considering these variables, clinicians can improve patient outcomes and accelerate recovery after surgery (Mustafa et al., 2025). Lastly, nothing is more important than individualized optimization regimens, particularly when it pertains to surgical interventions in patients post-weight loss. Since such patients typically present with unique anatomical and metabolic complications, there must be an individualized approach to managing the surgical planning. This can include staging procedures as necessary and setting realistic recovery and outcome expectations. Medication-assisted weight-loss patients, such as those on GLP-1 agonists, may require a specialty preoperative evaluation to address their distinct metabolic profile. Having a patient-led strategy not only improves surgical outcomes but also fosters a culture of teamwork in which patients are empowered to be active participants in their care plan. By prioritizing thorough preoperative assessments and specific optimization regimens, medical practitioners can significantly enhance the efficacy of surgical procedures and enhance patients' overall satisfaction and health outcomes (Giordano et al., 2025).

4.4.1. Preoperative Lifestyle Modifications

Preoperative lifestyle modification is significant for ensuring optimal patient outcomes during the perioperative period. They include nutritional modifications, increased physical activity, smoking cessation, and weight management, all of which may reduce surgical risk and optimize the healing process. Research suggests that prehabilitation with a structured program may physically and psychologically condition patients for surgery, thereby reducing postoperative complications and hospital stay. This proactive attitude, at the core of ERAS protocols, concentrates on using evidence-based strategies that promote patient resilience and overall health preoperatively (Michael et al., 2024). Modifying one's lifestyle in the weeks leading up to surgery can thus be a vital strategy for both optimizing acute surgical outcomes and optimal long-term recovery and well-being. It also incorporates lifestyle changes in psychosocial domains, which are so essential to optimal preoperative preparation. Education programs are encouraged that outline the importance of adhering to preoperative instructions, with an emphasis on how lifestyle changes can positively influence their surgical course. For instance, quitting smoking not only reduces the risk of respiratory problems but also enhances wound healing and overall recovery. Besides, stress reduction through techniques such as mindfulness or cognitive-behavioral therapies is capable of empowering the patients, increasing their mental preparedness for surgery. The changes enable patients to be actively involved in their healthcare choices and gain a sense of autonomy, which is beneficial during preoperative times (Michael et al., 2024). Thus, an integrated approach to preoperative lifestyle modification tremendously enhances patient involvement and satisfaction. Lastly, the contribution of interdisciplinary healthcare teams in education and the application of such lifestyle modifications cannot be overstated. Preoperative multidisciplinary teams, comprising surgeons, nurses, dietitians, and mental health professionals, are key to supporting patients throughout their preoperative journey. With the shared decision-making model, these teams can tailor preoperative interventions based on patient's requirements while providing constant support and motivation. Furthermore, teamwork can ensure communication and continuity of care, which are essential for adhering to preoperative guidelines. Effective assessment of such lifestyle determinants, coupled with appropriate interventions, not only complements the aim of personalized medicine but also significantly contributes to the overall outcome of surgical procedures, thereby complementing preoperative assessment and optimization within the surgical setting (Figure 4.9).

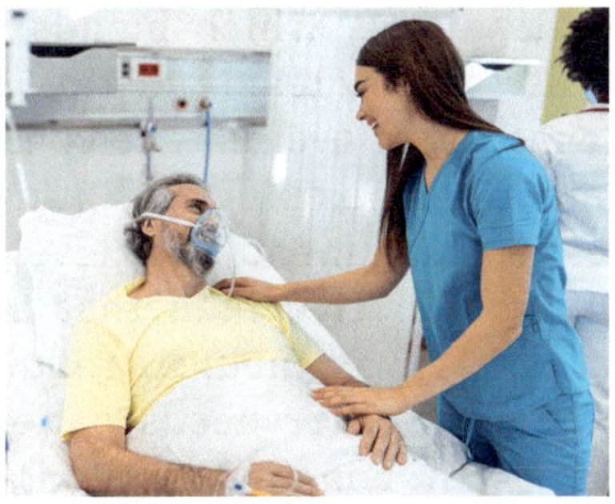

Figure 4.9. Preoperative lifestyle modifications.

Source: https://drramjimehrotra.com/wp-content/uploads/2024/03/MicrosoftTeams-image-70.png.

4.4.2. Management of Comorbid Conditions

Management of comorbid diseases is most important in preoperative assessment and optimization. Comorbidities like diabetes and obesity significantly complicate the surgical situation and are well known to affect the outcome of surgery adversely. For instance, diabetes mellitus has been associated with wound healing complications, infection, and hospital stay.

To prevent these risks, it is necessary to include an in-depth evaluation of patients' comorbidities and even an audit of their current management strategies. There is evidence that improving diabetes management through lifestyle modification, patient education, and medication optimization can advance surgical readiness. Specifically, in type 2 diabetic patients, the addition of sodium-glucose cotransporter 2 (SGLT2) inhibitors or glucagon-like peptide 1 (GLP-1) receptor agonists has been shown to have cardiovascular benefits, thereby influencing perioperative risk and outcomes (Melanie et al., 2018). Obesity presents an additional challenge in the preoperative management of patients. Surgeons usually encounter obese patients with multiple comorbidities, i.e., metabolic syndrome and cardiovascular disease. These conditions both heighten perioperative risk and mandate meticulous preoperative planning. A scrutinous assessment of obesity comorbidities, as well as risk stratification, is required to optimize patient results.

This entails meticulous assessments of cardiovascular status, pulmonary function, and metabolic control, particularly in thoracic surgery patients. Furthermore, a multifaceted treatment of the use of weight loss interventions, either behavioral modification or drug therapy, will improve patient readiness for surgery. Such interventions are key to minimizing the likelihood of postoperative complications, with implications for early consideration of these comorbidities before going under the knife (Douglas et al., 2017). Preoperative optimization methods should be guided by a detailed understanding of a patient's comorbid conditions and how they may affect the outcomes of surgery. Employment of an interdisciplinary team of medical doctors, surgeons, and dietitians facilitates individualized planning to maximize the patient's health status prior to surgery. Regular oversight of treatment programs, particularly for chronic illnesses like diabetes and obesity, is essential in achieving the optimal preoperative fitness state. In addition, enhanced patient education about these conditions can lead to improved self-management practices and a healthier overall state, which, in turn, equates to lower complication rates both before and after surgery. By prioritizing the management of comorbidities, healthcare practitioners can significantly enhance surgical outcomes and reduce lengths of stay, thereby helping both patients and healthcare systems (Douglas et al., 2017; Melanie et al., 2018).

4.4.3. Nutritional Assessment and Intervention

Among many factors that determine the optimal preoperative assessment, nutritional status is an important parameter that requires careful assessment. Malnutrition, generally characterized by inadequate nutrient intake, significantly hampers surgical outcomes and recovery. Preoperative patients, especially those with pre-existing conditions such as congenital heart disease, tend to have growth disorders alongside malnutrition due to chronic diseases, resulting in long-term food intake deficiency. A thorough nutritional assessment should incorporate a multidimensional process, i.e., dietary history, anthropometric measurements, and biochemical investigations. This extensive evaluation not only aids in the detection of nutritional deficiencies but also in the generation of an individualized intervention plan for the rehabilitation of nutritional status in a patient before surgery, ultimately benefiting their strength and recovery potential. A systematic process of nutritional care can have an increased impact on preoperative optimization. With standardized assessment methods, medical professionals can correctly diagnose nutritional deficiencies and provide specific interventions. In the case of undernourished children, as in research with such patients, it was stressed that following up on assessments from the bottom level using comprehensive medical history and face-to-face interviews is important in determining specific dietary needs. Interventions at that point may include dietary modification and vitamin supplementation. Continuing monitoring and evaluation of the patients' status ensures that health teams are in a position to alter interventions accordingly, thus contributing to improved clinical outcomes. Such active nutrition management not only enhances the physical status of the patients but also their psychological preparation for surgery. Furthermore, including nutritional assessment in preoperative care, which blends perfectly with multidisciplinary team practice, enhances patient management overall. The collaboration of surgeons, anesthesiologists, nutritionists, and nurses is instrumental in developing an integrated preoperative plan that addresses nutritional as well as medical requirements. For instance, high-order needs patients, such as patients with congenital heart disease, require careful monitoring to ensure that their nutritional needs are adequately provided for the surgical demand. Such measures as liberalizing fasting regimens and optimizing hydration can be integrated synergistically into nutritional therapies to reduce perioperative risks. The convergence of these interventions not only reduces the risk of surgical failure but also significantly improves patient satisfaction and overall treatment outcomes, underscoring the importance of an interdisciplinary approach to preoperative evaluation and optimization (Kuddah et al., 2025; Kamlesh et al., 2025) (Figure 4.10).

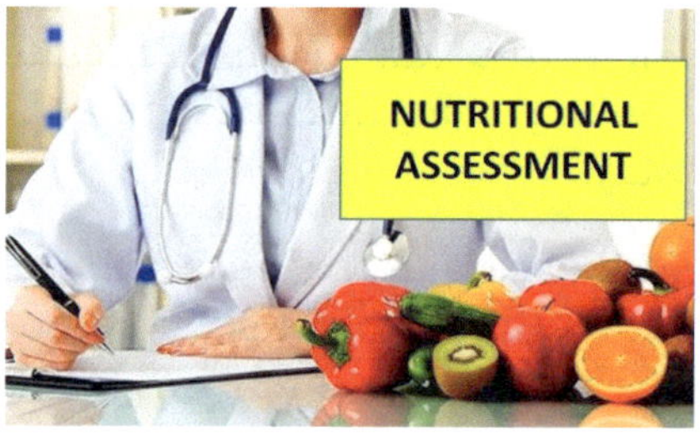

Figure 4.10. Nutritional assessment and intervention.

Source: https://i.ytimg.com/vi/ZFtWtZ4QWXg/hq720.jpg?sqp=-oaymwEhCK4FEIIDSFryq4qpAxMIARUAAAAAGAElAADIQj0AgKJD&rs=AOn4CLBPzs48-H9xJbLhF7CqG0zqcuWOkQ.

Test Your Knowledge

1. What preoperative optimization strategies can be implemented to reduce anesthetic risks in high-risk patients?
2. How do medical, nutritional, and lifestyle interventions improve patient outcomes before surgery and anesthesia?

4.5. Role of Multidisciplinary Teams

Learning Outcome

1. Collaboration among healthcare providers
2. Importance of communication in patient care
3. Case management and follow-up

The role of multidisciplinary teams (MDTs) during preoperative evaluation and optimization is key to providing comprehensive care for surgical patients. MDTs typically consist of surgeons, anesthesiologists, nurses, and other allied healthcare experts who consult together to assess and manage the patients' medical conditions before surgery. The collaboration enables the assembly of diverse expertise, which is essential for addressing a range of patient needs, particularly in complex cases. By considering a patient's overall health, MDTs can identify potential risk factors, optimize medical treatment, and align the surgical plan, thereby leading to better surgical outcomes and reduced complications. In addition, the use of formalized multidisciplinary assessment, such as frailty scoring, has been shown to significantly enhance surgical decision-making. According to current evidence, frail patients are at higher risk of postoperative complications, and it is crucial to detect them early and address interventions that MDTs alone can best provide. Specifically, assessment tools such as the Clinical Frailty Scale enable clinicians to individualize care pathways, including prehabilitation programs or surgical modality adjustments to minimize risk for these patients. Hence, the contribution of MDTs to facilitating preoperative assessments is one component that maximizes patient outcomes in the operating room, especially for high-risk patients. In addition to enhancing patient safety and recovery, multidisciplinary collaboration is crucial for addressing complications expected in surgical therapy. For instance, in maxillary sinus grafting, specialists in dentistry and otolaryngology play key roles in managing sinonasal complications. Effective preoperative evaluation by otolaryngologists can lead to better surgical planning and a lower risk of postoperative complications. Through concerted effort, MDTs ensure that potential complications are predicted and dealt with early on—highlighting the imperative for early detection and structured interdisciplinary approaches to improved patient care. Thus, the role of multidisciplinary teams cannot be overestimated; their combined efforts not only improve surgical outcomes but also optimize clinical efficiency and patient satisfaction.

4.5.1. Collaboration Among Healthcare Providers

Ideal coordination among health care professionals is necessary to optimize preoperative evaluation and optimization. The integration of various specialties enables a unified view of a patient's overall health, which is highly significant for minimizing surgical risks. Interdisciplinary groups of surgeons, anesthesiologists, and primary care physicians collaborate to screen patient histories, conduct corresponding screenings, and trigger preoperative optimization programs. These collaborations are encouraged by creating communication platforms that facilitate real-time information exchange, thereby easing decision-making processes. Furthermore, these collaborations help identify future complications in the early stages of the preoperative period, ultimately leading to improved surgical outcomes and patient satisfaction. The application of novel technologies significantly encourages the collaboration process among medical practitioners in the preoperative period. For instance, the incorporation of blockchain technology is emerging as a promising solution for secure sharing of patients' data among institutions. The decentralized nature of the system helps ward off threats associated with centralized data-sharing systems, such as unauthorized use and traceability concerns, as highlighted in recent studies. Through data provenance maintenance and the facilitation of transparent access structures, the technology allows providers to collaborate without compromise on Health Insurance Portability and Accountability Act (HIPAA) compliance. These developments usher in better preoperative evaluation, hence optimizing patient treatment and preoperative preparedness in general (Urs, 2025).

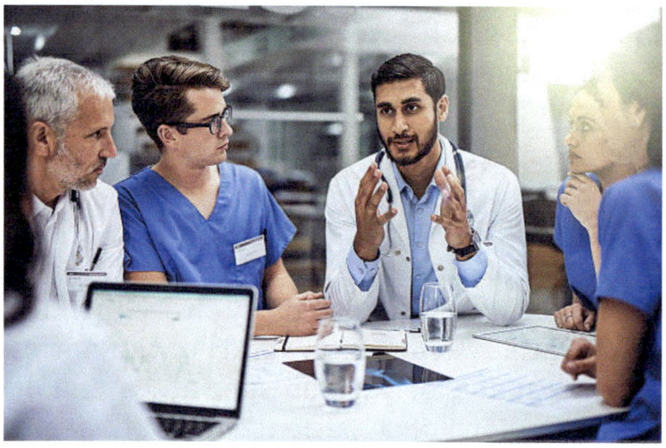

Figure 4.11. Collaboration among healthcare providers.

Source: https://wps03-media.cdn.ihealthspot.com/wp-content/uploads/sites/5/2023/07/istockphoto-638646884-612x612-1.jpg.

Secondly, the application of sophisticated analytical techniques such as deep learning has the potential to revolutionize the field of healthcare cooperation, especially when making preoperative diagnoses. Current studies underscore the role of Blockchain-Assisted technologies in protecting patient information and improving the efficacy of disease identification through collaborative analysis by healthcare professionals. By using advanced data models, groups can make educated predictions and iterate patient management strategy accordingly. The model proposed by these authors comprises several stages of preoperative assessment, from feature selection through classification to hyperparameter optimization, highlighting the value of multidisciplinary expertise in improving outcomes (Omar, 2025). Such advancements in collaborative procedures signal a revolutionary shift in how healthcare workers can work together to enhance preoperative procedures and ultimately, patient safety (Figure 4.11).

4.5.2. Importance of Communication in Patient Care

Good communication is the foundation for successful patient care, particularly preoperative evaluation. The ability to relay complex medical information to patients ensures they are aware of their procedures, risks, and expected outcomes. This type of communication is not only vital for overcoming patient fear but also for building trust with the healthcare provider. When fully informed, patients are likely to be engaged in their care, compliant with preoperative advice, and in the end, help positively with their postoperative rehabilitation. Failure to communicate may result in miscommunication, nonadherence, or complications, underscoring the importance of good conversations between patients and clinicians during the preoperative period. Piloting a variety of communication approaches can thus significantly enhance the quality of care during this pivotal time in patient care. Communication also goes beyond information exchange; it involves interpersonal interaction that can profoundly shape patient satisfaction and outcomes. Establishing rapport and communicating empathy creates a better supportive environment in which patients are heard and respected. In preoperative assessment, the healthcare practitioners are forced to heed the patient's complaints and wishes patiently, promoting collaboration in caring. Involving the patient in decision-making regarding their health status and surgical plan not only empowers patients but also makes it easier for them to adhere to medical recommendations, as they will follow dietary regimens or smoking cessation programs because they believe they are working with their health providers rather than against them. Through fostering such an environment, we are also enhancing the preoperative experience in general and, therefore, maximizing surgical outcomes, as the professionals' work in this field is put under the spotlight by the cases featured in Zeppenfeld et al. (2022) and Halvorsen et al. (2022).

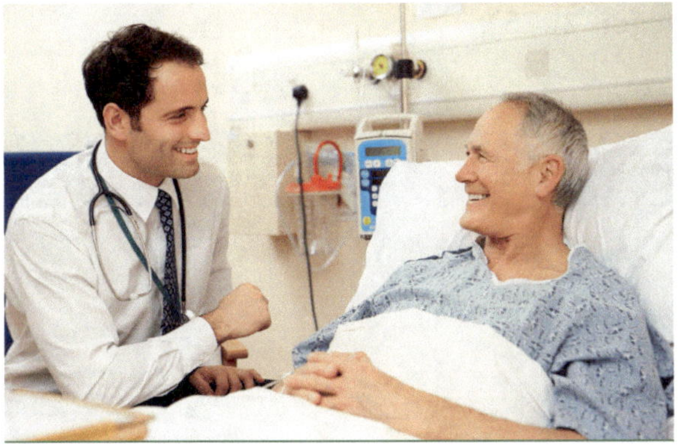

Figure 4.12. Importance of communication in patient care.

Source: https://www.capsahealthcare.com/wp-content/uploads/2024/07/6-Ways-to-Improve-Patient-Communication-Hero.png.

In addition to enhancing patient understanding and satisfaction, effective communication between the medical staff is also important. An orderly coordination of information among healthcare providers ensures that all participants in patient care are on the same page, thereby minimizing opportunities for errors or miscommunication. In preoperative assessment, this coordination aids in thorough assessments that consider all aspects of a patient's health—bodily, emotional, and social. This teamwork also identifies early potential complications and implements certain interventions to optimize patient readiness for surgery. Moreover, effective communication can enable the use of standardized processes, allowing every member of the team to practice best practices. Ultimately, the value of communication in patient care cannot be overemphasized; its effectiveness is directly linked to improved health outcomes, a principle well understood by contemporary healthcare professionals (Zeppenfeld et al., 2022; Halvorsen et al., 2022) (Figure 4.12).

4.5.3. Case Management and Follow-Up

Optimal follow-up and case management are essential components of preoperative optimization and evaluation. Care coordination between various health care providers facilitates patients having optimal, patient-specific strategies for their medical needs, risk factors, and preferences. Multidisciplinary team members involved in case management not only enhance communication but also maximize the quality of care provided. For instance, a surgical team, in collaboration with oncologists, physical therapists, and nutritionists, can best address the intricacies of preoperative optimization, especially for patients undergoing major surgery. Standard terminologies and documentation standards are of utmost importance because they facilitate better communication among clinicians and, consequently, improve clinical outcomes for surgically treated patients (Negoi, 2025). Besides, regular follow-up protocols need to be established to monitor patients' post-surgery and act early in the event of complications. Regular assessment through clinical examination and laboratory workup is crucial for identifying and addressing potential postoperative issues, such as infection, hemorrhage, or the need for further interventions. Best practice recommendations are that follow-up should include patient-reported outcomes and physical examination in an integrated monitoring process for recovery. Realignment of the management plan to future needs during this follow-up period can significantly affect recovery pathways and overall patient safety. Proactive intervention strategies and regular monitoring can mitigate risks within the healthcare system and ensure optimal recovery in the postoperative period (Abdulwahid et al., 2025). Case management and follow-up are therefore essential pillars of preoperative assessment and optimization. By designing structured care pathways that emphasize teamwork and communication among healthcare professionals, patients can be duly attended to according to their individual needs before and after surgery. Involvement of case management practices will likely rise individualized care plans that consider the patient's medical history and current health status, attaining the concept of patient-centered care. In doing so, healthcare providers cannot only enhance surgical outcomes but also the overall quality of the healthcare experience, positioning patients for successful recovery and improved long-term prognoses. Continued follow-up procedures also safeguard the significance of tracking patient progress, thereby ensuring the delivery of the highest possible levels of care throughout the surgical process (Negoi, 2025).

Test Your Knowledge

1. How does collaboration among anesthesiologists, surgeons, nurses, and other healthcare professionals improve patient safety and outcomes during anesthesia?
2. What specific roles do different members of the multidisciplinary team play in preoperative, intraoperative, and postoperative anesthetic care?

4.6. Challenges in Preoperative Assessment

Learning Outcome

1. Variability in patient presentations
2. Limitations of current assessment tools
3. Addressing patient anxiety and compliance

Preoperative assessment is riddled with challenges that can significantly influence surgical outcome. Among the significant challenges is variability in patients' medical histories and comorbidities, which require individualized assessments. Conditions such as diabetes, hypertension, and obesity, which are common among surgical candidates, must be assessed in detail to ensure maximum patient safety. Certain patients, particularly those who are to undergo body contouring in the aftermath of extensive weight loss, possess nuances in their physiological status that complicate surgical planning. These nuances necessitate that health care providers develop individualized preoperative assessments that account for unique medical histories and potential intraoperative complications. Comprehensive evaluations integrating medical history, current health status, and anticipated surgical requirements are required to eliminate surgical risks, thereby emphasizing the significance of a cautious approach in preoperative evaluations (Giordano et al., 2025). Added to individual patient evaluation challenges is the ongoing need for innovation in risk-stratification methods. Preoperative assessment typically struggles to strike a balance among the intricate interplay of surgical risk, medical stability, and individual patient factors. Patients with complex congenital heart disease (ACHD) present a unique group that necessitates advanced preoperative planning due to the risks of morbidity and mortality in non-cardiac surgery. These risk factors can arise with hemodynamic instability, arrhythmias, and thromboembolic events, which require careful management and multidisciplinary care. The use of risk assessment tools and protocols for high-risk patients will further assist in stratifying surgical candidates. Therefore, the use of these precise methodologies can make surgical procedures safer and more effective, representing a qualitative leap in preoperative assessment (Ladouceur et al., 2025). Preoperative assessment poses another challenge, as psychological factors can affect patient cooperation and surgical readiness. Both fear and anxiety about the operation process tend to keep patients away from engaging in their preoperative preparation, including basic lifestyle modifications and adherence to medical routines. Furthermore, the heavy emotional load placed upon patients undergoing complex surgical procedures warrants a holistic strategy for preoperative assessment, including attending to mental well-being as well as physical health. Offering psychological counsel or therapy may be paramount in countering preoperative anxiety, thereby enhancing patient outcomes and improving postoperative recovery rates. Finally, surmounting these psychological challenges in tandem with physical examination can lead to an improved optimization process, ensuring that patients are not only physically but also psychologically set to overcome the challenges of the surgical path before them (Giordano et al., 2025) (Figure 4.13).

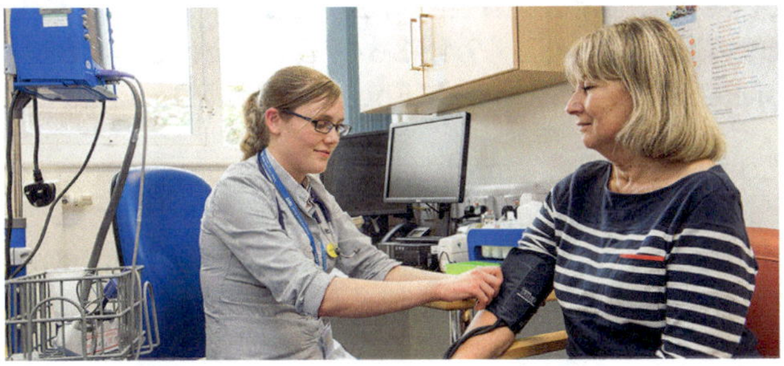

Figure 4.13. The preoperative assessment phase is fraught with numerous challenges that can significantly impact surgical outcomes.

Source: https://www.torbayandsouthdevon.nhs.uk/uploads/peripoperative_medicine_patient_having_blood_pressure_taken.jpg.

4.6.1. Variability in Patient Presentations

Interpatient variation in clinical presentation can significantly affect the preoperative assessment and optimization process. Each patient presents a unique collection of medical history, comorbidities, and physiological responses that dictate their surgical risk and recovery course. Variation in age, gender, and overall health status can produce a variety of clinical presentations. Older patients, for instance, come with several comorbidities such as hypertension or diabetes that may complicate their preoperative workups. Consequently, medical practitioners must modify their assessments to account for these differences so that a complete picture of the patient's health status is obtained prior to surgery. This level of personalized assessment is critical to minimizing complications and improving postoperative outcomes, underscoring the need for individualized assessment of each patient's distinct presentation. Issues arising from variability in patient presentation go beyond medical history and border on psychological and social problems as well. Psychological preparedness is also an essential factor in the recovery of patients; therefore, the assessment should include screening for mental status, anxiety levels, and social support systems. For example, a socially supported patient would recover more easily than an otherwise unsupported one. In addition, cultural factors can influence patient expectations and communication styles, thereby complicating preoperative optimization. Under these conditions, the providers of care are required to adopt a more integrated approach with simultaneous medical and psychosocial assessment. This broad-ranged assessment prevents formulating care plans not just medically suitable but also sensitive to patients' emotional and social conditions, which can significantly affect the results of surgery. Also, identification and control of variability in patient presentation are necessary given emerging surgical technologies and methods. With more frequent use of advanced technologies in minimally invasive techniques and robotic-assisted surgical techniques, variability in presentations requires continuous reevaluation of assessment protocols. The "2022 ACC/AHA Guideline for the Diagnosis and Management of Aortic Disease" illustrates this adaptability by issuing guidelines for varying clinical presentations, from asymptomatic to symptomatic conditions (Eric et al., 2022). This adaptability is important for accommodating patients with varying risks and treatment responses. By aligning preoperative evaluation with these guidelines, clinicians can better navigate the subtleties established by patient variability and ultimately enhance surgical safety and effectiveness. Addressing variability across the full range of capabilities ensures that each patient receives individually tailored care that accounts for their unique differences and establishes the basis for optimal surgical outcomes.

4.6.2. Limitations of Current Assessment Tools

In the realm of preoperative assessment and optimization, perhaps the most significant challenge for healthcare professionals is the limitations of current assessment instruments. Traditional methods, such as medical history processes and physical examinations, often fail to capture the complex, multifaceted nature of patient health. Application of generic risk-stratification instruments, for instance, is a prime example in which the instrument will not necessarily reflect the patient's individual clinical setting. These devices are likely to overlook important aspects such as patients' psychological status, socioeconomic status, and the specific needs of planned surgical procedures. As such, there has been increased demand for more sophisticated, personalized assessment tools that can overcome these limitations and support more informed surgical decisions, ultimately improving patient outcomes. Moreover, current tools fail to incorporate newer technologies that can enhance the preoperative assessment process. For instance, the use of artificial intelligence and machine learning in test procedures could perhaps enhance risk prediction models. However, the majority of instruments remain tied to traditional methods that prioritize standardization over individualization. While AI-based techniques ensure greater efficiency and responsiveness in assessing patients, they are also limited in use.

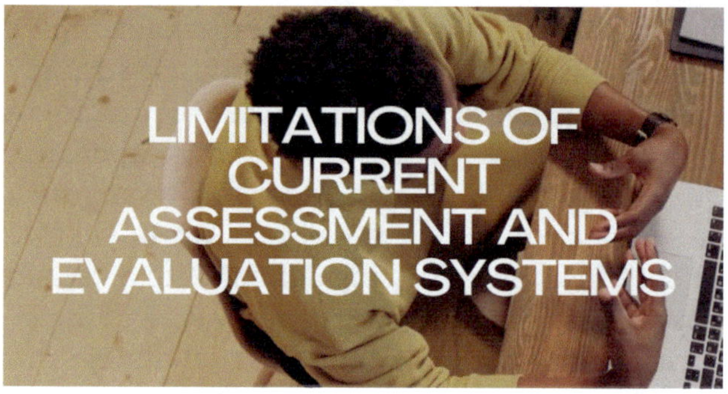

Figure 4.14. Limitations of current assessment tools.

Source: https://media.licdn.com/dms/image/v2/D5612AQEZhkdsZhlYuA/article-cover_image-shrink_720_1280/article-cover_image-shrink_720_1280/0/1714396979508?e=2147483647&v=beta&t=z8m-skP4SFizVi7J9XTe6xMFpe7BldTmiPDa-vzu270.

Complications such as false positives and restricted contextual understanding can hamper their effectiveness in application, and the suggestion is that current tools are not yet realizing the full potential of technology. The discrepancy underscores the need for ongoing research and innovation in preoperative assessment methods that leverage today's innovations to their fullest. Additionally, the functionality of preoperative assessment tools seems compromised by inconsistent application across healthcare settings. Variation in clinician training, compliance with protocols, and availability of resources could lead to disparate patient experiences and outcomes. For example, a review of current language assessment tools in language instruction suggests the potential benefits of blended assessment by incorporating traditional and new approaches to maximize breadth. This principle can be applied to the healthcare setting as well, where an interdisciplinary process—one that embraces both conventional instruments and emerging technologies—is critical to consistency and reliability. Thus, to get the most out of preoperative evaluations, it is absolutely critical that standardization be implemented in the use of such measures so that all patients receive the best and equitable care during the preoperative phase (Figure 4.14).

4.6.3. Addressing Patient Anxiety and Compliance

Preoperative anxiety among surgical patients is a significant concern that tends to have adverse effects on their short-term and long-term prognosis. Preoperation is a highly stressful time, and the majority of the patients are plagued by fear, uncertainty, and anxiety regarding undergoing the surgery. This mental stress can lead to noncompliance with preoperative instructions, which can undermine the effectiveness of subsequent recuperation procedures. Anxiety management is therefore a fundamental component of preoperative assessment and optimization. Constructing an understanding of the psychological problems at hand enables clinicians to implement interventions such as providing clear information about surgery, undertaking shared decision-making with the patient, and offering access to psychological assistance services. These measures, as well as addressing anxiety, also enhance patient compliance and engagement and improve patient-centered care, leading to the best surgical outcomes and better patient care (Carli et al., 2021). Multidisciplinary teams also contribute significantly to alleviating patient anxiety. Mental health professionals, surgeons, anesthesiologists, and nurses foster a team approach to patient care. With the inclusion of psychological testing in preoperative evaluations, teams can identify patients at high risk for anxiety and tailor interventions accordingly. This multidisciplinary model prioritizes emotional well-being as integral to physical health, thereby promoting an equitable approach to patient management. For instance, the roll-out of prehabilitation programs that encompass physical training alongside mental health support signifies a commitment towards improving both the psychological and physiological aspects of surgical care (Daniel et al., 2019).

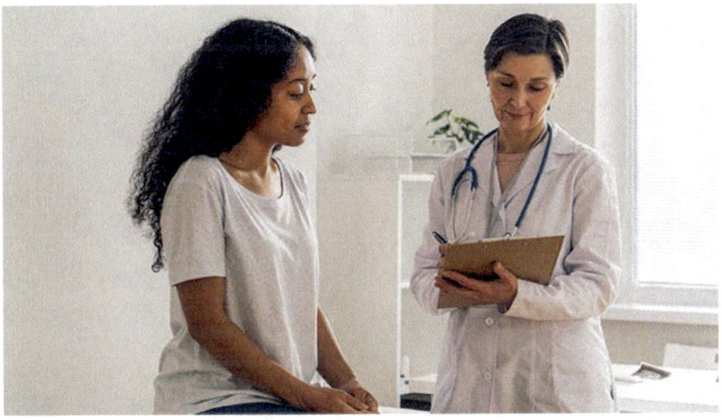

Figure 4.15. Addressing patient anxiety and compliance.

Source: https://www.apa.org/images/anxiety-tile_tcm7-310454.jpg.

Prehabilitation programs empower patients to take charge of their healing process, generating feelings of control and readiness that ultimately support medical advice and treatment adherence. Secondly, the establishing of clear lines of communication is necessary in the reduction of patient anxiety. Informed, active participants in their own care are more likely to comply with preoperative instructions and advice. Educational materials, such as information brochures or classes, can clarify the nature of surgery, the recovery time, and potential hazards, thereby removing ambiguity. Moreover, routine anxiety screenings, using standardized measures, allow clinicians to monitor and address emotional distress in a methodical way along the preoperative continuum. Besides facilitating this anticipatory process to customize patient care plans, it also enhances patients' therapeutic relationships with healthcare providers. Prioritizing mental health in the preoperative setting supports higher compliance rates and improves the likelihood of optimal postoperative outcomes (Carli et al., 2021) (Figure 4.15).

Test Your Knowledge

1. What are the common challenges faced during preoperative assessment, and how can they affect anesthesia planning?
2. How do patient-related factors, such as incomplete medical history or comorbidities, complicate preoperative evaluation and risk stratification?

SUMMARY

The optimization and preoperative evaluation process is of most significant value in the optimization of surgical outcomes and prevention of complications. Proper evaluation of a patient's overall health, including the detection of risk factors, is essential to surgical planning. Tools such as the Caprini risk score are valuable for stratifying patients by risk of venous thromboembolism (VTE) and thereby enabling individualized prophylactic therapy. As evidenced from recent studies, routine use of these risk assessment tools has been shown to significantly reduce the incidence of postoperative complications, including VTE, with effective intervention strategies (Gerhold et al., 2024). This underlines the relevance of systematic preoperative evaluation as a pillar of surgical practice. Organizational standards promulgated by organizations such as the European Society of Anaesthesiology and Intensive Care Medicine also support the preoperative evaluation framework. Clinical and organizational priorities in surgical care are promoted through orderly patient assessment by these standards. By incorporating the latest available evidence and expert consensus, practitioners are better positioned to address patient needs while minimizing surgical risks (Lamperti et al., 2024). As the surgical environment continues to change, the integration of new evaluation methods, including telemedicine and biomarkers that predict, can further optimize preoperative planning so that anesthesiologists may deliver the highest quality of care. In the end, a commitment to optimizing preoperative evaluations reflects a global philosophy of patient care and safety. By promoting teamwork among healthcare professionals, such as surgeons, anesthesiologists, and nurses, patients may benefit from a coordinated approach that addresses their specific risks and concerns. Enhanced communication and information availability, such as through electronic medical records, can help ensure that assessments are carried out smoothly, leading to better patient outcomes (Gerhold et al., 2024; Lamperti et al., 2024). In conclusion, a methodical and strict preoperative assessment not only enables detection of risks but also empowers patients by enabling informed decision-making, making the surgical process both safer and more efficient.

In pursuing quality preoperative assessment and optimization, several salient points underscore the value of this process in enhancing patient outcomes. To begin with, a thorough scrutiny of a patient's medical history and present status can uncover potential risk factors that may complicate surgeries. For instance, comorbidities such as cardiovascular disease or diabetes can help clinicians develop specially tailored anesthetic and surgical plans to mitigate risks. Furthermore, preoperative optimization, from lifestyle modification to proper medical care, can significantly help prepare patients for surgery. Anticipatory planning, backed by evidence from peer-reviewed articles, allows for the prevention of post-operative complications, resulting in improved recovery as well as reduced lengths of stay. Another important aspect of preoperative evaluation is that it helps stratify risk for certain patient groups, particularly the elderly. Literature calls out for the fact that older persons commonly present with geriatric frailties, whose enhancement of the complexity of surgical care and resultant effect on postoperative outcome cannot be overlooked. Identification of these frailties, through complete evaluations, enables the clinician to implement appropriate interventions that decrease the' risk of complications. For example, in the reports of geriatric patients undergoing CAR-T treatment, high-vulnerability patients had significant toxicity and unfavorable outcomes. This underscores the importance of a high-quality preoperative evaluation that considers not just standard medical assessment but also functional and psychosocial factors in tailoring surgical intervention to individual needs. Furthermore, the use of continuous surveillance and data collection within the preoperative process can go a long way in making patient care more efficient. With the use of systemic surveillance networks, such as the RespiVirNet surveillance system, medical professionals can gain information on disease epidemiological patterns, including seasonal influenza, which may affect surgical schedules and patient well-being. For instance, understanding the duration and severity of flu outbreaks can guide immunization policies that ultimately condition patients more effectively for surgery. Such types of interventions enable both the clinical and administrative aspects of surgical treatment to be handled in an integrated fashion. In conclusion, proper preoperative evaluation and optimization are critical to surgical outcomes, as they enable risks to be identified and addressed while also enabling individualized care strategies across various patient populations.

KEY TERMS FROM THIS CHAPTER

- Blood glucose
- Chronic health conditions
- Demographic
- Holistic approach
- Multidisciplinary surgical pause committees (MDSPCs)
- Phenotypic information
- Surgical intervention
- Chronic diseases
- Collaboration
- Healthcare professionals
- Mitigate postoperative anxiety
- Nutritional
- Psychological health
- Surgical site infections (SSI)

CRITICAL THINKING QUESTIONS

1. **What is the primary goal of preoperative assessment?**
   a. Diagnose underlying conditions
   b. Identify and optimize risk factors for surgery
   c. Reduce the duration of the surgery
   d. Choose the type of anesthesia to be used
2. **Which classification system is commonly used to assess a patient's physical status before anesthesia?**
   a. Glasgow Coma Scale
   b. ASA Physical Status Classification
   c. APACHE Score
   d. RASS Score
3. **Which of the following conditions is most critical to evaluate during a preoperative cardiac assessment?**
   a. Hypertension
   b. Coronary artery disease
   c. Varicose veins
   d. Tachycardia
4. **Which laboratory test is essential for a patient on anticoagulation therapy prior to surgery?**
   a. Complete blood count (CBC)
   b. Liver function tests (LFT)
   c. Prothrombin time (PT) and INR
   d. Serum electrolytes
5. **What is a key component of the airway evaluation during preoperative assessment?**
   a. Thyroid size
   b. Mallampati score
   c. Tracheal deviation
   d. Respiratory rate

Short Answer Questions

1. Explain the importance of preoperative assessment in ensuring patient safety and optimizing surgical outcomes.
2. Describe the American Society of Anesthesiologists (ASA) Physical Status Classification System and its relevance in preoperative evaluation.
3. What are the key components of a thorough preoperative history and physical examination?
4. Discuss the role of laboratory and diagnostic tests in preoperative assessment. Which tests are mandatory, and which are patient-specific?
5. Explain the significance of airway assessment in preoperative evaluation and the methods used to predict difficult intubation.
6. How are patients with diabetes mellitus managed preoperatively to reduce the risk of complications?

Answer to Critical Thinking Questions

1. (b); 2. (b); 3. (b); 4. (c); 5. (b)

REFERENCES

1. Ballacchino, M. M., McQuestion, C. C., Giuca, M. S., Dosluoglu, H. H., & Nader, N. D. (2024). The use of frailty scores for screening the surgical risk benefits. *Annals of Surgery*. https://doi.org/10.1097/sla.0000000000006452Boccalini, S., & Bechini, A. (2024). Assessment of epidemiological trend of influenza-like illness in Italy from 2010/2011 to 2023/2024 season: Key points to optimize future vaccination strategies against influenza. *Vaccines, 12*. https://www.semanticscholar.org/paper/f7bd71087eef5e21f2a609da4f21aedad9bfc362 (accessed on 28th June 2025).
2. Carli, F., Awasthi, R., Gillis, C., Baldini, G., Bessissow, A., Liberman, A. S., & Minnella, E. M. (2021). Integrating prehabilitation in the preoperative clinic: A paradigm shifts in perioperative care. *Anesthesia & Analgesia*. https://doi.org/10.1213/ane.0000000000005471 (accessed on 28th June 2025).
3. Davies, M. J., D'Alessio, D. A., Fradkin, J., Kernan, W. N., Mathieu, C., Mingrone, G., Rossing, P., et al. (2018). Management of hyperglycemia in type 2 diabetes, 2018: A consensus report by the American Diabetes Association (ADA) and the European Association for the Study of Diabetes (EASD). *Diabetes Care, 41*, 2669–2701. https://doi.org/10.2337/dci18-0033 (accessed on 28th June 2025).
4. Engelman, D. T., Ben Ali, W., Williams, J. B., Perrault, L. P., Reddy, V. S., Arora, R. C., Roselli, E. E., et al. (2019). Guidelines for perioperative care in cardiac surgery. *JAMA Surgery, 154*, 755–755. https://doi.org/10.1001/jamasurg.2019.1153 (accessed on 28th June 2025).
5. Englesbe, M., Friedman, J., Lussiez, A., Sullivan, C., et al. (2015). Implications of sarcopenia in major surgery. http://deepblue.lib.umich.edu/bitstream/2027.42/141677/1/ncp0175.pdf (accessed on 28th June 2025).
6. Fiddes, R. A., & McCaffrey, N. (2024). Preoperative smoking-cessation interventions to prevent postoperative complications: A quality assessment and overview of systematic review evidence. *Anesthesia & Analgesia, 140*, 1377–1387. https://www.semanticscholar.org/paper/1a2078ede6dfb82bea504a36e38f04bb58fa0450 (accessed on 28th June 2025).
7. Galieri, G., Orlando, V., Mazzucchi, E., Pignotti, F., Cusumano, D., Bazzu, P., Mantini, S., et al. (2025). Psychopathological influences on surgical and clinical outcomes in lumbar disk herniation: Prediction models and literature analysis. *Journal of Personalized Medicine, 15*. https://www.semanticscholar.org/paper/3edab640ab108def1706060841825ca90177ea43 (accessed on 28th June 2025).
8. Garousi, V., Joy, N., Jafarov, Z., Kelecs, A. B., Deugirmenci, S., Ozdemir, E., & Zarringhalami, R. (2024). AI-powered software testing tools: A systematic review and empirical assessment of their features and limitations. https://www.semanticscholar.org/paper/94f31fbe8a20d0e97bf489490e6af4d9c2b9b06f (accessed on 28th June 2025).
9. Gerhold, C., McLoughlin, L. T., Culpepper, B., Contractor, R. N., & Regan, T. (2024). Best practices for optimizing patients undergoing surgical procedures to prevent postoperative venous thromboembolism: A quality improvement project. *Cureus, 16*. https://www.semanticscholar.org/paper/73155ba3c609b41915495ee32ac96bee9d04faf1 (accessed on 28th June 2025).
10. Giordano, S., Salval, A., di Summa, P. G., & Oranges, C. M. (2025). Evolving body contouring strategies for patients after massive weight loss: Insights from bariatric and pharmacologic

interventions. *Surgeries*. https://www.semanticscholar.org/paper/97294c10d2de176fca612e3d2e94656e5c569838 (accessed on 28th June 2025).

11. Grant, M. C., Crisafi, C., Alvarez, A., Arora, R. C., Brindle, M. E., Chatterjee, S., Ender, J., et al. (2024). Perioperative care in cardiac surgery: A joint consensus statement by the Enhanced Recovery After Surgery (ERAS) Cardiac Society, ERAS International Society, and The Society of Thoracic Surgeons (STS). *The Annals of Thoracic Surgery, 117*, 669–689. https://doi.org/10.1016/j.athoracsur.2023.12.006 (accessed on 28th June 2025).
12. Halvorsen, S., Mehilli, J., Cassese, S., Hall, T. S., Abdelhamid, M., Barbato, E., De Hert, S., et al. (2022). 2022 ESC guidelines on cardiovascular assessment and management of patients undergoing non-cardiac surgery. *European Heart Journal, 43*, 3826–3924. https://doi.org/10.1093/eurheartj/ehac270 (accessed on 28th June 2025).
13. Hedrick, T. (2023). Perioperative assessment and optimization in major colorectal surgery. *Clinics in Colon and Rectal Surgery, 36*, 159–160. https://www.semanticscholar.org/paper/73355e56b3def232ed99af11f08a6d41c46e69ed (accessed on 28th June 2025).
14. Holubar, S. D., Lightner, A. L., Poylin, V., Vogel, J. D., Gaertner, W. B., Davis, B. R., Davis, K. G., et al. (2021). The American Society of Colon and Rectal Surgeons clinical practice guidelines for the surgical management of ulcerative colitis. *Diseases of the Colon & Rectum, 64*, 783–804. https://doi.org/10.1097/dcr.0000000000002037 (accessed on 28th June 2025).
15. Homaee, L. (2025). eP89 the role of frailty assessment in enhancing surgical outcomes in emergency general surgery. *British Journal of Surgery*. https://www.semanticscholar.org/paper/afbb5a3c46d5ddc0855a3ddf8941321803ff9900 (accessed on 28th June 2025).
16. Isselbacher, E. M., Preventza, O., Black, J. H., Augoustides, J., Beck, A. W., Bolen, M. A., Braverman, A. C., et al. (2022). 2022 ACC/AHA guideline for the diagnosis and management of aortic disease. *Circulation, 146*. https://doi.org/10.1161/cir.0000000000001106 (accessed on 28th June 2025).
17. Jalanko, T., Koskinen, I., Sammaltupa, H., Vasarainen, H., Hemminki, O., & Sairanen, J. (2025). IP24-16 Upgraded preoperative medical optimization and prehabilitation in ERAS radical cystectomy: A propensity scores matched analysis of clinical outcomes compared to basic ERAS and standard care protocols. *The Journal of Urology, 213*, e1269. https://www.semanticscholar.org/paper/b93aeda7346b82c93b002ff34b78c2e20d6e6c19 (accessed on 28th June 2025).
18. Jalanko, T., Sammaltupa, H., Koskinen, I., Vasarainen, H., Hemminki, O., & Sairanen, J. (2025). IP24-15 Upgraded preoperative medical optimization and prehabilitation in ERAS radical cystectomy: Preoperative test outcomes and risk factors for postoperative morbidity. *The Journal of Urology, 213*, e1269. https://www.semanticscholar.org/paper/1205eee2fe10d020f582765348f26e81d25919b1 (accessed on 28th June 2025).
19. Kamlesh, K., & Prajapati, H. (2025). Optimizing preoperative assessment and preparation for safe pediatric anesthesia. *International Journal of Anesthesiology Sciences*. https://www.semanticscholar.org/paper/4d9bc49ea5edc8d503ea095bb773f935556b5937 (accessed on 28th June 2025).
20. Kedar, P., Bhattacharya, S., Kanugo, A., & Prajapati, B. (2025). Novel strategies for the treatment of lung cancer: An in-depth analysis of the use of immunotherapy, precision medicine, and artificial intelligence to improve prognoses. *Current Medicinal Chemistry*. https://www.semanticscholar.org/paper/853db4e5b8034820218c92475fe44a3be47a7b80 (accessed on

28th June 2025).

21. Kim, D. H., Afilalo, J., Shi, S., Popma, J. J., Khabbaz, K. R., Laham, R. J., Grodstein, F., et al. (2019). Evaluation of changes in functional status in the year after aortic valve replacement. *JAMA Internal Medicine, 179*, 383–383. https://doi.org/10.1001/jamainternmed.2018.6738 (accessed on 28th June 2025).

22. Kuddah, N., & Sholehah, L. F. (2025). Standardized nutritional care process management of pediatric patients with congenital heart disease and malnutrition. *JURNAL KESMAS DAN GIZI (JKG)*. https://www.semanticscholar.org/paper/729abe652079483514cffc661ac8143bbc94aedc (accessed on 28th June 2025).

23. Ladouceur, M., Valacco, L., Ltaief, Z., Rutz, T., Hascoet, S., & Bouchardy, J. (2025). Perioperative risk in adults with congenital heart disease undergoing non-cardiac surgery: Challenges and tailored strategies. *Journal of Clinical Medicine, 14*. https://www.semanticscholar.org/paper/beef2a81d642fb44765a2f38830fe2fe11fd1556 (accessed on 28th June 2025).

24. Lamperti, M., Romero, C. S., Guarracino, F., Cammarota, G., Vetrugno, L., Tufegdzic, B., Lozsan, F., et al. (2024). Preoperative assessment of adults undergoing elective noncardiac surgery. *European Journal of Anesthesiology, 42*, 1–35. https://www.semanticscholar.org/paper/b393522135f88ca3555eccbfe8de1f54a6b49b6c (accessed on 28th June 2025).

25. Lepage, M. A., Lecavalier, A., Baldini, G., Sun, N. Z., & Bessissow, A. (2025). Preoperative risk assessment and optimization integrating surgical and anesthetic principles and practices: A national survey for internists. *Perioperative Medicine, 14*. https://www.semanticscholar.org/paper/82b4f2e40f545326bf52d56bbf9a320c6c15c160 (accessed on 28th June 2025).

26. Liou, D. Z., & Berry, M. F. (2017). Thoracic surgery considerations in obese patients. *Deleted Journal, 28*, 27–41. https://doi.org/10.1016/j.thorsurg.2017.09.004 (accessed on 28th June 2025).

27. Lyon, A. R., López-Fernández, T., Couch, L. S., Asteggiano, R., Aznar, M. C., Bergler-Klein, J., Boriani, G., et al. (2022). 2022 ESC guidelines on cardio-oncology developed in collaboration with the European Hematology Association (EHA), the European Society for Therapeutic Radiology and Oncology (ESTRO) and the International Cardio-Oncology Society (IC-OS). *European Heart Journal, 43*, 4229–4361. https://doi.org/10.1093/eurheartj/ehac244 (accessed on 28th June 2025).

28. Marchis, I. F., Negruț, M., Blebea, C., Crihan, M., Alexa, A., & Breazu, C. (2024). Trends in preoperative airway assessment. *Diagnostics, 14*. https://www.semanticscholar.org/paper/0e88e1669983a08e83ee6a3a3a0f2452fffdbe19 (accessed on 28th June 2025).

29. Mustafa, M. J., Abbas, F., Shah, S. H., Qureshi, M. B., Waqar, H., Sulaiman, M., & Adeel-ur-Rehman. (2025). Predictors of post-surgical pulmonary complications and strategies for risk reduction. *Insights-Journal of Life and Social Sciences*. https://www.semanticscholar.org/paper/0a545b6c4069ac5099884d345ed06c3bbbf33f68 (accessed on 28th June 2025).

30. Negoi. (2025). Guidance for the management of rectal cancer: An umbrella review of existing guidelines regarding surgical anatomy, adjuvant therapy, follow-up and surveillance, specific considerations, documentation, and palliative care. *Cureus, 17*. https://www.semanticscholar.org/paper/3769b53d1daf0646f4a0d0936023e161e5c53bb4 (accessed on 28th June 2025).

31. Omar, O. (2025). Blockchain assisted Al-Biruni earth radius optimization with deep learning model for sustainable healthcare disease detection. *Journal of*

Cybersecurity and Information Management. https://www.semanticscholar.org/paper/be52a370e900af50c032b9efc3b13cafb14dc43f (accessed on 28th June 2025).

32. Paluanova, K. (2024). Evaluating pragmatic competence in language learners through an assessment of current measurement tools. *Emergent: Journal of Educational Discoveries and Lifelong Learning (EJEDL)*. https://www.semanticscholar.org/paper/ed7aae21baa51d90d8b6754644b7cda78013760d (accessed on 28th June 2025).
33. Paredes, A. Z., Hyer, J. M., Díaz, A., Tsilimigras, D. I., & Pawlik, T. M. (2020). The impact of mental illness on postoperative outcomes among Medicare beneficiaries. *Annals of Surgery, 272*, 419–425. https://doi.org/10.1097/sla.0000000000004118 (accessed on 28th June 2025).
34. Poldermans, D., Bax, J. J., Boersma, E., De Hert, S., Eeckhout, E., Fowkes, G., Gorenek, B., et al. (2009). Guidelines for pre-operative cardiac risk assessment and perioperative cardiac management in non-cardiac surgery: The Task Force of the European Society of Cardiology (ESC), endorsed by the European Society of Anesthesiology (ESA). https://core.ac.uk/download/55798032.pdf (accessed on 28th June 2025).
35. Salih, A. M., Qaradakhy, A. J., Ahmed, S. F., Ali, R. M., Baba, H. O., Abdullah, A. M., Habibullah, I. J., et al. (2025). Primary thyroid non-Hodgkin B-cell lymphoma: A case series. *Barw Medical Journal*. https://www.semanticscholar.org/paper/2156fa9883910ee072db0818248bb045f9737b08 (accessed on 28th June 2025).
36. Savery, K. E., Kleiman, A., & Walters, S. M. (2023). Preoperative assessment and optimization of cardiopulmonary disease in noncardiac surgery. *Clinics in Colon and Rectal Surgery, 36*, 167–174. https://www.semanticscholar.org/paper/b1e1c073ed00418a5570f973fa9fb5c58f05a11d (accessed on 28th June 2025).
37. Sigurdardóttir, M., Sigurdsson, M., Vias, R. D., Ólafsson, Y., Gunnarsdottir, I., Sigurdsson, E. L., & Kárason, S. (2024). Preoperative optimization of modifiable risk factors is associated with decreased superficial surgical site infections after total joint arthroplasty: A prospective case-control study. *Acta Orthopaedical, 95*, 392–400. https://www.semanticscholar.org/paper/09b1a844fb54b4feeba4f50c8b51514b6f3f5f6f (accessed on 28th June 2025).
38. Turan, E. I., Baydemir, A. E., Şahin, A., & Özcan, F. G. (2025). Effectiveness of ChatGPT-4 in predicting the human decision to send patients to the postoperative intensive care unit: A prospective multicentric study. *Minerva Anesthesiologic*. https://www.semanticscholar.org/paper/81043ad93d473c393ed9288620b21f8fb8f0b840 (accessed on 28th June 2025).
39. Urs, A. D. (2025). Blockchain for secure 3D model sharing among healthcare providers: Exploring decentralized methods to prevent unauthorized access to medical models. *International Journal for Multidisciplinary Research*. https://www.semanticscholar.org/paper/7a2a964483ae0014d382cc481a3bee47c0c9a276 (accessed on 28th June 2025).
40. Vogel, J. D., Felder, S., Bhama, A. R., Hawkins, A. T., Langenfeld, S. J., Shaffer, V., Thorsen, A. J., et al. (2021). The American Society of Colon and Rectal Surgeons clinical practice guidelines for the management of colon cancer. *Diseases of the Colon & Rectum, 65*, 148–177. https://doi.org/10.1097/dcr.0000000000002323 (accessed on 28th June 2025).
41. Yates, S. J., Cursio, J., Artz, A. S., Kordas, K., Bishop, M. R., Derman, B., Kosuri, S., et al. (2024). Optimization of older adults by a geriatric assessment–guided multidisciplinary clinic before CAR T-cell therapy. *Blood Advances, 8*, 3785–3797. https://www.semanticscholar.org/paper/e097827d5d1472195c990b212c05e67040c11592 (accessed on 28th June 2025).

42. You, Y. T., Hardiman, K. M., Bafford, A. C., Poylin, V., Francone, T. D., Davis, K. G., Paquette, I. M., et al. (2020). The American Society of Colon and Rectal Surgeons clinical practice guidelines for the management of rectal cancer. *Diseases of the Colon & Rectum, 63*, 1191–1222. https://doi.org/10.1097/dcr.0000000000001762 (accessed on 28th June 2025).

43. Zeppenfeld, K., Tfelt-Hansen, J., Riva, M., Winkel, B. G., Behr, E. R., Blom, N. A., Charron, P., et al. (2022). 2022 ESC guidelines for the management of patients with ventricular arrhythmias and the prevention of sudden cardiac death. *European Heart Journal, 43*, 3997–4126. https://doi.org/10.1093/eurheartj/ehac262 (accessed on 28th June 2025).

AIRWAY MANAGEMENT IN ANESTHESIA

5

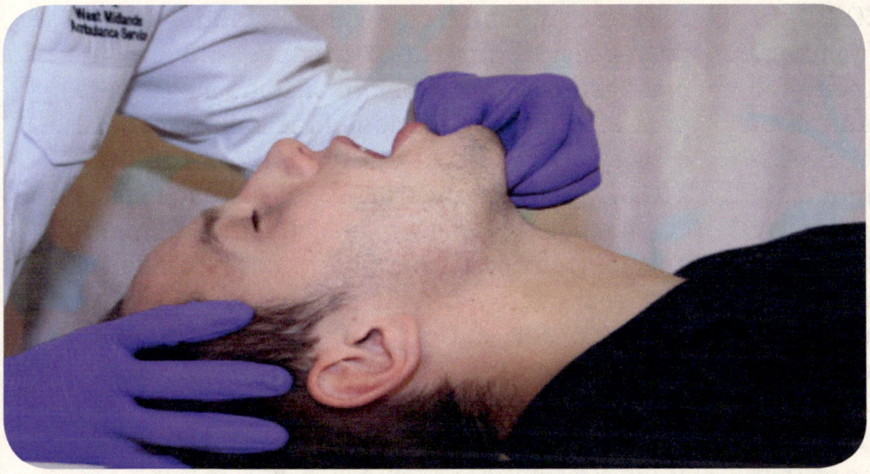

LEARNING OBJECTIVES

After studying this chapter, you will be able to:

1. Discuss the anatomy of the airway
2. Focus on the assessment of the airway
3. Explain the airway management techniques
4. Understand complications in airway management
5. Learn about advances in airway management
6. Explain the role of anesthesiologists in airway management

Introduction

Airway management in anesthesia is a core element of anesthetic care that directly affects patient safety and outcome. Sustained maintenance of an open airway is crucial for maximum benefit, particularly in the operating room setting, where patient physiology is deliberately manipulated by anesthesia. Airway management proves challenging across diverse patient populations, including adults and pediatrics, with its attendant baggage. Effective airway management methods involve both a well-defined set of protocols and the ability to support unforeseen events, typically determined by the patient's anatomy and the type of surgery. Thus, anesthesiologists must possess the knowledge and skills to make decisions to ensure proper airway support throughout the duration of an operation. Anesthesia procedures have evolved significantly over time and have made a significant contribution to airway management. In the past, inhalational anesthesia has been the norm, especially in pediatric airway surgery, where a balanced anesthetic condition is paramount. Recently, however, the advent of total intravenous anesthesia (TIVA) has fueled considerable debate within the medical community about its merits and demerits under different conditions. Providers often debate the effectiveness, safety, and cost-effectiveness of volatile anesthetics and TIVA to select the most appropriate agent for a given clinical scenario. Such ongoing review of anesthesia modalities is a demonstration of an adaptive practice environment in which evolving evidence and clinical experience shape decisions regarding airway management. In addition, emerging challenges, such as the COVID-19 pandemic, have reiterated the importance of new approaches to airway management for surgical interventions. The implementation of protection strategies, as demonstrated by Brown et al., has become paramount for minimizing the risk of viral transmission during airway manipulation procedures (Yang et al., 2020). These advancements have precipitated the sharing of clinical practices and modifications to enhance patient safety without diminishing employee protection. Airway management during anesthesia requires a nexus of traditional practices with contemporary innovations so that anesthesiologists can be prepared to counteract the challenges of varying clinical situations and deliver optimal patient care outcomes.

Definition of Airway Management

Maximum airway management is essential for anesthesia, which encompasses various airway procedures and techniques for ensuring airway patency during surgery. The primary purpose is the prevention of airway obstruction, enabling suitable ventilation and oxygenation of the patients. Maximized airway management not only minimizes the risk for respiratory complications but also promotes effective anesthetic delivery during the procedure. In this case, recognition of anatomical variation and potential challenges presented by a patient's airway is valuable to anesthesia providers. Preoperative assessment must include examination of the airway to identify any anatomical abnormalities so that the anesthesiologist is adequately prepared for potential difficulties with intubation or mask ventilation. Therefore, airway management is an active element of anesthetic care that requires both knowledge and technical expertise to address a range of clinical situations. In children, airway management assumes even greater significance, especially in relation to sedation management. The American Academy of Pediatric Dentistry and the American Academy of Pediatrics offer an orderly plan for the safe sedation of children, which includes many prerequisites for the procedure and airway management. Key elements include a complete pre-sedation examination of the child's medical history, with attention to potential airway pathology such as obstructive tonsils, and the use of age-specific airway management equipment. The ability to understand the pharmacokinetics and respiratory effects of selected drugs is essential for maintaining airway integrity during the process. Apart from these elements, good airway management enhances patient safety and minimizes the fear of anesthesia among practitioners and parents, making the surgical experience easier. In the realm of progressive challenges, airway management skills have also progressed over time to support contemporary clinical practices. Professionals are increasingly being asked to embrace holistic interventions that consider patient safety, speed of intervention, and efficiency of airway control methods in anesthesia. The use of advanced technology enables greater precision in assessing airway structures and responses, enhancing medical teams' capacity to respond quickly to complications. Furthermore, the need for multi-disciplinary coordination within surgical teams underscores the value of anesthesiologists in ensuring ongoing coordination of airway resources. Overall, organized airway management in the context of anesthesia is not just a technical skill profile but also involves a highly interactive understanding of patient-specific variables and cooperative dynamics that are inherent in current surgical practice, all of which are committed to ensuring optimal patient care under conditions of complexity in surgical procedures (Figure 5.1).

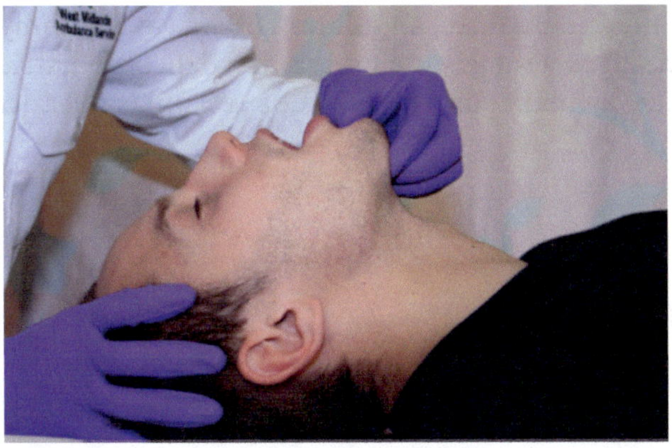

Figure 5.1. Airway management is essential in anesthesia.

Source: https://i0.wp.com/nursekey.com/wp-content/uploads/2017/05/fig1_5.jpg?w=960.

Importance in Anesthesia Practice

The significance of proper airway management in anesthesiology cannot be overstated, as it directly affects patient outcomes and the safety of healthcare providers. Anesthetists must have adequate knowledge of a range of airway management techniques, as they must tailor their practices to each patient's unique needs. During endotracheal intubation procedures, hazards related to aerosol-generating procedures, especially infectious diseases such as COVID-19, underscore the importance of stringent infection control measures. Through such awareness, healthcare workers minimize contact with potential pathogens and, therefore, ensure their own safety as well as that of patients. Effective airway management not only provides the smooth progression of surgical interventions but is also a part of the overall risk management strategy for the administration of anesthesia, stressing the importance of ongoing education and adherence to established guidelines, as mentioned in Chan et al. (2020), Beverley (2020). A critical aspect of airway management during anesthesia includes the application of proper protective measures to reduce the risk of cross-contamination. Given the particular challenges posed by respiratory diseases, including COVID-19, the use of personal protective equipment (PPE) has been prioritized. The World Health Organization and health agencies have emphasized that long-term strategies must include the proper use of PPE when performing high-risk procedures such as intubation.

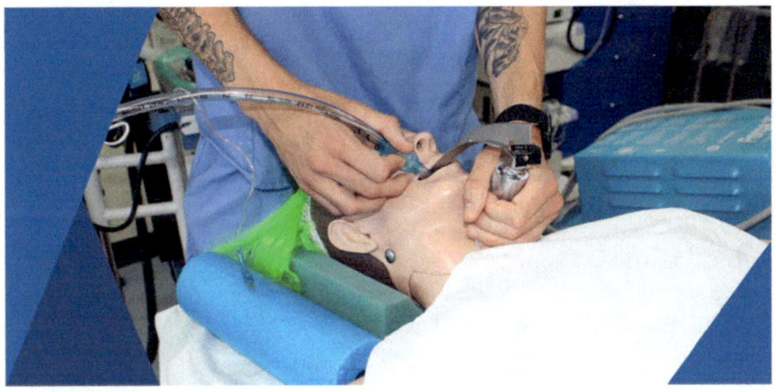

Figure 5.2. The significance of effective airway management in anesthesia practice.

Source: https://storage.googleapis.com/aims-edu/images/000/002/028/lead/01-Everything-you-should-know-before-becoming-an-anesthesia-technician.jpg.

Use of N95 respirators, face shields, and gowns recommendations are not just meant to protect the healthcare workers but also maximize patient safety. Implementation of proper airway management and PPE guidelines facilitates anesthesiologists to be sufficiently prepared to manage oncoming issues in their profession, thereby enhancing the quality and safety of care offered, according to Chan et al. (2020), Beverley (2020). In short, the critical importance of airway management in anesthetic practice is beyond technical competency in ventilation and intubation. It is a multifaceted intervention that entails the dissemination of information, adherence to infection control procedures, and the application of strict safety processes. The evolution of anesthetic practice, particularly in the face of changing health emergencies, is critical in encouraging continuous education and improvisation among anesthesiologists. The rapid exchange and implementation of updated guidelines help build healthcare systems to address potential hazards, underscoring the power of knowledge transfer to enhance patient care outcomes. Where anesthesiology grapples with challenges of airway management, it is apparent that emphasis on preventing infections and protecting workers remains the core, as reaffirmed in Chan et al. (2020), Beverley (2020) (Figure 5.2).

5.1. Anatomy of the Airway

Learning Outcome

1. Upper airway structures
2. Lower airway structures
3. Physiological considerations

Airway anatomy is highly relevant to anesthetic practice, demanding a broad knowledge base for airway management. The airway includes several structures extending from the nasal cavity to the lungs and comprises the pharynx, larynx, and trachea. Each part of the airway presents certain challenges, particularly in patients with unique anatomical differences, such as children and those with congenital abnormalities. Potential airway obstruction, especially in the case of sedation or anesthesia, emphasizes the importance of proper anatomical knowledge during preoperative assessment. Abnormalities such as large tonsils or a narrow airway can obstruct airflow and therefore require careful investigation and planning before any anesthetic intervention. Without accurate knowledge of these anatomical specifics, practitioners are at increased risk of airway management complications, underscoring the importance of comprehensive anatomical training in the clinical environment. Anatomical differences are more pronounced in pediatric cases, whose airways significantly differ from those of adults. Children have proportionally larger tongues and shorter, narrower tracheostomies, which make intubation and ventilatory support procedures difficult. Besides, angulation of airway anatomy changes with advancing age, and hence, pediatric airway management as a subspecialty is needed.

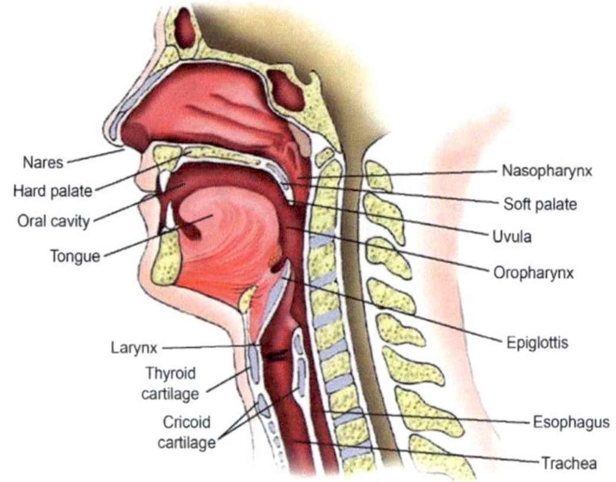

Figure 5.3. The anatomy of the airway plays a crucial role in the practice of anesthesia.

Source: https://i.pinimg.com/736x/36/a9/60/36a960f3afb5279af07d0b3211e4803b.jpg.

The latest literature focuses on the use of specialized techniques and equipment, especially to leverage the unique airway anatomy of children. A case in point is video laryngoscopy, which has been effective in maximizing rates of successful tracheal intubation in infants and improving the overall safety of airway management procedures. This targeted approach reflects growing recognition of the need to adopt pediatric-specific methods in anesthetic practice, with the risk of airway management morbidity remaining abysmally high in this age group (Hsu et al., 2021). The sequential strategy for sedation and airway management in pediatric patients also underscores the integration of anatomy into clinical standards. A thorough pre-sedation evaluation is essential to identify underlying medical issues and anatomical abnormalities that can increase a child's risk during sedation

(Charles et al., 2019). Anatomical peculiarities of patients are essential in individualized anesthesia management, establishing the depth of sedation, airway control, and application of proper pharmacological agents. Contributing to this complexity is the interface between anatomical abnormalities and the pharmacokinetics of sedative medications. Therefore, clear guidelines and protocols explicitly targeted towards the pediatric population are needed not only for effective airway management but also for perioperative safety in general, to allow practitioners to respond to the unique needs of their pediatric patients (Figure 5.3).

5.1.1. Upper Airway Structures

The upper airway structures play an important role in airway management during anesthesia, not only as conduits through which air can be introduced into the lungs but also as barriers against aspirated material. These include the nasal passages, oral cavity, pharynx, and larynx, all of which have unique contributions to respiration and phonation. Understanding of the anatomical and physiological characteristics of these structures is critical to anesthesiologists, since variations could influence ease of intubation and risk of procedural complications. Obesity or craniofacial deformities, for instance, could lead to alterations in these upper airway structures, which increase the risk of airway obstruction and subsequent selection of anesthetic techniques. The importance of such variations demands meticulous preoperative planning and evaluation to achieve optimal airway management with the lowest risk of anesthesia-related complications. In emergency circumstances or during unexpected intubation difficulties, the integrity of the upper airway structures is further highlighted. Professionals need to be proficient in both recognizing signs of airway compromise and using intervention modalities. As highlighted by recent findings, unrecognized esophageal intubation is a risk-prone phenomenon that can result in severe outcomes, including severe hypoxemia and brain damage. In an attempt to minimize such risks, anesthesiologists are mandated to use reliable detection methods, such as waveform capnography, to verify appropriate tracheal tube placement. This not only emphasizes the role of these structures in the upper airway for successful ventilation but also underscores the need for early and effective action in the event of potential failures in airway management (Chrimes et al., 2022).

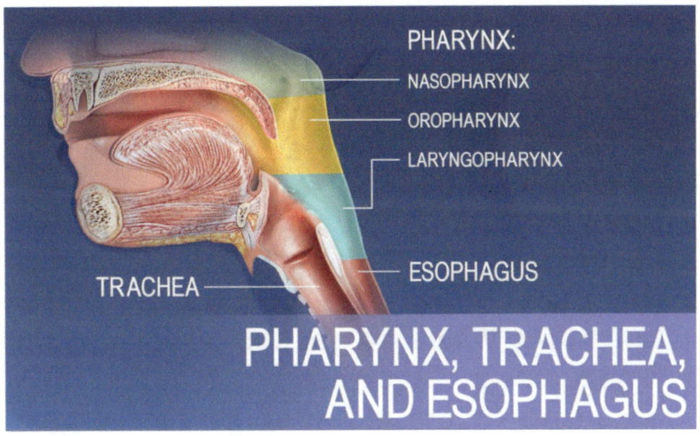

Figure 5.4. The upper airway structures play a vital role in the management of the airway during anesthesia.

Source: https://www.visiblebody.com/hs-fs/hub/189659/file-2560361987-jpg/Learn_Articles/Respiratory_System/Set_2_Upper_Respiratory_Sys/4BPharynxTracheaandEsophagus.jpg.

The anatomical features of the upper airways are pivotal to ensuring a successful anesthetic outcome, underscoring the need for ongoing education and training in airway management techniques. Practitioners should be aware of typical cognitive biases that can compromise decision-making under stress, particularly when faced with unplanned complications during intubation. In addition to technical competence, a thorough understanding of upper airway anatomy may improve overall performance in high-stakes scenarios. As practice guidelines evolve, they are based on evidence-supported approaches to airway management that combine cognitive and practical principles with the embedding of a culture of safety and readiness among anesthesia providers (Elliott et al., 2020). By focusing attention on an appreciation of upper airway anatomy and its application to anesthesia, clinicians can significantly reduce the incidence of airway complications and thus improve patient outcomes (Figure 5.4).

5.1.2. Lower Airway Structures

The lower respiratory tract holds primary structures essential to adequate ventilation and gas exchange. These are the trachea, bronchi, bronchioles, and ultimately the alveoli. The trachea is the central airway, branching into the left and right mainstem bronchi at the carina. Each bronchus further divides into smaller bronchi and bronchioles, culminating in the alveolar sacs, where oxygen and carbon dioxide exchange occurs. Anesthetic care necessitates an extensive understanding of these structures, particularly during mechanical ventilation and intubation, to avoid complications such as bronchial intubation or endobronchial blockade, which are detrimental to patient outcomes (Kogan et al., 2020). The lower airways' anatomical and physiological characteristics profoundly influence airway management skills in anesthesia. For instance, the length and diameter of the trachea vary widely between individuals, which affects the choice of endotracheal tube and the method of intubation employed. In addition, the airway must be made patent in patients with compromised respiratory status or existing pulmonary disease. Control is also effective when the risk of airway resistance is considered, which can be increased in conditions such as bronchospasm or profuse secretion. Thus, anesthesiologists must possess expertise in discerning these differences and challenges to enhance ventilation and minimize risk throughout surgery (Iorio et al., 2020). Also critical is maintaining the structure of the lower airway intact to prevent complications from the anesthetic agent. For example, certain inhalational anesthetics have the potential to irritate the airway or increase secretions, and thus there is a requirement for keen monitoring and management strategies. It is crucial to ensure that the lower airway remains unobstructed and that normal humidification and suctioning techniques are used where necessary. In addition, the complications of pneumonia or atelectasis can arise in the event that anesthesia techniques interfere with alveolar ventilation. Thus, an understanding of the finer details of lower airway structures enables anesthetists to implement integrative airway management strategies that enhance patient safety and outcomes during the perioperative period (Kogan et al., 2020) (Figure 5.5).

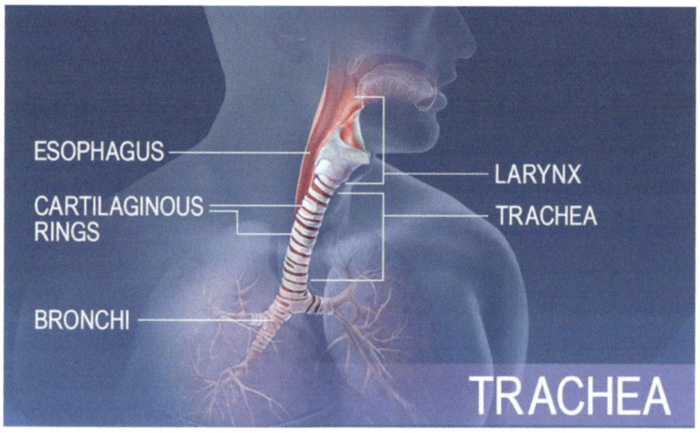

Figure 5.5. The lower airway comprises key structures essential for effective ventilation and gas exchange.

Source: https://www.visiblebody.com/hs-fs/hub/189659/file-2570898170-jpg/Learn_Articles/Respiratory_System/Set_3_Lower_Respiratory_Sys/2BTrachea.jpg.

5.1.3. Physiological Considerations

Successful airway management in anesthesia requires a thorough understanding of physiological parameters that influence patient outcomes. One of the significant challenges encountered during intubation is disruption of airway dynamics in critically ill patients.

Physiological alterations, such as edema, secretions, or anatomical abnormalities, can make glottic visualization challenging and interfere with first-pass success. These conditions increase the risk of hypoxia and are likely to bring about cardiovascular collapse during procedures, particularly in patients whose physiology is compromised. The evidence has shown that optimizing patient conditions can drastically reduce such risks. Such optimization interventions, for example, noninvasive ventilation prior to intubation, increase patient stability and make intubation safer (Myatra, 2020). Thus, professionals must be aware of such physiological variables so that they can appropriately alter their technique while managing the airway in susceptible populations. Moreover, the physiological effects of anesthetic drugs on respiratory function cannot be overlooked. The selection of neuromuscular blocking drugs rests primarily on a patient's general health condition because some conditions have a tendency to potentiate the action of these drugs. For instance, patients with compromised respiratory drive or elevated airway resistance will exhibit a prolonged neuromuscular blockade, causing unforeseen intraoperative complications in anesthetic management. In such scenarios, careful examination of drug pharmacodynamics is critical to avoid adverse consequences. Increasingly, the application of videolaryngoscopy and bougie instruments has been proposed, particularly in patients with difficult airway anatomy (Myatra, 2020). This is consistent with a conservative strategy to increase the success of the first intubation attempt, thereby minimizing the risk of mortality from repeated attempts. In addition to these, the onset of infectious diseases such as the 2019-nCoV has also introduced complications to airway management guidelines. Anesthesiologists must be especially mindful of the risk of airborne transmission, especially for procedures classified as aerosol-generating. This calls for implementing effective infection control measures, including the use of personal protective equipment (PPE) and environmental controls, to minimize exposure risk for healthcare workers and other patients. It is also crucial to understand the physiological susceptibility of infected patients, as they may have variable respiratory function, necessitating prompt treatment. Thus, the inclusion of these complex physiological factors in anesthetic practice is inevitable to enhance airway management and ensure patient safety in critical care settings.

Test Your Knowledge

1. What are the key anatomical structures of the upper and lower airway, and why is their knowledge critical for airway management during anesthesia?
2. How do variations in airway anatomy affect the choice of intubation techniques and airway devices in anesthetic practice?

5.2. Assessment of Airway

Learning Outcome

1. Preoperative evaluation techniques
2. Predictive factors for difficult intubation
3. Use of airway assessment tools

Assessment of the airway is a critical component of anesthesia care because it directly influences the effectiveness and safety of the anesthetic plan. Before any procedure, practitioners must conduct a thorough evaluation of the patient's airway characteristics, including assessing potential physical predictors of difficult ventilation and intubation. Standards advocated by the Canadian Airway Focus Group place strong emphasis on systematic airway evaluations, in which clinicians look for predictors such as the Mallampati score, neck mobility, and anatomical deformities. Predictors are used to organize the airway management strategy, ensuring that appropriate techniques and equipment are available when issues are anticipated. By establishing a documented plan based on a thorough evaluation, anesthesia providers can optimize safety and preparedness to address difficulties that may arise during airway intervention (Law et al., 2021). Furthermore, some patient groups, i.e., those with known risk factors, require individualized airway evaluation to account for their unique issues (Published by John Wiley and Sons Ltd.). For instance, mucopolysaccharidosis patients present unique challenges during anesthesia care, commonly characterized by impaired airway access and higher rates of complications. The literature reviews document the need for anesthesiologists to perform detailed preoperative workups, based on a vast array of case reports and clinical studies of such individuals. Use of procedures such as video laryngoscopy or fiberoptic bronchoscopy is advocated as an efficient alternative in such cases, enabling intubation procedures to take place, which could otherwise be impeded by variations in anatomy. Such interdisciplinary collaboration among care teams is important for ensuring optimal outcomes and for responding to the need to integrate specialist knowledge into the assessment process (Moretto et al., 2018). In addition, the dynamic nature of airway management demands that the assessment process not be a single event but an ongoing process that adapts to the patient's condition throughout the perioperative period. Things can turn around quickly after the induction of anesthesia, and frequent checks and re-evaluations of airway patency become important. Anesthesia personnel should always be vigilant and prepared to convert to backup methods in the event of a failure of the initial plan. Event-driven briefing and the use of challenging airway devices can significantly reduce risk in unpredictable situations. Lastly, the application of advanced assessment techniques, continuous monitoring, and an active approach to airway management offers a higher standard of safety and efficacy in anesthesiology practice, which is imperative for preserving patient well-being (Law et al., 2021) (Figure 5.6).

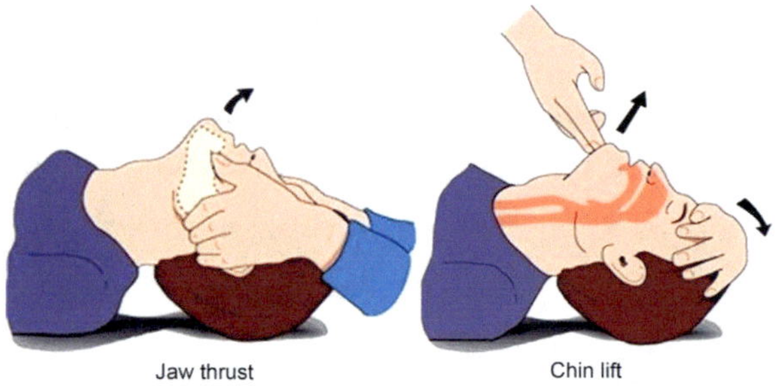

Figure 5.6. Airway assessment is a critical component of anesthesia management.

Source: https://s3.us-east-2.amazonaws.com/medictests/app/public/ckeditor_assets/pictures/522/content_headtilt_chinlift.jpg.

5.2.1. Preoperative Evaluation Techniques

Of critical importance in airway management during anesthesia is preoperative evaluation, the goal of which is to assess and minimize the risk associated with intubation and ventilation. Preoperative evaluation typically involves a complete history and physical examination to reveal anatomical variation, underlying disease, and comorbid conditions that may make airway management difficult. For example, individuals with diseases such as acromegaly pose unique challenges due to alterations in soft tissue and bony structures that may lead to airway compromise during intubation. Knowledge of these anatomical differences is important for the anesthetic team to prepare for. A thorough preoperative assessment not only facilitates predicting possible complications but also informs the choice of intubation techniques that may be necessary, such as video laryngoscopy or fiberoptic intubation, to ensure successful management of the patient in such complex cases (Mark et al., 2013). Apart from anatomical considerations, the inclusion of preoperative imaging investigations, such as cervical spine radiographs, is relevant for the determination of potential airway problems. Such imaging may uncover abnormalities that will exclude direct laryngoscopy or necessitate other methods of intubation. The experience gained in monitoring patients with rheumatoid arthritis is that radiographic findings are not sufficiently significant to change anesthesia delivery methods; nonetheless, complete assessments must still be performed. For instance, cervical spine abnormalities are present in most patients but need not be discovered preoperatively. Therefore, the anesthesiology team must balance imaging demand with clinical judgment to enhance airway management protocols and achieve the best possible outcomes for patients undergoing surgery (María et al., 2012). Moreover, advances in preoperative evaluation techniques have led to revisions in guidelines to encourage standardized airway management practices. These guidelines tend to emphasize a multidisciplinary approach, in which anesthesiologists work with surgeons and other professionals to gather in-depth patient information. In the same way that doing so in cases of complex surgical interventions can significantly reduce the incidence of unanticipated airway complications, involving patients in treatment decision-making further enhances the quality of the preoperative examination. Thus, an organized and informed preoperative assessment process is critical for effective airway management in anesthesia, ultimately resulting in improved patient outcomes and fewer perioperative complications (María et al., 2012; Mark et al., 2013).

5.2.2. Predictive Factors for Difficult Intubation

Effective airway management is critical in anesthetic practice, as difficulty with intubation can have devastating implications for patient safety. Predictive signs of difficult intubation have been extensively researched, with particular emphasis on preoperative assessment. A combination of various screening tests is strongly recommended to identify high-risk patients based on demographic and physiologic factors. These consist of age, gender, ethnicity, and systemic illness variables that have been associated with harder intubation. For instance, it was demonstrated in a research work that female patients, older adult patients, and those from some ethnic groups experienced a higher incidence of hard intubation. This reality highlights the need for tailored preoperative evaluation that considers these variations (Oria et al., 2022). This pre-emptive approach not only enhances safety but also prepares the anesthesia provider for any complications that can develop during the procedure. In addition to demographic predictors, some clinical predictors are important in predicting difficult intubation. Assessment of mouth opening, thyromental distance, and Mallampati classification are standard practices in the assessment process. For example, restricted mouth opening and decreased thyromental distance have been identified as strong predictors of intubation challenges. Additionally, patients categorized in higher Mallampati classes (classes III and IV) were found to experience greater difficulty during intubation attempts. The study findings all support the relationship between these physical characteristics and increased risk, suggesting that anesthesia practitioners should incorporate thorough airway evaluations into their practice (Oria et al., 2022). By doing so, anesthesia personnel are better able to anticipate and manage possible difficulties, ultimately perfecting airway management strategies. Furthermore, the airway management complications are particularly critical in specialized populations such as children with mucopolysaccharidoses or mucolipidoses. These subjects are at increased risk for perioperative complications, and therefore, it is crucial to determine their own predictive variables for difficult intubation. Research has established that some disease subtypes are associated with a higher incidence of adverse events attributed to airway management techniques. For instance, fiberoptic intubation through a supraglottic airway has been associated with fewer perioperative adverse events compared to direct laryngoscopy. This correlation underscores the importance of properly considering the anesthetic techniques in these high-risk patients, in which indirect techniques may be more suitable for anticipating difficult airway conditions. The integration of such information into clinical practice emphasizes the value of personalized airway management strategies to enhance patient outcomes (Figure 5.7).

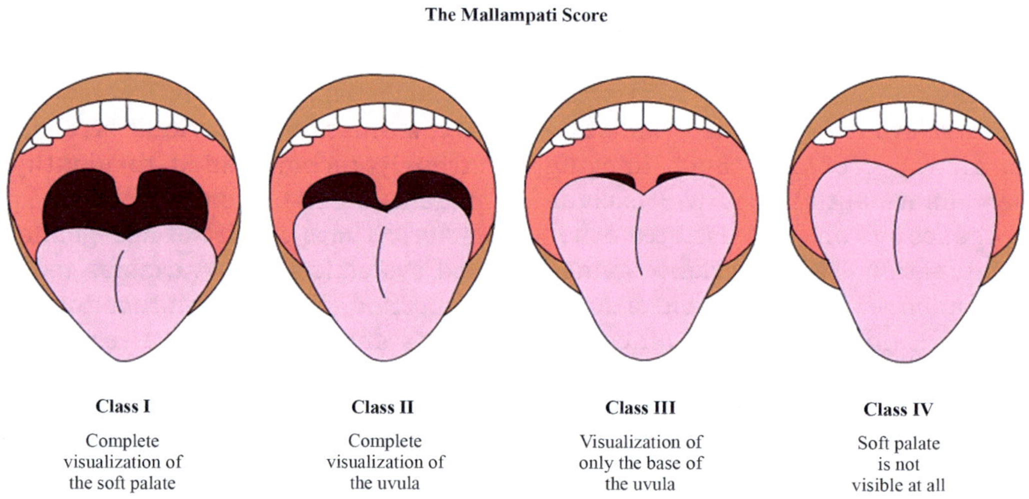

Figure 5.7. Predictive factors for difficult intubation.

Source: https://i0.wp.com/sleepworldmagazine.com/wp-content/uploads/2023/12/a7e2a-snag_38929a.png?resize=810%2C431&ssl=1.

5.2.3. Use of Airway Assessment Tools

In anesthesia airway management, airway assessment devices are key to identifying potential intubation and ventilation difficulties. The sensitivity of such devices can significantly contribute to patient safety and outcomes, as early identification of abnormalities is required. Classical measures such as Mallampati classification and thyromental distance are generally low in sensitivity and specificity, thus offering a relatively unreliable capacity to anticipate a difficult airway. The deficiencies built into the traditional measures necessitate the employment of new approaches, among which the utilization of ultrasound technology offers a non-invasive and rapid means of assessing airway anatomy and pathology (Zheng et al., 2019). By using newer imaging modalities, anesthesiologists can obtain accurate anatomical details, enhancing their ability to anticipate complications and optimize resource utilization during procedures. Ultrasound been a significant advancement in airway assessment practice, particularly in obstetric anesthesia, where physiological changes affect airway anatomy. Recent studies indicate that preoperative ultrasound evaluation can reveal important measurements of the upper airway, including soft tissue thickness at various anatomical landmarks (Zheng et al., 2019). These values can give predictive clues about intubation difficulty in parturient women, hence facilitating preoperative planning and decision-making. Such a capacity to visualize airway anatomy allows clinicians to tailor their management based on complete information, a dramatic improvement over the more subjective evaluations previously employed. The employment of ultrasound in airway evaluation thus not only enhances diagnostic accuracy but also increases safety and preparedness under anesthesia, reducing the rate of failed intubations. Additionally, systematic management of the airway requires careful, meticulous examination in both children and adults. Pediatric sedation guidelines emphasize the need for robust pre-sedation checks, with airway checks given anatomical variations and the presence of obstructions such as large tonsils. Exposure of practitioners to appropriate training and equipment is essential for effective airway management. This diverse preparation enhances the clinician's skill in effectively evaluating the airway, anticipating difficulties, and managing them safely. The inclusion of modern assessment instruments is a cornerstone of the overall approach to airway management, highlighting the benefits of multidisciplinary education programs and the implementation of best practices in anesthesia care (Figure 5.8).

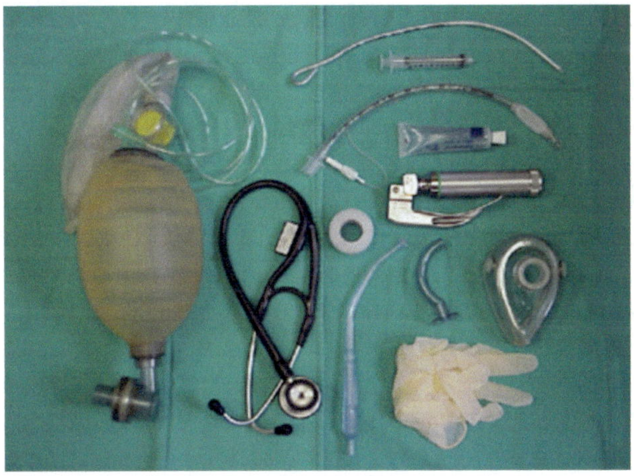

Figure 5.8. Use of airway assessment tools.

Source: https://www.professionalsuk.co.uk/uploads/assets/1707908431_65cc9d4f11390.png.

Test Your Knowledge

1. What methods and tools are used to assess a patient's airway preoperatively, and why is this assessment important for anesthesia planning?
2. How do predictors of a difficult airway influence the choice of airway management techniques during anesthesia?

5.3. Airway Management Techniques

Learning Outcome

1. Endotracheal intubation methods
2. Supraglottic airway devices
3. Bag-mask ventilation strategies

Effective airway management is crucial in anesthesia practice, as it is a sequence of techniques used to maintain oxygenation and ventilation during surgery. One of the significant ones is video laryngoscopy (VL), which is now becoming the method of choice because it offers advantages over direct laryngoscopy (DL). Evidence has shown that VL has invariably greater first-attempt success and fewer complications when compared with DL. Recommended by the Canadian Airway Focus Group (CAFG), VL works best when appropriately used blades are employed. The technique is achievable via improved visualization of the glottic opening, thus facilitating more effective tracheal intubations. Secondly, the CAFG guidelines specify a limit of three or fewer attempts to avoid patient distress and hypoxemia during airway intervention, underscoring the importance of strategic planning in airway management protocols (Law A et al., 2021). When tracheal intubation or insertion of a supraglottic airway (SGA) fails, it is paramount that anesthesia practitioners have an effective exit strategy. According to the CAFG guidelines, the priority should be to ensure ventilation and oxygenation, with the intention of limiting intubation attempts to a minimum before exploring alternative options. Alternative strategies to the intubation attempt include waking the patient, employing an SGA, or holding front-of-neck airway access (FONA) for urgent situations. This decision-making entails careful assessment of the patient's condition, particularly concerning the situation of imminent hypoxemia, which is a cannot ventilate, cannot oxygenate crisis. Through understanding and application of these approaches, anesthesia care providers maintain patient safety in times of crisis and strive for improved overall outcomes in airway management (Law et al., 2021). Pre-procedure airway assessment is yet another pillar of effective airway management. The CAFG points out that a preliminary assessment should explicitly designate predictors of potential difficulty with face-mask ventilation, tracheal intubation, and other airway maneuvers. Factors such as patient physiology, anatomical considerations, and environmental variables can provide invaluable data on probable difficulties. Following the development of anticipated complications, tailoring airway management plans to incorporate techniques such as awake tracheal intubation can offer an additional margin of safety. By attending thorough team briefings on contingency steps and having the necessary equipment at hand, anesthesia providers can reduce the risk of unforeseen complications. Proactiveness and a systematic approach to airway management make the team ready for challenges and are essential for maintaining patient safety throughout all stages of anesthesia (Figure 5.9).

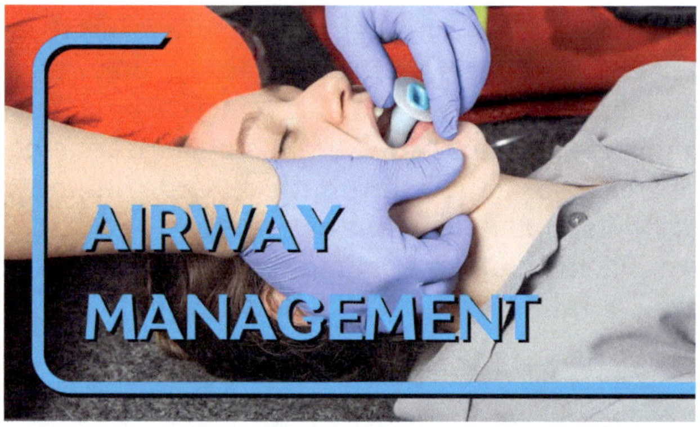

Figure 5.9. Effective airway management is critical in the practice of anesthesia.

Source: https://cdn.prod.website-files.com/63723fe799096ad12312edc2/65204fbf72a75899e9d9a585_airway%20management%20(1).webp.

5.3.1. Endotracheal Intubation Methods

Safe management of the airway is of utmost importance in the field of anesthesiology, and endotracheal intubation is the most common and valuable technique practiced. Intubation is a process of inserting a tube through the vocal cords into the trachea to ensure safe ventilation and oxygenation during surgery. There are various intubation techniques, and the choice is based on the patient's anatomy, the urgency of the case, and the likelihood of challenges such as a difficult airway. Traditional techniques, direct laryngoscopy being the most common, have long been the standard for intubation; yet newer technologies, such as video-assisted laryngoscopes and fiberoptic devices, have improved visualization and enabled navigation through the airway, thereby increasing success rates and reducing the risk of complications during this life-saving procedure. The advent of point-of-care ultrasound (POCUS) has opened a new avenue for managing the airway, particularly in challenging intubation. Because it can image airway structures in real time, ultrasound can identify anatomical barriers most likely to result in intubation complications. For example, ultrasound detection of the cricothyroid membrane has proven useful in guiding cricothyrotomy when traditional attempts at intubation fail. Apart from that, POCUS enhances the accuracy of endotracheal tube placement verification by separating clear respiratory indicators of successful intubation, such as bilateral lung sliding and the single bullet sign, from indicators of esophageal intubation. The application of ultrasound technology in this context is an excellent testimony to growing enthusiasm for integrating advanced imaging modalities during the perioperative period to enhance patient safety and outcomes (Kalagara et al., 2021). The significance of advanced and secure intubation is emphasized in the context of international health challenges, particularly in the light of the COVID-19 pandemic, highlighting aerosol-generating procedures for airway management. As the virus is transmitted through respiratory droplets, strict protocols during intubation are indispensable to protect healthcare workers. Protocols such as rapid sequence induction and keeping fewer individuals in the room are essential for reducing exposure during aerosol-generating procedures (David et al., 2020). Personal protective equipment (PPE) protocols have also been established to mitigate risks during intubation, emphasizing protection for healthcare teams while delivering the best patient care. The refinement of endotracheal intubation methods, along with strict adherence to safety protocols, is a testament to the ongoing progression of anesthesiology, which aims both to improve patient outcomes and to safeguard health professionals in an evolving clinical setting.

5.3.2. Supraglottic Airway Devices

Supraglottic airway devices (SGDs) application in anesthesia is very fashionable due to their advantages in airway management, particularly in situations where intubation is not possible. SGDs such as the laryngeal mask airway (LMA) offer an easy way to secure the airway with less damage to laryngeal structures. The anatomical configuration of such devices renders them blind-insertable, which, in most cases, can be effective; however, proper positioning is paramount to ensure proper functioning. Misplacement of SGDs will result in a high frequency of developing complications such as poor ventilation and aspiration. Therefore, understanding the relationship between SGD's anatomy and the laryngeal inlet is vital for practitioners to achieve the best outcomes in anesthesia management. Advances have introduced vision-guided insertion techniques that have enhanced the success of SGD placement. Video technology for SGD is a significant improvement over the conventional technique. The new technique enables immediate visualization of the device as it is inserted, allowing anesthesiologists to confirm proper positioning before proceeding with the procedure. By achieving the optimal fit at the proximal and distal seals, third-generation visualizing devices prevent complications such as gastric inflation and imperfect ventilation. Moreover, the enhanced facility of automatic documentation improves the quality of patient records, a requisite for contemporary clinical practice and future research, more strongly indicating the possibility of continued improvement in airway management practices of anesthetic care (André et al., 2024).

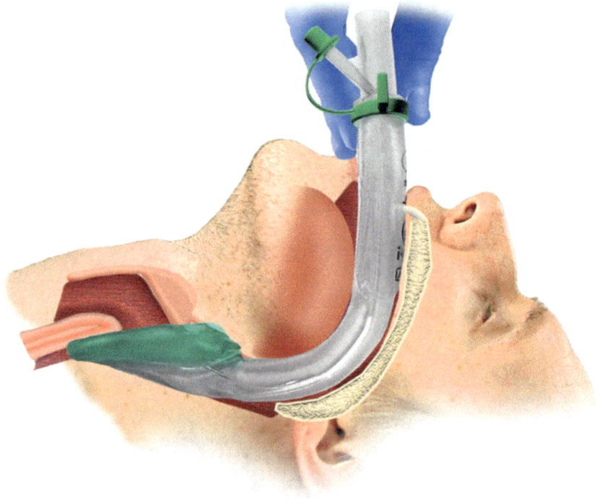

Figure 5.10. The use of supraglottic airway devices (SGDs) in anesthesia.

Source: https://www.jems.com/wp-content/uploads/2019/02/50087-1902JEMS-Holley.jpg.

In some surgical procedures, such as tracheal resection and anastomosis, SGDs may be used to enhance airway management outcomes. Anesthesiologists are faced with specific issues in managing the complexity of such procedures, where there is a need for a multifaceted preoperative plan aimed at successful airway strategies. Supraglottic airway devices are convenient in these cases, with alternatives to the use of the traditional endotracheal intubation method. More recent approaches integrating full airway support, including the provision of SGDs and adjunctive methods such as regional anesthesia, have emerged based on specific literature reports. These strategies require a collaborative, team-based approach from the surgical team to achieve the utmost patient safety and comfort (Marwaha et al., 2021). The ongoing development of SGD technology and training in its use have considerable potential to overcome existing issues in airway management in the anesthetic setting (Figure 5.10).

5.3.3. Bag-Mask Ventilation Strategies

Safe management of the airway in anesthesia is primarily based on the use of bag-mask ventilation maneuvers, particularly in the case of non-patent airway or respiratory failure. BMV is still a leading intervention for adjunct ventilation and oxygenation of patients where regular intubation fails short-term or is prudently postponed. The technique relies heavily on proper mask fit on the patient's face and positive pressure to force air from a resuscitation bag. Recent standards emphasize employing well-trained personnel with experience in BMV techniques, which has been associated with an increasing rate of successful ventilation and a decreasing rate of adverse effects, such as aspiration or inadequate oxygenation (Jeffrey et al., 2021). Awareness of the unique features of various types of masks and optimal positioning can further enhance these methods, making BMV a cornerstone in anesthetic technique. The only significant limitation in BMV is achieving a good seal between the patient's facial area and the mask to provide effective ventilation. Facial anatomy, facial or beard hair, and patient position can also become primary factors in determining whether BMV is helpful or not. The optimization of the mask fit is suggested by following a stepwise process that keeps adjustments to the patient's head position, the "sniffing position," and suitable mask sizes (Jeffrey et al., 2021). In addition, access to an assistant can enhance the success rate of ventilation attempts through concomitant airway maneuvers such as jaw thrusts, which maintain airway patency and aid mask application. Thus, through knowledge of mechanical principles and anatomic considerations, clinicians can optimize their proficiency at performing BMV and allow effective airway management during anesthesia. In light of the evolving health care landscape and the consequences of crises such as the COVID-19 pandemic for airway management models, BMV strategies must be revised to address emerging conditions. Physicians are urged to devise adaptive guidelines informed by evidence-based advice and to adjust to the particular circumstances posed by infectious respiratory disease. World Health Organization emphasizes timely revision and guidance for offering successful practice in an atmosphere of uncertainty. As a result, medical staff training courses must incorporate pandemic-response simulations, with special emphasis on teamwork and communication in high-stakes airway management. Therefore, BMV protocols remain significant in routine anesthesia and are even adapted to meet the demands of the crisis, underscoring the importance of ongoing learning and protocol adjustment (Figure 5.11).

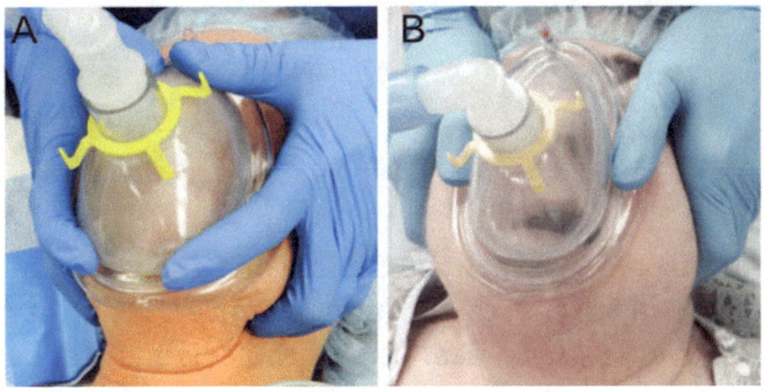

Figure 5.11. Bag-mask ventilation strategies.

Source: https://www.researchgate.net/profile/Daniel-Saddawi-Konefka/publication/283078174/figure/fig1/AS:666790074011651@1535986550893/Two-hand-bag-mask-ventilation-techniques-A-With-the-double-C-E-technique-each-thumb.ppm.

Test Your Knowledge

1. What are the different airway management techniques used in anesthesia, and in what clinical situations is each technique preferred?
2. How do advanced airway devices, such as laryngeal mask airways and video laryngoscopes, improve safety and effectiveness during anesthesia?

5.4. Complications in Airway Management

Learning Outcome

1. Common complications during intubation
2. Management of airway emergencies
3. Long-term effects of airway mismanagement

Airway management complications are a current problem in anesthetic practice, often resulting in adverse outcomes. One of the serious issues is failed intubation, in which the practitioner is unable to secure the airway after multiple attempts. Literature suggests that although traditional direct laryngoscopy has been the standard approach, video laryngoscopy (VL) is more beneficial, as it offers higher first-attempt success rates and lower complication rates. According to the Canadian Airway Focus Group, the introduction of VL has made it mandatory to use it to facilitate tracheal intubations in every clinical scenario. The professionals ought to have a systematized process with identifying when to discontinue attempts after unsuccessful ones and alter to other approaches, ensuring continuous ventilation throughout, thereby mitigating the dangers of an unsafe airway at critical phases of anesthesia induction (Law et al., 2021). In children, airway management complications can be especially disastrous due to characteristic physiological differences. The anatomical differences, combined with the lower reserve levels of the physiology, put them at higher risks for perioperative airway management. The implications can be life-threatening if airway obstruction is delayed. Pediatrics-specific protocols may not be available everywhere; available guidelines are usually adapted from adult frameworks, and even these may be suboptimal due to anatomical differences and varying degrees of development. Thorough management of such complications requires a focus on specific, rigorous training for clinicians in pediatric airway management. By establishing minimum standards for apparatus and personnel and conducting frequent practice drills, healthcare workers can minimize incidental complications related to airway obstruction in children (Engelhardt et al., 2019). Airway management complications are also typically caused by inadequate preparation and a lack of adherence to proper protocols. The use of an airway lead—a professional responsible for airway management—has been advocated to increase readiness and quality assurance in anesthetic practice. The role plays an important role in ensuring that all individuals are sufficiently trained and the necessary equipment is available. A systematic strategy, coupled with routine audits, simulation training, and feedback systems, can humanize the operation, allowing anesthesia teams to learn from past blunders and improve their approach to complications. Lastly, developing a culture of safety and continuous improvement in airway management methods is important for reducing morbidity and mortality from anesthesia, thereby providing a safer clinical environment for patients undergoing surgical procedures (Law et al., 2021).

5.4.1. Common Complications During Intubation

The complexities inherent with intubation can lead to a multitude of complications that may jeopardize patient safety and anesthetic success. Of these complications, failed intubation is of significant concern, especially in patients who present with an elevated body mass index (BMI) or who have anatomical considerations that render the airway more inaccessible. Critical review demonstrates that obese patients in particular are at increased risk for problematic intubation and subsequent complications because of their altered respiratory physiology and probable obstructive sleep apnea (Law et al., 2021). Failure to adequately secure the airway may produce hypoxia and necessitate rescue backup techniques, highlighting the significant need for proficiency in diverse intubation techniques among anesthetic providers. Thus, a thorough understanding of patient pathology and anatomy is essential in the prevention and management of these complications. Airway trauma is another common intubation complication that is triggered by direct and video laryngoscopy attempts. This is amplified when multiple attempts are made to intubate a patient, particularly in urgent or emergent conditions where time is of the essence. In all such attempts, one could end up inflicting laryngeal edema, vocal cord damage, or tracheal injury, which in turn could lead to serious long-term consequences (Law et al., 2021). Best practices advocate limiting attempts to three or fewer before opting for other airway management methods, so as not to increase chances of inflicting trauma. Secondly, the selection of the intubation device has the potential to influence significantly such injuries and, as a consequence, should be selected wisely by anesthesiologists such that it optimizes visualization and minimizes adverse effects. Lastly, incorrect ventilation settings upon using mechanical ventilation after intubation can generate additional complications, e.g., barotrauma or ventilator-associated lung injury. These are particularly important for patients with underlying respiratory illness or high-risk surgery (Bazurro et al., 2018). The anesthesia team will need to emphasize monitoring and titrating ventilation parameters to prevent overinflation of airway pressure and volume, which can injure lung function. Multimodal techniques, including opioid-sparing for analgesia and lung-protective ventilatory methods, can also provide optimization of patient outcomes during the post-intubation period. Therefore, careful ventilation management not only contributes importantly to the immediate success of anesthesia but also has significant effects upon the patient's postoperative course of recovery (Figure 5.12).

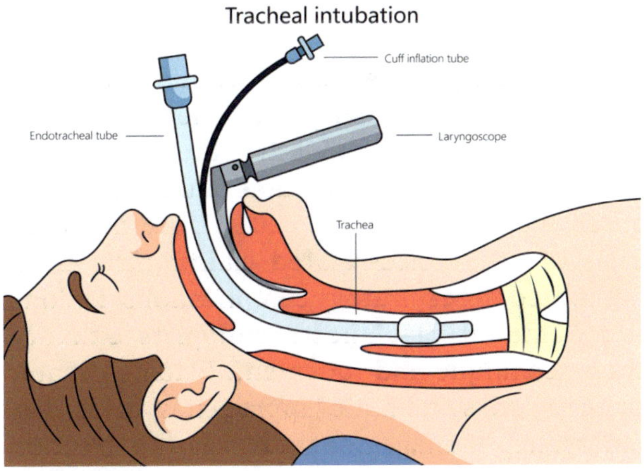

Figure 5.12. Common complications during intubation.

Source: https://hayekmedical.com/wp-content/uploads/2024/12/Tracheal-Intubation-1-1024x768.jpeg.

5.4.2. Management of Airway Emergencies

Effective management of airway emergencies is most critical in anesthetic care, as such emergencies can readily lead to catastrophic patient outcomes. Familiarity with airway anatomy, various intubation techniques, and the proper use of emergency airway devices is essential for anesthesiologists. Evidence-based implementation of protocols, e.g., preoperative airway assessment, is key to predicting potential issues during intubation. The increasing number of challenging airways necessitates frequent training and knowledge refresh to equip anesthesia experts with a prompt, effective remedy for any emerging complications. Besides, awareness of complications such as respiratory failure aggravated by infectious agents, such as 2019-nCoV, underscores the importance of preparedness in response to emerging medical issues, as outlined in critical emergency protocols established by health organizations (Randy et al., 2020). The analysis of past airway emergencies from closed-claims databases provides valuable information to inform airway management optimization. The claims often point to improper judgment and technique by anesthesia practitioners in difficult intubation cases, highlighting the importance of intensive training programs and competency assessment (Asai et al., 2019). As much as 85% of anesthesia-related claims have been attributed to respiratory complications, making it paramount that anesthesiologists enhance their technique and judgment. Placing greater priority on systematic approaches to airway emergency management, such as the creation of pre-plans for various intubation difficulties and early escalation to surgical treatment where needed, can mitigate risks. This proactive strategy ensures patient safety and reduces the risk of catastrophic events resulting from delayed airway management. Interprofessional teamwork in airway emergency management cannot be overemphasized. Anesthesiology, as a sequestered discipline, gains a lot from cooperative work with surgical and nursing staff in handling emergencies. Fostering common responsibility, especially for emergency airway care, favors a culture of safety and preparedness. Having readily accessible emergency airway carts, regular simulation practice, and developed communication among team members are critical components of an effective airway management plan. Also, removing systemic barriers, such as ensuring equipment is available and providing immediate access to surgical intervention when indicated, will be critical to improving airway outcomes. Lastly, establishing a multidisciplinary ethos ensures efficient and comprehensive management of airway emergencies in the anesthetic environment, as recommended by best practices in prior reviews and current guidelines (Asai et al., 2019).

5.4.3. Long-Term Effects of Airway Mismanagement

Poor airway management during the administration of anesthesia has long-term adverse effects on patients. The most prominent issue associated with poor airway management is hypoxia, which leads to irreversible injury of the brain. Prolonged hypoxia, particularly in susceptible groups such as in orthopedic or obstetric surgery, has been associated with cognitive dysfunction and neurological morbidity lasting for a long time after the procedure is done. The association of suboptimal airway management with adverse neurological outcome underscores the utmost importance of using established techniques and the latest technology to , develop, and maintain an adequate airway, particularly in high-risk patients. Accordingly, the implications of airway mishandling extend beyond overt perioperative problems, and a detailed understanding of its potential impact on patients' long-term health and well-being is required. Poor airway management also leads to other respiratory complications that can happen well after the postoperative period. Patients with airway mishandling end up suffering from chronic respiratory issues such as obstructive sleep apnea or recurrent pulmonary infections due to aspirated content. These events carry significant implications both for patient quality of life and healthcare systems that must contend with the long-term consequences of such complications. Adequate airway management may decrease the incidence of such chronic complications, thereby reducing health care costs and enhancing patient outcomes. It is crucial to understand the role of comprehensive airway management strategies, particularly in the context of such chronic respiratory complications, with special emphasis on prioritizing effective means to prevent complications arising from anesthesia treatment. Along with this, the psychological impact of mismanagement of airway can cause long-term problems for patients undergoing anesthesia. Traumatic experience of airway complications with the procedure can trigger symptoms of post-traumatic stress disorder (PTSD), delayed anxiety, and avoidance of subsequent medical interventions. The patient may suffer from increased fear associated with anesthesia or treatment, making subsequent therapies challenging. In addition, adverse consequences can undermine trust between patients and health professionals, disrupting subsequent healthcare interactions and reducing the use of required services. It is important for anesthesiologists to consider these potential long-term psychological effects so they can use effective communication and supportive measures pre- and postoperatively. By optimizing airway management techniques, anesthesiology professionals not only ensure patients' immediate safety but also eliminate potential long-term psychological effects resulting from prior airway mishandling, thereby facilitating a less stressful healthcare process overall (Figure 5.13).

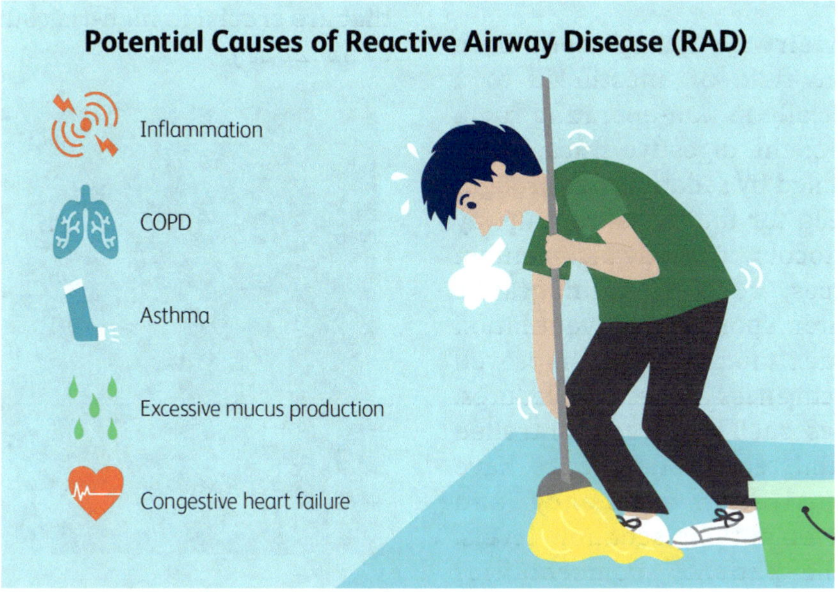

Figure 5.13. Long-term effects of airway mismanagement.

Source: https://www.verywellhealth.com/thmb/PieqR2M2Xo-BjMzPMVTytIZ0tRY=/1500x0/filters:no_upscale():max_bytes(150000):strip_icc()/what-is-reactive-airway-disease-200611_final-01-c2d275164fa3440ca2517699d292c134.jpg.

Test Your Knowledge

1. What are the common complications that can arise during airway management, and how can they be prevented or managed?
2. How do patient-specific factors and anatomical variations increase the risk of airway complications during anesthesia?

5.5. Advances in Airway Management

Learning Outcome

1. Technological innovations in devices
2. Simulation training for practitioners
3. Evidence-based guidelines and protocols

Advancements in airway management have revolutionized the field of anesthesia to a great extent, especially in non-operating room areas. Endoscopy of the digestive tract, which is mainly accompanied by sedation, has brought to the fore the need for individualized airway management protocols. The advancement in monitoring devices, such as capnographs modified to monitor spontaneous ventilation and bispectral index monitors, has improved the safety and effectiveness of these procedures. Further, techniques such as target-controlled infusion for administering anesthetics have improved administration efficiency and improved control of patient sedation levels. Understanding the patients' comorbidities and evaluation of risk of aspiration of gastric content are essential in making effective anesthetic plans, therefore pointing to the importance of advanced preparations in airway management (Pardo et al., 2022). This meticulous approach not only ensures patient safety but also enables more sophisticated endoscopic techniques, reflecting advances in airway management in anesthesiology. New airway devices and techniques have also revolutionized management in more complex surgical cases, particularly in tracheal surgery. Tracheal resection anastomosis is a complex group of anesthetic challenges due to anatomical conditions and potential complications of such procedures. New technologies, ranging from supraglottic airway devices to extracorporeal support devices, have expanded the options available to anesthesiologists for managing these complex situations. Techniques like cross-field ventilation with endotracheal intubation and jet ventilation remain standard but require meticulous preoperative planning and effective intraoperative communication within the surgical team. The development of these innovative airway management methods not only improves surgical outcomes but also enhances safety protocols by investigating both airway preservation and ventilation methods that are crucial in high-risk surgeries (Marwaha et al., 2021).

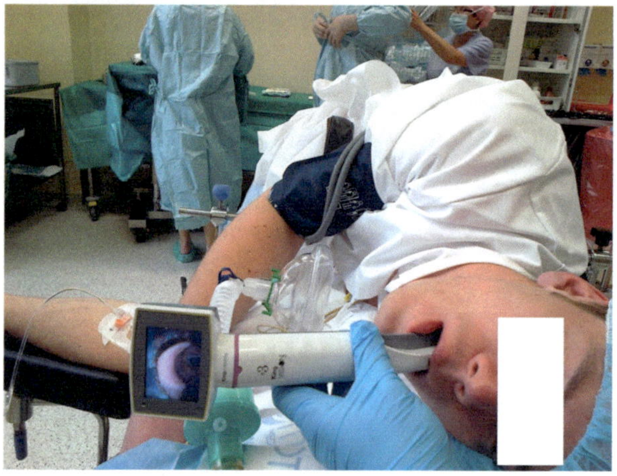

Figure 5.14. Advancements in airway management have significantly transformed the landscape of anesthesia.

Source: https://pub.mdpi-res.com/healthcare/healthcare-11-02468/article_deploy/html/images/healthcare-11-02468-g007.png?1698215235.

Furthermore, the incorporation of enhanced training and guidelines for airway management has become central to modern anesthetic practice. With progress still underway, anesthesiologists must continue to stay current not only with technical knowledge but also with how these advances affect patient care as a whole. Emerging anesthetic drugs and techniques, paired with extensive knowledge of airway management, require ongoing education and practice development. This continuous evolution, aligned with the broad patterns of anesthesia, aims to minimize risk of airway-related complications and improve patient outcomes. The need for proper training and expertise in information on recent developments in airway management cannot be overstated, since it largely sets the course for safe anesthesia practice in various clinical settings (Marwaha et al., 2021; Pardo et al., 2022) (Figure 5.14).

5.5.1. Technological Innovations in Devices

In anesthesia, technological advancements in airway management devices have introduced significant practice changes that enhance patient safety and procedural efficiency. The introduction of high-end visualization technology, such as video laryngoscopes, has changed the process of airway securing by anesthesiologists, particularly for patients with challenging anatomical variations. The devices provide a magnified view of the airway, allowing practitioners to perform intubations more conveniently and accurately. Also, with the use of artificial intelligence, such equipment is evolving to deliver instant feedback and assistance, significantly reducing major complications associated with difficult intubations. This shift highlights the importance of continued investment in technology to improve surgical outcomes and to enable training for anesthesiology specialists, as elaborated in recent reviews on the benefits of innovative airway management strategies (Jarosław et al., 2022). One of the most significant breakthroughs is the use of 3D printing technology, which is on the cutting edge of bespoke medical device production. The technology itself enables the creation of patient-specific airway models to maximize preoperative preparation and simulation. By using 3D-printed reproductions of a patient's anatomy, anesthesiologists can more clearly visualize specific airway difficulties and rehearse difficult intubation scenarios before the procedure. This proactive approach not only improves clinicians' confidence but is also associated with reduced procedural times and better patient outcomes. Studies indicate that such innovations not only facilitate the easy practice of complex procedures but are also revolutionizing medical education for future anesthesiologists, validating the necessity for innovative solutions in airway management (Jarosław et al., 2022). Aside from this, the COVID-19 pandemic has introduced telehealth technology, prompting a reassessment of traditional anesthesiology standards, especially in airway management. Remote monitoring devices have gained popularity, enabling remote monitoring of patients' respiratory parameters and airway conditions. This is especially applicable to reducing exposure risk in aerosol-generating procedures, highlighting the dual advantage of technology in enhancing patient safety and operational efficacy. The pandemic has accelerated advances in digital technologies, resulting in a paradigm shift in surgical strategies, including those for airway management. As anesthesiologists increasingly embrace these technologies, they must also contend with the attendant issues of data privacy and integration with current health infrastructure to optimize their contributions to patient care.

5.5.2. Simulation Training for Practitioners

Simulation training has been witnessed to become a significant solution to the issues practitioners face in airway management in anesthesia. The training enables doctors to develop technical and non-technical skills in a simulation environment, boosting their confidence and ability to perform high-stakes procedures. Anesthesia professionals are typically unprepared by conventional training for unforeseen circumstances and challenging situations like difficult tracheal intubation, where quick decision-making and correct action are critical in maintaining patient safety. Simulation training, therefore, not only reinforces procedural skills but also enhances critical thinking, communication, and interdependent team behavior of the team members, ultimately enhancing patient care as a whole. Secondly, the simulated setting allows for understanding through errors without risking patient lives, thereby enabling practitioners to better appreciate the intricacies of airway management and the nuances of various techniques and equipment used in this regard. Finally, simulation training allows practitioners to become acclimatized with newer airway management devices and techniques. As noted in clinical publications, airway management complications remain one of the leading causes of anesthesia-related morbidity and mortality, and demands for continuing skill acquisition remain unabated (Asai et al., 2019). Simulation facilitates experts in translating theory into practice by conducting repeated drills on new equipment, thereby equipping them to handle real challenges. For example, "cannot intubate, cannot oxygenate" scenarios for simulation training are valuable practices to validate a practitioner's ability to make quick decisions, such as the fast formation of a surgical airway (Asai et al., 2019). Repeated practice of these emergent scenarios diminishes fear and increases competence, enabling clinicians to better manage airway difficulties in their daily practice. Furthermore, an ordered approach to anesthesia training—on the model of procedures adopted by aviation—can further improve airway management outcomes. In aviation, repeated simulation and practice have been essential in maintaining high standards of crisis management. By extension, it can be understood that effective airway management is a matter of having a well-thought-out protocol that includes rigorous simulation training so that all anesthesia personnel are adequately skilled and judicious. This training must also include assessing equipment availability and functionality to prevent systemic failures that are often at the root of adverse outcomes (Asai et al., 2019). Through a common curriculum that includes simulation and standardized practice, anesthesia providers are better able to anticipate challenges, improve their response times, and ultimately increase patient safety during airway management cases (Figure 5.15).

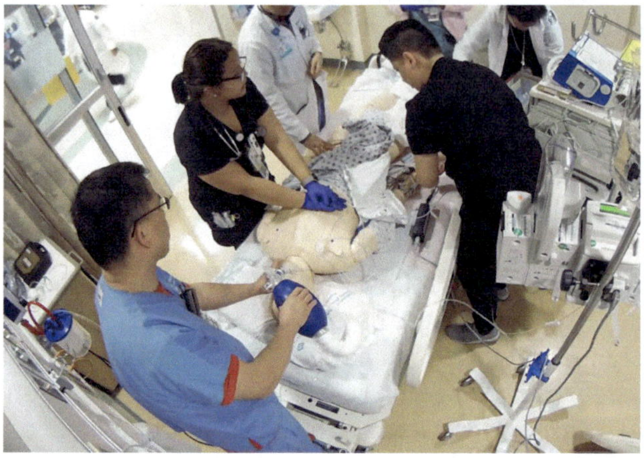

Figure 5.15. The implementation of simulation training has emerged as an essential component in addressing the challenges practitioners face during airway management in anesthesia.

Source: https://ems-works.com/wp-content/uploads/2023/07/MicrosoftTeams-image-12-1-1024x733.jpg.

5.5.3. Evidence-Based Guidelines and Protocols

The evolution of evidence-based guidelines and protocols in airway management has significantly influenced clinical practice in anesthesia. At its core is the widening evidence base that drives best practice, whereby recommendations by groups like the Canadian Airway Focus Group (CAFG) are crucial to contemporary anesthetic practice. The newer guidelines from the CAFGs emphasize the greater efficacy of video laryngoscopy over direct laryngoscopy, with particular emphasis on higher first-pass success rates and lower airway management-related complications. The article grounds the use of video laryngoscopy with suitably selected blades to achieve successful tracheal intubation, thereby enhancing patient safety and procedure success.

Moreover, the CAFG guidelines highlight the need for formal protocols that help practitioners make decisions about exit plans after failed intubation attempts, thereby ensuring the use of standard procedures to minimize risks in airway emergencies (Law et al., 2021). Implementation of evidence-based practices not only improves outcomes in airway management but also enhances anesthesia professionals' training and expertise. As airway situations have grown in complexity, education about airway protocols has become important. The CAFG suggests that facilities appoint an "airway lead" to manage the use of these protocols, ensuring trained personnel and available equipment. Participation in routine education about such guidelines helps anesthesia professionals cope with complex airway cases more effectively, fosters a culture of critical thinking and responsiveness, and aligns with the broader trend towards competency-based education in medicine. It emphasizes the importance of integrating updated guidelines into institutional practice to enhance patient safety and optimize care delivery within the perioperative setting (Mahmood et al., 2016). The evidence-based guideline process also comprehensively addresses the use of perioperative ultrasound, which is on the rise as a promising airway management tool. A few recent publications report deficiencies in ultrasound education among anesthesia providers and urge the establishment of standardized education protocols that address the various uses of ultrasound in the perioperative environment. The integration of ultrasonography into anesthesiology training is not only vital for assessing airway structures but also for simplifying procedures such as tracheal intubation and regional anesthesia. The development of a balanced curriculum that integrates ultrasound encourages evidence-based practice across all phases of anesthesia care, from airway assessment to emergencies. As the technology becomes more sophisticated, highly specialized training programs will be instrumental in obtaining anesthesiologists' skill levels to utilize these devices properly, further entrenching evidence-based practices as a mainstay of modern airway management (Mahmood et al., 2016).

Test Your Knowledge

1. What recent technological and procedural advances have improved the safety and effectiveness of airway management in anesthesia?
2. How have devices such as video laryngoscopes, supraglottic airways, and fiberoptic bronchoscopes changed airway management practices?

5.6. Role of Anesthesiologists in Airway Management

Learning Outcome

1. Responsibilities during surgical procedures
2. Collaboration with surgical teams
3. Continuous education and training

The role of the anesthesiologists in airway management is crucial, especially when used for anesthesia delivery in surgical procedures. The anesthesiologists have the responsibility of ensuring a patient's airway safety during the time they are under anesthesia. This involves assessing the airway before surgery, which may be done by thoroughly examining the patient to identify any anatomic or physiologic features that may inhibit airway entry. With the use of various methods, such as intubation and advanced airway device placement, anesthesiologists can manage routine and difficult airway cases with ease. In emergencies and special cases, the need to make well-informed decisions about airway management is always greater, as the anesthesiologists' skills directly impact patient safety and outcomes. The recent pandemics, particularly COVID-19, have made airway management highly important and challenging within the practice of anesthesiology. The rapid spread of the coronavirus has accelerated protocol and practice changes in intubation and ventilation, compelling anesthesiologists to adopt guidelines that prioritize patient and healthcare worker safety. For example, the Pediatric Difficult Intubation Collaborative (PeDI-C) met consensus guidelines for conducting pediatric airway procedures in the face of airborne infection, emphasizing strategies such as avoiding aerosol generation and restricting the number of individuals present in the room during procedures. Such evolution of practice reflects anesthesiologists' resilience in coping with the complexities of the latest health crises while maintaining high standards of care throughout airway management (Matava et al., 2020). Besides direct airway intervention, the anesthesiologists' work also entails continuous education and the development of evidence-based guidelines that enhance patient safety. This education is critical, particularly for evolving respiratory viruses that pose particular challenges in the operating room. Through collaboration with infection control professionals and the use of advanced monitoring technologies, anesthesiologists can improve the safety and efficacy of airway management practices. Practices such as the use of video laryngoscopy and rapid sequence induction have become increasingly common, highlighting the need for continued learning and adaptation in the field. As noted by experts during the SARS epidemic, effective communication among healthcare workers on the best airway management techniques can significantly reduce the risk of aerosol-generating procedures (Beverley, 2020). Anesthesiologists thus have a crucial role in shaping the future of airway management techniques under changing clinical settings (Figure 5.16).

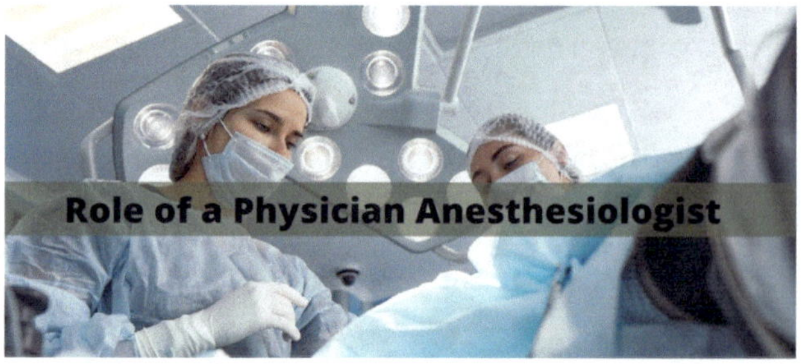

Figure 5.16. The role of anesthesiologists in airway management is critical.

Source: https://www.brainwonders.in/blog_feature_images/2022/05/2022-05-16-12-35-50Role_of_a_Physician_Anesthesiologist.jpg.

5.6.1. Responsibilities During Surgical Procedures

In the complex scenario of a surgical procedure, responsibilities are assigned to various members of the surgical team to work together toward the global aim of patient safety and optimal outcomes. The most significant responsibility of the anesthesiologist is airway control, one of the most important elements of anesthesia care. This charge includes not only the selection of appropriate techniques for airway management, such as intubation or supraglottic airway device placement, but also actively anticipating potential complications. They must have clear communication with the surgical team in order to make synchrony in critical points, such as induction and extubation, possible. Furthermore, with the ever-present problem of transmissible infections in the modern age, especially with moments of heightened sensitivity like the COVID-19 pandemic, the practice of anesthesiology must also adapt to encompass rigorous aseptic practice and more frequent use of personal protective gear to safeguard both the medical staff and the patient undergoing procedures (Liang et al., 2020). Also essential is the surgical team's requirement to stay within guidelines designed to reduce risks associated with airway management. This includes the provision of in-depth checklists before the procedure, which serve as a guarantee against potential lapses. Members should also be skilled at outfitting themselves with the required protective gear, particularly in cases where patients would remain asymptomatic carriers of infectious agents. Role definition is important: while the anesthesiologist focuses on airway management, the assistant and the surgeon must be prepared to respond immediately if an airway emergency arises during surgery. Compliance with these roles on a day-to-day basis instills a culture of responsibility among the surgical team, which ultimately leads to better patient outcomes and fewer risks (Soh et al., 2020). Postoperative responsibility is not limited to the smooth completion of the surgical procedure but goes deeper, as it involves monitoring recovery and addressing potential postoperative airway management complications. The anesthesiologist must maintain vigilance throughout recovery, ensuring airway patency and any respiratory distress nipped in the bud. This observation is particularly crucial for patients who may have had procedures that predispose them to postoperative complications such as airway edema or aspiration. Good communication remains a priority at this time because the anesthesiologist must communicate with the recovery nursing staff regarding the patient's airway status. Through a coordinated approach and adherence to clearly defined roles throughout the surgical process, the health care team can deliver optimal care in airway management (Liang et al., 2020) (Figure 5.17).

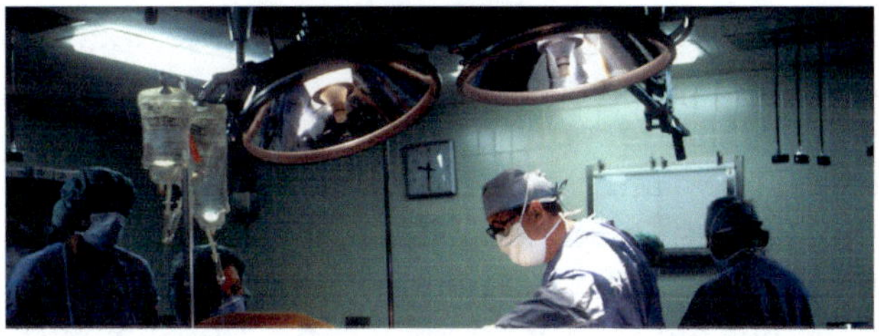

Figure 5.17. Responsibilities during surgical procedures.

Source: https://images.unsplash.com/photo-1579154491915-611e891d3a5b?crop=entropy&cs=srgb&fm=jpg&ixid=M3w0MjA4MDF8MHwxfHNlYXJjaHw3fHxwaGFybWFjeSUyMGRydWclMjBhZG1pbmlzdHJhdGlvbiUyMG1lZGljaW5lJTIwaGVhbHRoY2FyZXxlbnwxfDB8fHwxNzAzODY5NTI2fDA&ixlib=rb-4.0.3&q=85&w=800&fit=crop&h=300&q=75&fm=webp.

5.6.2. Collaboration with Surgical Teams

Effective collaboration between anesthesiologists and surgical teams is essential for optimal airway management, particularly in procedures involving general anesthesia. Through this collaboration, the patient's airway is effectively preoperatively assessed, which is central to anticipating potential complications. Through their expertise in airway anatomy and physiology, anesthesiologists work closely with surgical teams to develop a coordinated plan tailored to the patient's unique needs. This collaboration not only enhances surgical efficiency but also significantly reduces intraoperative emergency risk. Utilizing the best of both expertise, patient safety, and outcomes for patients who are to undergo surgery are enhanced, leading to an optimal approach of addressing challenging airway conditions that may arise during surgeries. Respect for a team-oriented, disciplined approach is essential in managing the difficult airway patient. Perioperative teams have valuable information to share about the anatomy-specific challenges of specific procedures to help anesthesiologists create tailored strategies for managing the airway. Effective preoperative planning, with open communication regarding patient positioning, exposure, and contingency planning, sets the stage for success. This is augmented by fresh guidelines, as evidenced by the top anesthesiology societies, where multidisciplinary collaboration in caring for difficult airways is emphasized to be of paramount importance (Jeffrey et al., 2021). This minimizes disruption to surgery and fosters an active culture in which patient outcomes remain a responsibility for both surgeons and anesthesiologists, thereby fortifying patient safety as a shared priority across professions. Against the background of shifting circumstances, such as the COVID-19 pandemic, coordination between operating teams is highlighted as essential. Call for strict protocols and the sharing of resources is essential, as highlighted in the new guidelines on surgical management of patients with COVID-19 (Coccolini et al., 2020). Anesthesiologists must work closely with the surgical team to develop procedures that not only ensure successful airway management but also protect the safety and health of every member of the team. The collaboration must minimize the risk of infection and ensure continuity of surgical services, even in emergencies. Through such cooperation, healthcare providers are better positioned to navigate the complexities of airway management, ultimately leading to improved patient outcomes and a united front against the unprecedented hurdles confronting the healthcare system.

5.6.3. Continuous Education and Training

Continuous education and training are part of proper airway management in anesthesia, reflecting the ever-changing nature of medical practice and patient safety protocols. With an increasingly expanding anesthesiology branch due to technological advances and practices, anesthesiologists must adopt a lifelong learning pattern to stay abreast of airway management. This commitment includes attending workshops, simulations, and continuing medical education (CME) courses specifically focusing on the latest advances in airway devices and complex airway management. In addition, a solid educational background allows anesthesiologists to integrate evidence-based practice tailored to the complexity of individual patients, thus enhancing the quality of care and diminishing perioperative airway management-related complications. In this case, formal training being integrated into clinical practice is of utmost importance for guarding patients' welfare and achieving the optimal outcomes inside the operating room. In addition to technical competence, ongoing education facilitates a balanced understanding of the interdisciplinary approach to anesthesia care. understanding of the bigger picture of health care reinforces anesthesiologists' abilities to manage patients' airway management practices effortlessly, as well as coordinate with the smooth working relationship of surgical teams, nurse anesthetists, and other health professionals to make sure that airway management habits are strictly adhered to along the perioperative course. Interprofessional working becomes increasingly vital as the healthcare system transitions towards value-based practice, where the outcome is prioritized. Through active participation in cross-disciplinary education and training, anesthesiologists are better able to address the challenges of airway management, thereby improving their practice and fostering a culture of safety and quality among medical teams. The balanced strategy for continuous education ensures that all parties are moving in the same direction toward common goals that benefit the patient. Implementing structured training programs in airway management is crucial, as health care systems struggle to keep pace with demand driven by changing patient populations and complex surgical procedures. According to the literature, novel approaches such as simulation-based training can significantly improve anesthesiologists' responses to airway emergencies, thereby enhancing patient outcomes and minimizing complications. In addition, regular evaluations of training efficacy are needed to guide and modify educational materials so that they are consistent with modern practice and current problems in airway management. Organizations should recognize the resources necessary for ongoing education to reemphasize the critical role of thoroughly trained anesthesia personnel in providing quality care. Satisfying these educational needs straight away aligns with the broader goal of improving surgical outcomes and patient safety in the perioperative period, as evidenced by the pressing measures outlined in José et al. (2023) and Gottumukkala et al. (2023).

Test Your Knowledge

1. What are the key responsibilities of anesthesiologists in ensuring safe and effective airway management before, during, and after anesthesia?
2. How do anesthesiologists assess, plan, and respond to difficult or emergency airway situations?

SUMMARY

In discussing airway management during anesthesia, it is crucial to highlight the importance of personalized approaches tailored to patient groups and surgical requirements. Efficient airway management not only guarantees the safety of anesthetic procedures but also considerably influences postoperative outcomes. By combining state-of-the-art techniques and careful observation, anesthetists can minimize risks of airway compromise, especially in vulnerable groups such as infants and children. Airway management complexity necessitates practitioners staying up to date with evolving guidelines and emerging research to incorporate evidence-based practices into their anesthetic care protocols. Lastly, a thorough appreciation of airway dynamics equips anesthetists with skills necessary to address complexities in a variety of clinical scenarios, maintaining responsibility for patient safety and quality of care. The literature identifies that airway management techniques and strategies are the major determinants of patient outcome. There are a number of studies that illustrate the relationship between choice of airway device and the occurrence of complications during anesthesia. As an illustration, the latest statistics show that while the use of general anesthesia remains common for experts, other methods, such as regional anesthesia, should be duly addressed, particularly in young patients undergoing outpatient procedures. In this case, the findings presented by McCann et al. (2019) warrant careful scrutiny of the risks associated with different types of anesthesia to prevent potential adverse effects on neurodevelopment during early childhood. All of these should inform clinical practice, leading to varied airway management approaches to ensure the health and safety of patients of any age. Furthermore, ongoing professional development and adherence to up-to-date clinical guidelines remain critical to enhancing airway management practices. As illustrated by Rosen et al. (2018), the convergence of expert opinion and present evidence from various studies permits the development of standardized protocols that can contribute significantly to improving the quality of care. The dynamic nature of anesthesia necessitates that practitioners not only remain current with technological advances and medical developments but also participate in peer debates and with professional organizations. This collaborative effort fosters safety and excellence in culture within anesthesia, ultimately enhancing patient care. Overall, well-executed airway management, based on the latest evidence and continuous education, is essential to the success of anesthetic practice and to overall patient outcomes.

Good airway management during anesthesia is a key component of surgical procedures, ensuring patient safety and optimum outcomes. Key issues regarding airway management include the necessity for a complete preoperative assessment to identify likely difficulties, such as anatomical abnormalities or known medical illness, which can lead to intubation problems. Such an appraisal is crucial to the development of a personal airway plan in accordance with the patient's individual requirements. Furthermore, the professionals must stay up to date with the operation of various airway devices, both standard and non-standard, to secure the airway successfully. Continued training in advances in airway management techniques is important, as it equips anesthesiologists to handle more complex cases, thereby keeping complications that occur during anesthesia induction and maintenance as low as possible. Apart from patient-related information, technology use in airway management has taken center stage. New imaging technologies, such as ultrasound guidance, improve visualization of airway anatomy, enabling more precise intubation procedures. These technologies complement existing technologies, providing practitioners with a more comprehensive arsenal to handle diverse airway conditions. Moreover, the development of centers with expertise in complex airway procedures allows for the standardization of treatment and better patient outcomes. Such facilities can facilitate knowledge exchange between practitioners, which, in turn, is translated into the optimization of airway practice and protocols. This strategic collaboration ensures that clinicians are adequately equipped to handle challenging airway cases, which ultimately enhances the safety of general anesthesia. Finally, an interdisciplinary approach towards airway management also involves constant monitoring and readjustment within the perioperative setting. Anesthesiologists must monitor patients carefully for potential airway-related complications during and after surgery. This includes assessment of respiratory function and the adequacy of postoperative ventilation strategies. Current evidence identifies the key role for surgical and anesthetic teams' collaboration and communication in the resolution of airway management dilemmas, complicated cases such as neoplastic tracheobronchial resections. Developing a collaborative anesthetic-surgical plan is imperative in that it allows for a patient-specific airway management strategy that can dynamically respond to intraoperative challenges and preserve patient safety and welfare while undergoing anesthesia and surgical intervention (Stoica et al., 2019; Chen et al., 2020).

KEY TERMS FROM THIS CHAPTER

- Airway management
- Body mass index (BMI)
- Circumstances
- Inhalational anesthesia
- Oxygenation
- Personal protective equipment (PPE)
- Robust safety
- Technical skill
- Bag-mask ventilation (BMV)
- Bronchospasm
- Healthcare systems
- Larynx
- Pediatric airway management
- Pharynx
- Surgical protocols
- Trachea

CRITICAL THINKING QUESTIONS

1. **Which of the following is the most reliable method to confirm endotracheal intubation?**
   a. Auscultation of breath sounds
   b. Visualization of the tube passing through the vocal cords
   c. Chest rise observation
   d. End-tidal CO_2 detection
2. **Which of the following is not a predictor of difficult mask ventilation?**
   a. Age > 55 years
   b. Presence of a beard
   c. High BMI
   d. Hypotension
3. **The "sniffing position" improves airway patency by:**
   a. Extending the neck
   b. Flexing the head and extending the neck
   c. Hyperextending the neck
   d. Keeping the head in a neutral position
4. **Which device is most commonly used for securing an emergency airway in a patient with cervical spine injury?**
   a. Supraglottic airway device
   b. Cricothyrotomy
   c. Nasopharyngeal airway
   d. Video laryngoscope
5. **What is the primary function of a stylet in endotracheal intubation?**
   a. To guide the tube during insertion
   b. To clear airway obstructions
   c. To measure endotracheal tube pressure
   d. To assist in mask ventilation

Short Answer Questions

1. Describe the anatomy of the upper airway and its significance in airway management.
2. Discuss the indications, techniques, and complications of endotracheal intubation.
3. What are the predictors of a difficult airway, and how is it managed in anesthesia practice?
4. Explain the use of supraglottic airway devices (SGAs) in anesthesia.
5. What are the key components of the ASA Difficult Airway Algorithm, and how is it applied in clinical scenarios?

Answer to Critical Thinking Questions

1. (d); 2. (d); 3. (b); 4. (d); 5. (a)

REFERENCES

1. Apfelbaum, J. L., Hagberg, C. A., Connis, R. T., Abdelmalak, B. B., Agarkar, M., Dutton, R. P., Fiadjoe, J. E., Greif, R., Klock, P. A., Mercier, D., Myatra, S. N., O'Sullivan, E. P., Rosenblatt, W. H., Sorbello, M., & Tung, A. (2021). 2022 American Society of Anesthesiologists Practice Guidelines for Management of the Difficult Airway *. *Anesthesiology*, *136*(1), 31–81. https://doi.org/10.1097/aln.0000000000004002Asai, T., & Hillman, D. R. (2019). Current difficult airway management—Not good enough! *Anesthesiology, 131*, 774–776. https://doi.org/10.1097/aln.0000000000002885 (accessed on 28th June 2025).
2. Aslanidis, T., Darcy, C., Alves Bersot, C. D., Barros, V. G., Carlos, D., Bersot, G., Dhir, M., et al. (2023). Airway management in emergency medicine. *IntechOpen eBooks*. https://doi.org/10.5772/intechopen.110971 (accessed on 28th June 2025).
3. Aziz, S., Arabi, Y. M., Alhazzani, W., Evans, L., Citerio, G., Fischkoff, K., Salluh, J. I., et al. (2020). Managing ICU surge during the COVID-19 crisis: Rapid guidelines. *Intensive Care Medicine, 46*, 1303–1325. https://doi.org/10.1007/s00134-020-06092-5 (accessed on 28th June 2025).
4. Bazurro, S., Ball, L., & Pelosi, P. (2018). Perioperative management of obese patient. *Current Opinion in Critical Care, 24*, 560–567. https://doi.org/10.1097/mcc.0000000000000555 (accessed on 28th June 2025).
5. Chan, A. K. M., Nickson, C. P., Rudolph, J. W., Lee, A., & Joynt, G. M. (2020). Social media for rapid knowledge dissemination: Early experience from the COVID-19 pandemic. *Anesthesia, 75*, 1579–1582. https://doi.org/10.1111/anae.15057 (accessed on 28th June 2025).
6. Chen, C., Gao, G., Xu, Y., Pu, L., Wang, Q., Wang, L., Wang, W., et al. (2020). SARS-CoV-2–positive sputum and feces after conversion of pharyngeal samples in patients with COVID-19. *Annals of Internal Medicine, 172*, 832–834. https://doi.org/10.7326/m20-0991 (accessed on 28th June 2025).
7. Chrimes, N., Higgs, A., Hagberg, C. A., Baker, P., Cooper, R. M., Greif, R., Kovács, G., et al. (2022). Preventing unrecognized esophageal intubation: A consensus guideline from the Project for Universal Management of Airways and international airway societies. *Anesthesia, 77*, 1395–1415. https://doi.org/10.1111/anae.15817 (accessed on 28th June 2025).
8. Coccolini, F., Perrone, G., Chiarugi, M., Di Marzo, F., Ansaloni, L., Scandroglio, I., Marini, P., et al. (2020). Surgery in COVID-19 patients: Operational directives. *World Journal of Emergency Surgery, 15*. https://doi.org/10.1186/s13017-020-00307-2 (accessed on 28th June 2025).
9. Coté, C. J., & Wilson, S. (2019). Guidelines for monitoring and management of pediatric patients before, during, and after sedation for diagnostic and therapeutic procedures. *Pediatrics, 143*. https://doi.org/10.1542/peds.2019-1000 (accessed on 28th June 2025).
10. Crouser, E. D., Maier, L. A., Wilson, K. C., Bonham, C. A., Morgenthau, A. S., Patterson, K., Abston, E., et al. (2020). Diagnosis and detection of sarcoidosis: An official American Thoracic Society clinical practice guideline. *American Journal of Respiratory and Critical Care Medicine, 201*, e26–e51. https://doi.org/10.1164/rccm.202002-0251st (accessed on 28th June 2025).
11. Dohrmann, T., Muschol, N., Sehner, S., Punke, M. A., Haas, S., Roeher, K., Breyer, S., et al. (2019). Airway management and perioperative adverse events in children with mucopolysaccharidoses and mucolipidoses: A retrospective cohort study. *Pediatric Anesthesia, 30*, 181–190. https://doi.org/10.1111/pan.13787 (accessed on 28th June 2025).

12. Engelhardt, T., Fiadjoe, J. E., Weiß, M., Baker, P., Bew, S., Echeverry Marín, P., & von Ungern-Sternberg, B. S. (2019). A framework for the management of the pediatric airway. *Pediatric Anesthesia, 29*, 985–992. https://doi.org/10.1111/pan.13716 (accessed on 28th June 2025).

13. Friedel, M. E., Johnston, D. R., Singhal, S., Al Khalili, K., Farrell, C., Evans, J. J., Nyquist, G., et al. (2013). Airway management and perioperative concerns in acromegaly patients undergoing endoscopic transsphenoidal surgery for pituitary tumors. *Otolaryngology, 149*, 840–844. https://doi.org/10.1177/0194599813507236 (accessed on 28th June 2025).

14. Gerbershagen, M. U., & Baagil, H. (2024). Caesarean delivery: A narrative review on the choice of neuraxially administered opioid and its implications for the multimodal peripartum pain concept. *Medicina, 60*, 358. https://doi.org/10.3390/medicina60030358 (accessed on 28th June 2025).

15. Gottumukkala, V., Vetter, T. R., & Gan, T. J. (2023). Perioperative medicine: What the future can hold for anesthesiology. *Anesthesia & Analgesia, 136*, 628–635. https://doi.org/10.1213/ane.0000000000006412 (accessed on 28th June 2025).

16. Healy, D. W., Cloyd, B. H., Brenner, M., Kupfer, R. A., Anam, K. S., & Schechtman, S. A. (2020). The COVID-19 pandemic: Implications for the head and neck anesthesiologist. *Journal of Head & Neck Anesthesia, 4*, e26. https://doi.org/10.1097/hn9.0000000000000026 (accessed on 28th June 2025).

17. Hsu, G., von Ungern-Sternberg, B. S., & Engelhardt, T. (2021). Pediatric airway management. *Current Opinion in Anesthesiology, 34*, 276–283. https://doi.org/10.1097/aco.0000000000000993 (accessed on 28th June 2025).

18. Iorio-Morin, C., Hodaie, M., Sarica, C., Dea, N., Westwick, H. J., Christie, S., McDonald, P. J., et al. (2020). Letter: The risk of COVID-19 infection during neurosurgical procedures: A review of severe acute respiratory distress syndrome coronavirus 2 (SARS-CoV-2) modes of transmission and proposed neurosurgery-specific measures for mitigation. *Neurosurgery, 87*, E178–E185. https://doi.org/10.1093/neuros/nyaa157 (accessed on 28th June 2025).

19. Joglar, J. A., Chung, M. K., Armbruster, A. L., Benjamin, E. J., Chyou, J. Y., Cronin, E. M., Deswal, A., et al. (2023). 2023 ACC/AHA/ACCP/HRS guideline for the diagnosis and management of atrial fibrillation: A report of the American College of Cardiology/American Heart Association Joint Committee on Clinical Practice Guidelines. *Circulation, 149*. https://doi.org/10.1161/cir.0000000000001193 (accessed on 28th June 2025).

20. Kalagara, H., Coker, B. J., Gerstein, N. S., Kukreja, P., Deriy, L., Pierce, A., & Townsley, M. M. (2021). Point-of-care ultrasound (POCUS) for the cardiothoracic anesthesiologist. *Journal of Cardiothoracic and Vascular Anesthesia, 36*, 1132–1147. https://doi.org/10.1053/j.jvca.2021.01.018 (accessed on 28th June 2025).

21. Kogan, M., Klein, S. E., Hannon, C. P., & Nolte, M. T. (2020). Orthopedic education during the COVID-19 pandemic. *Journal of the American Academy of Orthopedic Surgeons, 28*, e456–e464. https://doi.org/10.5435/jaaos-d-20-00292 (accessed on 28th June 2025).

22. Lauder, G., Thomas, M., von Ungern-Sternberg, B. S., & Engelhardt, T. (2019). Volatiles or TIVA: Which is the standard of care for pediatric airway procedures? A pro-con discussion. *Pediatric Anesthesia, 30*, 209–220. https://doi.org/10.1111/pan.13809 (accessed on 28th June 2025).

23. Law, J. A., Duggan, L. V., Asselin, M., Baker, P., Crosby, E. T., Downey, A., Hung, O., et al. (2021). Canadian Airway Focus Group updated consensus-based recommendations for management of the difficult airway: Part 1. Difficult airway management encountered in an unconscious patient. *Canadian Journal of Anesthesia/Journal Canadine Anesthesia, 68*, 1373–1404. https://doi.org/10.1007/s12630-021-02007-0 (accessed on 28th June 2025).

24. Law, J. A., Duggan, L. V., Asselin, M., Baker, P., Crosby, E. T., Downey, A., Hung, O., et al. (2021). Canadian Airway Focus Group updated consensus-based recommendations for management of the difficult airway: Part 2. Planning and implementing safe management of the patient with an anticipated difficult airway. *Canadian Journal of Anesthesia/Journal Canadine Anesthesia, 68*, 1405–1436. https://doi.org/10.1007/s12630-021-02008-z (accessed on 28th June 2025).

25. Liang, Z., Chong, M., Sim, M. A., Lim, J. L., Castañeda, P., Green, D. W., Fisher, D., et al. (2020). Surgical considerations in patients with COVID-19. *Journal of Bone and Joint Surgery, 102*, e50. https://doi.org/10.2106/jbjs.20.00513 (accessed on 28th June 2025).

26. López-Olivo, M. A., Andrabi, T. R., Palla, S. L., & Suarez-Almazor, M. E. (2012). Cervical spine radiographs in patients with rheumatoid arthritis undergoing anesthesia. *JCR Journal of Clinical Rheumatology, 18*, 61–66. https://doi.org/10.1097/rhu.0b013e318247bb0d (accessed on 28th June 2025).

27. Lu, A. C., Cannesson, M., & Kamdar, N. (2020). The tipping point of medical technology: Implications for the post pandemic era. *Anesthesia & Analgesia, 131*, 335–339. https://doi.org/10.1213/ane.0000000000005040 (accessed on 28th June 2025).

28. Mahmood, F., Matyal, R., Skubas, N. J., Montealegre-Gallegos, M., Swaminathan, M., Denault, A., Sniecinski, R. M., et al. (2016). Perioperative ultrasound training in anesthesiology: A call to action. *Anesthesia & Analgesia, 122*, 1794–1804. https://doi.org/10.1213/ane.0000000000001134 (accessed on 28th June 2025).

29. Marwaha, A., Kumar, A., Sharma, S., & Sood, J. (2021). Anesthesia for tracheal resection and anastomosis. *Journal of Anesthesiology Clinical Pharmacology, 38*, 48–57. https://doi.org/10.4103/joacp.joacp_611_20 (accessed on 28th June 2025).

30. Matava, C., Kovatsis, P. G., Lee, J. K., Castro, P., Denning, S., Yu, J., Park, R., et al. (2020). Pediatric airway management in COVID-19 patients: Consensus guidelines from the Society for Pediatric Anesthesia's Pediatric Difficult Intubation Collaborative and the Canadian Pediatric Anesthesia Society. *Anesthesia & Analgesia, 131*, 61–73. https://doi.org/10.1213/ane.0000000000004872 (accessed on 28th June 2025).

31. McCann, M. E., de Graaff, J. C., Dorris, L., Disma, N., Withington, D. E., Bell, G., Grobler, A., et al. (2019). Neurodevelopmental outcome at 5 years of age after general anesthesia or awake-regional anesthesia in infancy (GAS): An international, multicenter, randomized, controlled equivalence trial. *The Lancet, 393*, 664–677. https://doi.org/10.1016/s0140-6736(18)32485-1 (accessed on 28th June 2025).

32. Meyer-Szary, J., Souza Luis, M., Mikulski, S., Patel, A., Schulz, F., Tretiakow, D., Fercho, J., et al. (2022). The role of 3D printing in planning complex medical procedures and training of medical professionals—Cross-sectional multispecialty review. *International Journal of Environmental Research and Public Health, 19*, 3331. https://doi.org/10.3390/ijerph19063331 (accessed on 28th June 2025).

33. Moretto, A., Bosatra, M. G., Marchesini, L., & Tesoro, S. (2018). Anesthesiologic risks in mucopolysaccharidoses. *The Italian Journal of Pediatrics, 44*. https://doi.org/10.1186/s13052-018-0554-1 (accessed on 28th June 2025).

34. Myatra, S. N. (2020). Airway management in the critically ill. *Current Opinion in Critical Care, 27*, 37–45. https://doi.org/10.1097/mcc.0000000000000791 (accessed on 28th June 2025).

35. Oria, M. S., Halimi, S. A., Negin, F., & Asady, A. (2022). Predisposing factors of difficult tracheal intubation among adult patients in Aliabad Teaching Hospital in Kabul, Afghanistan–A prospective observational study. *International Journal of General Medicine, 15*, 1161–1169. https://doi.org/10.2147/ijgm.s348813 (accessed on 28th June 2025).

36. Orser, B. A. (2020). Recommendations for endotracheal intubation of COVID-19 patients. *Anesthesia & Analgesia, 130*, 1109–1110. https://doi.org/10.1213/ane.0000000000004803 (accessed on 28th June 2025).

37. Pardo, E., Camus, M., & Verdonk, F. (2022). Anesthesia for digestive tract endoscopy. *Current Opinion in Anesthesiology, 35*, 528–535. https://doi.org/10.1097/aco.0000000000001162 (accessed on 28th June 2025).

38. Rosen, R., Vandenplas, Y., Singendonk, M., Cabana, M. D., DiLorenzo, C., Gottrand, F., Gupta, S. K., et al. (2018). Pediatric gastroesophageal reflux clinical practice guidelines. *Journal of Pediatric Gastroenterology and Nutrition, 66*, 516–554. https://doi.org/10.1097/mpg.0000000000001889 (accessed on 28th June 2025).

39. Soh, T. L. T., Ho, S. W. L., Yap, W. M., & Oh, J. Y. L. (2020). Spine surgery and COVID-19. *Journal of Bone and Joint Surgery, 102*, e56. https://doi.org/10.2106/jbjs.20.00503 (accessed on 28th June 2025).

40. Stoica, R., Cordoş, I., & Popescu, W. M. (2019). Anesthetic considerations for tracheobronchial resection in oncologic surgery. *Current Opinion in Anesthesiology, 33*, 55–63. https://doi.org/10.1097/aco.0000000000000821 (accessed on 28th June 2025).

41. van Zundert, A., Gatt, S. P., Van Zundert, T. C. R. V., Hagberg, C. A., & Pandit, J. J. (2024). Supraglottic airway devices: Present state and outlook for 2050. *Anesthesia & Analgesia, 138*, 337–349. https://doi.org/10.1213/ane.0000000000006673 (accessed on 28th June 2025).

42. Wax, R. S., & Sandrock, C. (2020). Practical recommendations for critical care and anesthesiology teams caring for novel coronavirus (2019-nCoV) patients. *Canadian Journal of Anesthesia/Journal Canadine Anesthesia, 67*, 568–576. https://doi.org/10.1007/s12630-020-01591-x (accessed on 28th June 2025).

43. Yang, Y. L., Huang, C. H., Luk, H. N., & Tsai, P. B. (2020). Adaptation to the plastic barrier sheet to facilitate intubation during the COVID-19 pandemic. *Anesthesia & Analgesia, 131*, e97–e99. https://doi.org/10.1213/ane.0000000000004923 (accessed on 28th June 2025).

44. Zheng, B., Zheng, H., & Lin, X. (2019). Ultrasound for predicting difficult airway in obstetric anesthesia. *Medicine, 98*, e17846. https://doi.org/10.1097/md.0000000000017846 (accessed on 28th June 2025).

TECHNIQUES OF ANESTHESIA

6

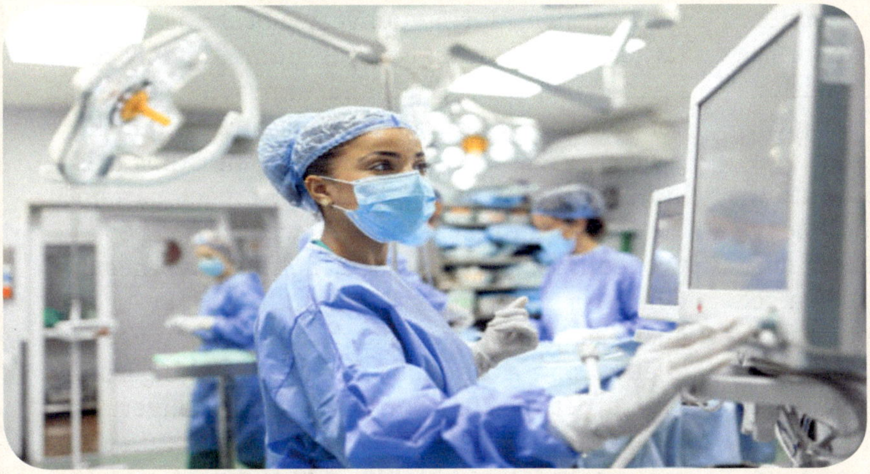

LEARNING OBJECTIVES

After studying this chapter, you will be able to:

1. Discuss the general anesthesia
2. Explain the regional anesthesia
3. Focus on local anesthesia
4. Understand sedation techniques
5. Know anesthesia in special populations
6. Describe the advances in anesthesia technology

Introduction

The art of anesthesia encompasses a tremendous range of techniques and styles that constitute the crux of modern medicine, particularly in surgical procedures. Anesthesia not only suppresses pain but also provides security and comfort to the patient, thereby facilitating complex surgeries. As technology and pharmacology have advanced, anesthesia techniques have evolved significantly to provide varying levels of sedation and analgesia tailored to the needs of the procedure and the patient. The precise balance between the safety and efficacy of anesthesia requires thorough knowledge of pharmacokinetics and pharmacodynamics so that the medical practitioner does not make decisions about the application of anesthetic agents in a blind manner. The application of protocols and guidelines, such as the updated Dutch protocol for treating craniosynostosis (Mathijssen, 2020), also underscores the need for evidence-based practice to achieve optimal outcomes for patients. In addition to pharmacological interventions, anesthesia methods are also regulated by patient profiles, including age, history, and comorbidities. This broad scope of variation demands thorough analysis by anesthesiologists, who are particularly responsible for determining the optimum technique for pain and sedation management. Techniques range from general anesthetics that render patients' unconscious to regional and local anesthetics that target specific areas to prevent pain from procedures. Patient safety is always of utmost importance, particularly given the complexity and increasing diversity of surgical procedures. Recent studies have explored the relationships of early detection and referral patterns in craniosynostosis treatment, as evidenced by the coordination of anesthetic approaches and overall surgical results (Mathijssen, 2020). Such consideration underscores the value of multimodal education and continued learning among the anesthesiology field. Beyond that, developments in anesthesia techniques are coupled with growing reliance on technology to optimize patient monitoring and anesthetic delivery further. Technologies such as ultrasound-assisted regional anesthesia and machine-learning algorithms for pain control demonstrate the integration of new methods into practice, with the latter enabling anesthesiologists to adapt their approach in real time based on patient responses to improve safety and efficiency. For instance, the use of machine-learning algorithms in pain research sheds light on the intricate interaction between multidimensional drivers of pain phenotype and anesthetic efficacy. With the evolving field of anesthesiology, it becomes crucial for practitioners to stay up to date on advancements in methods and knowledge to provide quality care that meets the needs of increasingly diverse patient populations.

Definition of Anesthesia

Anesthesia, in the broadest sense, is a state of medicine that suppresses sensation and consciousness to enable the carrying out of surgical and diagnostic manipulations without inflicting pain or distress on the patient. It is a complex pharmacologic intervention that plays a significant role in contemporary medicine, enabling both invasive and non-invasive procedures to be performed safely and efficiently. Anesthesia can be further categorized into general, regional, and local anesthesia, each with its own specific aims and mechanisms of action. General anesthesia induces complete unconsciousness and lack of sensation in all parts of the body, while regional anesthesia removes sensation in one area, e.g., an epidural for the relief of pain during delivery. Local anesthesia targets small, localized sites, numbing only the region of a procedure and improving patient compliance without discomfort throughout the process. The manner in which anesthesia is administered can significantly impact patient outcomes and even the success of surgical procedures. For instance, spinal anesthesia, which is commonly used in orthopedic or obstetric procedures, has been noted to cause hypotension, a common side effect resulting from sympathetic vasomotor block, and is dangerous to the mother and infant during labor. Current recommendations highlight the importance of understanding the pharmacological effect of drugs given with anesthesia, such as ephedrine and phenylephrine, with varied influences on maternal hemodynamics and fetal outcome. The selection of a vasopressor to correct hypotension is significant, as evidenced by the finding that phenylephrine administration can be associated with improved fetal acid-base status compared to ephedrine, illustrating that anesthetic management must account for the patient's physiology and the specific procedural demands (Kinsella et al., 2017). Besides, the practice of anesthesia has also evolved through systematic reviews and meta-analyses, underscoring the need for robust evidence in guideline development and in anesthetic techniques used across clinical settings. The efficacy of anesthetic strategies can be influenced by body mass index, labor, and the type of procedure, reflecting the complexity of anesthesia. Despite technological progress, the anesthetic community remains burdened by publication bias, which distorts the evidence-based critical understanding needed for safe practice. Continued investigation and adherence to practices that minimize reporting bias can enhance the quality of anesthetic evidence and eventually improve patient care outcomes. With the growing emphasis on individualized anesthetic practices, further refining the definition and concept of anesthesia through rigorous scientific research remains imperative (Jarrod et al., 2016) (Figure 6.1).

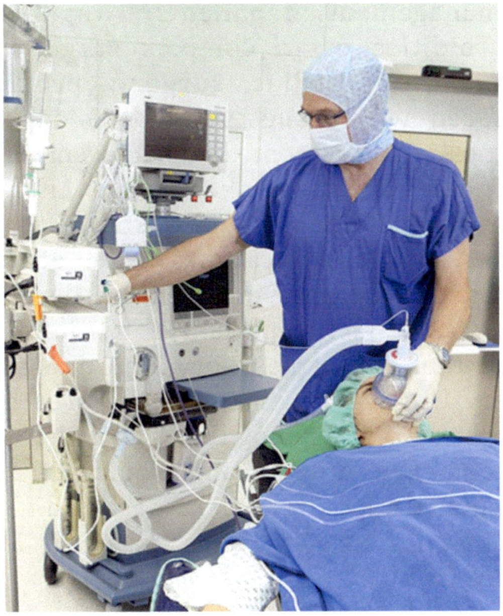

Figure 6.1. The field of anesthesia encompasses.

Source: https://staticnew-prod.topdoctors.co.uk/files/Image/large/5ad42457ea060d3bd53a6472111c44fd.jpg.

Importance in Medical Procedures

The contributions of anesthesia procedures during surgery cannot be ignored, as they are key to successful and safe surgery. Anesthesia allows patients to withstand potentially invasive or painful procedures without sensation or consciousness, thereby limiting the psychological and physiological trauma caused by surgery. This role is especially critical during lengthy procedures, where minimal discomfort could cause patients to experience traumatic reactions leading to complications. In addition, proper anesthesia application enables greater surgical precision by allowing surgeons to focus on their procedures without distraction from patient movement or discomfort. With diversification and transformation in procedures comes the necessity for evolution in anesthesia techniques to uphold comfort and safety for the patient during the entire surgical process. In the world of modern medical complications, anesthesia also plays a role in critical care settings, thus establishing its place among medical procedures. Anesthesiologists increasingly become directly engaged in treating patients with severe disease, such as those with respiratory illness or requiring close monitoring. For instance, during the COVID-19 pandemic, anesthesia experts emphasized the importance of specialized ventilation and intubation techniques to prevent the spread of viruses while ensuring patient care. Aligning with new recommendations, the use of personal protective equipment (PPE) and aerosol-generating procedure planning reflects advancements in anesthesia practice for meeting urgent medical needs. Thus, the evolution of anesthetic techniques in response to contemporary healthcare environments is a typical representation of their fundamental role in facilitating optimal patient outcomes and improved surgical safety (Beverley, 2020). Also, the application of ultrasound technology in anesthesia represents a significant advancement that maximizes procedural efficiency and safety. Perioperative ultrasound enables anesthesiologists to visualize real-time anatomy, thereby facilitating more accurate interventions, such as regional anesthesia blocks and vascular access. This decreases complications, makes patients more comfortable, and ultimately leads to quicker recoveries. The rising demand for competence in ultrasound-guided procedures makes official inclusion of this training in residency curricula an imperative, as highlighted in recent controversies in anesthesiology education (Mahmood et al., 2016). As the field of medicine continues to advance, embracing new anesthesia methodologies further underscores its integral role in enhancing surgical practice and patient care across diverse medical fields.

Overview of Anesthesia Techniques

The development of anesthesia techniques has significantly transformed surgical operations, alongside enhancing patient comfort and safety. Among the techniques, general anesthesia remains the foundation, resulting in loss of sensation and consciousness. It is commonly performed through intravenous or inhalational drugs, with profound relaxation of the muscles and shielding of the pain sensation. However, the selection of an anesthetic technique often depends on a range of variables, including the type of procedure, the patient's health status, and comorbidities. Some procedures, particularly in cardiac surgery, require fastidious anesthetic care to maintain hemodynamic stability and facilitate the rapid therapeutic intervention of any intraoperative morbidities. On this point, the role of the anesthesiologist becomes pivotal in using suitable anesthetic techniques desirable to the surgical objectives and health of the patient, as elaborated in the case of cardiothoracic surgeries (Anastsiia et al., 2024).

Augmenting general anesthesia, regional anesthetic techniques—such as nerve blocks and epidurals—have grown more central over the last few years. These techniques have the potential to provide pain relief directed to the surgical area but restrict systemic action and opioid use, hence promoting improved recovery from surgery. As emphasized in studies on transplantation, regional anesthesia has been adequate, both for managing pain after surgery and improving patient hemodynamics as well as reducing the need for supplemental analgesics. The Society for the Advancement of Transplant Anesthesia encourages the use of uniform techniques across transplant centers, reasoning that regional anesthetic techniques should be employed as integral components of the perioperative regimen. There are differences in the implementation of these methods, but their potential benefits make them still worthy of investigation and reporting in the anesthetic literature (Ander et al., 2024). The spectrum of anesthesia techniques also extends to patient safety and the management of potential complications.

Anesthesiologists will have to perform under a range of conditions, particularly in the management of patients with multiple comorbidities or in complex surgery. For instance, in cardiac surgery, providers are faced with issues related to depth of anesthesia management, fluid management, and prevention of thromboembolic events. Literature underscores the importance of staying vigilant against such complications while ensuring that the approaches employed are developed to address specific patient conditions. The contribution of anesthesiology towards ensuring surgery becomes safer cannot be overstated, considering that ongoing research and practice development aims to maximize outcomes while minimizing anesthesia risks across different specialties of surgery (Anastsiia et al., 2024) (Figure 6.2).

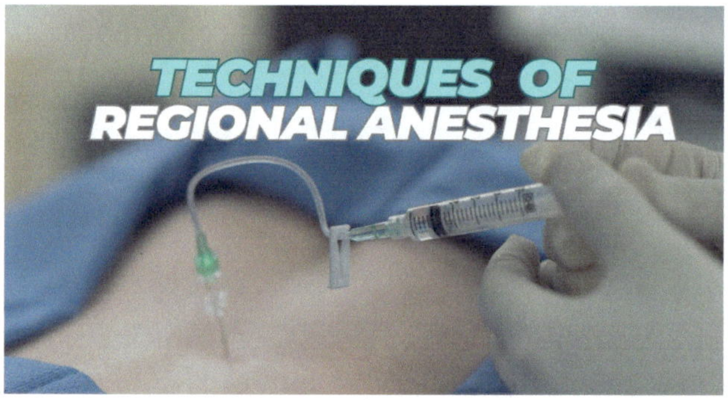

Figure 6.2. The evolution of anesthesia techniques.

Source: https://i.ytimg.com/vi/uH52H7GSrLE/maxresdefault.jpg.

6.1. General Anesthesia

Learning Outcome

1. Mechanism of action
2. Indications for use
3. Risks and complications

General anesthesia is a crucial element of contemporary surgical practice that renders patients entirely unconscious and pain-insensitive during invasive procedures. The method is primarily based on a synergistic combination of intravenous and inhalational drugs to produce rapid onset of deep sedation. One advantage of general anesthesia is that it can facilitate long-duration procedures under precise control of anesthetic depth, thereby preventing patient movement and improving operating conditions. It is required in the management of complex and painful procedures when local anesthesia itself cannot be effective.

The patient's history determines the agents employed, the type of surgery, and the anticipated length of procedure, a rationale for individualized anesthetic plans to ensure optimal patient safety and comfort. Despite its widespread application, general anesthesia is not without risks. Complications associated with the administration of anesthetic agents include cardiovascular instability and anesthetic-related responses. Recent studies emphasize the importance of constant monitoring throughout the process to avoid such complications. For example, various studies have found that general anesthesia, when performed by experienced anesthesiologists at highly specialized centers, is generally safe; however, patient age and prior medical conditions can significantly influence outcomes. Intriguingly, comorbid patients, particularly those with ASA physical status ≥ III, may require closer monitoring and other types of anesthesia to avoid adversity. This is particularly so in vulnerable populations, such as pediatrics, where outcomes following exposure to anesthetics are quite predictable and thus require constant caution and accommodative measures in the practice of anesthesia (Amornyotin et al., 2012). Yet another issue about general anesthesia is its potential impact on neurodevelopment in kids. Fresh evidence suggests that exposure to anesthetic agents during critical periods of brain growth may lead to undesirable outcomes like learning disabilities and abnormalities in neurobehavior.

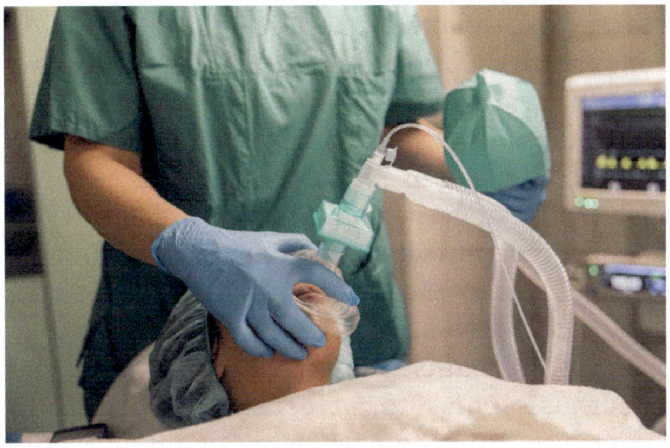

Figure 6.3. General anesthesia represents a critical component of contemporary surgical practices.

Source: https://www.nysora.com/wp-content/uploads/2025/01/general-anesthesia.jpg.

A review of studies reveals that anesthetics, particularly those possessing NMDA receptor antagonist activity, may initiate neurodegenerative processes in developing brains (Robert et al., 2009). While research with animal models has identified concerns about potential neurodevelopmental effects, extending this information to human populations is complex. Appreciation of the delicate balance between the necessity for general anesthesia for definitive surgical procedures and potential long-term effects on the developing brain is critical for anesthesiologists. Thus, clinicians are also encouraged to consider alternative modes of anesthetizing, especially in children, and to have well-prepared discussions with family members regarding the implications and risks associated with general anesthesia (Figure 6.3).

6.1.1. Mechanism of Action

In anesthesiology, an understanding of how anesthetic drugs work is necessary to optimize patient care and improve surgical outcomes. Anesthetic drugs primarily act by altering neuronal function in the central nervous system to produce and sustain states of unconsciousness, during which sensory perception is reduced. They do this through various mechanisms, including the strengthening of inhibitory neurotransmission and the blocking of excitatory transmission. For instance, propofol drugs enhance the activity of GABA-A receptors, leading to increased chloride ion influx into the neuron, hyperpolarization, and, ultimately, sedation and anesthesia. This kind of mechanistic information enables the anesthesiologist to select the appropriate agent based on the patient's individual profile and the type of surgery, reducing the risk of complications and speeding recovery (Bradley et al., 2018). In addition, anesthetic drug pharmacodynamics reveal the relationship among drug concentration, brain site of action, and clinical effect. The lipid solubility theory is especially significant: higher concentrations of lipid-soluble drugs permeate the central nervous system more readily, resulting in a rapid onset of anesthesia. The blood-to-gas partition coefficient is also of significance because it determines the rate at which inhalational anesthetics become active. Lower coefficients signify a quicker onset and recovery, allowing greater control over the depth of anesthesia during surgery. These features emphasize the importance of a thorough understanding of anesthetic pharmacokinetics in delivering balanced anesthesia, characterized by rapid induction and plateaued maintenance throughout surgery (Bradley et al., 2018). In addition, the mechanism of action is relevant to postoperative complications, particularly for analgesics used in the perioperative period. Opioids, for example, exert their effects by binding to mu-opioid receptors, modifying pain perception, and modulating ascending pain pathways. The efficacy and safety of these medications require appropriate consideration of their mechanisms to avoid side effects such as respiratory depression and sedation. Besides, evidence-based guidelines for the application of multimodal analgesia are under development, bringing together different agents with dissimilar mechanisms of action. Not only does this enhance pain control, but it also decreases opioid intake, soothing the present worry with opioid side effects in clinical settings. Last but not least, thorough knowledge of the mechanisms engaged permits the development of more effective anesthetic techniques, individually tailored to the needs of a patient (Mahmood et al., 2016).

6.1.2. Indications for Use

The variety of different anesthesia techniques depends only on their indications of use to guide clinicians in selecting the most appropriate method for the management of pain and anesthesia in various clinical conditions. Among the available techniques, the erector spinae plane block has been an effective tool for managing acute and chronic pain, particularly in the thoracic and abdominal cavities. This interfascial block is used to administer analgesia through the delivery of local anesthetic within the anatomical interfascial space between the erector spinae muscles and the vertebrotransverse process. Evidence shows that success with the ESP block can reduce opioid consumption by a significant level, providing the advantage of reducing risk from opioid side effects while guaranteeing excellent pain relief (Cassai AD et al., 2019). Further, the uses of the ESP block also involve postoperative recovery after thoracic and abdominal surgeries because it falls under enhanced recovery. It has been matched with equal effectiveness to routine epidural analgesia, so that it allows clinicians to administer an alternative which is less complicated, for instance, a possible infection due to epidural catheterization. Successful pain control can reduce hospital stay and hasten recovery for patients, making the ESP block a worthwhile skill in the anesthesiologist's arsenal. Effective use of the ESP block has been documented in various operations in a retrospective review, vindicating its expanding relevance to contemporary anesthesia practice (Tulgar et al., 2019).

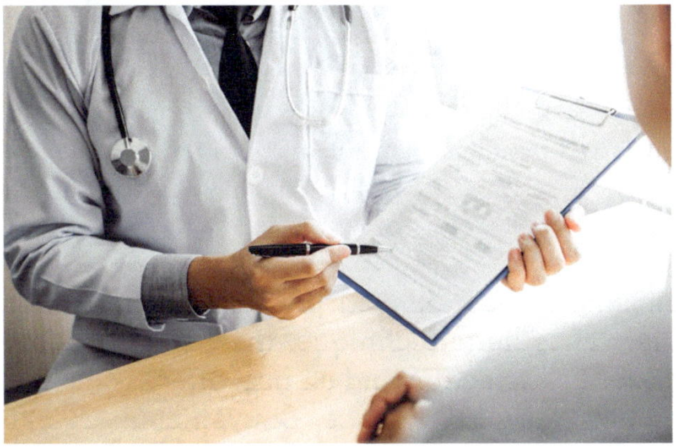

Figure 6.4. The application of various anesthesia techniques.

Source: https://osteoboost.com/wp-content/uploads/2024/08/Osteoboost-Indications-for-Use.jpeg.

While the reports of ESP block use are promising, there is clear recognition of the need to act as an aid to other studies to fully characterize mechanisms of action, safety profiles, and individual efficacy compared with available regional anesthetic techniques. While it is welcome in light of what currently prevails in the literature, proof is required for adequate randomized controlled trials to provide credible information on the complication rate and the clinical effects of the ESP block. Such studies would further establish it as a normative practice in anesthesia, thereby enabling its wider application among healthcare providers. They will be compelled to weigh advantage against potential risk, but further investigation into ESP block will yield useful insights for optimizing anesthetic technique and patient care (Figure 6.4).

6.1.3. Risks and Complications

Anesthesia administration, while generally safe, carries inherent risks and complications that must be addressed with care by the medical community. Of these risks, post-operative complications arise typically, with more reference to the technique employed. Comparative analysis of total intravenous anesthesia (TIVA) and inhalational anesthesia (IA) showed that TIVA provided a more comfortable recovery experience for patients, with 77.8% satisfaction compared to 62% for IA. And yet, postoperative nausea and vomiting were common complications in both groups, affecting 22.2% of patients receiving TIVA and 20% of patients receiving IA, demonstrating that despite advances, anesthetic methods are not free of difficulty (Tahir et al., 2025). Knowledge of complications enables practitioners to make informed choices during anesthetic planning and ensures patient safety remains a top priority at all stages of the perioperative process. Geriatric patients are a high-risk population when it comes to anesthesia administration. Physiologic alterations and the increased prevalence of comorbidities in elderly patients amplify the risk of surgical complications by a large margin. In a retrospective study, cardiovascular events were the most common reported complication and occurred in 35% of geriatric patients. This was followed by respiratory complications in 20% of the cases and drug-related complications in 15% (Yadav et al., 2024). The findings support the need for individualized management protocols in the treatment of elderly patients undergoing anesthesia. The implementation of complete preoperative evaluation and close intraoperative monitoring prevents such risks and overall improves outcomes for this population, as techniques in anesthesia are optimized according to their respective health conditions and needs. Apart from physiological issues related to anesthetic modalities, anesthesia choice also relies on balancing intraoperative complications. As a case in point, while TIVA has been promising for recovery time and patient satisfaction, its implication with higher postoperative pain scores makes consideration of it during anesthesia planning a requirement. The mean pain scores documented in the study indicated statistically significant variation, with TIVA at 4.06 and IA at 3.71 (Tahir et al., 2025). This aspect of anesthesia demonstrates a complex interplay among efficacy, safety, and patient comfort and further underscores the need for individualized anesthesia regimens. Lastly, prevention and awareness of these risks by proper patient evaluation and technique selection are critical in maximizing surgical results and maintaining patient welfare.

Test Your Knowledge

1. What are the main goals and components of general anesthesia, and how is it achieved pharmacologically?
2. What factors influence the choice of general anesthetic agents and techniques for different surgical procedures?

6.2. Regional Anesthesia

Learning Outcome

1. Types of regional anesthesia
2. Applications in surgery
3. Benefits and limitations

The application of regional anesthesia has revolutionized pain management in the operating room, providing targeted analgesia with little systemic impact from general anesthesia. Irradiating specific nerve tracts, techniques such as epidural anesthesia and nerve blocks can cause potent analgesia confined to the operative site. This targeted method not only enhances patient comfort but also reduces the requirement for opioids, which are generally associated with the potential of unwanted side effects such as respiratory depression as well as longer recovery times. Due to this, regional anesthesia is particularly beneficial in high-risk patient populations, such as cancer surgery patients, where controlling pain is effective in significantly influencing postoperative recovery results. The development of regional anesthesia has allowed practitioners to tailor their anesthetic technique, thereby improving patient satisfaction and clinical effectiveness in modern surgical practice (Bhuyan et al., 2024). Regional anesthesia is also crucial to multimodal pain management strategies, which enable accelerated recovery across various surgical scenarios. ERAS pathways have progressively added regional techniques to optimize results in patients, especially for high-risk procedures like organ transplantation. Reduction of perioperative opioid use not only prevents the side effects generally associated with the use of opioids but also promotes a quicker recovery towards baseline function in the patient. Regional anesthesia can provide deep analgesia while maintaining hemodynamic stability, a vital factor in procedures that are subject to extreme physiological stress. Despite the proven advantages, the absence of clear guidelines for regional anesthesia in certain surgical specialties, such as transplantation, underscores a void that warrants further investigation and the dissemination of best practices among clinical professionals (Ander et al., 2024). Regional anesthesia in oncology has implications beyond immediate alleviation of pain and can, in theory at least, influence long-term cancer outcomes in patients. The available evidence suggests that regional anesthesia may influence immune function and reduce cancer recurrence rates, a consideration when managing patients who are facing resection of a tumor. Techniques such as paravertebral blocks and intrathecal anesthesia have shown promise in minimizing the surgery-induced stress response and thereby enhancing recovery, with the potential to impact the pathophysiology of cancer growth. Future research aims to elucidate these correlations and ultimately inform clinical decision-making in surgical oncology. As regional anesthesia continues to advance and evolve in the complex context of cancer care, its inclusion in surgical management could substantially enhance patient care, not only promoting short-term postoperative symptom relief but also offering long-term survival benefits (Bhuyan et al., 2024) (Figure 6.5).

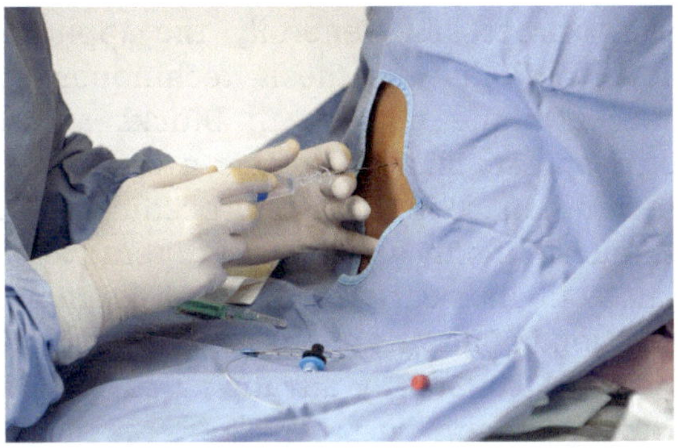

Figure 6.5. The application of regional anesthesia.

Source: https://www.verywellhealth.com/thmb/YwoG7Rb7TaAEUUS1pxNEMCUEcvQ=/1500x0/filters:no_upscale():max_bytes(150000):strip_icc()/GettyImages-154725435-59a034a50d327a001006171b.jpg.

6.2.1. Types of Regional Anesthesia

The practice of regional anesthesia offers several techniques to enhance surgical outcomes while minimizing patient discomfort. Among the most prevalent are peripheral nerve blocks, spinal anesthesia, and epidural anesthesia. Peripheral nerve blocks are performed by targeted injection of anesthetic near specific nerves to produce numbness in a localized area. This method is particularly ideal for limb surgery and is favored for its rapid recovery and lower incidence of systemic effects compared to general anesthesia. The advantages of peripheral nerve blocks have driven the development of ultrasound guidance, enabling more precise needle placement and further guaranteeing patient safety and overall satisfaction in surgery. Spinal anesthesia is remarkable for its efficacy in procedures in the lower body, such as orthopedic and gynecological procedures. The technique involves the injection of local anesthetics into the cerebrospinal fluid, thereby creating deep and instant anesthesia from the abdominal region below. Spinal anesthesia is characterized by fewer postoperative pain and reduced narcotic use, leading to better recovery outcomes. Evidence shows that patients undergoing surgery under spinal anesthesia report lower pain scores, especially in the immediate postoperative period, thus facilitating earlier mobilization and quicker discharge from hospital units. As with all regional anesthetic techniques, training and practice are key to achieving optimal outcomes, underscoring the importance of formal education in the specialty. Epidural anesthesia is another frequently utilized regional anesthetic with continuous pain control, particularly valuable in labor and long abdominal operations. With the placement of a catheter within the epidural space, anesthetic drugs may be infused, providing prolonged analgesia based on the patients' needs. This flexibility is also found to be of particular value for the comfort of the patients, both during and post-surgery, as adjustments can be made in the anesthetic dosage based on fluctuating pain. Clinicians who receive hands-on education in methods such as ultrasound-guided regional anesthesia are shown to have greater confidence and skills in administering such blocks, which ultimately lead to improved patient outcomes and satisfaction (Theodoraki et al., 2021). As diverse as these methods of regional anesthesia are, they all share a common goal: enhancing patient care and minimizing the physiological discomfort of surgery (Figure 6.6).

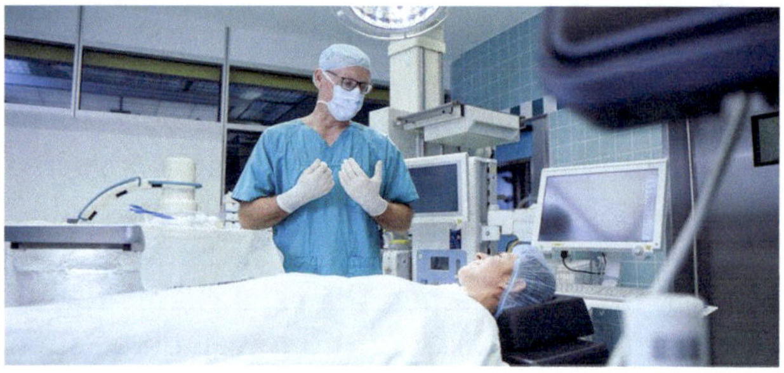

Figure 6.6. The realm of regional anesthesia offers various techniques that enhance surgical outcomes while minimizing patient discomfort.

Source: https://pajunk.com/fileadmin/_processed_/f/c/csm_pa_hero_RA_News_8bab2fd295.jpg.

6.2.2. Applications in Surgery

The employment of regional anesthesia techniques in surgery has been of keen interest in current times, particularly as an effective means of managing postoperative pain and improving patient outcomes. The employment of fascial plane chest wall blocks in cardiac surgical procedures is one such innovation that has become more relevant as part of optimized recovery after surgery (ERAS) protocols. The blocks provide effective analgesia, allowing patients to experience less postoperative pain and discomfort. Although early evidence indicates promising efficacy across varied cardiac surgery settings, there remains much to be desired in terms of high-quality evidence on their efficacy and safety. It is thus crucial that anesthesiologists familiarize themselves with the associated fascial plane anatomy and techniques so that patients experience faster recoveries and improved functional outcomes from minimally invasive cardiac procedures (Kelava et al., 2020). Another significant advancement in anesthetic methods for surgical application is the erector spinae plane block. Historically, regional anesthesia for posterior thoracic operations has been limited mainly to neuraxial and paravertebral blocks; however, with the ESP block, the dorsal rami of spinal nerves at the posterior thoracic wall are blocked, thereby offering a new alternative. The successful application of the ESP block in a pediatric surgical case illustrates its advantages, as it provided optimal postoperative pain relief and hemodynamic stability, with decreased systemic analgesic requirements. The patient experienced rapid postoperative functional recovery, which emphasizes the role of this method in enhancing discharge routines and overall patient satisfaction (Maria et al., 2017). The erector spinae plane block is just one indicator of the evolving character of anesthetic techniques, which offer specialized solutions for specific surgical needs and help achieve smoother recovery processes. Generally, the application of novel regional anesthesia techniques, such as fascial plane chest wall blocks and the erector spinae plane block, is a reflection of their significance in surgical procedures. These techniques not only enhance postoperative pain, but also enhance early recovery and functional restoration in patients after extensive surgeries. As with the constantly advancing surgical and anesthetic techniques, further research is required to investigate mechanisms of action, optimal dosing regimens, and comparative effectiveness of these new blocks. In this manner, anesthesiology can ensure that patient outcomes are enhanced consistently, leading to reduced opioid use and a better perioperative experience (Kelava et al., 2020; Maria et al., 2017).

6.2.3. Benefits and Limitations

The use of multimodal pain control methods in anesthesia has several major benefits, particularly in orthopedic surgery. By combining pharmacologic and non-pharmacologic methods, multimodal pain management provides effective relief across multiple pain pathways. The best benefit is perhaps the substantial reduction in opioid usage, critical in an era plagued by the opioid crisis. Multimodal strategies have been demonstrated through research to result in less severe postoperative pain and better patient' outcomes, as an indicator of improved patient satisfaction and enabling early mobilization post-surgery (Machado et al., 2025). Besides decreasing pain, it also allows the reduction of hospital stays, hence maximizing healthcare resource utilization. Although these advantages exist, it is also important to note that the use of multimodal protocols can be resource-sucking, demanding complete knowledge of many agents and their interactions, which may be difficult in clinical practice. In contrast, the drawbacks of existing anesthetic practices, particularly environmental impacts, should not be neglected. Use of inhaled anesthetics such as desflurane and nitrous oxide has raised a lot of concern due to their high global warming potentials (GWPs). A large percentage of the greenhouse gas emissions of the healthcare sector come from anesthesia, making the profession consider changing its practices (Cappellini et al., 2024). Even though many anesthetics have effectively managed perioperative pain, the environmental impacts are a good reason to move towards greener agents. In addition, technological limitations and the medical profession's reluctance render it challenging to adopt environmentally friendly practices. Both factors call for reconciling patient safety through appropriate analgesia and responding to the pressing need for environmental accountability within the healthcare system. In light of these benefits and limitations, the future of anesthesia practice must lean toward sustainability while ensuring that patient care remains the top priority. The application of anesthetics with lower GWPs, combined with innovations such as low-flow anesthesia and intravenous techniques, can significantly reduce environmental impact without compromising the quality of pain relief (Cappellini et al., 2024). However, the realization of these green practices is contingent upon integral education, lobbying, and robust policy frameworks to drive changes in practice. Collaboration among anesthesiologists, policymakers, and environmental stakeholders is essential in crafting a framework that prioritizes both patient safety and environmental well-being. Ultimately, reconciling the benefits and limitations of anesthesia practices not only improves patient outcomes but also forms a healthcare strategy that supports global sustainability goals, upholding the health of generations to come.

Test Your Knowledge

1. What are the different types of regional anesthesia, and how do they differ in terms of the area of the body they anesthetize?
2. How do techniques such as spinal, epidural, and peripheral nerve blocks differ in administration, onset, and duration of anesthesia?

6.3. Local Anesthesia

Learning Outcome

1. Common agents used
2. Techniques for administration
3. Patient considerations

Local anesthesia is a key procedure in modern medical practice, particularly in surgery and dentistry. Its primary function is to temporarily anesthetize a local area of the body, inhibiting pain perception without sedating the patient. This local approach eliminates the systemic side effects of general anesthesia, hence being the mode of choice for patients and practitioners alike. Effective local anesthetics such as lidocaine and bupivacaine may have a rapid onset of analgesia and an unpredictable duration of action, depending on the requirements of the procedure. Local anesthesia thus not only serves the purpose of pain management but also aids the overall surgical process by allowing shorter recovery times and less postoperative pain. The proper use and choice of the local anesthetic drugs remain the cornerstone to achieving maximum success with procedures ranging from a minor skin excision to intricate dental procedures. With all its benefits, however, local anesthesia is not without risk and has certain considerations to keep in mind. Rebound pain is a significant problem a clinician may encounter; it is transient, acute pain that occurs after discontinuation of the sensory blockade. Rebound pain may not have a significant impact on global patient satisfaction or opioid consumption, but it is clinically meaningful and must be treated within perioperative management. Prevention is achieved through the implementation of a multimodal analgesic regimen as well as educating patients extensively regarding the expectation of postoperative pain. Moreover, techniques that prolong the duration of local anesthesia, such as continuous catheter techniques, may reduce rebound pain. Understanding these nuances is essential in providing comprehensive surgical care so that patients' comfort is maintained throughout the perioperative period (Mu Fñoz-Leyva et al., 2020). Recent advancements in regional anesthesia techniques further illustrate the evolving landscape of local anesthetic application. The erector spinae plane block is a new method that identifies the function of local anesthetic extension beyond standard uses. By delivering anesthetic into the fascial plane of the erector spinae muscle, efficacy in controlling acute and chronic pain has been demonstrated, with a good safety record. Further studies indicate its use in various clinical contexts and circumstances. Nonetheless, even though single-shot usage is the most common, further study would be valuable to determine its benefits and refine its use. In line with the transition to progress in local anesthesia methods, ongoing research must be conducted to develop improved pain management techniques that align with shifting patient populations' needs (Kot et al., 2019) (Figure 6.7).

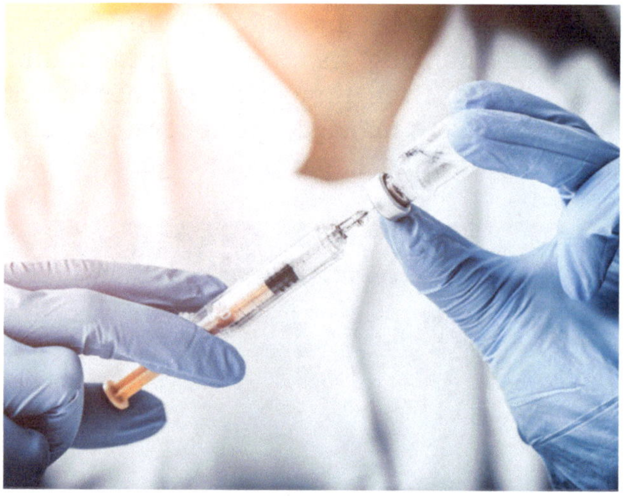

Figure 6.7. A medical professional is preparing an injection with a syringe and a vial.

Source: https://madeforthismoment.asahq.org/wp-content/uploads/2017/10/iStock-627196908.jpg.

6.3.1. Common Agents Used

The selection of the most frequently used agents in anesthesia plays a crucial role in maintaining patient safety and the effectiveness of surgical procedures. Isoflurane and sevoflurane are among the most frequently used agents in current anesthetic practice. Isoflurane, with its rapid onset and recovery, facilitates immediate adjustments in anesthetic depth, which are required at various stages of surgery. Similarly, sevoflurane is used for its smooth induction and rapid elimination from the body, making it a favorite for outpatient surgeries. Both drugs have exhibited an excellent safety profile, going a long way in enhancing the quality of anesthetic care. Besides, these inhalational agents provide control of anesthetic depth, a critical factor in avoiding anesthesia-related complications during surgery, thereby highlighting their application in modern anesthesia practice (Oh et al., 2024). Besides inhalational agents, intravenous agents are also crucial in the armamentarium of anesthetics. Agents such as propofol and etomidate are widely used owing to their immediate onset of action and comparatively short action time. Propofol, an agent with sedative-hypnotic effects, has rapid recovery and is therefore particularly well adapted for ambulatory surgery, where patient turnover is of primary concern. Etomidate, on the other hand, is to be employed in those situations where cardiovascular stability is paramount because it has the least hemodynamic effect. The judicious application of these intravenous anesthetics demonstrates the anesthesiologist's skill at tailoring anesthetic protocols to an individual patient's requirements and unique surgical circumstances. These individualized approaches are as essential to optimizing patient outcomes as they are to pushing the lofty standards of anesthesia practice (Sasangohar et al., 2020). Preoperative administration of adjunct medications also significantly enhances the efficacy of the anesthetic agents employed. Analgesics such as NSAIDs and opioids are presently routine in anesthesia regimens to affect pain relief and reduce the total anesthetic need. By treating pain preoperatively, clinicians can enhance patients' comfort and facilitate a more straightforward postoperative recovery. NSAIDs, for instance, are effective in the prevention of inflammation and pain without the adverse effects of opioid administration, such as respiratory depression. This multimodal approach emphasizes how generic agents of anesthesia are combined with broader pain management strategies to ultimately enhance patient satisfaction and clinical results. The wise application and blending of anesthetic medications reflect the evolving nature of anesthetic techniques, with the aim of greater safety and effectiveness in the operating theatre (Oh et al., 2024).

6.3.2. Techniques for Administration

Anesthesia administration methods are core to delivering both effectiveness and patient comfort during medical procedures. One important consideration in such methods is the use of local anesthesia, which is widely employed in dentistry and minor surgical procedures. The method of administration has a significant influence on patients' anxiety and pain sensitivity. Techniques involving distraction strategies, such as virtual reality, have emerged as new methods for reducing the fear and distress of the procedure. In a review of the impact of virtual reality on children receiving buccal infiltration anesthesia, results indicated an anxiety reduction, no matter whether the distraction was visual or auditory, an indication of the requirement for psychological attention in the administration process (Osama et al., 2021). These findings suggest that combining technological innovation with standard practice enhances patient experience during the administration of anesthesia. Another key feature of anesthesia administration is the process and timing of care delivery. The relationship between intervals and outcomes has been widely documented, most notably in acute conditions such as stroke therapy. For example, in the ESCAPE trial, every additional 30 minutes of augmentation of the interval between computed tomography and reperfusion adversely affected the likelihood of favorable recovery (Bijoy et al., 2016). This underscores the need to expedite anesthesia administration without compromising safety in emergency care. Understanding the impact of time on anesthesia administration can assist healthcare professionals in maximizing their procedures and workflows, ultimately leading to improved patient outcomes. This time management illustrates how anesthesia administration methods can significantly affect the quality and timeliness of care. Also, the choice of anesthetic agents and delivery routes is at the core of administration. Intravenous (IV) sedation, local infiltration, and general anesthesia are techniques used to accommodate individual patient and surgical needs. The choice of technique has a significant impact on both procedure outcome and patient comfort. For instance, while IV sedation is dominated by its quick onset and easy titration, general anesthesia is used for complex operations that involve higher levels of sedation. Studies have also shown that general anesthetic patients experience longer delays in certain care intervals, therefore impacting efficiency overall (Bijoy et al., 2016). Ultimately, careful selection of agents and techniques not only determines the anesthetic experience but also points to the necessity to tailor administration methods to specific patients' circumstances.

6.3.3. Patient Considerations

Patient considerations in anesthesia encompass a variety of factors that must be handled with care in the general management plan to ensure the most favorable outcomes for patients undergoing surgical procedures. The patient's medical history is an essential factor, including underlying conditions that may influence anesthesia safety and effectiveness. Respiratory-compromised or cardiovascular-compromised patients, for instance, need customized anesthetic techniques to prevent injury during surgery. The importance of an adequate preoperative assessment becomes obvious, as it enables physicians to identify risks and formulate appropriate anesthetic regimens to ensure safety and the effective performance of procedures. By knowing these factors ahead of time, the risk of complications can be significantly reduced, enhancing the overall quality of care administered to patients. The activity of selecting anesthetics based on individual physiological and psychological profiles is another important patient factor. Different patients exhibit varying responsiveness to anesthetics, necessitating a nuanced understanding of pharmacodynamics and pharmacokinetics to administer drugs. For example, pediatric or complex regional pain syndrome patients, as in the case of diseases in young children, require practitioners to apply specialized techniques, such as lumbar sympathetic blocks under general anesthesia, to treat distinct pain management problems (Amany et al., 2024). These personalized settings not only optimize anesthesia but also improve recovery outcomes. Thus, a tailored anesthetic approach according to age, weight, and medical background is of utmost importance to optimize patient safety and comfort under anesthesia. Patient monitoring and safeguarding during anesthesia are also of utmost importance, especially for procedures that require advanced interventions, such as whole-lung lavage (WLL) for pulmonary alveolar proteinosis (PAP). Clinicians must employ careful intraoperative monitoring to detect complications such as hypoxemia or fluid overload that can arise during operations involving the delivery of high volumes of fluids (Sikachi et al., 2024). Intraoperative eventual complications are managed and patient safety ensured by a multidisciplinary team involving anesthesiologists, surgeons, and nurses. Continuous monitoring not only facilitates timely intervention but also fosters trust with patients and their kin towards the procedural processes engaged. Overall, incorporating these patient considerations into anesthesia practice plays a significant role in improving surgical outcomes and building trust in healthcare providers (Figure 6.8).

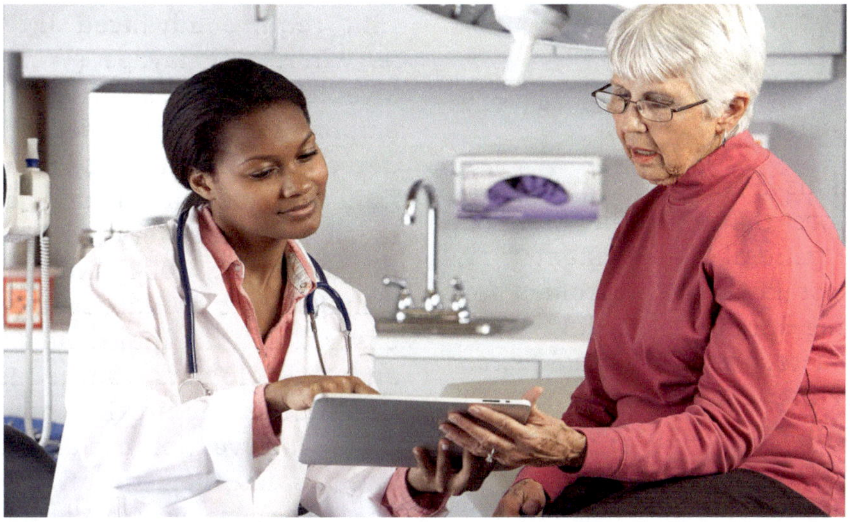

Figure 6.8. Patient considerations in anesthesia.

Source: https://pcna.net/wp-content/uploads/2024/12/Counseling-patient-scaled-1.jpg.

Test Your Knowledge

1. What is local anesthesia, and how does it produce loss of sensation in a specific area without affecting consciousness?
2. What are the common types of local anesthetic agents, and how do their onset, duration, and toxicity profiles differ?

6.4. Sedation Techniques

Learning Outcome

1. Levels of sedation
2. Monitoring during sedation
3. Applications in dentistry and minor procedures

Patient considerations in anesthesia encompass a variety of factors that must be handled with care in the general management plan to ensure the most favorable outcomes for patients undergoing surgical procedures. The patient's medical history is an essential factor, including underlying conditions that may influence anesthesia safety and effectiveness. Respiratory-compromised or cardiovascular-compromised patients, for instance, need customized anesthetic techniques to prevent injury during surgery. The importance of an adequate preoperative assessment becomes obvious, as it enables physicians to identify risks and formulate appropriate anesthetic regimens to ensure safety and the effective performance of procedures. By knowing these factors ahead of time, the risk of complications can be significantly reduced, enhancing the overall quality of care administered to patients. The activity of selecting anesthetics based on individual physiological and psychological profiles is another important patient factor. Different patients exhibit varying responsiveness to anesthetics, necessitating a nuanced understanding of pharmacodynamics and pharmacokinetics to administer drugs. For example, pediatric or complex regional pain syndrome patients, as in the case of diseases in young children, require practitioners to apply specialized techniques, such as lumbar sympathetic blocks under general anesthesia, to treat distinct pain management problems (Amany et al., 2024). These personalized settings not only optimize anesthesia but also improve recovery outcomes. Thus, a tailored anesthetic approach according to age, weight, and medical background is of utmost importance to optimize patient safety and comfort under anesthesia. Patient monitoring and safeguarding during anesthesia are also of utmost importance, especially for procedures that require advanced interventions, such as whole-lung lavage (WLL) for pulmonary alveolar proteinosis (PAP). Clinicians must employ careful intraoperative monitoring to detect complications such as hypoxemia or fluid overload that can arise during operations involving the delivery of high volumes of fluids (Sikachi et al., 2024). Intraoperative eventual complications are managed and patient safety ensured by a multidisciplinary team involving anesthesiologists, surgeons, and nurses. Continuous monitoring not only facilitates timely intervention but also fosters trust with patients and their kin towards the procedural processes engaged. Overall, incorporating these patient considerations into anesthesia practice plays a significant role in improving surgical outcomes and building trust in healthcare providers (Figure 6.9).

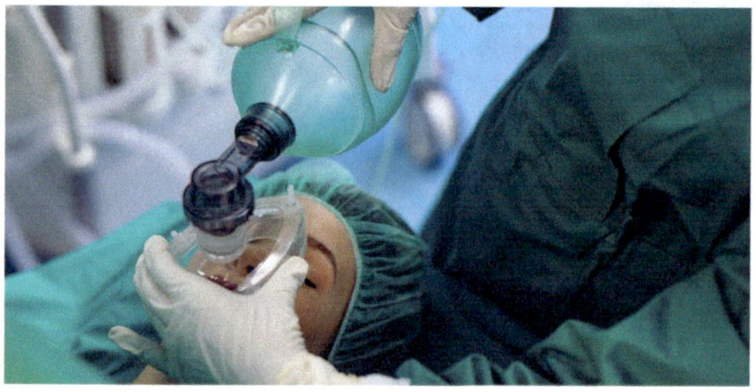

Figure 6.9. Sedation techniques play a crucial role in anesthesia.

Source: https://www.discoverdentalrocklin.com/wp-content/uploads/2024/02/Sedation-Techniques-Used-in-Dentistry.jpg.

6.4.1. Levels of Sedation

Sustaining the correct level of sedation is an essential component of anesthesia techniques, particularly in dental procedures where the cooperativeness and anxiety levels of the patient might be pretty diverse. Sedation is classified into four levels: minimal, moderate, deep, and general anesthesia. Minimal sedation, which is usually achieved by using oral agents such as nitrous oxide, allows the patient to be alert but relaxed and ensures effective communication throughout the procedure. Moderate sedation is a more profound state in which patients can respond to verbal commands intentionally but may or may not recall the episode. It is particularly beneficial in patients who require extensive treatments, since the combination of limited amnesia and anxiety reduction offers better productivity in the treatment setting. The value of procedures like nitrous oxide sedation underscores how minimal to moderate sedation can be highly effective in reducing patient distress, underscoring its vital role in the range of dentistry sedation practices (Mourad et al., 2022). As we consider deeper levels of sedation, moderate and deep sedation are top of mind, with each presenting drawbacks and advantages of its own. Deep sedation renders patients unresponsive to verbal command and demands close monitoring of such vital signs as blood pressure, heart rate, and oxygen saturation. Benzodiazepines like midazolam are typical for the induction of deep sedation, and appropriate titration is generally necessary to find a balance between safety and efficacy. It has been proven by research that midazolam is able to cause a greater incidence of moderate to deep sedation compared to diazepam, and this makes procedures feasible that otherwise call for general anesthesia (Zanette et al., 2013). It is, however, important to mention that deeper stages of sedation, while increasing procedural comfort, also involve possible complications that have to be judiciously watched out for by well-trained staff. The careful selection of sedation levels, therefore, mirrors the overall clinical practice of anesthesia, in which patient safety and effectiveness are assured. In conclusion, modulation of the complexity of sedation methods is crucial for individualizing anesthesia to the patient. The judicious application of levels of sedation—minimal, moderate, deep—allows the practitioner to treat varying degrees of anxiety and pain response effectively. For instance, the exceptionally high success rate of nitrous oxide sedation in pediatric dental patients shows that there is the promise of significantly reducing dependency upon more invasive treatment, such as general anesthesia. This is a paradigm shift in the manner in which dental practitioners can treat anxious or noncompliant children; minimizing the interventions needed for anesthesia can lead to improved treatment outcomes. Ultimately, the complexity of identifying sedation levels enhances not just procedural outcomes but also patient satisfaction and safety, making sedation an anchor of contemporary-day anesthetic practice in both dental and broader medical settings (Mourad et al., 2022) (Figure 6.10).

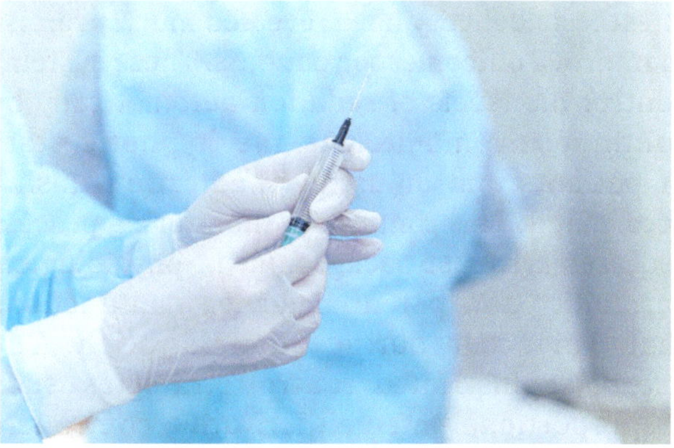

Figure 6.10. An anesthesiologist preparing a syringe for administration.

Source: https://www.anesthesiaserviceswi.com/wp-content/uploads/2023/10/levelssedationanesthesia.jpeg.

6.4.2. Monitoring During Sedation

Monitoring during sedation is a critical aspect of anesthesia techniques because it directly impacts patient safety and the success of the procedure. Effective monitoring enables healthcare providers to assess a patient's vital signs throughout, thereby enabling them to intervene appropriately when physiological adaptations occur. The necessity for vigilant observation is clearly emphasized in procedures with inherent respiratory complications where inappropriate handling can lead to severe complications, including death or neurological damage. For purposes of limiting such risks, practitioners are encouraged to utilize stringent monitoring protocols, including physiological parameters, as well as applying crisis resource management principles to foster improved decision-making in the event of a possible crisis. The overall strategy has also become highly significant owing to the complexity that shrouds sedation in various clinical settings, especially outside of traditional operating rooms (Tanoubi et al., 2022). The advancement of technology has significantly influenced the methods used to monitor under sedation. Emerging technologies in closed-loop systems of anesthesia delivery have revealed much promise to improve outcomes for patients. These systems control the levels of sedation automatically by continuously monitoring the hypnotic state of patients and adjusting medication dosing accordingly. This continuous monitoring process requires a robust background in physiological variability and potential device malfunctions that can occur during administration. The use of sophisticated control strategies, such as proportional-integral-derivative controllers and sliding-mode controllers, also enhances the accuracy of sedation control. Indeed, the application of in-silico strategies enables experts to simulate the performance of such monitoring systems in an integrated manner, leading to a more effective and safer sedation process for patients undergoing various medical interventions (Alshalalfah et al., 2020). Besides, training and education in proper monitoring are crucial for healthcare providers who administer sedation. Simulation courses have now become an innovative mode of education, providing hands-on experience in technical skills and CRM principles to learners. These are typically practice situations resembling real life, promoting critical thinking and decision-making under pressure. Such trainees demonstrate significantly better performance in confidence and competence when complications arise during sedation. As more medical specialties embrace such high-fidelity simulation programs, they pave the way for a better-skilled workforce able to recognize and meet the challenges of sedation. Beyond patient safety, this engaged education fosters a culture of continuous professional development in anesthesia (Tanoubi et al., 2022).

6.4.3. Applications in Dentistry and Minor Procedures

In dentistry, the application of anesthetic techniques is most important to provide a pain-free environment and successful procedural outcomes. Local anesthesia is applied ubiquitously in the many procedures of dental treatments, including fillings, extractions, and root canal surgeries. By targeting specific nerve pathways, these anesthetics enable dentists to perform complex procedures with minimal patient distress, thereby enhancing the patient's experience. Anesthetic choice is important and depends to a great extent on the complexity of the procedure, the patients' medical history, and personal anxiety. Furthermore, improvements in local anesthetic drugs and drug delivery systems continue to enhance efficacy and safety, thereby boosting patient satisfaction in dental clinics. In pediatric dentistry, anesthesia administration is multifaceted and meets a precarious balance of appreciating pharmacological principles and the individual needs of children. In consideration of their stages of development, youth patients tend to have increased anxiety levels that require sedation approaches to be handled with care to enable dental treatments. Practitioners are required to conduct proper pre-sedation assessments, about medical conditions that may increase the risks of sedating drugs. The intricacies of pediatrics also include determining appropriate fasting regimens and coordinating airway management for children with anatomical abnormalities. As outlined in professional association guidelines, such as those of the American Academy of Pediatrics and the American Academy of Pediatric Dentistry, adherence to systemic approaches ensures that sedation attempts are safe and successful in these risk groups (Charles et al., 2019). Beyond regular dental treatment, developments in anesthesia techniques enhance the feasibility of minor procedures within dental clinics. Procedures such as soft tissue biopsies, frenectomies, or dental implants are commonly supplemented with local anesthesia and sedation. These give dental practitioners the option of treating conditions that were previously the sole preserve of the surgical environment, thereby reducing the complexity of patient treatment and increasing patient access to required therapies. Good pain and anxiety control during these procedures can play an immense role in patient compliance and rates of recovery. Also, the integration of monitoring technologies into these minor procedures ensures that patients are maintained at adequate levels of consciousness and physiological stability, thereby improving the quality and safety of minor dental procedures (N/A, 2018) (Figure 6.11).

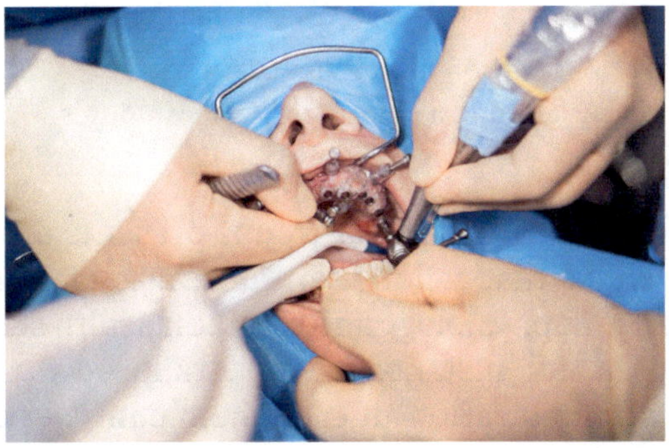

Figure 6.11. Applications in dentistry and minor procedures.

Source: https://drquadri.com/wp-content/uploads/2022/08/Which-Type-of-Anesthesia-Is-Used-for-This-Dental-Surgery.jpg.

Test Your Knowledge

1. What vital signs and clinical parameters should be continuously monitored during sedation to ensure patient safety?
2. How does monitoring during sedation help in the early detection and management of complications such as respiratory depression or hypotension?

6.5. Anesthesia in Special Populations

Learning Outcome

1. Pediatric anesthesia considerations
2. Geriatric anesthesia challenges
3. Anesthesia for patients with comorbidities

Anesthesia in the special groups presents unique challenges that call for careful consideration of variance in physiology and common health status. Children, for instance, require tailored dosage and administration due to their compact size and altered metabolism. Anesthesiologists must take into account varying pharmacodynamics and pharmacokinetics when administering anesthetic medication to children, as responses may variably deviate from adult responses. Also, the elderly patient usually presents with a myriad of comorbidities and altered organ function, which demands precise anesthetic management. Patient-specific care in this way ensures proper pain control while minimizing complications like postoperative cognitive dysfunction, which are linked with anesthesia in the geriatric population. By grasping these nuances, anesthesiologists can better prepare for cases and improve patient outcomes overall, underlining the need for ongoing education within this high-specialty domain of anesthesia (Marinkovic et al., 2018). Obese or metabolically abnormal patients also present a large special population that resists standard anesthesia techniques. Obesity's physiologic alterations, including changes to airway anatomy, respiratory physiology, and drug distribution, require adjustments in anesthesia. Anesthesiologists must provide diligent preoperative assessment to determine appropriate monitoring techniques and dosing schedules in these patients. Topical issues regarding positioning and airway management are also pertinent, as additional tissue may compromise the airway or hinder ventilation. The rising prevalence of obesity further emphasizes the necessity for targeted investigation into anesthesia's effects upon these patients, given that standard protocols are not necessarily translatable from normal-weight subjects. Understanding this population is the basis of the application of clinical guidelines and contributes to patient safety in operative procedures (Schober et al., 2018). Furthermore, patients with robust psychosocial factors, including anxiety disorders or trauma histories, can present special challenges during the course of anesthesia. Anesthesiologists frequently encounter patients whose psychological status can complicate perioperative management and anesthesia delivery. This underscores the importance of establishing rapport and practicing effective communication strategies to alleviate patients' anxiety and build their confidence. Strategies such as relaxation techniques, preoperative counseling, and integrating patient preferences into the anesthetic plan are critical to enhancing the experience. Treating the psychological dimension of anesthesia enables practitioners to bond more effectively with patients, ultimately resulting in increased patient satisfaction and surgical outcomes. As the art of anesthesia evolves, an understanding of the intricate relationship between physiological and psychological elements in special populations is needed for optimal care (Marinkovic et al., 2018).

6.5.1. Pediatric Anesthesia Considerations

In pediatric anesthesia, certain issues must be considered to ensure the safety and efficacy of anesthetic techniques. Children differ considerably from adults anatomically, physiologically, and pharmacologically, necessitating an approach tailored to their needs. For instance, the respiratory system of children is more prone to airway obstruction, whereas their cardiovascular system is less tolerant to hemodynamic changes due to significant variations in blood flow and heart rate. Correct management of these peculiar features is crucial, particularly during the process of creating surgical procedures for congenital heart disease, which involves selective anesthesia regimens. As noted in a pediatric cardiac anesthesia review, understanding the developmental processes of the cardiovascular system and congenital heart disease, and their implications, is important for optimal anesthetic management of such patients (Ayşe et al., 2025). The selection of anesthetic drugs is another key element of pediatric anesthesia. Due to the changing physiology of children, certain anesthetics that are safe in adults may be potentially dangerous in the pediatric population. For instance, those with a prolonged half-life or those that may hurt neurodevelopment must be used cautiously. Additionally, there is a possibility of anesthetic-induced complications such as postoperative vomiting and nausea, which may be greater in children. This demands rigorous preoperative assessments and personalized anesthetic protocols, taking into consideration the specific health status and surgical requirements of each child patient. The enhancement of anesthesia techniques via technological and procedural advances can strengthen not just safety but also recovery, hence making it mandatory for practitioners to stay current with the latest trends in pediatric anesthesiology (Rahib et al., 2024). Preoperative care in pediatrics must also incorporate the psychological aspects of surgery because younger patients tend to be very anxious or fearful of surgery. Effective communication among the patient, child, and parents is essential for reducing anxiety about anesthesia and surgery. Preoperative visits can be employed as an avenue to educate families and familiarize children with the operating room setting, which should ease anxiety. Moreover, an effective anesthesia plan can involve the administration of premedication to induce sedation and comfort. Perioperative monitoring and care are essential to enable early detection and management of potential complications. By addressing both psychological and physical health concerns, anesthesiologists can improve the experience for pediatric patients and their families (Ayşe et al., 2025) (Figure 6.12).

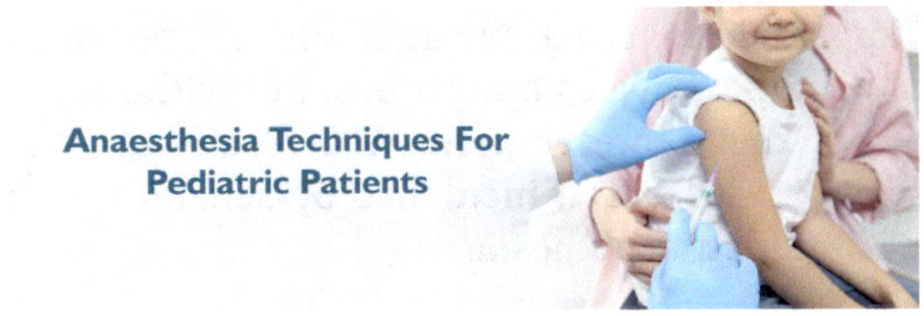

Figure 6.12. Pediatric anesthesia considerations.

Source: https://www.medicoverhospitals.in/images/articles/anaesthesia-techniques-for-pediatric-patients-challenges-and-considerations.webp.

6.5.2. Geriatric Anesthesia Challenges

As the population ages, anesthesiologists face the challenge of administering anesthesia to elderly patients. These patients typically have more than one comorbid condition, altered pharmacokinetics, and heightened sensitivity to the anesthetic drugs, and it is challenging to manage anesthesia in these. Among the considerations is the increased postoperative delirium and cognitive dysfunction, illnesses that are exceedingly prevalent among older individuals. Recent studies emphasize the link between deep anesthesia and poor postoperative outcomes, casting doubt on the long-held notion that lighter levels of anesthesia can lead to improved recovery pathways. According to Cottrell and Hartung, it is backed by abundant evidence that shallower anesthesia would decrease delirium and cognitive dysfunction risks in elderly patients, a huge paradigm shifts in elderly anesthetic practice in jeopardy (Bradley et al., 2020). Anesthetic depth assessment in elderly patients involves using several monitoring tools, including bispectral index (BIS) and electroencephalogram (EEG). These devices help balance the needs of proper anesthesia without the risks of excessive depth, which can cause problems. The Electroencephalography Guidance of Anesthesia to Alleviate Geriatric Syndromes trial introduced a new idea by showing that deeper stages of EEG suppression were associated with higher rates of postoperative complications. But without the aid of these interventions, the results did not support decreased incidence of delirium with EEG-guided anesthesia.

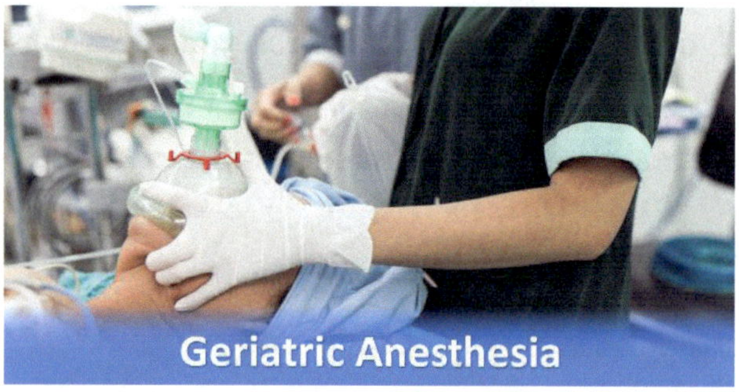

Figure 6.13. Geriatric anesthesia challenges.

Source: https://cdn.docplexus.com/117/7/4/954083c2-1749-44e8-962a-2907042a0908_t.jpg.

Even in the EEG-monitored group, patients still exhibited an excess of unwanted intraoperative movement, and queries concerning the safety of anesthesia, an issue of utmost concern in elderly patients at risk of intraoperative awareness (Troy et al., 2019). Finally, geriatric anesthesia challenges demand a more advanced understanding of patient factors that influence anesthetic outcome. Clinicians must cope with the limitations offered by each patient's unique medical background and experience of anesthesia. Maximizing patient safety and minimizing postoperative complications are essential goals for geriatric anesthesia practice, and evidence-based guidelines are therefore necessary. The up-to-date understanding of anesthesia's impact on the elderly highlights that further randomized controlled trials are required to further determine the causal determinants for anesthetic depth and postoperative complications. A balanced approach supports reflection on patient welfare by integrating technological advancements in monitoring and deeper knowledge of geriatric physiology, with the aim of ensuring that older patients receive anesthetic care tailored to their distinctive needs (Bradley et al., 2020) (Figure 6.13).

6.5.3. Anesthesia for Patients with Comorbidities

Anesthetic management of comorbid patients presents a difficult challenge to anesthesiologists in terms of optimization of surgical outcome and minimization of perioperative risks. Comorbid diseases, such as cardiovascular disorders, diabetes, and chronic respiratory diseases, can provide significant levels of added complexity in the administration and maintenance of anesthesia. The presence of such diseases usually necessitates tailored anesthetic regimens that neutralize certain frailties in the patient. For instance, some of the anesthetic medications may be contraindicated in seriously ill cardiac patients and thus need careful consideration of the pharmacodynamics involved. Moreover, precise preoperative assessment using indices such as the Charlson comorbidity index (CCI) can clarify the degree of risk associated with anesthesia in such a patient, inform the anesthetic management plan, and anticipate potential intraoperative and postoperative complications (Mathew et al., 2023). Application of regional anesthesia techniques could be particularly beneficial in comorbid patients, as these techniques can lower systemic drug exposure and reduce the risk of respiratory complications. Regional anesthesia could result in faster recovery and lower rates of postoperative pain, so it is an appropriate choice for frail elderly who are likely to have multiple morbidities. The success of such techniques rests on the demand for tailored skill sets and accurate anatomical data, focusing on training and expertise among anesthesiologists.

Further, innovations in predictive analytics, notably machine-learning approaches, offer new horizons for predicting perioperative adverse events, such as hypotension, which can significantly influence patient management across diverse comorbidities (Kendale et al., 2018). This indicates the potential of technology to streamline decision-making processes and improve patient outcomes in anesthesia clinics. Continuous monitoring after operation is essential in comorbid patients to monitor recovery of function and identify early complications. Studies have identified frail patients to be at significantly higher risk for death and poor functional recovery after surgery, so a complete postoperative care plan must be implemented that includes serial monitoring of vital signs and activities of daily living. By adding the appropriate safety nets and multidisciplinary team care, these patients are more appropriately managed during recovery by medical providers. Moreover, specialized postoperative care, including telemedicine services, can facilitate ongoing monitoring of comorbidity management—emphasizing that anesthesia planning and delivery in comorbid patients must extend beyond the operating room to ensure optimal long-term outcomes (Mathew et al., 2023).

Test Your Knowledge

1. What considerations must be taken into account when administering anesthesia to special populations such as pregnant women, the elderly, and patients with comorbidities?
2. How do physiological differences in special populations affect anesthetic drug selection, dosing, and monitoring?

6.6. Advances in Anesthesia Technology

Learning Outcome

1. Role of anesthesia machines
2. Development of new anesthetic agents
3. Impact of technology on patient safety

The evolution of anesthesia technology has had a profound impact on patient outcomes and clinical anesthesiology practice. Advances such as ultrasound-guided regional anesthesia enhanced pain management accuracy and minimized potential complications associated with traditional practice. Through real-time imaging, anesthesiologists can delineate nerves with precision, thereby administering anesthetic agents precisely where they are needed. This innovation not only increases the efficacy of anesthesia but also reduces the hazards of drug injection in the wrong places, thereby improving patient safety during surgery. Moreover, the incorporation of computerized systems for anesthesia delivery enables precise drug administration, offering individualized anesthetic regimens tailored to the specific requirements of individual patients. These devices play a key role in improving recovery patterns after surgery, underscoring the significance of technological developments in the practice of anesthesia. Recent research has highlighted the importance of combined methods, especially with regard to obstetrics, and has pointed to developments such as combined spinal-epidural anesthesia. This has been recognized as a promising and highly effective approach to pain management during labor. A comparative research confirmed that women treated with this method had comparatively lower pain scores compared to those who received conventional natural delivery procedures. In addition, the research indicated improved postpartum recovery and lactation in women who underwent painless delivery through advanced anesthesia technology. Specifically, Group B, receiving combined spinal-epidural anesthesia, experienced improved outcomes in both pain relief and recovery indicators compared with their peers in the control group, ultimately signaling a shift towards patient-centered practices in maternal care (Shen, 2024).

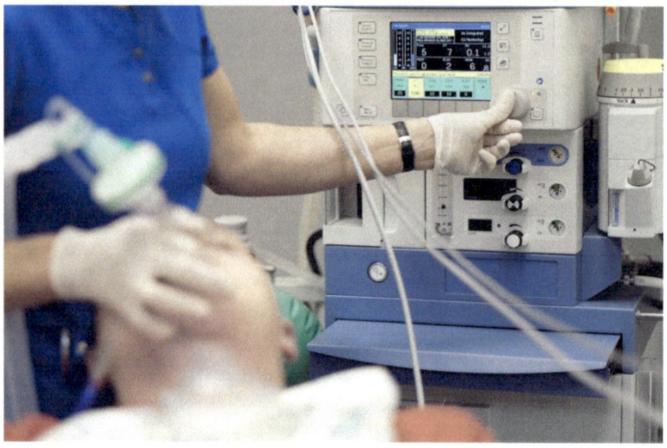

Figure 6.14. The evolution of anesthesia technology has significantly transformed clinical practices.

Source: https://news.mit.edu/sites/default/files/images/202202/anesthesia.jpg.

In doing so, such developments not only advance maternal experience but also foreshadow broader application to other medical interventions. Also, the inclusion of enhanced recovery protocols within operating rooms reflects shifting trends in anesthesia. For instance, the use of regional anesthesia in transplant surgeries has become more common, aimed at optimizing postoperative pain management and reducing opioid dependence. The Society for the Advancement of Transplant Anesthesia mandates a systematic review of current literature to empower practitioners to incorporate these techniques effectively. Findings confirm the efficacy of regional anesthesia in diverse transplant procedures, positively affecting patient hemodynamics and recovery patterns. As the widespread use of regional anesthesia in the perioperative period continues to increase, the potential for improved patient satisfaction and outcomes increases. This means not only a paradigm shift in surgical practice but also a more strategic development of pain management, underscoring the central role of anesthesia technology in current medical practice (Ander et al., 2024) (Figure 6.14).

6.6.1. Role of Anesthesia Machines

Anesthesia machines are central to modern surgery and critical to delivering anesthesia to patients. The very sophisticated machines guarantee precise delivery of anesthetic gases, promoting patient safety and comfort during the procedure. The machines include components such as gas flowmeters, vaporizer systems, and ventilators, which collectively control the inhalation of anesthetic agents. With constant levels of anesthetics and oxygen, anesthesia machines enable the clinician to monitor and regulate the patient's respiratory status in real time. With advances in surgery, the need for new ways has increased dramatically, underscoring the significance of delivering anesthetics. In line with the increase in minimally invasive surgical interventions, anesthesia machines have also evolved to provide tailored delivery systems that align with diverse surgical requirements, thereby becoming an integral part of contemporary anesthesia practice (Mohankumar et al., 2023). Anesthesia technology has also advanced in tandem with the development of surgical procedures, adapting to the growing complexity of the procedure and ensuring better patient care. Anesthesia machines have undergone significant evolution, resulting in greater accuracy, dependability, and simplicity. Modern machines come with advanced monitoring systems that provide real-time data, allowing anesthesiologists to make informed decisions based on a patient's vital signs and responses during the operation. Safety mechanisms are also integrated into the machines, minimizing the likelihood of anesthetic overdose or machine failure and thereby improving patient safety in the operating room. The anesthetic machines also have the ability to interface with electronic health records, allowing patient information to be added seamlessly and assisting anesthesiologists in formulating personalized anesthesia plans that take into account the patient's medical history and surgical situation (Iorio et al., 2020). Further, as anesthesia technology continues to evolve, the function of anesthesia machines is no longer confined to drug delivery; they are now a critical part of patient benefit through more effective monitoring, greater individualization, and the capacity to adapt to various surgical conditions. For instance, the application of machine learning and artificial intelligence to anesthetic devices could revolutionize anesthesia administration by recommending dosage adjustments based on real-time monitoring of physiological parameters. This can lead to more tailored regimens of anesthesia that are adjusted according to each patient's requirements, minimizing the risks of anesthetic administration. In this evolving situation, the role of anesthesia machines is not just to deliver agents but to encompass a broader category of patient management during complex procedures, ensuring safety and effectiveness in the evolving era of surgery (Mohankumar et al., 2023).

6.6.2. Development of New Anesthetic Agents

The creation of anesthetic agents has been a significant focus of research in anesthesia, both to increase efficacy and to minimize side effects. Introduction of new agents is often warranted due to the limitations of the existing anesthetics, including their neurotoxicity, particularly among vulnerable populations like children and infants. Research has shown that exposure to anesthetics early in life may harm neurodevelopmental outcomes, which led to serious assessments of the methods currently being employed in the surgical community. For instance, the U.S. Food and Drug Administration issued a warning regarding the administration of certain anesthetics among young patients, which led to questioning about balancing the need for surgery with long-term cognitive impairment. Thus, the challenge is to develop anesthetic drugs that are effective yet safe for patients and as risk-free as possible, particularly in pediatric anesthesiology (László et al., 2019). To address concerns about neurotoxicity, studies still aim to refine anesthetic drugs and discover newer techniques that have shorter exposure durations or involve less toxic materials. One new approach is the shift from general to regional techniques, which may pose fewer risks to younger patients. Recent studies, for instance, the GAS trial, have provided strong evidence that exposure to such drugs as sevoflurane, even for brief periods, is not responsible for substantial neurodevelopmental injury (László et al., 2019). Such observations support further investigation into new types of anesthetics and their applications to ensure they can be safely implemented in at-risk populations. While research on safer agents proceeds, interdisciplinary communication will be crucial for optimizing their production and utilization and, ultimately, enhancing anesthetic regimens. Also, technological and methodological advances have begun to play a key role in the development of new anesthetic drugs. Techniques such as electroencephalography (EEG) are increasingly employed to enhance our understanding of anesthetic depth and transitions, thereby enabling more advanced approaches to patient monitoring during surgery. New methods from neuroscience, including applications of network science and artificial intelligence, are enhancing our capacity to assess the effects of various anesthetics on brain dynamics and consciousness. By combining these new analytical approaches with conventional methods, scientists are not only encouraging a tailored approach to anesthesia but also enhancing the safety and efficacy of anesthetic care across diverse patient groups. This convergence of pharmacology and technology is a revolutionary era in anesthetic development, ensuring that safety and efficacy remain top priorities in clinical practice.

6.6.3. Impact of Technology on Patient Safety

The use of technology in anesthesia practice has greatly helped ensure patient safety by enabling more monitoring and management during procedures. Advanced monitoring equipment, such as multi-parameter monitors and real-time data analysis, enables anesthesiologists to closely monitor critical signs and take action as changes occur. Ongoing monitoring reduces the risk of complications, particularly in complex procedures where patients' physiological stability is critical. Moreover, technological advances enable anesthesiologists to make evidence-based decisions, thereby improving clinical outcomes. Evidence suggests that as reliance on high-tech monitoring and decision-support systems increases, the safety profile of anesthesia practice in general has been improved, demonstrating the contribution of technology to patient safety with continuing operative care (Lori et al., 2021). The development of artificial intelligence (AI) in anesthesia is a thrilling innovation with the potential to make patients even safer. By applying machine learning algorithms, A.I. can analyze vast amounts of information from multiple sources to predict patient responses and detect anomalies before they become serious issues. For instance, algorithms can review oxygen saturation, heart rate, and blood pressure data, alerting clinicians to potential complications such as hemorrhagic shock or respiratory distress. The potential of A.I. to augment clinical judgment underpins more precise and timely interventions, although its current applications are largely experimental. Fostering cooperation between anesthesiologists and data scientists is paramount to integrating these tools into daily clinical practice, thereby advancing the efficiency and safety of anesthesia care (Lonsdale et al., 2020). Despite technological advances that enable safer anesthesia, integrating these advances into clinical practice remains challenging. One such critical concern is the adequate training of all health care personnel in the usage of sophisticated monitoring systems and A.I. Failure to provide expertise may lead to misinterpretation of information, compromising patient safety rather than enhancing it. Furthermore, existing barriers in technology standardization across different clinical settings render universal adoption of innovations challenging. Hence, frequent and stringent training coupled with ongoing research into successful technology implementation is mandatory. The commitment to maintaining patient safety as the priority, despite these challenges, by integrating technology will shape the future of anesthesia practice (Lori et al., 2021).

Test Your Knowledge

1. How do anesthesia machines contribute to the safe and precise delivery of anesthetic gases and vapors during surgery?
2. What monitoring and safety features of anesthesia machines help prevent complications such as hypoxia or overdose?

SUMMARY

The examination of varying approaches to anesthesia reveals an ever-changing profile shaped by technological innovation and advances in physiological process knowledge. The role of systematic reviews and meta-analyses, stressed in recent research, underscores the necessity of a scientific method for integrating across studies. These reviews provide clarity on the effectiveness of different anesthesia methods, though they also raise concerns such as publication bias, which can distort perceived effects. As stated, the troubling statistics on the measurement of publication bias indicate that the community of anesthesia researchers must do better at evaluating published studies (Jarrod et al., 2016). By addressing these methodological deficits, practitioners can better hone their understanding of anesthesia procedures and outcomes. Furthermore, the use of ultrasound-guided regional anesthesia has introduced new avenues for optimizing nerve localization and minimizing complications. The evidence supporting such advances, as documented in recent assessments, identifies both the technological developments and the clinical uses of ultrasound. Despite clear advantages such as reduced risk of local anesthetic systemic toxicity and improved block characteristics, the clinical significance of these differences must be interpreted guardedly. Practitioners should evaluate these results in a balanced context, keeping in mind that the relative merits of techniques are a function of patient populations and specific clinical scenarios (Joseph et al., 2015). Therefore, the discussion of ultrasound guidance remains critical to further defining anesthesia practices. Finally, the necessity of increased educational efforts and clear reporting criteria cannot be overemphasized. As anesthesia methods progress, there must be an environment that promotes critical appraisal and publication of all research results, positive or negative. This will not only improve the quality of research but also provide the practitioner with comprehensive information to make well-informed decisions. Compliance with established guidelines, such as the PRISMA method, will enable a more standardized evaluation of systematic reviews. Designing precise avenues for reporting negative studies is also crucial in mitigating the current bias towards positive findings. In summary, encouraging the practice of anesthesia involves both methodological rigor and mutual commitment to transparency, leading to improved patient outcomes and practice integrity.

In anesthesia, several techniques improve patient comfort and safety during surgery. One of these techniques, the application of regional anesthesia, including spinal and epidural blocks, has become more prominent because it is highly effective for pain relief and offers quicker recovery compared to general anesthesia. Regional methods can reduce systemic side effects and minimize the requirement of narcotics after surgery, thus improving patient satisfaction. Moreover, developments in ultrasound technology have improved the accuracy of regional anesthesia delivery, enabling efficient nerve blocks and reducing the risk of injury. Such advances in techniques set a platform where anesthesiologists can customize anesthesia plans according to patients' needs, thereby allowing for better outcomes across various surgical disciplines, reaffirming the relevance of ongoing integration of technology into anesthesia practice (Bogo et al., 2024). General anesthesia remains a perioperative care foundation, granting surgeons access for invasive procedures while offering patient immobility and amnesia. Induction is typically with agents such as propofol or inhalational anesthetics that permit an extremely rapid onset of unconsciousness. Recent pharmacological advances, especially in formulations that promote rapid recovery and prevent postoperative nausea and vomiting, have made general anesthesia more contemporary. Techniques such as total intravenous anesthesia (TIVA) are particularly worth mentioning, as they provide continuous infusion of anesthetic drugs, thereby avoiding variation in anesthetic depth. This is beneficial in outpatient procedures where the patient's turnaround time is critical, as patients can be sent home faster without compromising safety (Anania et al., 2024). Development of monitoring equipment is also another significant aspect of general anesthesia delivery, enabling clinicians to monitor patient physiological responses during surgery. Furthermore, the use of artificial intelligence (AI) in anesthesiology has already begun to transform traditional practices, particularly in preoperative assessment and intraoperative management. AI-based algorithms can process large volumes of data to predict patient-specific risks and customize drug dosing, thereby enhancing the precision of anesthesia delivery. Technologies such as machine learning have been promising for maximizing postoperative care by estimating patient recovery time, thereby efficiently utilizing hospital resources. For instance, predictive models can estimate length of stay (LoS) following operations, enabling efficient planning of logistical services for healthcare facilities (Bogo et al., 2024). This changing scenario underscores the need for ongoing research and the adaptation of technological innovation in anesthesia methods to enable patient care to keep pace with current medical challenges while maintaining high safety standards (Anania et al., 2024).

KEY TERMS FROM THIS CHAPTER

- Anesthesia community
- Craniosynostosis
- Hypotension
- Opioid consumption
- Potential complications
- Regional anesthesia
- Anesthesiology
- Erector spinae plane (ESP)
- Inhalational anesthesia (IA)
- Patient safety
- Potential neurodevelopmental
- Surgical interventions

CRITICAL THINKING QUESTIONS

1. **What is the primary goal of balanced anesthesia?**
    a. To achieve a state of analgesia only
    b. To use a combination of drugs for optimal effects
    c. To avoid the use of general anesthesia
    d. To induce unconsciousness alone
2. **Which of the following is NOT a technique of regional anesthesia?**
    a. Spinal anesthesia
    b. Epidural anesthesia
    c. Nerve block
    d. Inhalational anesthesia
3. **Which induction agent is most commonly used for rapid sequence induction?**
    a. Ketamine
    b. Etomidate
    c. Propofol
    d. Thiopental sodium
4. **In spinal anesthesia, where is the local anesthetic injected?**
    a. Subarachnoid space
    b. Epidural space
    c. Intramuscular
    d. Intravenous
5. **What is the advantage of using epidural anesthesia over spinal anesthesia?**
    a. Faster onset
    b. Longer duration of analgesia
    c. No risk of hypotension
    d. Single shot administration

Short Answer Questions

1. What are the primary goals of pre-anesthetic assessment, and which key patient factors should be evaluated?
2. Explain the mechanism of action of propofol and discuss its advantages and disadvantages in induction of anesthesia.
3. Describe the Mallampati classification and its relevance in airway assessment.
4. Discuss the role of local anesthetics in regional blocks. Include the pharmacology and potential toxic effects of bupivacaine.
5. How do volatile anesthetics like sevoflurane and isoflurane differ in terms of solubility, MAC values, and recovery times?
6. Explain the principles and clinical importance of neuromuscular blockade monitoring.

Answer to Critical Thinking Questions

1. (b); 2. (d); 3. (c); 4. (a); 5. (a)

REFERENCES

1. Alam, F., & Matava, C. (2022). A new virtual world? The future of immersive environments in anesthesiology. *Anesthesia & Analgesia, 135*(2), 230–238. https://doi.org/10.1213/ane.0000000000006118Alshalalfah, A. L., Hamad, G. B., & Mohamed, O. (2020). System-level analysis of closed-loop anesthesia control under temporal sensor faults via UPPAAL-SMC. *2020 42nd Annual International Conference of the IEEE Engineering in Medicine & Biology Society (EMBC).* https://www.semanticscholar.org/paper/d9f8ee23f1a294108ab2322497f13d4314c22e46 (accessed on 28th June 2025).
2. Amornyotin, S., & Kongphlay, S. (2012). Esophagogastroduodenoscopy procedure in sick pediatric patients: A comparison between deep sedation and general anesthesia technique. *Journal of Anesthesia & Clinical Research, 03.* https://doi.org/10.4172/2155-6148.1000185 (accessed on 28th June 2025).
3. Anania, G., Chiozza, M., Pedarzani, E., Resta, G., Campagnaro, A., Pedon, S., Valpiani, G., et al. (2024). Predicting postoperative length of stay in patients undergoing laparoscopic right hemicolectomy for colon cancer: A machine learning approach using SICE (Società Italiana di Chirurgia Endoscopica) CoDIG data. *Cancers, 16.* https://www.semanticscholar.org/paper/52e6320bb52a4d54516ac0da47b17c1d95aaf24c (accessed on 28th June 2025).
4. Ander, M., Mugve, N., Crouch, C. E., Kassel, C. A., Fukazawa, K., Isaak, R., Deshpande, R., et al. (2024). Regional anesthesia for transplantation surgery–A white paper part 2: Abdominal transplantation surgery. *Clinical Transplantation, 38.* https://www.semanticscholar.org/paper/6ea4636ca79319ca207d8fef0940196f41432907 (accessed on 28th June 2025).
5. Ayad, A. E., Agiza, N. A., Elrifay, A. H., Mortada, A. M., Girgis, M. Y., & Varrassi, G. (2024). Lumbar sympathetic block to treat CRPS in an 18-month-old girl: A breaking barriers case report and review of literature. *Pain and Therapy, 13*, 1325–1334. https://www.semanticscholar.org/paper/82dc6b872fe261812f4d8359aec2d8b4f5adfb01 (accessed on 28th June 2025).
6. Bhuyan, S., Bhuyan, D., & Rahane, S. (2024). Optimizing regional anesthesia for cancer patients: A comprehensive review of current practices and future directions. *Cureus, 16.* https://www.semanticscholar.org/paper/020a48f6a8c0739b0c50baa4be57cd0a405372cb (accessed on 28th June 2025).
7. Bogoń, A., Górska, M., Ostojska, M., Kałuża, I., Dziuba, G., & Dobosz, M. (2024). Artificial intelligence in anesthesiology–a review. *Journal of Pre-Clinical and Clinical Research.* https://www.semanticscholar.org/paper/f0675c7d4ce9e68003a85b778c5e4c0872e48443 (accessed on 28th June 2025).
8. Cappellini, E. S. (2024). Bridging anesthesia and sustainability: A special article for a path towards eco-conscious practice. *Anesthesia Research.* https://www.semanticscholar.org/paper/d43042caf6dd30fae658600927cedbcf2433e5cc (accessed on 28th June 2025).
9. Carmichael, J. C., Keller, D. S., Baldini, G., Bordeianou, L., Weiss, E. G., Lee, L., Boutros, M., et al. (2017). Clinical practice guidelines for enhanced recovery after colon and rectal surgery from the American Society of Colon and Rectal Surgeons and Society of American Gastrointestinal and Endoscopic Surgeons. *Diseases of the Colon & Rectum, 60*, 761–784. https://doi.org/10.1097/dcr.0000000000000883 (accessed on 28th June 2025).

10. Chow, C. L., Siu, Y., Ma, C., & Lui, T. (2024). Ultrasound-guided regional anesthesia by orthopedic surgeons in fixation of distal radius fracture. *Journal of Orthopedics, Trauma and Rehabilitation, 32*, 9–13. https://www.semanticscholar.org/paper/7dd9a360a08b23f2b5304fce93167637424fe693 (accessed on 28th June 2025).

11. Claassen, J. A. H. R., Thijssen, D. H. J., Panerai, R. B., & Faraci, F. M. (2021). Regulation of cerebral blood flow in humans: Physiology and clinical implications of autoregulation. *Physiological Reviews, 101*, 1487–1559. https://doi.org/10.1152/physrev.00022.2020 (accessed on 28th June 2025).

12. Coté, C. J., & Wilson, S. (2019). Guidelines for monitoring and management of pediatric patients before, during, and after sedation for diagnostic and therapeutic procedures. *Pediatrics, 143*. https://doi.org/10.1542/peds.2019-1000 (accessed on 28th June 2025).

13. Dalton, J. E., Bolen, S., & Mascha, E. J. (2016). Publication bias: The elephant in the review. *Anesthesia & Analgesia, 123*, 812–813. https://doi.org/10.1213/ane.0000000000001596 (accessed on 28th June 2025).

14. Davis, B. R., Lee-Kong, S. A., Migaly, J., Feingold, D. L., & Steele, S. R. (2018). The American Society of Colon and Rectal Surgeons clinical practice guidelines for the management of hemorrhoids. *Diseases of the Colon & Rectum, 61*, 284–292. https://doi.org/10.1097/dcr.0000000000001030 (accessed on 28th June 2025).

15. De Cassai, A., Bonvicini, D., Correale, C., Sandei, L., Tulgar, S., & Tonetti, T. (2019). Erector spinae plane block: A systematic qualitative review. *Minerva Anesthesiologic, 85*. https://doi.org/10.23736/s0375-9393.18.13341-4 (accessed on 28th June 2025).

16. Eagleman, S. L., & Drover, D. R. (2018). Calculations of consciousness. *Current Opinion in Anesthesiology, 31*, 431–438. https://doi.org/10.1097/aco.0000000000000618 (accessed on 28th June 2025).

17. Felemban, O. M., Alshamrani, R. M., Aljeddawi, D. H., & Bagher, S. M. (2021). Effect of virtual reality distraction on pain and anxiety during infiltration anesthesia in pediatric patients: A randomized clinical trial. *BMC Oral Health, 21*. https://doi.org/10.1186/s12903-021-01678-x (accessed on 28th June 2025).

18. Fritz, B. A., Budelier, T. P., Ben Abdallah, A., & Avidan, M. S. (2020). The unbearableness of being light. *Anesthesia & Analgesia, 131*, 977–980. https://doi.org/10.1213/ane.0000000000004814 (accessed on 28th June 2025).

19. Fu, G., Xu, L., Chen, H., & Lin, J. (2025). State-of-the-art anesthesia practices: A comprehensive review on optimizing patient safety and recovery. *BMC Surgery, 25*. https://doi.org/10.1186/s12893-025-02763-6 (accessed on 28th June 2025).

20. Hernandez, M. A., Palazzi, L., Lapalma, J., Forero, M., & Chin, K. J. (2017). Erector spinae plane block for surgery of the posterior thoracic wall in a pediatric patient. *Regional Anesthesia & Pain Medicine*. https://doi.org/10.1097/aap.0000000000000716 (accessed on 28th June 2025).

21. Iorio-Morin, C., Hodaie, M., Sarica, C., Dea, N., Westwick, H. J., Christie, S., McDonald, P. J., et al. (2020). Letter: The risk of COVID-19 infection during neurosurgical procedures: A review of severe acute respiratory distress syndrome coronavirus 2 (SARS-CoV-2) modes of transmission and proposed neurosurgery-specific measures for mitigation. *Neurosurgery, 87*, E178–E185. https://doi.org/10.1093/neuros/nyaa157 (accessed on 28th June 2025).

22. Islam, R. K., Tong, V. T., Robicheaux, C., Tageant, H., Haas, C. J., Kline, R. J., & Islam, K. N. (2024). The impact of anesthesia on dermatological outcomes: A narrative review. *Cureus, 16*. https://www.semanticscholar.org/paper/8e56fe6bcf52fd98948309e41ac01c50cfc4322b (accessed on 28th June 2025).

23. Kelava, M., Alfirevic, A., Bustamante, S., Hargrave, J., & Marciniak, D. (2020). Regional anesthesia in cardiac surgery: An overview of fascial plane chest wall blocks. *Anesthesia & Analgesia, 131*, 127–135. https://doi.org/10.1213/ane.0000000000004682 (accessed on 28th June 2025).

24. Kendale, S., Kulkarni, P., Rosenberg, A. D., & Wang, J. (2018). Supervised machine-learning predictive analytics for prediction of postinduction hypotension. *Anesthesiology, 129*, 675–688. https://doi.org/10.1097/aln.0000000000002374 (accessed on 28th June 2025).

25. Kinsella, S., Carvalho, B., Dyer, R. A., Fernando, R., McDonnell, N., Mercier, F. J., Palanisamy, A., et al. (2017). International consensus statement on the management of hypotension with vasopressors during caesarean section under spinal anesthesia. *Anesthesia, 73*, 71–92. https://doi.org/10.1111/anae.14080 (accessed on 28th June 2025).

26. Kot, P., Rodríguez, P., Granell, M., Cano, B., Rovira, L., Morales, J. E., Broseta, A., et al. (2019). The erector spinae plane block: A narrative review. *Korean Journal of Anesthesiology, 72*, 209–220. https://doi.org/10.4097/kja.d.19.00012 (accessed on 28th June 2025).

27. Lerner, L. B., McVary, K. T., Barry, M. J., Bixler, B. R., Dahm, P., Das, A. K., Gandhi, M. C., et al. (2021). Management of lower urinary tract symptoms attributed to benign prostatic hyperplasia: AUA guideline part II—Surgical evaluation and treatment. *The Journal of Urology, 206*, 818–826. https://doi.org/10.1097/ju.0000000000002184 (accessed on 28th June 2025).

28. Lonsdale, H., Jalali, A., Gálvez, J. A., Ahumada, L., & Simpao, A. F. (2020). Artificial intelligence in anesthesiology: Hype, hope, and hurdles. *Anesthesia & Analgesia, 130*, 1111–1113. https://doi.org/10.1213/ane.0000000000004751 (accessed on 28th June 2025).

29. Lötsch, J., & Ultsch, A. (2017). Machine learning in pain research. *Pain, 159*, 623–630. https://doi.org/10.1097/j.pain.0000000000001118 (accessed on 28th June 2025).

30. Machado, V. G., de Figueiredo Azevedo, A. C., Dutra Alves, B. P. S., Valadares, J. F. M., Dias, M. T. H., Souza, L. D. Q., Tiveron, E., et al. (2025). Anesthesiology in multimodal pain management for orthopedic patients. *Journal of Medical Science and Evidences*. https://www.semanticscholar.org/paper/9e60e7ee3b0d370d0bda26992541dc0677837045 (accessed on 28th June 2025).

31. Mahmood, F., Matyal, R., Skubas, N. J., Montealegre-Gallegos, M., Swaminathan, M., Denault, A., Sniecinski, R. M., et al. (2016). Perioperative ultrasound training in anesthesiology: A call to action. *Anesthesia & Analgesia, 122*, 1794–1804. https://doi.org/10.1213/ane.0000000000001134 (accessed on 28th June 2025).

32. Marchis, I. F., Negruţ, M. F., Blebea, C. M., Crihan, M., Alexa, A. L., & Breazu, C. (2024). Trends in preoperative airway assessment. *Diagnostics, 14*, 610. https://doi.org/10.3390/diagnostics14060610 (accessed on 28th June 2025).

33. Marinkovic, A., & Lee, S. M. (2018). Interviewing in social science research: A relational approach. *Anesthesia & Analgesia, 127*, e13–e14. https://doi.org/10.1213/ane.0000000000003462 (accessed on 28th June 2025).

34. Mathew, A., Lukachan, G. A., Varughese, D., Raju, N. K. K., Mathai, A. S., & Johnson, A. (2023). Impact of frailty and comorbidity index on postoperative complications and functional

outcomes among elderly patients undergoing hip fracture surgeries under regional anesthesia techniques. *Anesthesia Pain & Intensive Care, 27*, 161–169. https://doi.org/10.35975/apic.v27i2.2132 (accessed on 28th June 2025).

35. Mathijssen, I. M. J. (2020). Updated guideline on treatment and management of craniosynostosis. *Journal of Craniofacial Surgery, 32*, 371–450. https://doi.org/10.1097/scs.0000000000007035 (accessed on 28th June 2025).

36. Menon, B. K., Sajobi, T. T., Zhang, Y., Rempel, J., Shuaib, A., Thornton, J., Williams, D., et al. (2016). Analysis of workflow and time to treatment on thrombectomy outcome in the Endovascular Treatment for Small Core and Proximal Occlusion Ischemic Stroke (ESCAPE) randomized, controlled trial. *Circulation, 133*, 2279–2286. https://doi.org/10.1161/circulationaha.115.019983 (accessed on 28th June 2025).

37. Mohankumar, A., & Rajan, M. (2023). Role of hyaluronidase as an adjuvant in local anesthesia for cataract surgery. *Indian Journal of Ophthalmology, 71*, 2649–2655. https://doi.org/10.4103/ijo.ijo_2515_22 (accessed on 28th June 2025).

38. Mourad, M. S., Splieth, C. H., Al Masri, A., & Schmoeckel, J. (2022). Potential for nitrous oxide sedation in pedodontics practice to reduce the need for dental general anesthesia. *PubMed, 53*, 598–606. https://doi.org/10.3290/j.qi.b3044863 (accessed on 28th June 2025).

39. Muñoz-Leyva, F., Cubillos, J., & Chin, K. J. (2020). Managing rebound pain after regional anesthesia. *Korean Journal of Anesthesiology, 73*, 372–383. https://doi.org/10.4097/kja.20436 (accessed on 28th June 2025).

40. N/A. (2018). Practice guidelines for intravenous conscious sedation in dentistry (Second Edition, 2017). *Anesthesia Progress, 65*, e1–e18. https://doi.org/10.2344/anpr-65-04-15w (accessed on 28th June 2025).

41. Neal, J. M., Brull, R., Horn, J. L., Liu, S. S., McCartney, C. J. L., Perlas, A., Salinas, F. V., et al. (2015). The second American Society of Regional Anesthesia and Pain Medicine evidence-based medicine assessment of ultrasound-guided regional anesthesia. *Regional Anesthesia & Pain Medicine, 41*, 181–194. https://doi.org/10.1097/aap.0000000000000331 (accessed on 28th June 2025).

42. Novikova, A. I., Lyubushkin, V. E., Studenikina, A. V., Albotova, D. Kh., Bakhmeteva, P. I., Torchinova, D. A., Chkareuli, D. N., et al. (2024). The role of anesthesiology in modern cardiac surgery: Overview of key techniques and issues. *CARDIOMETRY*. https://www.semanticscholar.org/paper/e9ca845a8de28a31fca089396b62598feac4a104 (accessed on 28th June 2025).

43. Oh, S. S., & Narver, H. L. (2024). Mouse and rat anesthesia and analgesia. *Current Protocols, 4*. https://doi.org/10.1002/cpz1.995 (accessed on 28th June 2025).

44. Orser, B. A. (2020). Recommendations for endotracheal intubation of COVID-19 patients. *Anesthesia & Analgesia, 130*, 1109–1110. https://doi.org/10.1213/ane.0000000000004803 (accessed on 28th June 2025).

45. Saraçoğlu, A. G., & Salman, N. (2025). Anesthetic management in pediatric cardiac surgery. *Surgery on Children*. https://www.semanticscholar.org/paper/a33b953df052e40acf0bfce05ee778cb14a6e41f (accessed on 28th June 2025).

46. Sasangohar, F., Jones, S. L., Masud, F., Vahidy, F., & Kash, B. A. (2020). Provider burnout and fatigue during the COVID-19 pandemic: Lessons learned from a high-volume intensive care

unit. *Anesthesia & Analgesia, 131*, 106–111. https://doi.org/10.1213/ane.0000000000004866 (accessed on 28th June 2025).

47. Schober, P., Boer, C., & Schwarte, L. A. (2018). Correlation coefficients: Appropriate use and interpretation. *Anesthesia & Analgesia, 126*, 1763–1768. https://doi.org/10.1213/ane.0000000000002864 (accessed on 28th June 2025).

48. Shen, D. (2024). Analysis of the application effect of painless delivery technology in clinical obstetrics. *Advances in Obstetrics and Gynecology Research*. https://www.semanticscholar.org/paper/b52175f2b0fa74b401f5cbc64cdb0636d80dd4f3 (accessed on 28th June 2025).

49. Sikachi, R., & Anders, M. (2024). Whole lung lavage: Considerations from the anesthesiology perspective. *Current Opinion in Pulmonary Medicine, 31*, 53–58. https://www.semanticscholar.org/paper/97c0348b6191f59a26a31106b004ca386ceacc35 (accessed on 28th June 2025).

50. Tahir, M. F., Ahmad, W., Ahmad, N., Waseem, N., Naz, A., & Shahzad, H. (2025). Comparison between TIVA and inhalational anesthetics, risks and benefits. *Insights–Journal of Health and Rehabilitation*. https://www.semanticscholar.org/paper/801d8c6e24ea5506c6df8a2307152c7edc3cfc34 (accessed on 28th June 2025).

51. Tanoubi, R. P., Bélanger, M.-È., Georgescu, M., Robitaille, A., & Drolet, P. (2022). High-fidelity simulation-based education: Description of an original crisis resource management and sedation learning for dental surgeons. *European Journal of Investigation in Health, Psychology and Education, 12*, 91–97. https://www.semanticscholar.org/paper/136df832dbcbf7fa8b8d8343aee2ed98c620180c (accessed on 28th June 2025).

52. Theodoraki, K., Moka, E., Makris, A., & Stavropoulou, E., On behalf of ESRA Hellas Working Group. (2021). A survey of regional anesthesia uses in Greece and the impact of a structured regional anesthesia course on regional techniques knowledge and practice. *Journal of Clinical Medicine, 10*. https://www.semanticscholar.org/paper/bd51c335e162abad14f56b850b6890adf55463b8 (accessed on 28th June 2025).

53. Tulgar, S., Selvi, O., Şentürk, Ö., Şerifsoy, T. E., & Thomas, D. T. (2019). Ultrasound-guided erector spinae plane block: Indications, complications, and effects on acute and chronic pain based on a single-center experience. *Cureus*. https://doi.org/10.7759/cureus.3815 (accessed on 28th June 2025).

54. Vutskits, L., & Culley, D. J. (2019). GAS, PANDA, and MASK. *Anesthesiology, 131*, 762–764. https://doi.org/10.1097/aln.0000000000002863 (accessed on 28th June 2025).

55. Wilder, R. T., Flick, R. P., Šprung, J., Katusic, S. K., Barbaresi, W. J., Mickelson, C., Gleich, S. J., et al. (2009). Early exposure to anesthesia and learning disabilities in a population-based birth cohort. *Anesthesiology, 110*, 796–804. https://doi.org/10.1097/01.anes.0000344728.34332.5d (accessed on 28th June 2025).

56. Wildes, T. S., Mickle, A. M., Ben Abdallah, A., Maybrier, H., Oberhaus, J., Budelier, T. P., Kronzer, A., et al. (2019). Effect of electroencephalography-guided anesthetic administration on postoperative delirium among older adults undergoing major surgery. *JAMA, 321*, 473–473. https://doi.org/10.1001/jama.2018.22005 (accessed on 28th June 2025).

MONITORING IN ANESTHESIA

7

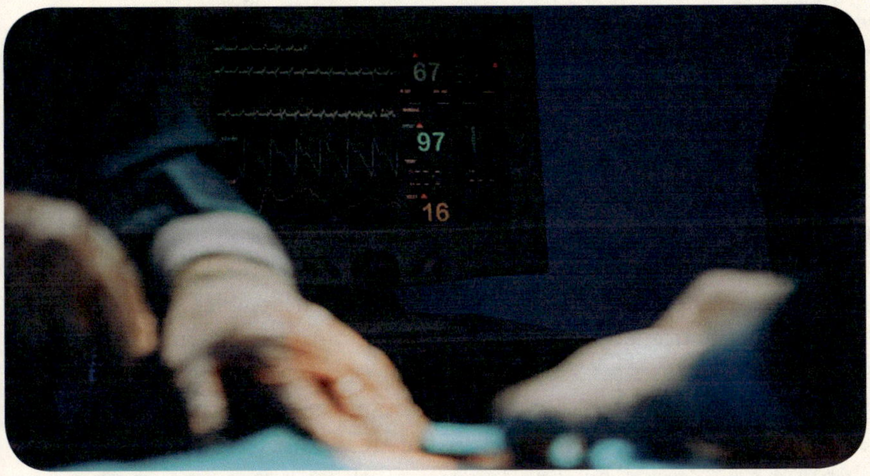

LEARNING OBJECTIVES

After studying this chapter, you will be able to:

1. Discuss the types of anesthesia
2. Explain the physiological parameters monitored
3. Focus on monitoring equipment and technology
4. Describe the role of anesthesia providers
5. Explain the risks and complications
6. Understand advances in monitoring techniques

Introduction

With the evolving landscape of anesthesia, monitoring equipment is at the vanguard of patient safety and best outcomes. Anesthesia practice has also seen tremendous transformations, underscoring the importance of robust monitoring systems that provide real-time information to anesthesiologists. All this is essentially a product of technological breakthroughs, particularly the emergence of artificial intelligence and machine learning technologies. These technologies have the potential to enhance monitoring capabilities by sifting through seas of information to predict potential complications and to improve clinical decision-making. The integration of such innovations into daily practice, however, is complex and fraught with challenges, including the need for anesthesiologists and data scientists to collaborate to harmonize technological advancements with clinical relevance (Lonsdale et al., 2020). The stringent demand for monitoring anesthesia is brought home by the criticality of perioperative care, where failures as minute as one would have critical consequences. Monitoring is not limited to basic vital signs; it encompasses a spectrum of parameters that would indicate patient status and potential anesthetic complications. While anesthesiologists strive to maintain homeostasis and accommodate physiological changes in the moment, interest in applying sophisticated technologies and simulation to optimize training and performance is growing. For instance, combining virtual reality and high-fidelity simulation in residency training can assist in the acquisition of surgical and anesthesia skill that translates directly into improved patient outcomes (Badash et al., 2016). Further, such advancements can also aim to solve the complexity of patient safety in the operating room, requiring higher standards of training protocols and everyday practice. Advances in monitoring are encouraging but also imply a need for practical evaluation and testing of new technologies in clinical settings. Current literature suggests an implementation gap between the theoretical potential of artificial intelligence solutions and their actual adoption in anesthesiology. For instance, while there exists a large body of literature on the development of machine-learning algorithms, few have demonstrated that they function in real-world clinical workflows. Thus, anesthesiology must ride the Gartner Hype Cycle—beyond early enthusiasm about A.I. possibilities to a stage of cautious integration that focuses on empirical evidence and patient outcomes. The future of anesthetic monitoring thus depends not only on technological advancement but also on a commitment to strict research, ethical conduct, and collaboration among multidisciplinary staff (Lonsdale et al., 2020). Such a focus will ultimately ensure that monitoring development optimizes patient safety and the quality of anesthetic care.

Definition of Anesthesia Monitoring

Anesthesia monitoring is paramount in surgical operations, where the efficiency of anesthesia delivery and the safety of the patient are the primary concerns. Monitoring procedure involves continuous monitoring of physiological parameters to assess a patient's vital signs and general condition during the course of anesthetic administration. Typically, the parameters monitored include oxygen saturation, blood pressure, heart rate, and respiratory rate, as well as more advanced measures such as end-tidal carbon dioxide and neuromuscular function. By taking these measures together, the clinicians can detect early trends of complications or distress and be in a position to intervene in a manner that might minimize risks of anesthesia. In addition, effective monitoring is responsible for optimizing anesthetic depth, which is critical for both surgical success and patient comfort. Therefore, anesthesia monitoring is not merely an administrative necessity but an essential component that ensures the safe delivery of anesthesia across various medical settings, thereby enhancing patient outcomes. Anesthesia monitoring's sophistication also increases when it comes to specific populations, such as children or those with prior medical conditions. In these cases, a more discreet method is required, taking into consideration possible factors that will result in sedation or anesthesia complications. An example is an extensive presedation evaluation that reviews medical history and anatomy so that in the event of airway obstruction or drug interaction, preparations are made (Charles et al., 2019). This tailored approach to monitoring likewise highlights the need for training and equipotential resources for anesthesia providers, particularly when performing procedures involving greater risk, such as those conducted under deep sedation or general anesthesia. Flexibility in monitoring practice is thus paramount to ensuring the unique dangers presented by heterogeneous patient populations are met with nonetheless ensuring safety overall. In the field of medical technology, anesthesia monitoring is undergoing rapid improvements that enhance both efficacy and precision. More advanced monitoring technologies, including hemodynamic monitoring equipment and combined monitoring devices, provide more in-depth analysis of a patient's physiological condition. Not only does this integration simplify the monitoring process, but it also permits anesthesia providers to make evidence-based decisions based on real-time information. Moreover, anesthetic pharmacokinetics and drug research form the basis for protocols for individualized dose adjustment, facilitating enhanced knowledge of responses to anesthesia on a patient-specific basis (Calkins et al., 2017). Synergy between technological advances and evidence-based practice in monitoring anesthesia improves not only safety but also overall patient care quality. As a result, continuous updates in monitoring protocols and technological implementations are crucial as the field of anesthesia advances (Figure 7.1).

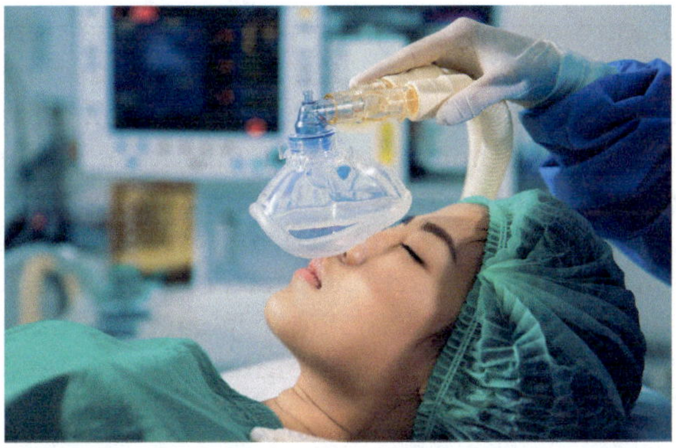

Figure 7.1. Anesthesia monitoring is essential in the context of surgical procedures.

Source: https://cdn-assets.leister.com/pim/medias/11/89/89/118989.jpg.

Importance of Monitoring in Anesthesia

Intra-anesthetic monitoring is for patient safety and to allow for the optimal clinical outcome. Anesthesia induces profound physiological changes in patients that profoundly affect cardiovascular, respiratory, and neurological functions. Continuous monitoring, therefore, allows anesthesiologists to detect deviations from normal values and respond instantly to any emerging complication. Of note, adequate monitoring ensures the appropriate depth of anesthesia, minimizes the risk of awareness under anesthesia or over-sedation, and impacts patient satisfaction and the duration of recovery. Studies have demonstrated that the conscious, wakeful state requires ongoing maintenance, underscoring the value of monitoring systems for assessing consciousness and depth of anesthesia during procedures (Leandro et al., 2019). Furthermore, advances in monitoring technology have changed the practice of anesthesia to encompass real-time monitoring of vital signs and cerebral function. Capnography, pulse oximetry, and electroencephalography are a few of the new technologies of contemporary monitoring, each providing special information about patient well-being during anesthesia. Capnography allows one to measure carbon dioxide exhaled from the breath as an indirect confirmation of successful ventilation, and pulse oximetry allows one to monitor oxygen saturation in real-time. The integration of these technologies ensures that anesthesiologists can monitor trends and make decisions promptly, and hence reduce the risk of adverse effects and enhance patient safety. Monitoring is especially critical in high-risk populations, in which comorbidities complicate anesthetic management and necessitate increased vigilance regarding physiological stability (Calkins et al., 2017). Summing up, monitoring is not only essential in anesthesia, but also the very foundation of safe anesthetic practice and optimal patient outcomes. Good monitoring systems not only keep patients in desired anesthetic levels, but also help to institute timely interventions against physiological derangements. The role of ongoing technological innovations is to enhance further the precision and reliability of such monitoring systems, which can facilitate more personalized and adaptive anesthesia care. Consequently, the benefits of a widespread monitoring approach are improved patient safety, reduced intraoperative complications, and higher-quality recovery experiences, rendering it essential in modern anesthesia practice and patient care standards (Leandro et al., 2019).

7.1. Types of Anesthesia

Learning Outcome

1. General anesthesia
2. Regional anesthesia
3. Local anesthesia

Anesthesia is a broad category with many distinct forms, all designed for specific medical settings and patient needs. General anesthesia is probably the most recognized category, characterized by reversible unconsciousness, analgesia, and muscle relaxation. This is generally closely watched for cardiovascular and respiratory side effects such as hypotension or airway obstruction. By contrast, regional anesthesia involves the selective blockade of nerves, resulting in relief of pain in specific regions of the body without rendering the patient unconscious. Techniques such as epidurals and nerve blocks have been effective in managing pain during and after surgery, with the resultant reduction of systemic opioids, which also possess side effects. Hence, an understanding of the distinctions between regional and general anesthesia is imperative for monitoring protocols, as they dictate different approaches to maintaining patient safety throughout the surgical process. Local anesthesia is yet another equally significant category with the impact of numbing a small portion of the body without affecting consciousness. This procedure is widely employed in minor surgery and in outpatient clinics to enable a speedy recovery with minimal disruption to the patient's daily life. Although local anesthesia is safer than general or regional forms, it also requires close observation, particularly in monitoring the patient's reaction to both the anesthetic drug and to the operative stimulus. Ultrasound guidance for enhancing the accuracy of local anesthetic delivery and monitoring has become increasingly common, boosting patient safety and comfort. Besides, the role of the anesthesia practitioner can extend beyond agent delivery to encompass real-time monitoring of physiological responses, as outlined in recent innovations in perioperative ultrasound education, which has significantly broadened the scope of perioperative management (Mahmood et al., 2016). In intraoperative neurophysiologic monitoring (IONM), the choice of anesthetic is particularly crucial due to its potential impact on surgical outcomes, especially for delicate neural structures. Repeated motor-evoked potentials (MEPs) monitoring is utilized throughout spinal surgery to ascertain any damage to motor tracts. Since anesthetic drugs significantly affect MEP monitoring, especially when neuromuscular blocking agents are present, anesthesia needs to be carefully controlled to ensure accurate interpretation of neuromuscular function during surgery. The necessity of a multidisciplinary approach, involving collaboration between anesthesia experts and neurophysiologists, has been stressed to achieve better outcomes for patients undergoing major surgical procedures. By integrating these monitoring strategies with knowledge of the different types of anesthesia, clinicians can optimize the safety and effectiveness of surgical interventions and minimize the risks of anesthesia complications (Alan et al., 2016).

7.1.1. General Anesthesia

General anesthesia is a crucial aspect of modern surgery, enabling patients to be operated on in a state of unconsciousness and freedom from pain. The key to successful general anesthesia is the vigilant monitoring of its multiple components under the operating conditions. The three significant anesthesia domains—hypnosis, analgesia, and muscular relaxation—must be continuously assessed to keep the patient in the optimal state. While measuring muscular relaxation has been standardized using techniques such as the train-of-four, measuring hypnosis and analgesia is much harder. The complexity of the brain and the overlap of various physiological systems complicate the development of useful depth-of-anesthesia monitoring devices. Thus, technological advancement is essential to enhance patient safety and anesthetic care during surgery. In a longstanding debate regarding anesthesia techniques, total intravenous anesthesia (TIVA) through target-controlled infusion (TCI) has been identified for its potential advantages over inhaled techniques. The advocates of TIVA tout it under processed electroencephalogram (pEEG) monitoring for minimizing postoperative morbidity such as nausea and vomiting, with improved emergence from anesthesia. But that approach calls for a deep act of faith on the part of those accustomed to the real-time assurance provided by declining gas concentration measurements of inhalational anesthesia. As outlined in an up-to-date Pro-Con debate, the choice between TIVA and inhaled anesthetics can substantially impact patient outcomes, prompting anesthetists to weigh the benefits of pEEG-guided anesthesia against standard monitoring techniques that provide immediate assurance of adequate drug delivery (Johnson et al., 2023). The importance of systematic monitoring under general anesthesia cannot be overemphasized as it is the foundation of maintaining patient well-being. Objective measurement of a patient's status at any point during surgery is crucial for managing the three general pillars of anesthesia: hypnosis, analgesia, and muscular relaxation. Additionally, despite tremendous advances in technology for assessing muscular paralysis, it has been challenging to achieve a similar degree of standardization in measuring the depth of hypnosis and analgesia (Martinez-Vazquez et al., 2022). Various monitoring methods of nociception emphasize the utmost importance of the clinicians being responsive and attentive, as the patients' unique physiological responses can directly impact anesthetic depth and safety. Successful integration of such monitoring techniques can lead to enhanced patient outcomes and experience, constructing the foundation of safe anesthetic practice (Figure 7.2).

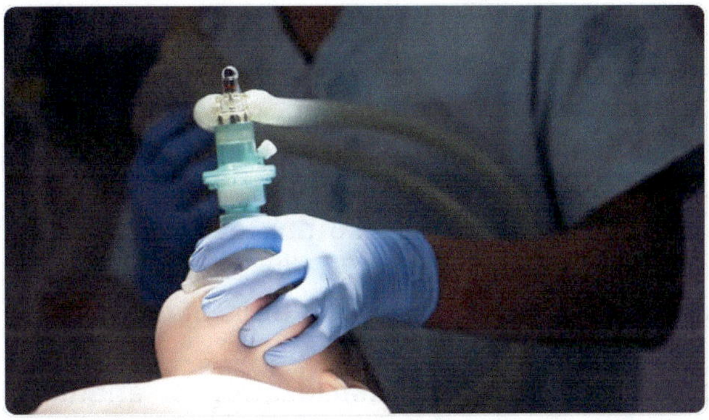

Figure 7.2. General anesthesia represents a crucial component of modern surgical practice.

Source: https://www.news-medical.net/image-handler/picture/2017/8/shutterstock_526251763.jpg.

7.1.2. Regional Anesthesia

Within anesthesia, regional anesthesia is an important practice that highlights the importance of targeted pain relief with minimal systemic effects. The technique involves administering anesthetic medication to targeted nerve regions to effectively shut off sensation in a specified region, which is immensely beneficial during surgical procedures on the limbs or lower limbs. Regional anesthesia not only enhances patient comfort and reduces postoperative pain but also aids in optimizing recovery periods and reducing analgesic needs after surgery. With the inclusion of sophisticated monitoring techniques, anesthetists can closely observe vital parameters and regional efficacy, thereby safeguarding patients under operative settings. As noted in recent literature, improvements in anesthesia monitoring technologies have transformed the practice, enabling anesthetists to make optimally informed decisions that maximize patient outcomes and enhance safety in surgery. Specifically, surgeries requiring maximum focus on regional blocks have been maximized by such improvements (e.g., Durrani, 2024). The importance of vigilant monitoring of regional anesthesia is immense, as it greatly minimizes potential complications from nerve blocks. Anesthetists must be vigilant for any evidence of adverse effects, such as hematoma formation or nerve damage, which can result from needle placement error or accidental administration. These conditions not only demand extensive training of skills but also the incorporation of imaging modalities, such as ultrasound guidance, which have changed the administration of regional blocks. Utilization of these technologies facilitates enhanced visualization of anatomy, enabling precise needle placement and providing real-time feedback intraoperatively. Understanding hemodynamic stability and the dynamics of cerebrovascular function is significant; for instance, monitoring regional cerebral oxygen saturation prevents cognitive dysfunction associated with compromised blood flow during operations, a topic of increasing concern in innovative and intricate operations (Daabiss et al., 2024). Additionally, regional anesthesia imposes significant effects on postoperative pain management and recovery. With regional techniques, clinicians can enable a more rapid transition into the postoperative period, allowing individuals to engage in rehabilitation without the limitations of systemic analgesia. Not only does this enable a quicker return to normal function, but it also supports the new emphasis on multimodal analgesia, which encourages diverse strategies for pain management. Continual monitoring of patient responses through sophisticated systems allows anesthetists to adjust anesthetic regimens as needed, including changes in patients' responses to drugs and tolerances to procedures. Lastly, the implementation of stringent monitoring protocols, along with the strategic use of regional anesthesia, indicates a paradigm shift toward more effective, safer, and patient-centered surgical care (Durrani, 2024).

7.1.3. Local Anesthesia

Local anesthesia plays a critical role in modern surgical practice, particularly as we look for the comfort of the patient along with adequate pain control. Using local anesthetic drugs, surgeons can perform many procedures without general anesthesia, which is riskier. The application of local anesthesia allows for a more precise approach, isolating the area of operation from sensory nerve conduction and rendering it insensitive to pain while leaving the patient aware. Not only does this technique minimize physiological effects that accompany general anesthesia, but it also enables speedy recovery, something which makes it particularly useful in outpatient procedures. Also, ongoing improvements in local anesthetic formulations and techniques strengthen the efficacy and safety profiles of local anesthesia, ensuring better outcomes for patients during surgical interventions. For anesthesia monitoring, local anesthesia requires an independent approach to vigilance, as patients are awake and remain highly aware of their surroundings. Continuous observation of vital signs, i.e., oxygen saturation and heart rate, should be performed to identify early warning signs of complications such as LAST. Clinicians must utilize both visual and auditory feedback to monitor the patient's comfort and response during the procedure. According to current evidence, the use of monitoring devices such as capnography is a practical method for immediately ascertaining respiratory complications and implementing prompt intervention. This monitoring element underscored the twofold role of anesthesiologists: they must ensure patient safety and establish a calming ambiance that alleviates worry, as patients may feel uneasy because they are awake during the procedure. The integration of monitored anesthesia care (MAC) with local anesthesia further enhances the level of patient care in the operating room. With the integration of local anesthetic techniques and sedative medications, anesthesiologists can achieve a sedation level that decreases anxiety without compromising the patients' response to verbal commands. This enhances patients' satisfaction, as they can give commands to the operating team while remaining relaxed during the procedure. It has been reported in studies that drug protocols, including drugs like dexmedetomidine, not only enhance sedation but also reduce dosages required of older drugs, thereby reducing side effects. The advent of MAC has been discovered to be a revolutionary procedure in anesthesia, resulting in a safer environment for patients through thorough monitoring and instant modification based on any change in patient status or vital signs, thus exhibiting local anesthetics' adaptability in current surgical practices (Das et al., 2015; Prontera et al., 2017) (Figure 7.3).

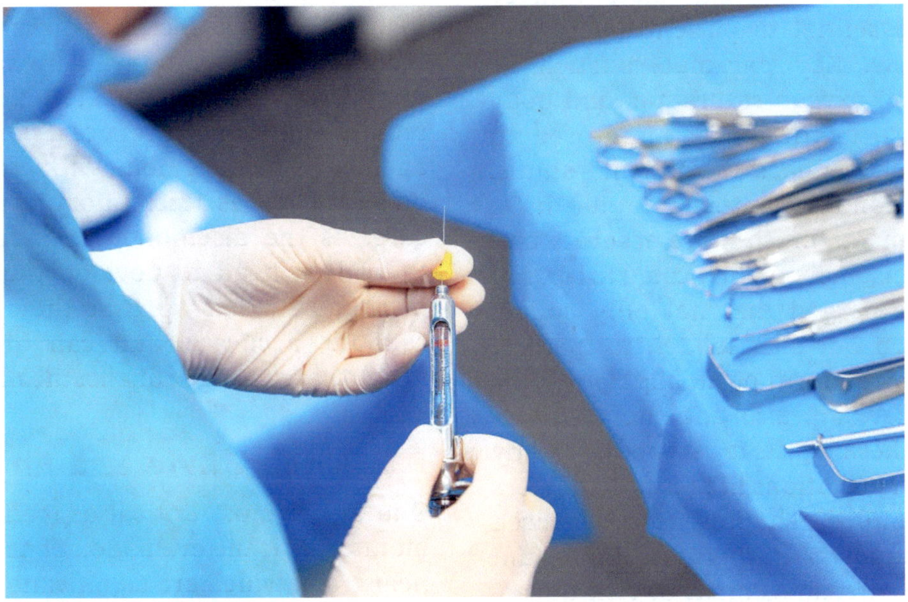

Figure 7.3. Local anesthesia plays a critical role in modern surgical practices.

Source: https://antalyadentsmile.com/wp-content/uploads/2023/05/Local-Anesthesia-Injection.jpg.

Test Your Knowledge

1. What is regional anesthesia, and how does it differ from general and local anesthesia in terms of mechanism and clinical application?
2. What are the common types of regional anesthesia, and what factors determine the choice of technique for a specific surgical procedure?

7.2. Physiological Parameters Monitored

Learning Outcome

1. Heart rate and rhythm
2. Blood pressure
3. Oxygen saturation levels

Monitoring of physiological parameters under anesthesia is essential to patient safety and surgical success. Key parameters such as heart rate, blood oxygen saturation, and body temperature are continuously monitored to provide real-time feedback of a patient's status. Advances in monitoring technologies have made measurements much more accurate and accessible. For instance, sophisticated IoT-based systems have emerged that not only collect vital information but also send it to medical professionals in the form of mobile apps. This enables immediate appraisal and interventions, equipping anesthesiologists to respond promptly to any abnormal deviations in these parameters (Bashkaran et al., 2025). The presence of advanced monitoring equipment is therefore important to the preemptive management of risk during anesthesia and general surgical procedures. In the post-anesthesia care unit (PACU), continued monitoring of physiological status remains central to identifying complications in the postoperative setting. During this recovery phase, patients are particularly vulnerable to the adverse consequences of anesthesia, requiring increased vigilance to ensure the safe reversal of consciousness. Equipped with cameras and advanced monitoring algorithms, contemporary PACUs use cutting-edge technologies to record and obtain physiological data from patient monitors. Specifically, video analysis techniques, such as those employing the FC-YOLOv4-tiny network and the PP-OCR model, have been developed to observe vital signs with high accuracy (Wang et al., 2024). This mechanical process of extraction is less susceptible to human error, which is absolutely vital in high-stress situations when medical staff can tire and become diverted. In addition, the incorporation of full-scale monitoring systems not only improves patient safety but also enhances the quality of healthcare services in operating rooms. Through remote monitoring and real-time observation, medical professionals can maintain a constant vigil over a patient's vital signs from a distance as well. Real-time data transfer of this nature allows anesthesiologists to make effective decisions promptly, which may further translate into saving lives through timely interventions. The physiological parameter monitoring changes reflect a paradigm shift in anesthesia management, with greater emphasis on technology as a facilitator of enhanced patient care. As the discipline continues to advance, there is a need to develop these monitoring methods further so that they become more reliable, accurate, and can offer important insights at all stages of anesthesia management.

7.2.1. Heart Rate and Rhythm

One of the most critical aspects of anesthesia monitoring is the evaluation of heart rhythm and heart rate, which are significant predictors of a patient's cardiovascular stability during surgery. The autonomic nervous system response, as reflected in heart rate variability (HRV), can indicate the body's capacity to recover from surgical stress. Abnormal HRV values during anesthesia have been linked with increased postoperative complications such as cardiac events or hospital prolongation. A comparative analysis shows that patients under general anesthesia will exhibit significant decreases in HRV parameters such as SDNN and pNN50 by the end of the interventions, whereas in regional anesthesia cases, HRV returns to baseline levels (Ushnevych et al., 2025). Understanding these dynamics enables anesthesiologists to more effectively predict and manage potential complications while ensuring patient safety and optimal recovery outcomes. In addition to traditional monitoring methods, new technologies such as photoplethysmography (PPG) are also explored for real-time heart rate monitoring during anesthesia. PPG technology, particularly smartphone-based models, presents a non-invasive means of real-time monitoring of heart rate. Recent studies indicate that PPG can obtain heart rate in AF patients, who are prevalent in the operating room. However, PPG accuracy may decrease in some situations, particularly during AF episodes, when the device occasionally underestimates heart rate (Gruwez et al., 2024). This highlights the need to use multiple monitoring methods to ensure accurate heart rate control, particularly in critically ill patients. These advances can enhance the anesthesiologist's capability of predicting arrhythmias or wild fluctuations during the intraoperative course. Implementation of heart rate and rhythm monitoring has a direct impact that extends beyond intraoperative care to postoperative management and outcomes. Variations in heart rate under anesthesia are indicative of occult cardiovascular instability and require additional assessment and control. Continuous heart rate data allow for early detection of tachycardia or bradycardia, conditions that may necessitate immediate medical interventions to avoid serious complications. In addition, more profound understanding of HRV behavior during various methods of anesthesia serves to individualize anesthetic treatment based on patient profiles. By applying autonomic response monitoring using heart rate parameters, anesthesiologists are better able to manage patients with pre-existing cardiovascular pathology and, ultimately, improve the efficacy and safety of surgery (Ushnevych et al., 2025). This multidimensional monitoring of heart rate and rhythm is required for enhancing the quality of anesthesia services in all surgical settings (Figure 7.4).

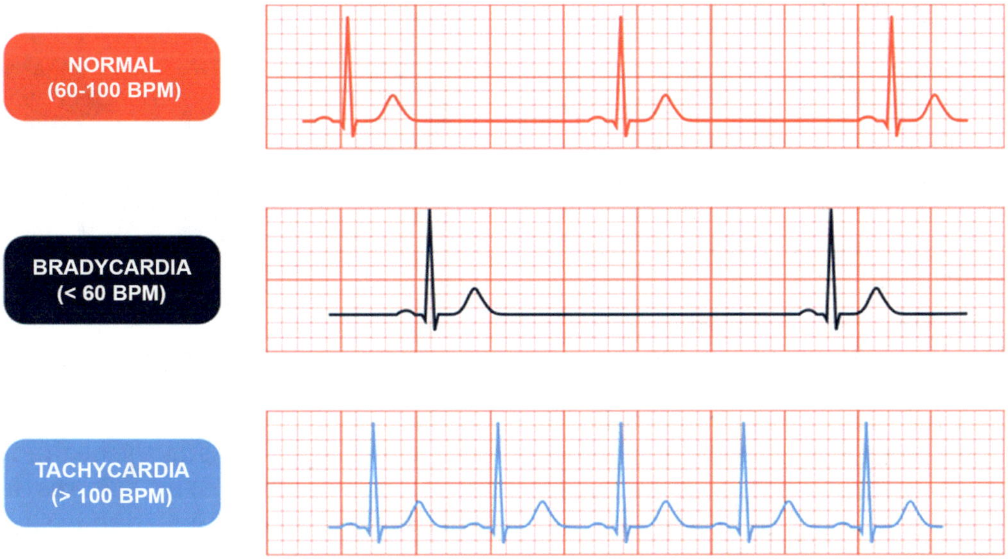

Figure 7.4. An integral aspect of monitoring in anesthesia is assessing heart rate and rhythm.

Source: https://d1z8zkw1yi6kd7.cloudfront.net/uploads/ckeditor/pictures/data/000/001/303//content/rate.jpeg.

7.2.2. Blood Pressure

Optimal blood pressure maintenance under anesthesia is crucial both for surgical success and patient safety. Under general anesthesia, the cardiac effect of anesthetic agents can cause hypotension, and this can compromise organ perfusion and worsen adverse outcomes. Ongoing monitoring and proper intervention are needed to manage blood pressure. Devices such as non-invasive oscillometric devices or continuous arterial waveforms allow anesthesiologists to measure systolic, diastolic, and mean arterial pressures precisely. This monitoring is particularly useful in obstetric surgery, where spinal anesthesia may lead to profound hypotension and maternal and fetal complications. New guidelines recommend administering prophylactic vasopressors such as phenylephrine or ephedrine to mitigate the risk of severe hypotension during spinal anesthesia, reflecting a better understanding of maternal hemodynamics during surgery (Kinsella et al., 2017). Intraoperative clinical management of hypotension during anesthesia needs to treat the problem from a multidirectional angle, encompassing pharmacologic and non-pharmacologic maneuvers. Pharmacologically, the vasopressors play a central role in countering hypotension but must be selected carefully based on their cardiovascular effects. Although ephedrine, for instance, can increase cardiac output and rate, it has side effects that can negate the benefit to the fetus during obstetric intervention. Phenylephrine, however, maintains maternal blood pressure with little impact on fetal circulation. Non-drug therapy may include preloading or co-loading with fluid, positional maneuvering to prevent inferior vena cava compression, and avoiding extremity venous pooling. More highly recommended is controlling systemic vascular resistance by titrating blood pressure and cardiac output with caution, thereby creating a protocol that addresses the dynamic nature of intraoperative physiology (N/A, 2012). Anesthesia blood pressure management also has to consider patient profiles. Pre-existing hypertension, patient positioning, and body mass index play critical roles in the incidence and severity of perioperative hypotension. Between-groups variability in hemodynamic responses has been established in observational trials, and individualized management methods are therefore necessary in anesthesia. An example is women undergoing elective cesarean section, who represent a high-risk group due to the profound influence of physiological changes during pregnancy and spinal anesthesia. Understanding the nuances of such clinical variables enables anesthesiologists to risk-stratify more effectively and apply preventive measures successfully. Overall, maintaining blood pressure at a target level not only enhances maternal safety but also optimizes fetal outcome, reiterating the utmost significance of vigilant monitoring in the art of anesthesia (Kinsella et al., 2017) (Figure 7.5).

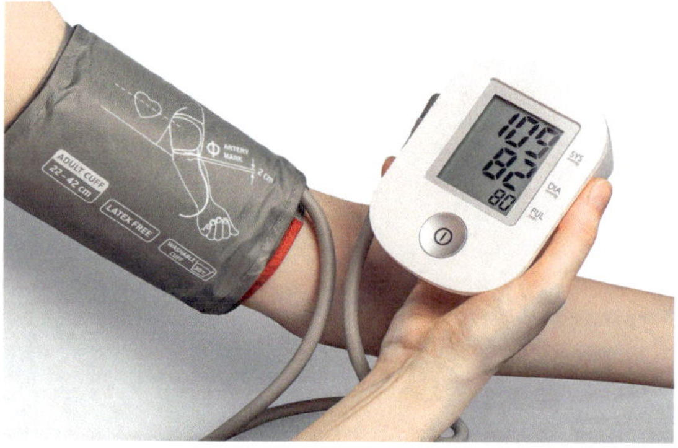

Figure 7.5. Maintaining optimal blood pressure during anesthesia.

Source: https://www.stmaryshealthcaresystem.org/sites/default/files/hg_features/hg_post/9294418e9f995caec5529e32d0b6cc2a.jpg.

7.2.3. Oxygen Saturation Levels

Oxygen saturation levels are of keen interest in the world of anesthesia monitoring because they provide very valuable information about a patient's respiratory function during the course of an operation. An oxygen saturation report, typically obtained with pulse oximetry, provides the percentage of hemoglobin molecules available in the bloodstream that are filled with oxygen. An adequate level of oxygen saturation is necessary to ensure the organs and tissues are adequately oxygenated, thus preventing hypoxia. Anesthesia can cause decreased oxygen saturation (hypoxemia) due to airway obstruction, inadequate ventilation, or the administration of certain anesthetic agents. Therefore, continuous monitoring of oxygen saturation is important, allowing anesthesiologists to respond promptly to any deviation from normal and make appropriate compensatory adjustments in ventilation or oxygen delivery to maintain patient well-being. Further, studies have underscored the importance of oxygen saturation monitoring in other clinical of settings, regarding patient anxiety and pain perception during procedures. For instance, research has indicated that even though patients undergoing procedures such as root canal may become physiologically changed in heart rate from stress, oxygen levels remain stable, and with a reassuring marker of respiratory status (Singh et al., 2025). This stability is especially significant because it suggests that, though perhaps there will be changes in a patient's state of anxiety, the inherent respiratory condition can be maintained with proper monitoring and interventions. Anesthesiologists can more effectively assess global patient stability and comfort by relating oxygen saturation to other physiological parameters. This maximizes both safety and procedural success. In addition, the interaction between oxygen saturation and the autonomic function of the nervous system underscores the importance of complete monitoring in anesthesia. Changes in oxygen saturation have been reported to occur in patients suffering from respiratory disease, namely chronic obstructive pulmonary disease (COPD), and influence global morbidity and mortality (Jeena et al., 2025). In those with compromised pulmonary reserve, tight monitoring of oxygen saturation is essential, as even small changes may indicate deterioration in respiratory status. This emphasizes the need for anesthesiologists to integrate advanced monitoring technologies to allow real-time assessment of not just oxygen saturation but also related parameters such as heart rate variability. These whole-brain approaches can augment management strategies and improve patient outcomes, demonstrating the critical interconnection between oxygen monitoring and patient safety throughout the anesthesia continuum (Figure 7.6).

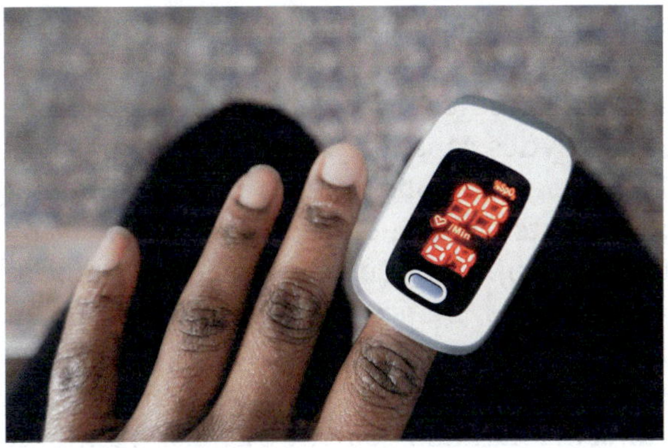

Figure 7.6. Oxygen saturation levels play a critical role in the realm of anesthesia monitoring.

Source: https://www.health.com/thmb/m6LJzmgvc6wRy2KM5hLfTgKJL_4=/4000x0/filters:no_upscale():max_bytes(150000):strip_icc()/GettyImages-1292318009-91773f45006a4cb7a75a785f412519bb.jpg.

Test Your Knowledge

1. What are the key physiological parameters monitored during anesthesia, and why is each important for patient safety?
2. How does continuous monitoring of parameters such as heart rate, blood pressure, oxygen saturation, and respiratory rate help prevent anesthetic complications?

7.3. Monitoring Equipment and Technology

Learning Outcome

1. Electrocardiogram (ECG)
2. Pulse oximeter
3. Capnometer

Anesthetic practice has been dramatically improved by the availability of monitoring equipment and technology, critical in the protection of patient safety during operating conditions. In contemporary practice, multi-parameter monitoring machines allow anesthesiologists to track real-time vital signs such as heart rate, blood pressure, and oxygen saturation. With such instant feedback, the healthcare team can easily adjust anesthetic depth and dosage. The incorporation of electronic medical records (EMRs) and patient data analytics capability further supports these monitoring functions. With predictive modeling, anesthetists can pre-empt likely complications, such as respiratory compromise or thrombotic complications, before they even develop, thus enabling early interventions. These anticipatory measures have not only improved the outcomes of anesthesia management but also reinforced the culture of safety in operating rooms, as highlighted in recent studies on pediatric anesthesia management (Shrivastava et al., 2025). The combination of cutting-edge radiological technologies with anesthesia monitoring devices significantly enhances surgical precision and patient safety. Modern anesthesia machines not only provide immediate feedback on a patient's physiological state but also fulfill an ancient role in reducing infection risk on the operating table. Operating teams benefit from enhanced field visualization, especially in minimally invasive techniques. Imaging modalities contribute to planning procedures by providing superior anatomical data, enabling surgeons to tailor their approach to each patient's individualized needs. Thus, the incorporation of these sophisticated monitoring devices and radiological tools supports optimized surgical results and minimized healing times. Thus, the relationship among these technologies is crucial for revolutionizing surgical procedures and achieving their combined impact on patient safety and procedure effectiveness (Al-Zamanan et al., 2024). Despite the apparent benefits provided by existing monitoring technologies, difficulties persist in their adoption in clinical settings. Diversity in technology implementation, particularly across different healthcare organizations, is likely to lead to inconsistent patient experience and outcomes. Training, resource availability, and institutional processes can limit the smooth incorporation of advanced monitoring devices into anesthesia practice. Furthermore, hesitancy among some health professionals to embrace new technologies can delay innovation and hinder the delivery of quality care. Overcoming these impediments will require further education, budget support, and commitment to establishing standard procedures that capitalize on recent advances in monitoring technology. As the art of anesthesia advances, it is essential that the medical fraternity unite to integrate these advances into an approach that achieves both safety and efficacy in the treatment of patients (Shrivastava et al., 2025).

7.3.1. Electrocardiogram (ECG)

The ECG is the mainstay of anesthesia monitoring, providing invaluable data regarding a patient's cardiac function intraoperatively. By capturing the electrical activity of the heart, an ECG allows anesthesiologists to detect such arrhythmias, ischemic changes, and other cardiac derangements as could occur with anesthetic agents or with surgical-related physiological stress. These intraoperative measurements not only support hemodynamic stability but are also crucial for guiding intervention in the event of cardiac complications. Moreover, preoperative ECG monitoring enables clinicians to assess baseline cardiac function, thereby supporting evidence-based decision-making regarding anesthetic management and risk stratification for patients with pre-existing cardiovascular disease. Appreciation of the value of ECG during anesthesia drives recommendations such as those in the 2023 ACC/AHA/ACCP/HRS Guideline for the Diagnosis and Management of Atrial Fibrillation, which underscore the necessity of meticulous cardiac assessment in procedure rooms.

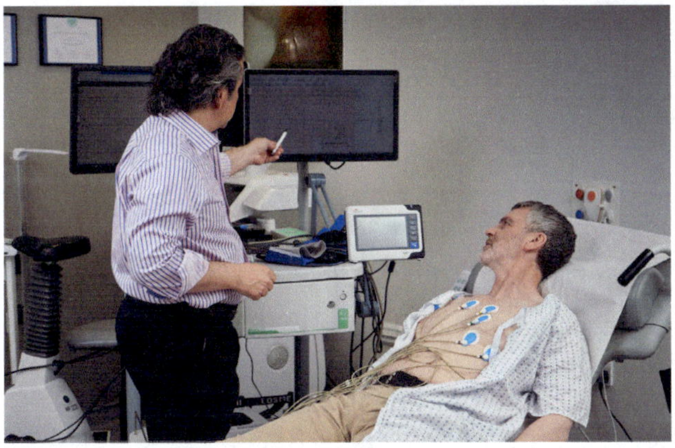

Figure 7.7. The Electrocardiogram (ECG) serves as a fundamental tool in the realm of anesthesia monitoring.

Source: https://onewelbeck.com/media/2xmjcxte/1wel_hh_0350.jpg.

Guidelines emphasize the necessity of detecting arrhythmias that imperil patient safety and surgical success. Specifically, the identification of atrial fibrillation and other high-impact rhythm disorders can prompt adequate interventions, thus preventing periprocedural risks associated with anesthesia. remain current with evolving guidelines, as these may influence the use of ECG monitoring and interpretation criteria in the operating room, directly affecting patient care and outcomes. In addition to ECG, a comprehensive monitoring plan during anesthesia can involve monitoring of other vital signs and other factors. This multi-modal monitoring plan enhances understanding of the immediate physiological status of a patient and helps in the prevention of complications that may arise. However, ECG interpretation must be placed in the context of anesthetic care as a whole, taking into account factors such as the type of anesthetic drugs employed, patient comorbidities, and the nature of surgical intervention. The dynamic nature of anesthesia necessitates an elastic monitoring approach, such that the ECG remains a core component of real-time evaluation of cardiac status, de facto safeguarding patient well-being throughout the complex interplay between surgery and anesthetic intervention (Figure 7.7).

7.3.2. Pulse Oximeter

In anesthesiology, adequate oxygenation is paramount, and the pulse oximeter is a very useful tool in perioperative care. By measuring arterial oxygen saturation (SpO2), pulse oximeters provide immediate information necessary for identifying hypoxemia during surgery and in recovery. This ability is especially important in situations involving general anesthesia, where patients' respiratory function is dramatically altered and can contribute to inadequate oxygen delivery. The real-time monitoring achieved through pulse oximetry can allow clinicians to take early intervention measures, even preventing serious postoperative complications like hypoxia, which has been associated with poor recovery outcomes. Further, the role of pulse oximetry extends beyond the intraoperative period, as it remains vital during postoperative recovery, where patient monitoring helps ensure that early postoperative hypoxemia (EPH) risks are averted (Ryan et al., 2025). However, the function of pulse oximeters is not universally available, particularly in resource-limited settings. Inequalities in the use of pulse oximetry and in proper training in its application can result in significant differences in patient care, especially in low- and middle-income economies. One such study performed in Guatemala accounted for these limitations, reporting a high rate of EPH among patients undergoing surgery despite the use of pulse oximetry. The majority of health care providers in these facilities report a need for additional monitoring capabilities and for establishing specialized post-anesthesia care units.

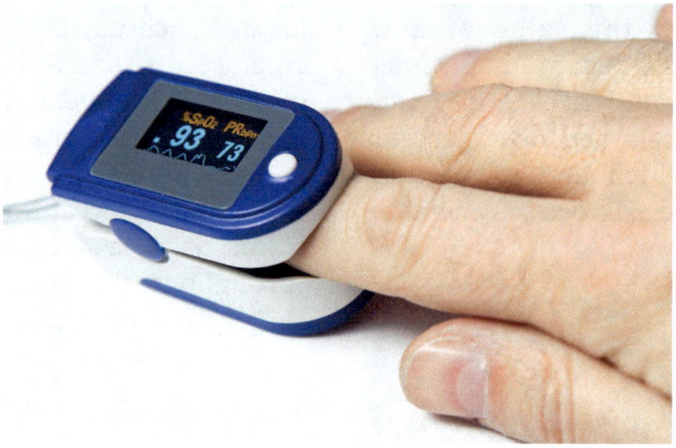

Figure 7.8. Pulse oximeter.

Source: https://healthnewshub.org/wp-content/uploads/2020/06/Newspulseoximeter.jpg.

This indicates that, despite the fact that pulse oximeters play a vital role in improving patient safety and monitoring during anesthesia, systemic impediments still hinder their full potential in clinical practice (Ryan et al., 2025). The future of pulse oximetry in anesthesia also encompasses innovation in remote monitoring, potentially further expanding the care. Recent research has established the clinical benefit of incorporating home-based pulse oximetry into longstanding care plans for chronically ill patients, demonstrating an emerging trend toward more completely integrated monitoring solutions. These technologies could enable predictive control of oxygen saturation levels and identify trends that enable proactive intervention before patients even present for additional clinical management. Widespread application of remote monitoring technology may thus revolutionize the quality of anesthesia care by extending the monitoring horizon beyond traditional hospital settings, making pulse oximetry an even more useful device for both acute and chronic patient management.

7.3.3. Capnometer

A capnometer is also an important part of modern anesthetic monitoring, particularly in assessing a patient's respiratory status in the operating room. By monitoring the concentration of CO_2 in expired air in real time, the capnometer provides immediate feedback on the body's respiratory exchange. This is crucial since existing monitoring modalities, such as pulse oximetry, often lag in detecting respiratory depression until considerable hypoxemia has occurred. Research has shown that capnography can identify respiratory issues much earlier, thereby enhancing patient safety during anesthesia. By identifying changes in CO2 levels, clinical professionals can respond quickly, potentially reducing the risk of complications and optimizing postoperative recovery. This underscores the value of incorporating innovative monitoring technologies in clinical practice, enabling anesthesiologists to respond to patient demand rapidly and efficiently. A quality improvement project emphasized the usefulness of capnography in postoperative settings, with an increase in usage following targeted educational interventions among PACU nurses. Initial data indicated that capnography monitoring was present only 0.38% of the time before education interventions, but this more than doubled to 1.3% following interventions, with a striking change in practice ($p = 0.02$). Even though there was a slight improvement in scores of nurse knowledge, it reflects the complexity of translating knowledge into practice. Effective capnography monitoring is not merely reliant on technical know-how in operating the device but also on understanding its implications for patient care. Generally, these findings suggest that, as knowledge increases, surmounting implementation issues is an important objective for realizing capnometer benefits in clinical practice (Mueller, 2024). The growing emphasis on anesthesia monitoring using capnography is in line with more extensive educational efforts to improve patient safety and quality of care. As stated in the complete resource for Clinical Anesthesia residents, understanding the fundamental aspects of monitoring, i.e., capnography, is important in developing mastery over anesthesiology (George et al., 2016). This is because effective monitoring will have a direct influence on patient outcomes in the operating room. Second, the capacity of continuous CO_2 monitoring to aid earlier detection of respiratory distress highlights its ability to reduce postoperative complications. Training of anesthesia personnel in the value and significance of capnography promotes a culture of vigilance that is critical to minimizing risk in anesthesia. Future efforts must encompass technical training as well as an operational incorporation of capnography into practice so that its value is utilized throughout the treatment of patients (Figure 7.9).

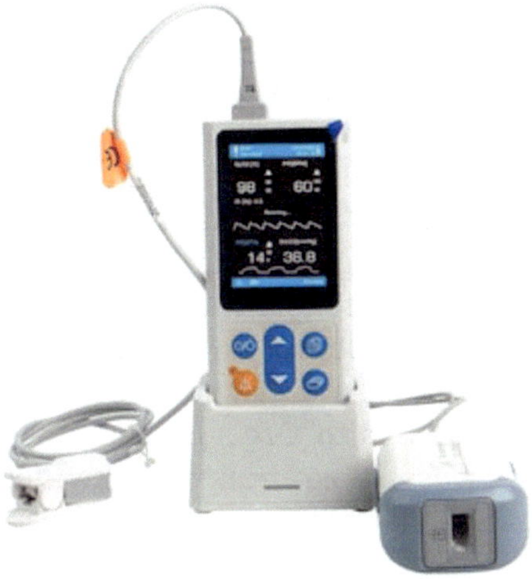

Figure 7.9. The capnometer plays a pivotal role in modern anesthetic monitoring.

Source: https://content.jdmagicbox.com/quickquotes/images_main/super-amoled-capnometer-803140506-8zsh3bxz.jpg?impolicy=queryparam&im=Resize=(360,360),aspect=fit.

Test Your Knowledge

1. What types of monitoring equipment are commonly used during anesthesia, and how do they assist in assessing a patient's vital functions?
2. How have advances in monitoring technology improved the safety and effectiveness of anesthetic care?

7.4. Role of Anesthesia Providers

Learning Outcome

1. Anesthesiologist responsibilities
2. Nurse anesthetist roles
3. Collaboration with the surgical team

Anesthesia providers play a critical role on the surgical team, not only providing anesthesia but also monitoring patients continuously and regulating their condition throughout the operative process. Their functions are not just limited to keeping patients' pain-free; they encompass uninterrupted monitoring of vital signs and physiologic status to detect any signs of distress or adverse effect. As noted by the World Health Organization, anesthesia service success is naturally intertwined with best-practice patient safety, highlighting the need for well-trained anesthesiologists with adequate monitoring equipment and skills to safely care for both simple and complex cases. The vigilant monitoring of anesthesia allows practitioners to make real-time changes, responding promptly to changes in a patient's status, thus minimizing anesthesia-related risks in surgery and facilitating optimal results for patients undergoing various procedures (Khan et al., 2023). Additionally, where anesthesia practitioners are working affects their ability to deliver safe and effective care. Issues such as inadequate resources, particularly in low- and middle-income nations, can hinder the quality of anesthesia care and negatively affect patient safety. Inadequately trained personnel and equipment can render it unsafe where the effectiveness of monitoring is questionable, leading to complications. Coordination of services among anesthesiologists, nurses, and operating rooms in these environments becomes imperative, given that they all work under the limitations of available infrastructure to promote patient health. Training and equipment investments become paramount to enable these services, ensuring anesthesia providers have the training and equipment necessary to provide high-quality care and avoid perilous breakdowns in patient monitoring and safety (Khan et al., 2023). The anesthetists' role has also evolved significantly with the issues of global health challenges, as experienced during the COVID-19 pandemic. As the number of patients increased and danger risks grew, these experts had to adapt rapidly to optimize monitoring while protecting themselves from contracting the virus. These occupational fatigue and burnout issues have also been raised and impact the mental health and performance of the healthcare providers, including the anesthesia providers. The situation underscores the need for holistic support systems to ensure the physical and psychological well-being of these vital health care providers. Through increased communication, resource management, and organizational adaptability, anesthesia professionals are in a better position to surf the waves of modern surgical practice, landing much more effectively at maintaining an eye on patient safety and continuing high standards of practice even in difficult times.

7.4.1. Anesthesiologist Responsibilities

In anesthesia practice, anesthesiologists play significant roles in patient safety and procedure outcomes. They play perioperative leadership roles by conducting extensive preoperative assessments for the identification of potential risks and pathologies that could complicate anesthesia management. Preoperative assessment includes reviewing a patient's history, evaluating the patient's present state of health, and determining appropriate anesthetic modalities to be employed. Anesthesiologists should also set preoperative fasting protocols for specific patient needs, as non-compliance can have terrible adverse effects during sedation. Patient safety starts with this complete basis, upon which previous conditions are managed before administering sedating drugs. During the operation, the role of the anesthesiologists continues to monitor the patient's physiologic state, including vital signs and oxygen saturation levels.

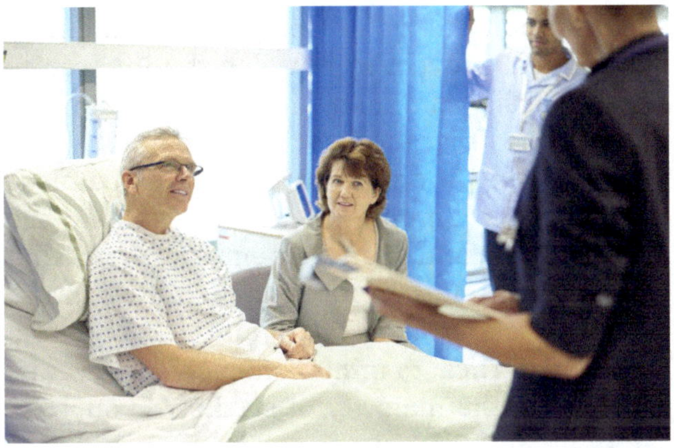

Figure 7.10. The realm of anesthesia, anesthesiologists carry substantial responsibilities.

Source: https://cdn-prod.medicalnewstoday.com/content/images/articles/287/287857/anesthesiologist.jpg.

They monitor the depth of anesthesia and make momentary medication adjustments based on real-time feedback from surgical stimuli. Such a dynamic environment compels anesthesiologists to demonstrate acute technical and decision-making skills in airway management, especially for complex patients, e.g., those with anatomic variations (Sasangohar et al., 2020). The requirement to balance appropriate anesthesia with risk factors, particularly in children, highlights their adaptability and expertise. By effective management of the level of sedation, anesthesiologists not only ensure patient comfort but also the success of the surgical procedure as a whole, thereby demonstrating the vital nature of their work as monitors under anesthesia. Post-operatively, anesthesiologists continue their role in ensuring timely, issue-free patient recovery. They monitor patients in the recovery areas, assessing levels of consciousness and ensuring individuals return to preoperative status before discharge. Effective pain management strategies are employed to reduce postoperative pain, which is crucial for patient satisfaction and recovery times. Furthermore, anesthesiologists provide important discharge information to patients, ensuring that patients comprehend postoperative care procedures and identify warning signs of potential complications. This final stage of monitoring reinforces their role in the middle of the care continuum, with the imperative for not just administrative expertise but also integrative management of the patient throughout the operation (Sasangohar et al., 2020). Ultimately, the responsibilities of anesthesiologists encompass the full continuum of care, ensuring patient safety and well-being from preoperative evaluation to postoperative recovery (Figure 7.10).

7.4.2. Nurse Anesthetist Roles

In the practice of anesthesia, nurse anesthetists or certified registered nurse anesthetists (CRNAs) are integral components of perioperative care. CRNAs' roles are not limited to administering anesthesia; they also directly participate in monitoring, preoperative evaluation, and postoperative care. CRNAs are engaged in close collaboration within interprofessional teams, contributing rich information to decision-making that makes anesthesia management safe and efficient. Their expertise allows them to closely monitor patients' vital signs during the surgical process, which is most important for identifying and resolving potential complications. As depicted in the team dynamics literature, effective communication and coordination among CRNAs, anesthesiologists, and other healthcare providers significantly enhance patient outcomes and optimize the utilization of available resources in clinical practice (Kleinpell et al., 2021). Because medication management is integrated into anesthesia care, nurse anesthetists must be pharmacology experts, especially regarding anesthetic drugs.

CRNAs assess each patient's unique risk and tailor anesthesia plans to their medical history and procedures. They also closely monitor patients' responses to pharmacotherapeutics intraoperatively. For instance, adjusting drug dosages based on real-time assessments and titrating medications are their tasks. This anticipatory role not only enhances patient safety but also underlines the necessity of constant vigilance in anesthesia practice. The activity of CRNAs has become more specialized, especially in critical care settings, where their work contributes disproportionately to the care of patients in high-risk environments, as observed through adaptations required during health crises such as the COVID-19 pandemic (Thomas et al., 2020). In addition to clinical responsibilities, CRNAs also participate in educational programs that teach nursing staff, anesthesiology residents, and allied health professionals best practices in anesthesia. Their ability to educate and guide others is crucial in a constantly evolving healthcare system, where optimal provision of efficient and effective anesthesia services is necessary. Such commitment to education guarantees continuity of excellent standards of care and enhances a learning culture, facilitating professional growth. Aside from that, CRNAs are integral to fostering patient safety and improving practice quality through their involvement in multi-disciplinary teams with a focus on quality improvement initiatives. Their actions not only contribute to the overall performance of anesthesia departments but also enhance their critical role within the broader healthcare context, which emphasizes teamwork as the driver of optimal patient outcomes (Kleinpell et al., 2021).

7.4.3. Collaboration with Surgical Team

Teamwork among the surgical team is essential to ensure optimal patient outcomes, especially in monitoring anesthesia. Having anesthesiologists as part of the surgical team introduces a dynamic working relationship that enhances patient safety during the perioperative period. Surgeons and anesthesiologists both have integral roles outside their own domain that involve open communication and an implicit understanding of the other's role. Successful collaboration allows not only management of the surgical procedure but also the intricacies of anesthesia administration and monitoring. Where the high-stakes environment, like the operating room, is in question, seamless coordination among members enables the identification and management of any arising complications. It therefore enhances the culture of shared responsibility and joint participation, which are critical to minimizing adverse events, as noted in the majority of studies on surgical safety guidelines (Jain et al., 2025).

Periodic communication among surgical team members has a profound impact on the degree of coordination and efficacy of monitoring patients during surgery. The implementation of standardized checklists, such as the WHO surgical safety checklist, illustrates why standardized communication within the operating room is critical (Nene et al., 2024). This checklist is a touchstone that inspires discussion among surgeons, anesthesiologists, and nurses at critical moments: preoperatively, intraoperatively, and postoperatively.

Reviewing the key points—such as patient identification, site marking, and anesthesia preparation—systematically, team members carefully consider each detail of the surgical process. This structured communication is not only procedural in nature; it is concurrent with establishing trust and rapport, which are foundations of effective teamwork. As research indicates, establishing team cohesion can actually go a significant way in preventing communication breakdowns, which typically lead to undesirable outcomes (Nene et al., 2024). Further, enhanced collaboration between the operating room team requires a focus on continuous education and respect among all team players. The evolution of surgical care has highlighted the importance of advancing the relationship between the anesthesiologist and surgeon so that there can be a proper response to the complexity of the surgical procedure. Interprofessional training sessions and informal opportunities to interact beyond the operating room can help solidify these relationships and lead to improved understanding of individual roles and expectations. Involvement in collaborative learning environments allows for knowledge sharing, ultimately refining the general knowledge base underpinning the decision-making processes of surgery and anesthesia monitoring. According to research, these ongoing interactions not only support better patient care but also promote a more collaborative work environment, with a focus on team welfare and professional growth (Jain et al., 2025) (Figure 7.11).

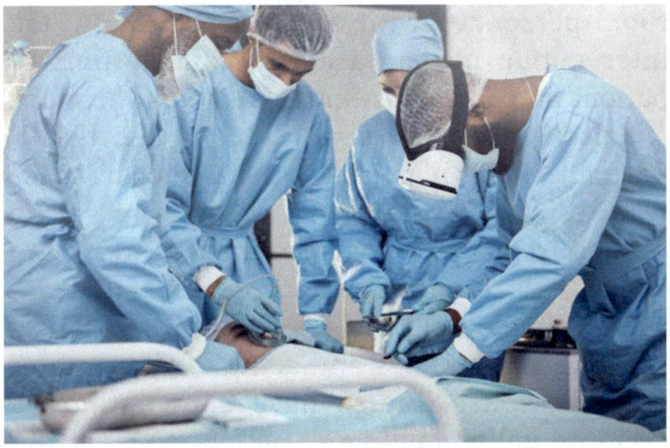

Figure 7.11. Collaborative efforts within the surgical team.

Source: https://img.freepik.com/premium-photo/doctors-surgery-collaboration-with-medicine-team-scrubs-operating-man-patient-hospital-doctor-nurse-teamwork-with-medical-group-clinic-perform-operation_590464-121160.jpg.

Test Your Knowledge

1. What are the primary responsibilities of an anesthesiologist before, during, and after surgery to ensure patient safety and effective anesthesia?
2. How does the anesthesiologist coordinate with the surgical team and other healthcare professionals to manage perioperative care and handle emergencies?

7.5. Risks and Complications

Learning Outcome

1. Potential complications of inadequate monitoring
2. Patient safety concerns
3. Legal implications of monitoring failures

In the instance of anesthesia, monitoring plays a critical part in patient safety, given the enormity of risks and complications involved in diverse types of surgery. The effect of anesthetic drugs on the respiratory function is also a significant consideration, particularly among patients with pre-existing conditions such as obesity. Research has indicated that patients who are obese are at increased risk of developing postoperative pulmonary complications owing mainly to issues like challenging intubation and obstructive sleep apnea. Effective perioperative risk stratification would enable detection of such patients and thereby maximize monitoring and employ tailored measures to mitigate potential complications during and after surgery (Bazurro et al., 2018). Awareness of potential risks is most important for anesthesiologists and operating room personnel, with early identification and intervention playing a key role in optimizing patient outcomes. Cardiovascular complications are also a significant concern during anesthesia, particularly for high-risk patients such as those who require undergoing catheter ablation procedures. The intricacy that comes with catheter ablation, for instance, necessitates close hemodynamic monitoring since the procedure can provoke arrhythmias and acute cardiovascular complications. Studies have shown that an accurate understanding of patient-specific risk factors, such as left atrial size, can help with prognostic assessment and risk stratification for complications. This understanding is important because complications like stroke, heart failure, or arrhythmias can lead to long-term morbidity. To achieve this goal, the creation of monitoring devices has become a practice that allows clinicians to better predict and handle these cardiovascular hazards in the process (Calkins et al., 2017). The postoperative course is also significant with regard to monitoring because prior anesthetic processes may trigger adverse reactions. Side effects such as prolonged neuromuscular blockade or recovery from anesthesia can be of critical risk, especially in comorbid patients. Continuous monitoring of PACU is crucial for early recognition and management of such complications, ultimately preventing delayed recovery and enhancing patient safety. Moreover, the use of multimodal monitoring techniques can provide a holistic picture of the patient's status, hence supporting better decision-making. Therefore, an understanding of the variety of anesthesia complications and risks is paramount to optimizing monitoring approaches and improving outcomes in a wide range of patient populations (Bazurro et al., 2018).

7.5.1. Potential Complications of Inadequate Monitoring

Inadequate monitoring of anesthesia can lead to a wide range of serious complications, significantly impacting patient outcomes. One of the most serious risks is failure to recognize and correct respiratory complications promptly, such as airway obstruction or inadequate ventilation. For instance, for a patient with a complex history of disease or genetic syndrome like CLIFAHDD, the postoperative course can be beset with trouble, as is clear from a report detailing a child with recurrent episodes of apnea after extubation despite intraoperative stability. This scenario requires strict postoperative monitoring to detect and address breathing difficulties early, thereby preventing respiratory failure and extended hospital stays (Jessica et al., 2025). Such scenarios highlight the importance of specific guidelines for monitoring patients depending on their individual needs, particularly those with unusual anatomical or physiological considerations. Another major source of concern regarding inadequate monitoring is the risk of occult hemodynamic instability. In situations where vital signs, such as blood pressure and heart rate, are not closely monitored, clinicians may miss early signs of decline, which can transform into catastrophic states like shock or cardiac arrest. Advanced technologies have evolved for the detection of organ function, particularly in the context of anesthetic management. These technologies can provide critical information about hemodynamic status and enable more accurate real-time monitoring. Yet, the central nervous system is most often the least monitored system under anesthesia, despite being a critical component of patient safety. The volatility of sedative and hypnotic effects in critically ill patients increases the risk of complications when monitoring is suboptimal. Therefore, there is a need for more aggressive neuromonitoring practices, as they may help prevent such complications and optimize patient outcomes (Romagnoli et al., 2024). Furthermore, inadequate monitoring extends beyond acute physiological indicators to encompass the possibility of prolonged neurological injury. Postoperative cognitive impairment and other neurological dysfunction can occur in anesthetized patients, particularly among the elderly or those with predisposing medical conditions. Lacking proper monitoring of brain function during and after surgery, clinicians may be unable to detect changes in consciousness or awareness that may indicate underlying issues. The lack of objective ways to ascertain brain activity is especially a problem, since it could lead either to an inadequate amount of sedation or to excessive anesthetic delivery, both of which have been linked to poor neurological outcomes. Standardization of neuromonitoring protocols and offering guarantees for the implementation of non-invasive technology can go a long way towards preventing such complications, ensuring adequate anesthetic care for the patient without causing long-term cognitive effects (Romagnoli et al., 2024) (Figure 7.12).

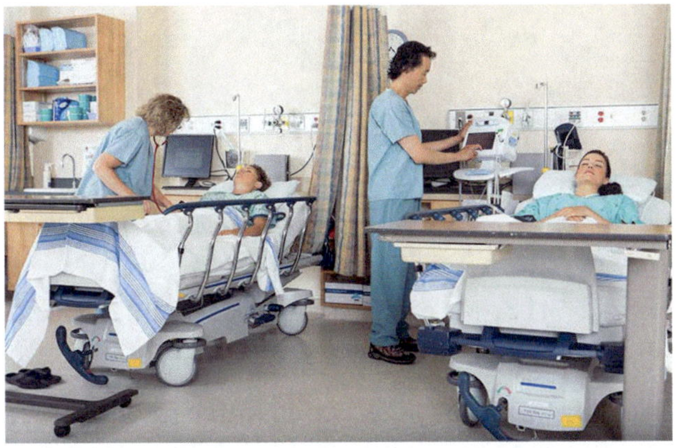

Figure 7.12. Potential complications of inadequate monitoring.

Source: https://ausmed-images.s3-ap-southeast-2.amazonaws.com/ausmed.com/ausmed-articles/20200911_r_body_3.jpg.

7.5.2. Patient Safety Concerns

In anesthesia, though, patient safety comes first because of the complex interplay of physiological factors throughout surgery. Anesthetic drug choice is most important, particularly in patient populations like those undergoing cardiac surgery, in whom risks to the cardiovascular system are multiplied. Research indicates that newer induction agents, e.g., propofol and etomidate, are effective in providing cardiovascular stability, while agents like isoflurane and sevoflurane are amenable to hemodynamic control. These advances are not only technical but are significant in minimizing complications and optimizing patient safety. The use of state-of-the-art monitoring technologies, such as transesophageal echocardiography, has been proven to be vital in offering real-time assessment of hemodynamic status and thereby significantly improving surgical outcomes (Ahmed et al., 2025). Hence, a fundamental understanding of such dynamics is necessary for anesthesiologists to navigate the complexities of patient management during surgical interventions. Further, the use of regional anesthesia techniques has become increasingly prevalent in modern surgical practices, particularly due to their association with improved pain control and faster recovery. However, patient safety remains a principal concern when employing these techniques, especially in patients on anticoagulation therapy or with other comorbidities. Current guidelines emphasize the importance of appropriate evaluation and risk assessment before employing neuraxial blocks in such individuals. A guideline practice, as suggested by specialist panels, provides anesthesiologists with evidence-based guidelines to mitigate regional anesthesia risks. In particular, adherence to guidelines that consider the application of dual guidance in peripheral nerve blocks enhances procedural effectiveness and patient safety (Torrano et al., 2025). A systematic and standardized approach, therefore, needs to be achieved to cross the complex nature of regional anesthesia, attaining maximum gain for patients in every clinical situation. Another challenge to patient safety under anesthesia is the increasing record of postoperative cognitive dysfunction, particularly among vulnerable populations such as elderly patients. Diagnosis of the condition necessitates a more sensitive approach to anesthetic management. Innovative techniques such as target-controlled infusion anesthesia (TIVA) have shown promise in reducing postoperative cognitive side effects. Coupled with advanced monitoring, these techniques allow for a more personalized approach that may adapt to individual patient needs during surgery. Analogously, enhanced recovery strategies and multimodal analgesia protocols underscore the need for a holistic vision of patient safety that extends beyond the operating room. With evolving trends in anesthesia, continuous research is necessary to advance these practices further, with the utmost regard for patient safety as the foremost element in anesthetic practice (Ahmed et al., 2025; Torrano et al., 2025). Prioritization of these concerns in monitoring will therefore be crucial for maximizing patient outcomes in anesthesia.

7.5.3. Legal Implications of Monitoring Failures

Failure in anesthesia monitoring can have substantial legal implications, primarily on account of negligence and malpractice concerns. If anesthesia monitoring systems fail to report proper and timely data, clinicians are at higher risk of encountering adverse events that threaten patient safety. In this regard, informed consent is operative, as patients are to be made aware not only of the procedure's risks but also of potential technological breakdowns that could disrupt their treatment. Anesthesiologists risk being sued if monitoring shortcomings result in patient harm, underscoring the need for strict monitoring equipment and technique standards. In addition, the evolving era of anesthesia technology demands that clinicians not only understand the capabilities of their monitoring devices but also be aware of the legal consequences of relying on such equipment for critical surgeries (Char et al., 2020). The legal responsibility of anesthesiologists goes beyond actual patient care since their interaction with machine learning (ML) and automatic technologies imposes additional aspects of responsibility. With the incorporation of ML technologies into clinical practice, liability issues arise when such systems malfunction or provide incorrect recommendations. This problem is dramatically evident in the Boeing 737 Max crashes, where the misuse of automation led to disastrous consequences.

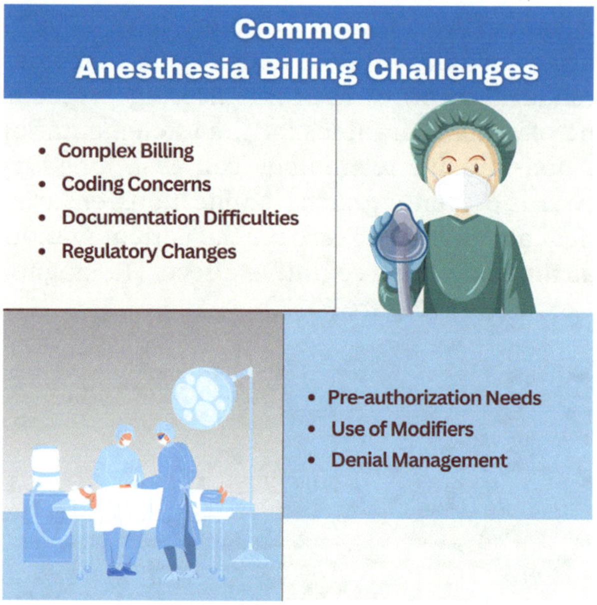

Figure 7.13. Monitoring failures in anesthesia can lead to significant legal implications.

Source: https://www.outsourcestrategies.com/wp-content/uploads/2024/06/common-anesthesia-billing-challenges.png.

Therefore, anesthesiologists need to balance the dual mandate of patient protection with awareness of the operational limitations of the technology employed in their own practice. Lack of clear regulatory guidelines to ensure accountability for ML outcomes also makes legal cases more complicated, placing additional burden on clinicians to develop competence in the strengths and weaknesses of these innovative technologies in an attempt to minimize potential legal repercussions (Robert, 2016). With greater demands for open disclosure and safety standards, the legal basis of anesthesia practice is poised to evolve. Anesthesiologists need to be attuned to how monitoring failures overlap with emerging legal frameworks, particularly those addressing patient data privacy and machine learning regulation. Vigilant efforts to revise regulatory guidelines, such as those from the FDA, will play a pivotal role in developing protocols to safeguard patients and clinicians in the event of monitoring failure. Ultimately, establishing a culture of accountability in anesthesia practice will involve not only complying with existing law but also actively promoting patient safety and ethics by lobbying. There will need to be providers willing and able to navigate legal systems to remain committed to delivering high-quality anesthesia monitoring, thereby minimizing liability and maximizing patient outcomes (Char et al., 2020) (Figure 7.13).

Test Your Knowledge

1. What are the common risks and complications associated with anesthesia, and how can healthcare providers minimize these risks?
2. How do patient-specific factors and intraoperative monitoring contribute to identifying and managing potential safety concerns during anesthesia?

7.6. Advances in Monitoring Techniques

Learning Outcome

1. Development of non-invasive monitoring
2. Integration of technology in monitoring
3. Future trends in anesthesia monitoring

The evolution of monitoring technology throughout the discipline of anesthesia has had a profound impact on surgical outcomes and patient safety. Advances such as continuous and non-invasive monitoring have facilitated real-time understanding of the patient's physiology. For instance, technology such as impedance cardiography and continuous non-invasive arterial pressure monitoring allows anesthesiologists to quantify cardiovascular stability without the risks associated with the invasive method. Through the integration of these focused approaches, clinicians can tailor anesthetic management and fluid therapy protocols to dynamic clinical scenarios. This transition toward more sophisticated monitoring enables more effective perioperative care, thereby reducing the frequency of complications and aiding recovery (Bharadwaj, 2025). As a result, individualized anesthesia care becomes increasingly feasible, leading to enhanced patient experiences and optimized surgical outcomes. Moreover, advancements in artificial intelligence (AI) and machine learning have increasingly revolutionized anesthesia monitoring methods. The use of AI-based analytics enables practitioners to predict adverse events and patient deterioration and intervene in time. For instance, real-time data analysis with wearable biosensors enables sustained monitoring of vital signs and immediate alerts for any threatening changes in patient status. Such predictive capabilities not only enhance safety in the intraoperative period but also streamline postoperative recovery paths by enabling proper monitoring of recovery parameters (Bharadwaj, 2025). The challenge comes in implementing such advanced technologies in routine clinical practice because factors such as cost, training, and the availability of administrative support are critical to tapping their full potential to enhance patient care. Finally, the future of anesthesia monitoring strategies looks bright, particularly given the ongoing development of closed-loop systems that automatically adjust anesthetic delivery upon detection of patient response. Closed-loop systems aim to completely eliminate human error and variation in consistency when administering anesthetics, using a single mode of patient management. Finally, the use of real-time technical feedback loops incorporated into surgical procedures can enhance surgeons' situational awareness. As additional evidence proves the effectiveness and efficiency of such newer paradigms of monitoring, evidence-based practice will guide implementation in the clinical setting. Battling the implementation barriers, such as training and infrastructure development, will be essential in capitalizing on these innovations and transforming the practice environment of anesthesia monitoring (Bosso et al., 2025) (Figure 7.14).

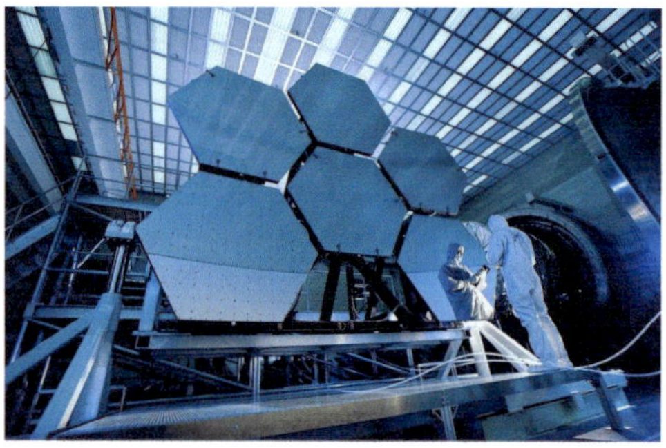

Figure 7.14. The evolution of monitoring techniques within the realm of anesthesia.

Source: https://cdn.thenewstack.io/media/2021/08/83510fc2-telescopic-mirror-74034_1280-1024x681.jpg.

7.6.1. Development of Non-Invasive Monitoring

The development of non-invasive monitoring equipment is a significant advancement in anesthesia, enhancing patient well-being and safety during surgery. Traditional methods, such as the oscillometric blood pressure (BP) cuff, have certain limitations, particularly when ongoing surveillance is necessary. Modern developments in the application of pulse wave analysis (PWA) and photoplethysmography (PPG) are extremely encouraging, as they are cost-effective and readily adhered to by patients. In particular, PPG-based PWA of oBPM™ has been shown to have promise for enabling effective continuous BP monitoring during the induction of anesthesia. The method offers continuous measurement without the hassles of oscillometric cuffs, thus facilitating a better overall patient experience in the operating room. Further, the algorithm for oBPM™ has also been robustly tested, ensuring its stability and reliability in correlating estimated BP values with traditional measurements, offering a better alternative for both clinicians and patients (Proença et al., 2019). The resurgence of interest in non-intubated methods in thoracic surgery is another evidence of the necessity to develop non-invasive monitoring technologies. This technique, which permits spontaneous ventilation without subjecting patients to intubation or the risks of positive-pressure ventilation, provides an unimpeded field of operation. Advances in anesthetic and monitoring techniques have made such procedures not only feasible but increasingly so safe for both patient and physician. The flexibility offered by non-invasive monitoring devices allows anesthesiologists to maintain close monitoring of vital parameters even as they support the unique requirements of non-intubated procedures. With multiple anesthetic approaches, the ability to monitor patients comfortably and precisely is paramount, particularly as the sophistication of cases continues to rise (Coley et al., 2017). As monitoring devices become less invasive, they provide an opportunity to expand their use in a variety of surgical pathologies, with beneficial effects on patient outcomes. Ongoing algorithm development and equipment, as well as intense training of anesthesiologists, get the medical teams ready for responding more readily to trends in surgical methods. The advantages of these new technologies extend beyond comfort; accurate monitoring is essential for avoiding complications and maintaining patient safety.

With the advancement of the specialty, more rigorous studies are required to establish standardized protocols and best practices for non-invasive monitoring during anesthesia. Ongoing research will illuminate the clinical community regarding the optimal technique and applications, so that someday non-invasive methods become integral to modern anesthetic practice (Proença et al., 2019).

7.6.2. Integration of Technology in Monitoring

The integration of technology into anesthetic monitoring has revolutionized patient care, primarily through the advent of artificial intelligence (AI) and advanced data analysis. It begins in the preoperative phase, where AI is employed to create individualized risk assessment and personalize anesthesia planning by predicting appropriate drug dosages based on a patient's specific needs. These technologies are designed to examine large datasets from previous cases and thereby enhance anesthesiologists' decision-making, ultimately resulting in improved patient outcomes. It is certain that as the field of anesthesia continues to evolve with advances in technology, the application of AI in clinical practice will transform standards of care and improve efficiency, safety, and accuracy in patient monitoring during surgery (Singam, 2023). During the intraoperative time, technology continues to support monitoring with state-of-the-art anesthesia monitoring systems and closed-loop control systems. Real-time data are used by these systems to continuously track a patient's vital signs, drug effects, and physiological responses, so that anesthesiologists can make real-time adjustments to the delivery of an anesthetic. Another such breakthrough is the use of robotics in the operating room, which allows for greater precision and control for delicate procedures. Adaptive algorithms for monitoring systems learn from the patient's data, leading to more sophisticated monitoring methods that actively avoid potential complications. Not only does the data-driven approach increase the level of efficiency of operation within the operating room, but it also increases healthcare practitioners' confidence level in managing issues related to anesthesia during procedures (Singam, 2023).

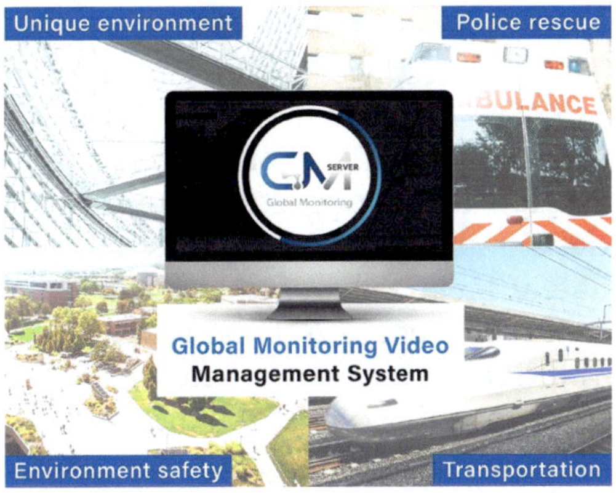

Figure 7.15. The integration of technology in monitoring during anesthesia.

Source: https://www.securityworldmarket.com/media/b5077fc0-5ec8-4ed0-953f-e8910f89fe63/V4uoDA/Images/NewsImages/Archive/Global2022PaidContent/Nov/TSSIA_2nd/FDB65C6B-605F-4699-B1CB-C7B5E8925083.jpeg?w=1000&action=fill&sh=79c80.

During the postoperative stage, technology's role in monitoring is to facilitate a smooth recovery and prevent complications. Advanced postoperative monitoring systems can detect early warning signs of adverse events by continuously monitoring patients' vital signs and recovery indicators. They also use artificial intelligence in forecasting potential postoperative complications, thereby enabling timely interventions. The COVID-19 pandemic emphasized the need to collect data and make healthcare systems interoperable, as hospitals needed new ways to address the influx of patients while maintaining safety standards. The use of electronic health records (EHR) and information technologies to improve data sharing reflects the need for combined monitoring measures across institutions, presenting an opportunity for anesthesiology to leverage technology to refine patient recovery procedures and elevate the quality of care provided (Figure 7.15).

7.6.3. Future Trends in Anesthesia Monitoring

The future of anesthesia monitoring will witness revolutionary changes driven by technological innovation, with artificial intelligence (AI) taking center stage. Current practices are hindered by traditional monitoring techniques that may not adequately meet the dynamic complexities of intraoperative management. AI has the potential to revolutionize these practices through real-time analysis and personalized interventions for patients undergoing procedures. The integration of AI into anesthetic monitoring systems has the potential to harmonize intraoperative pain management through data-driven analysis, facilitating real-time improvements in patient safety and satisfaction. This focus on individualized care aligns with the evolving mission of healthcare to offer safer, more efficient anesthesia practice. Implementation of this technological shift will require extensive educational initiatives for anesthesiology professionals to enhance their awareness and expertise regarding AI deployment in clinical settings, as shown by findings from recent quality improvement studies (Diaz et al., 2024). Another trend with immense potential in anesthesia monitoring is the greater use of perioperative transesophageal echocardiography (TEE), especially for cardiac operations. TEE enhances intraoperative monitoring by providing real-time data about cardiac function and hemodynamics. With cardiovascular disease remaining a leading global health concern, incorporating TEE to enhance surgical outcomes through accurate monitoring has become vital. In addition to facilitating preoperative planning, the use of TEE also aids intraoperative decision-making and postoperative assessment. Besides, technological progress in AI offers new opportunities for TEE image interpretation, improving diagnostic accuracy and providing real-time support for anesthesiologists. As stakeholders call for standardized training protocols to counteract the challenges of TEE implementation, its integration into routine anesthesia monitoring is set to revolutionize the quality of patient care in operating rooms (Liang et al., 2025). The convergence of these technological advances creates a unique opportunity to move forward with anesthesia monitoring by a more integrated approach that combines several modalities. Improvements in non-invasive monitoring technologies, such as wearable sensors, enable continuous measurement of vital signs without increasing patient discomfort. As the future unfolds, these technologies will be supplemented with robust data management systems capable of assimilating information from multiple sources and providing an overview of a patient's physiological state. This integrative approach to monitoring not only anticipates complications before they arise but also facilitates collaborative decision-making by multidisciplinary groups of caregivers. As education systems evolve to incorporate these new technologies, anesthesia professionals will find it easier to access their potential, ultimately enhancing patient care and streamlining the healthcare model.

Test Your Knowledge

1. What emerging technologies and innovations are expected to improve anesthesia monitoring and patient safety in the future?
2. How might artificial intelligence, wearable devices, and advanced sensors transform real-time monitoring and decision-making during anesthesia?

SUMMARY

The application of sophisticated monitoring techniques in anesthesiology practice can significantly enhance patient safety and treatment outcomes. The application of artificial intelligence-based tools in systematic reviews has led to considerable improvements in decision-making capabilities across many fields of anesthesiology, including monitoring depth of anesthesia and risk prediction. With the application of AI systems, anesthesiologists can enhance diagnostic quality through real-time modifications that minimize the risk of adverse events while maximizing analgesic infusion. Research findings under consideration indicate that AI-enhanced monitoring is not only promising but also increasingly superior to traditional methods, thereby confirming the central role that such technologies play in anesthetic care today (Lopes et al., 2023). Another essential parameter of anesthesia monitoring worthy of attention is nociception-guided management. As indicated by available evidence, the application of nociception monitoring can lead to more individualized approaches in the application of opioids, potentially reducing intraoperative opioid consumption. Heterogeneity between procedures and anesthetic techniques implies that additional evidence is necessary to assure the above before recommending nociception monitoring for routine practice. While some of the nociception monitors have yielded promising results, the overall consensus remains reserved, and more extensive research is needed to establish definite outcomes in pain management and the efficacy of some monitoring equipment (Meijer et al., 2019). Ultimately, the establishment of anesthetic monitoring systems marks a paradigm shift toward increased patient-centricity in perioperative care. As the profession adopts new technologies, professionals are charged with ensuring that such innovation is channeled into concrete benefits for patients. This entails not just the evolution of surgical methods and postoperative care but also a commitment to ongoing research and education in the profession. The sophisticated nature of anesthetic monitoring necessitates an integrated effort among healthcare professionals, technology firms, and researchers to foster an ecosystem that supports innovation while prioritizing patient safety and best practices in pain management (Meijer et al., 2019; Lopes et al., 2023).

Monitoring anesthesia is a multidisciplinary area in which intraoperative ideal decision-making is critically important to maintain patient safety. The use of artificial intelligence (AI) in this field has come to the forefront, as AI can significantly contribute to anesthesiologists' work by maximizing decision-making processes involved in the delivery and control of anesthesia. AIs' ability to support monitoring responsibilities, as laid out in a comprehensive paper, transcends various types, including anesthesia depth and event prediction by employing advanced algorithms and statistical tools (Hashemi et al., 2024). This systematic approach highlights the revolutionary capability of AI since it enables anesthesiologists to reduce complications and optimize the efficacy of their interventions, thereby improving patient outcomes. To AI's contribution, anatomical structure knowledge, particularly fascia, is paramount to effective techniques of anesthesia administration, such as fascial plane blocks. These blocks are essential in modern anesthesia practice and are commonly used to augment pain relief during procedures as part of a shift in the regional anesthesia paradigm. However, their efficacy remains in doubt due to the varied outcomes arising from their anatomical intricacy and differences in technique application (Chien-Chung et al., 2020). Improved knowledge of the anatomy of fascia and how local anesthetics interact with the various structural complexities may lead to improved block success rates as per the literature. This highlights the need for rigorous anatomical studies to establish and standardize optimal techniques for such procedures, minimizing variability and ensuring maximum clinical effectiveness. More importantly, the diverse factors influencing the spread of local anesthetics also must be explored. Variations in tissue structure, patient position, and other technical aspects have been reported to influence the results of fascial plane blocks significantly. These factors introduce a degree of uncertainty in anesthetic distribution, and it is hard for practitioners to ensure consistent and reliable anesthesia. Current research indicates that an understanding of these complexities is essential for shaping anesthetic protocols and achieving optimal patient care (Nicholas et al., 2020). So, the future of anesthesia and monitoring is in the convergence of new technology, anatomical knowledge, and an integrated model for perfection of procedures. This evolution is not just aiming for better techniques but also for enhancing the entire anesthetic process for patients who are to undergo surgery.

KEY TERMS FROM THIS CHAPTER

- Anesthesia monitoring
- Fatigue
- Intraoperative neurophysiologic monitoring
- Motor-evoked potentials (MEPs)
- Oxygen saturation
- Post-anesthesia care unit (PACU)
- Total intravenous anesthesia (TIVA)
- Artificial intelligence
- Hemodynamic
- Monitored anesthesia care (MAC)
- Multimodal analgesia
- Pharmacokinetics
- Target-controlled infusion (TCI)
- Local anesthetic systemic toxicity (LAST)

CRITICAL THINKING QUESTIONS

1. **Which of the following is NOT part of the ASA minimum monitoring standards during general anesthesia?**
   a. Pulse oximetry
   b. Blood pressure
   c. Capnography
   d. Central venous pressure
2. **What does pulse oximetry primarily measure?**
   a. PaO_2
   b. Hemoglobin concentration
   c. Arterial oxygen saturation (SpO_2)
   d. Mixed venous oxygen saturation
3. **A sudden drop in end-tidal CO_2 ($ETCO_2$) to near zero likely indicates:**
   a. Hyperventilation
   b. Hypothermia
   c. Pulmonary embolism or disconnection of the circuit
   d. Increased metabolic rate
4. **The Bispectral Index (BIS) monitor is used to assess:**
   a. Blood pressure variability
   b. Pain perception
   c. Depth of anesthesia
   d. Respiratory rate
5. **Which of the following conditions can cause falsely low SpO_2 readings?**
   a. Anemia
   b. Hypothermia
   c. Carbon monoxide poisoning
   d. Motion artifact

Short Answer Questions

1. Describe the principles of pulse oximetry and identify common causes of inaccurate readings.
2. Explain how capnography works and interpret the significance of a rising end-tidal CO_2 ($ETCO_2$) level during anesthesia.
3. What are the indications for invasive arterial blood pressure monitoring, and how does it differ from non-invasive blood pressure measurement?
4. How is depth of anesthesia monitored, and what are the roles of BIS (Bispectral Index) and other EEG-based monitors?
5. Describe the use of central venous pressure (CVP) monitoring. What does CVP indicate, and in what clinical scenarios is it useful?

Answer to Critical Thinking Questions

1. (b); 2. (d); 3. (c); 4. (a); 5. (a)

REFERENCES

1. Ahmed, M. a. K., Bahurmuz, M. A., & Muthanna, F. M. (2025). General Anesthesia in Cardiac Surgery: A Narrative Review for Evolving Techniques and Patient-Centered Best Practices. *Yemeni Journal for Medical Sciences, 19*(2). https://doi.org/10.20428/yjms.v19i2.2696Alonso, L. M., Solovey, G., Yanagawa, T., Proekt, A., Cecchi, G., & Magnasco, M. O. (2019). Single-trial classification of awareness state during anesthesia by measuring critical dynamics of global brain activity. *Scientific Reports, 9*. https://doi.org/10.1038/s41598-019-41345-4 (accessed on 28th June 2025).
2. Al-Zamanan, H. M. Z., Alarjani, B. M. H., Al Rapaiyei, F. S. M., Alshagaih, B. N., Al Monajam, N. Y., AlShehri, S. A., Al Omar, M. M., et al. (2024). Comprehensive review of anesthesia monitoring systems and radiological tools in complex surgical interventions. *Journal of Eco Humanism*. https://www.semanticscholar.org/paper/f065d57748f5d707f16da3425ebe5aa6541dead4 (accessed on 28th June 2025).
3. Badash, I., Burtt, K. E., Solorzano, C., & Carey, J. (2016). Innovations in surgery simulation: A review of past, current and future techniques. *Annals of Translational Medicine, 4*, 453. https://doi.org/10.21037/atm.2016.12.24 (accessed on 28th June 2025).
4. Barth, S., Edwards, C., Borton, R., Beever, D., Adams, W., Jenkins, G., Pizzo, E., et al. (2024). REMOTE-ILD study: Description of the protocol for a multicenter, 12-month randomized controlled trial to assess the clinical and cost-effectiveness of remote monitoring of spirometry and pulse oximetry in patients with interstitial lung disease. *BMJ Open Respiratory Research, 11*. https://www.semanticscholar.org/paper/41a13f92e6cbabacf1e77aea93372e883bb4737e (accessed on 28th June 2025).
5. Bashkaran, K., Kamatchi, M., Biruntha, R., & Kavya, M. (2025). Anesthesia machine monitoring and controlling system with IoT integration. *International Research Journal on Advanced Engineering Hub (IRJAEH)*. https://www.semanticscholar.org/paper/10c118f4025545950729811260516d72bd3dced9 (accessed on 28th June 2025).
6. Bazurro, S., Ball, L., & Pelosi, P. (2018). Perioperative management of obese patient. *Current Opinion in Critical Care, 24*, 560–567. https://doi.org/10.1097/mcc.0000000000000555 (accessed on 28th June 2025).
7. Bharadwaj, A. (2025). Revolutionizing perioperative medicine: Technological advancements for enhanced recovery. *Serbian Journal of Anesthesia and Intensive Therapy*. https://www.semanticscholar.org/paper/b03fdb09a017d1a6a3471ea560d0564ba80ad208 (accessed on 28th June 2025).
8. Black, N. D., Stecco, C., & Chan, V. (2020). Fascial plane blocks: More questions than answers? *Anesthesia & Analgesia, 132*, 899–905. https://doi.org/10.1213/ane.0000000000005321 (accessed on 28th June 2025).
9. Bosso, H., Araújo, T. A., Maluf, E. S., Mateus, M., et al. (2025). Advanced hemodynamic monitoring in polytraumatized patients: A comprehensive review. *Journal of Medical Science and Evidences*. https://www.semanticscholar.org/paper/ea32219474a2324856917957bcb001a1b041766e (accessed on 28th June 2025).
10. Calkins, H., Hindricks, G., Cappato, R., Kim, Y. H., Saad, E., Aguinaga, L., Akar, J. G., et al. (2017). 2017 HRS/EHRA/ECAS/APHRS/SOLAECE expert consensus statement on catheter

and surgical ablation of atrial fibrillation: Executive summary. *Journal of Arrhythmia, 33*, 369–409. https://doi.org/10.1016/j.joa.2017.08.001 (accessed on 28th June 2025).

11. Char, D., & Burgart, A. M. (2020). Machine-learning implementation in clinical anesthesia: Opportunities and challenges. *Anesthesia & Analgesia, 130*, 1709–1712. https://doi.org/10.1213/ane.0000000000004656 (accessed on 28th June 2025).
12. Coley, E., & Irons, J. (2017). Non-intubated anesthetic techniques for thoracic surgery. *2*, 69. https://www.semanticscholar.org/paper/019648d18f08abcdefd5a5f92a38e39d55d64150 (accessed on 28th June 2025).
13. Coté, C. J., & Wilson, S. (2019). Guidelines for monitoring and management of pediatric patients before, during, and after sedation for diagnostic and therapeutic procedures. *PEDIATRICS, 143*. https://doi.org/10.1542/peds.2019-1000 (accessed on 28th June 2025).
14. Daabiss, M., Otaibi, R. A., Otaibi, M. A., Shalaan, O., Shah, S., & Sharif, M. A. (2024). The impact of various anesthetic techniques on cerebral oxygenation during spinal surgery performed in a prone position with controlled hypotension. *Anesthesia and Critical Care Medicine Journal*. https://www.semanticscholar.org/paper/3aaee09267a39f7bb2c7756f0397ea0807d1a7a5 (accessed on 28th June 2025).
15. Das, S., & Ghosh, S. (2015). Monitored anesthesia care: An overview. *Journal of Anesthesiology Clinical Pharmacology, 31*, 27. https://doi.org/10.4103/0970-9185.150525 (accessed on 28th June 2025).
16. Diaz, V. J., et al. (2024). Utilization of artificial intelligence algorithms in the perioperative management and reduction of pain: An evidence-based educational module. https://core.ac.uk/download/622984193.pdf (accessed on 28th June 2025).
17. Durrani, R. (2024). Specialist training in anesthesia around the world. *Anesthesia, Pain & Intensive Care*. https://www.semanticscholar.org/paper/dcc49dba80a52593986c239acff87f708017d1fe (accessed on 28th June 2025).
18. Gruwez, H., Ezzat, D., Van Puyvelde, T., Dhont, S., Meekers, E., Wouters, F., Kellens, M., et al. (2024). Real-world validation of smartphone-based photoplethysmography for heart rate monitoring in atrial fibrillation. *Europace, 26*. https://www.semanticscholar.org/paper/4d30953f3d19e1aa192556449a1c06f2412bea34 (accessed on 28th June 2025).
19. Han, D. H., Kim, K. H., Nam, K. H., Lee, J. I., Kim, K. H., Park, J. H., & Ahn, H. S. (2024). Human-robot interaction and social robot: The emerging field of healthcare robotics and current and future perspectives for spinal care. *Neurospine, 21*, 868–877. https://www.semanticscholar.org/paper/aabe95c7d78dd82b9cc9be29826742e258322325 (accessed on 28th June 2025).
20. Hashemi, S., Yousefzadeh, Z., Abin, A. A., Ejmalian, A., Nabavi, S., & Dabbagh, A. (2024). Machine learning-guided anesthesiology: A review of recent advances and clinical applications. *Deleted Journal, 9*. https://doi.org/10.5812/jcma-145369 (accessed on 28th June 2025).
21. Jain, M., Sakale, H., & Shyam, A. (2025). Safe surgery is everyone's responsibility. *Journal of Orthopedic Case Reports, 15*, 1–3. https://www.semanticscholar.org/paper/ca300531416f19249d095f79c8d508ed0b2ff3b7 (accessed on 28th June 2025).
22. Jeena, P. A., Mohideen, B., Ashraf, A. R., Thaha, S. M., Shajahan, M. A., Nazar, I., Nair, R. G., et al. (2025). Heart rate variability and peripheral oxygen saturation levels in chronic obstructive pulmonary disease. *Cureus, 17*. https://www.semanticscholar.org/paper/dcfd4271830ef873c9b20f7a07bcf91f66f3ba5f (accessed on 28th June 2025).

23. Joglar, J. A., Chung, M. K., Armbruster, A. L., Benjamin, E. J., Chyou, J. Y., Cronin, E. M., Deswal, A., et al. (2023). 2023 ACC/AHA/ACCP/HRS guideline for the diagnosis and management of atrial fibrillation: A report of the American College of Cardiology/American Heart Association Joint Committee on Clinical Practice Guidelines. *Circulation, 149*. https://doi.org/10.1161/cir.0000000000001193 (accessed on 28th June 2025).

24. Johnson, K., & Egan, T. (2023). In total intravenous anesthesia we trust: Building confidence in total intravenous anesthesia techniques. *Anesthesia & Analgesia, 137*, 559–564. https://www.semanticscholar.org/paper/d3ccaf3b91292e1a8fa23a00ea123fad6fe501e2 (accessed on 28th June 2025).

25. Khan, I. A., & Karim, H. M. R. (2023). Anesthesia services in low- and middle-income countries: The fragile point for safe surgery and patient safety. *Cureus*. https://doi.org/10.7759/cureus.43174 (accessed on 28th June 2025).

26. Kinsella, S., Carvalho, B., Dyer, R. A., Fernando, R., McDonnell, N., Mercier, F. J., Palanisamy, A., et al. (2017). International consensus statement on the management of hypotension with vasopressors during caesarean section under spinal anesthesia. *Anesthesia, 73*, 71–92. https://doi.org/10.1111/anae.14080 (accessed on 28th June 2025).

27. Kleinpell, R., Grabenkort, W. R., Boyle, W. A., Vines, D., & Olsen, K. M. (2021). The Society of Critical Care Medicine at 50 years: Interprofessional practice in critical care: Looking back and forging ahead. *Critical Care Medicine, 49*, 2017–2032. https://doi.org/10.1097/ccm.0000000000005276 (accessed on 28th June 2025).

28. Kuck, K., Lofgren, L. R., & Lybbert, C. (2024). Anesthesia patient monitoring 2050. *Anesthesia & Analgesia, 138*, 273–283. https://www.semanticscholar.org/paper/191b50c7d0e0b47310f1cab0b08b987ad4bcdc5e (accessed on 28th June 2025).

29. Legatt, A. D., Emerson, R. G., Epstein, C. M., MacDonald, D. B., Deletis, V., Bravo, R., López, J., et al. (2016). ACNS guideline. *Journal of Clinical Neurophysiology, 33*, 42–50. https://doi.org/10.1097/wnp.0000000000000253 (accessed on 28th June 2025).

30. Liang, G., Liang, J., & Ma, X. (2025). Transesophageal echocardiography: Revolutionizing perioperative cardiac care. https://core.ac.uk/download/644449667.pdf (accessed on 28th June 2025).

31. Lonsdale, H., Jalali, A., Gálvez, J. A., Ahumada, L., & Simpao, A. F. (2020). Artificial intelligence in anesthesiology: Hype, hope, and hurdles. *Anesthesia & Analgesia, 130*, 1111–1113. https://doi.org/10.1213/ane.0000000000004751 (accessed on 28th June 2025).

32. Lopes, S., Rocha, G., & Guimarães-Pereira, L. (2023). Artificial intelligence and its clinical application in anesthesiology: A systematic review. *Journal of Clinical Monitoring and Computing, 38*, 247–259. https://doi.org/10.1007/s10877-023-01088-0 (accessed on 28th June 2025).

33. Mahmood, F., Matyal, R., Skubas, N. J., Montealegre-Gallegos, M., Swaminathan, M., Denault, A., Sniecinski, R. M., et al. (2016). Perioperative ultrasound training in anesthesiology: A call to action. *Anesthesia & Analgesia, 122*, 1794–1804. https://doi.org/10.1213/ane.0000000000001134 (accessed on 28th June 2025).

34. Martinez-Vazquez, P., & Jensen, E. (2022). Different perspectives for monitoring nociception during general anesthesia. *Korean Journal of Anesthesiology, 75*, 112–123. https://www.semanticscholar.org/paper/b8346c622d8e8f2fac329c3d8f048a1c034b8a08 (accessed on 28th June 2025).

35. Meijer, F., Niesters, M., van Velzen, M., Martini, C. H., Olofsen, E., Edry, R., Sessler, D. I., et al. (2019). Does nociception monitor-guided anesthesia affect opioid consumption? A systematic review of randomized controlled trials. *Journal of Clinical Monitoring and Computing, 34*, 629–641. https://doi.org/10.1007/s10877-019-00362-4 (accessed on 28th June 2025).

36. Miller, T. R., & Radcliff, T. A. (2020). Economic shocks from the novel COVID-19 pandemic for anesthesiologists and their practices. *Anesthesia & Analgesia, 131*, 112–116. https://doi.org/10.1213/ane.0000000000004882 (accessed on 28th June 2025).

37. Mueller, R. (2024). Capnography monitoring in the PACU: Improving patient safety through education. https://libres.uncg.edu/ir/uncg/f/R_Mueller_Paper_2024.pdf (accessed on 28th June 2025).

38. Nene, B. S., Sriramka, B., Jain, M., Biswal, P., & Shyam, A. (2024). Partners in precision: Cultivating trust and respect in the surgeon–anesthetist dynamics. *Journal of Orthopedic Case Reports, 14*, 3–5. https://www.semanticscholar.org/paper/08a11297e596fc2f311fc388ad3c6593358b0104 (accessed on 28th June 2025).

39. O'Reilly-Shah, V. N., Gentry, K. R., Van Cleve, W., Kendale, S., Jabaley, C. S., & Long, D. R. (2020). The COVID-19 pandemic highlights shortcomings in US health care informatics infrastructure: A call to action. *Anesthesia & Analgesia, 131*, 340–344. https://doi.org/10.1213/ane.0000000000004945 (accessed on 28th June 2025).

40. Proença, M., Bonnier, G., Ferrario, D., Verjus, C., & Lemay, M. (2019). PPG-based blood pressure monitoring by pulse wave analysis: Calibration parameters are stable for three months. *2019 41st Annual International Conference of the IEEE Engineering in Medicine and Biology Society (EMBC)*. https://www.semanticscholar.org/paper/a92747db50ff58961ea20eb85b662bca8a24978c (accessed on 28th June 2025).

41. Prontera, A., Baroni, S., Marudi, A., Valzania, F., Feletti, A., Benuzzi, F., Bertellini, E., et al. (2017). Awake craniotomy anesthetic management using dexmedetomidine, propofol, and remifentanil. *Drug Design Development and Therapy, 11*, 593–598. https://doi.org/10.2147/dddt.s124736 (accessed on 28th June 2025).

42. Romagnoli, S., Lobo, F. A., Picetti, E., Rasulo, F. A., Robba, C., & Matta, B. (2024). Non-invasive technology for brain monitoring: Definition and meaning of the principal parameters for the International PRactice On TEChnology neuro-moniToring group (I-PROTECT). *Journal of Clinical Monitoring and Computing, 38*, 827–845. https://www.semanticscholar.org/paper/064ecdb2264717564d311ff6406b84972c749690 (accessed on 28th June 2025).

43. Sands, B. E., Peyrin-Biroulet, L., Loftus, E. V., Danese, S., Colombel, J. F., Törüner, M., Jonaitis, L., et al. (2019). Vedolizumab versus adalimumab for moderate-to-severe ulcerative colitis. *New England Journal of Medicine, 381*, 1215–1226. https://doi.org/10.1056/nejmoa1905725 (accessed on 28th June 2025).

44. Santos, J. G., & Buffon, A. C. (2025). Anesthetic management of a 9-year-old girl with congenital contractures of the limbs and face, hypotonia, and developmental delay syndrome: Airway difficulties and postoperative apnea during tendon surgery. *Anesthesia and Pain Medicine, 20*, 46–49. https://www.semanticscholar.org/paper/284032ed7827167f5ae9ae4a1272681a3f2698f2 (accessed on 28th June 2025).

45. Sasangohar, F., Jones, S. L., Masud, F., Vahidy, F., & Kash, B. A. (2020). Provider burnout and fatigue during the COVID-19 pandemic: Lessons learned from a high-volume intensive care

unit. *Anesthesia & Analgesia, 131*, 106–111. https://doi.org/10.1213/ane.0000000000004866 (accessed on 28th June 2025).

46. Shrivastava, N., Verma, A., & Saikia, K. (2025). Advances in pediatric anesthesia: Safety protocols and emerging practices. *International Journal of Research in Medical Sciences.* https://www.semanticscholar.org/paper/20ebc78cf6120b2a5b5a0c95ef2485ebaf2e1708 (accessed on 28th June 2025).
47. Sikes, R. S. (2016). 2016 Guidelines of the American Society of Mammalogists for the use of wild mammals in research and education. *Journal of Mammalogy, 97*, 663–688. https://doi.org/10.1093/jmammal/gyw078 (accessed on 28th June 2025).
48. Singam, A. (2023). Revolutionizing patient care: A comprehensive review of artificial intelligence applications in anesthesia. *Cureus*. https://doi.org/10.7759/cureus.49887 (accessed on 28th June 2025).
49. Singh, S., Pandey, P., Jasrasaria, N., Bharti, R., & Pandey, R. (2025). Monitoring patient anxiety, pain, and physiological responses during root canal treatment: An observational study. *The Journal of Contemporary Dental Practice, 26(3)*, 244–249. https://www.semanticscholar.org/paper/e8c9e464f3f51031896731c530d6f84ebbabdcda (accessed on 28th June 2025).
50. Torrano, V., Anastasi, S., Balzani, E., Barbara, E., Behr, A., Bosco, M., Buttarelli, C., et al. (2025). Enhancing safety in regional anesthesia: Guidelines from the Italian Society of Anesthesia, Analgesia, Resuscitation and Intensive Care (SIAARTI). *Journal of Anesthesia, Analgesia and Critical Care, 5.* https://www.semanticscholar.org/paper/8b297b59de82635e69e23ead62f109565c272746 (accessed on 28th June 2025).
51. Turner, R. A., Simmons, C. G., Ramirez, S., & Gamboa, J. E. (2025). Hypoxemia and postoperative monitoring after anesthesia: A prospective observational study using portable pulse oximetry in a resource-limited setting in Guatemala. *Cureus, 17.* https://www.semanticscholar.org/paper/f9953ff9c6418c400e4678cd800d5cd3c0e7f672 (accessed on 28th June 2025).
52. Ushnevych, Z. O., & Harbar, M. (2025). Dynamics of heart rate variability depending on the type of anesthesia during surgery for anterior abdominal wall hernias. *Emergency Medicine.* https://www.semanticscholar.org/paper/6694b01f89a740c8371525eb5637f7f5b73d2127 (accessed on 28th June 2025).
53. Wang, Z., Cheng, Z., Wang, C., Wu, Z., Wang, S., & Xu, H. (2024). A method for extracting physiological parameters of anesthetic patients based on video. *Proceedings of the 2024 4th International Conference on Bioinformatics and Intelligent Computing.* https://www.semanticscholar.org/paper/c89c15bbb4186714ce33914cedeae3e4b095e88d (accessed on 28th June 2025).
54. Williams, G. W., & Williams, E. S. (2016). *Basic Anesthesiology Examination Review.* https://ndl.ethernet.edu.et/bitstream/123456789/91547/1/Williams%2C%20Erin%20Scott_%20Williams%2C%20George%20W%20-%20Basic%20anesthesiology%20examination%20review%20%282016%2C%20Oxford%20University%20Press%29%20-%20libgen.lc.pdf#page=66 (accessed on 28th June 2025).

FLUID, ELECTROLYTE, AND BLOOD MANAGEMENT

8

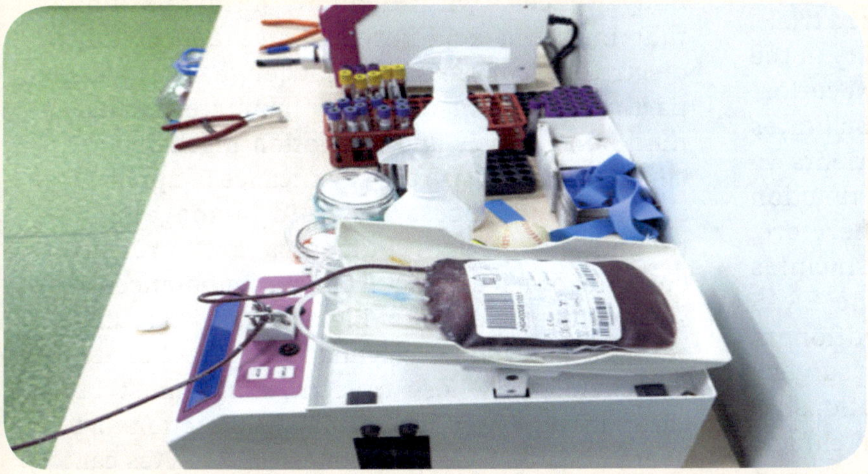

LEARNING OBJECTIVES

After studying this chapter, you will be able to:

1. Discuss the fluid balance
2. Explain the electrolyte homeostasis
3. Focus on blood components
4. Understand blood transfusion practices
5. Know fluid therapy
6. Learn about electrolyte replacement

Introduction

Fluid, electrolyte, and blood management is a critical aspect of perioperative care with a significant impact on patient outcomes in all areas of the medical environment. Optimal fluid balance and electrolyte homeostasis is complex in nature and specifically of concern in surgical patients, where surgery and anesthetic requirements can significantly change body fluid dynamics. It is through understanding these changes that clinicians can initiate effective management protocols that maintain patients in physiological equilibrium. Integration of all the best available current evidence-based practices is important in addressing the challenges posed by intraoperative and postoperative fluid management, which, if not managed, lead to complications like hypovolemia, electrolyte imbalance, or even cardiac dysrhythmias. Thus, research into fluid, electrolyte, and blood management practices constitutes a vital foundation for improved surgical outcomes and enhanced patient care. Enhanced recovery pathways have been more thoroughly profiled in recent years, particularly emphasizing the importance of multimodal, evidence-based strategies in perioperative fluid management. Organizational leadership efforts, such as the Enhanced Recovery After Surgery (ERAS) Society, offer comprehensive evidence-based guidelines that incorporate best practices in fluid and electrolyte management tailored to the specific needs of individual patients. As emphasized by ERAS guidelines, all the suggestions for protocol items are based on critical summaries of current literature, i.e., meta-analyses and randomized controlled trials, and therefore there is excellent reliability in the execution of such measures. Such execution, besides minimizing complications, facilitates quicker recovery times, allowing patients to return to their pre-surgical baseline function earlier (Gustafsson et al., 2018). Therefore, understanding the underpinning principles of fluid and electrolyte balance in the ERAS environment is worthwhile for practitioners committed to maximizing the delivery of surgical care. Additionally, the interactive relationship between fluid treatment and broader clinical recommendations, such as those produced by the European Society of Cardiology (ESC), underscores the need for practitioners to integrate a wide range of clinical decisions into practice. The ESC Guidelines emphasize that healthcare professionals must weigh evidence against individual patient circumstances, ensuring that therapeutic strategies remain up to date with the latest scientific findings while meeting established ethical and professional standards (Kirchhof et al., 2016). Application of guidelines in fluid and electrolyte management requires sensitivity to an individual patient's physiological condition, thereby facilitating individualized care. Herein, the fluid, blood product, and electrolyte management does not just reveal itself as a technical aspect of surgical recovery but is also a fundamental building block of overall patient care strategies attempting to optimize health outcomes in increasingly complex medical environments.

Definition of Fluid, Electrolyte, and Blood Management

Fluid, electrolyte, and blood management is an important clinical practice domain that involves the regulation and balance of fluids, electrolytes, and blood products within the human body. It is crucial because these components are involved in numerous physiological processes such as circulation, homeostasis, and metabolic function. The fluids are compartmentalized into various body spaces, with dynamic interrelations that maintain acid-base balance and steady electrolyte content. As knowledge advances, particularly from advances in microvascular fluid homeostasis and regulation mechanisms, clinicians emphasize the significance of applying an orderly process in fluid management to enhance patient outcomes and prevent complications arising from an imbalance in such critical elements. Electrolytes, including sodium, potassium, calcium, and bicarbonate, are chemicals whose concentrations must be carefully regulated for normal cell function and overall health. Dysregulation of electrolytes can lead to pathological states, as in the instance of hyperkalemia or hyponatremia, that lead to acute complications, like cardiac arrest or neurological dysfunction. Furthermore, the kidney function plays the most important role in fluid and electrolyte management as it is the kidney that has the responsibility of maintaining the balance by filtration and reabsorption (Daniel et al., 2018). With acute kidney injury, it becomes important to measure the requirement of fluid accurately because incorrect management exacerbates kidney damage and jeopardizes recovery. Thus, awareness of electrolyte dynamics forms a foundation for effective management measures in patient treatment. At the same time, blood management involves balancing the use of blood products in fields such as surgery, trauma, and hematologic malignancy. Demand can arise for red blood cells, platelets, or plasma products from acute blood loss or chronic anemia, which triggers a thoughtful assessment of the patient's status. Furthermore, advancements in treatment, such as CAR T cell therapy, have introduced new considerations in the management of blood, particularly regarding the risk of cytokine release syndrome and its complications (Daniel et al., 2018). This points to the necessity of applying standard protocols and grading systems to control these complex interactions in fluid, electrolyte, and blood management as therapists approach evidence-based practice to improve patient outcomes (Figure 8.1).

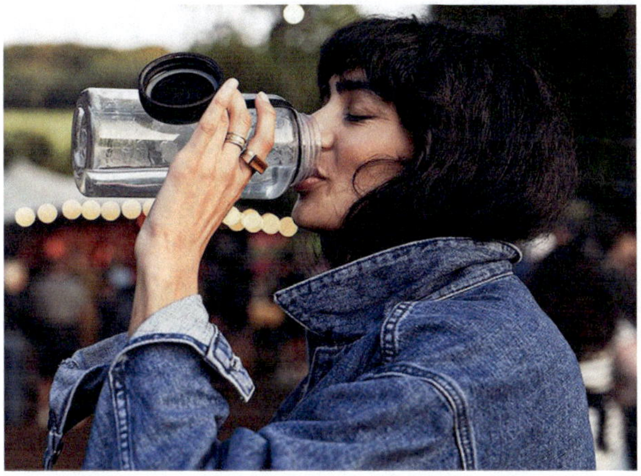

Figure 8.1. Fluid, electrolyte, and blood management is an essential area of clinical practice that addresses the balance and regulation of fluids.

Source: https://media.post.rvohealth.io/wp-content/uploads/sites/3/2024/11/what-electrolytes-GettyImages-2039421115-Thumb.jpg.

Importance in Clinical Settings

Fluid, electrolyte, and blood management play a very important role in clinical settings, particularly in patients with liver disease, where ascites and hepatorenal syndrome (HRS) complications are common. Ascites could be a sign of significant impairment of the liver, which usually results in a sudden reduction of the survival rate of the patient, from 80% to as low as 30% within five years (Scott et al., 2021). Optimal management in these cases involves ongoing assessment of fluid balance, diuretics, dietary adjustment, and, if severe, referral for liver transplantation. Also, to prevent complications such as infection and renal dysfunction, clinicians should adopt an integrated strategy that includes vigilant monitoring of renal function, serum electrolytes, and the patients' overall clinical status. This comprehensive management regime underlines the imperative importance of electrolyte and fluid homeostasis in optimizing patient outcomes in challenging clinical scenarios. Effective fluid management and electrolyte protocols are particularly vital in intensive care units, where rapid patient deterioration is a possibility. For instance, hyponatremia diagnosis and treatment in patients with chronic liver disease are paramount, as it may lead to serious complications such as hepatic encephalopathy and acute kidney injury (Scott et al., 2021). Treatment regimens such as sodium limitation, fluid management, and adequate drug therapy in such patients may have a direct influence on the patients' recovery patterns. Moreover, continued patient education regarding the risks of hyponatremia and importance of follow-up assessment can enable timely intervention and improved overall health outcomes. An integrated approach that tackles these various aspects of fluid and electrolyte regulation is crucial to optimize care in patients with severe health conditions. Lastly, fluid, electrolyte, and blood factor management entails complex interactions requiring a multidisciplinary strategy in clinical practice. The entry of new therapies like those in immunotherapy for hematologic malignancies emphasizes the changing fluid management risks, namely cytokine release syndrome (CRS) and immune effector cell-related neurotoxicity. As popularity increases, uniform grading and evaluation criteria of adverse effects in the context of clinical trials and after product licensure are increasingly necessary. The application of an evidence-based system can facilitate more effective communication among healthcare teams, ensuring better collaborative decision-making. It is through such collaborative efforts that healthcare providers can ensure effective fluid and electrolyte management, thereby improving patient safety and treatment outcomes across various clinical settings (Figure 8.2).

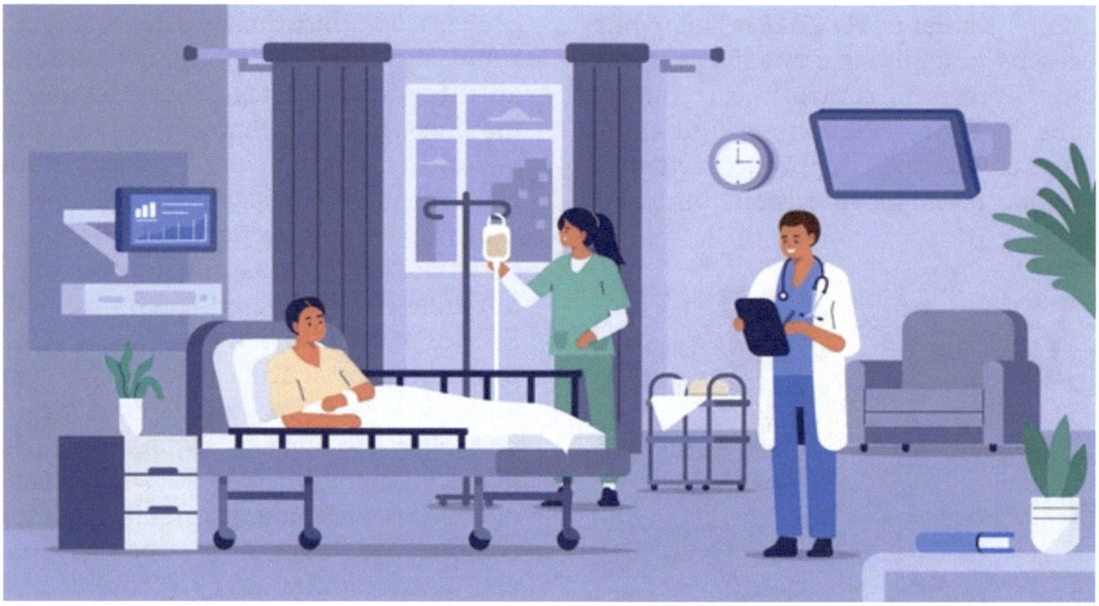

Figure 8.2. Importance in clinical settings.

Source: https://www.shutterstock.com/image-vector/hospitalized-patient-lying-hospital-bed-600nw-1592852215.jpg.

Overview of Key Concepts

Fluid, electrolyte, and blood management are core aspects of medical practice, particularly in acute and critical care. The foundation for effective management rests on knowledge of the body's fluid compartments, which are primarily divided into intracellular and extracellular fluids. All these compartments play a pivotal role in the attainment of homeostasis as well as the physiological processes of cells. Patients, especially those with severe health conditions, may express disturbances in these compartments depending on various factors such as hemorrhage, dehydration, or renal failure. Therefore, clinicians must examine electrolyte imbalance and fluid loss to manage these compartments in line in order to provide therapeutic care according to the patient's individual requirements. Electrolyte balance is equally crucial as electrolytes have a fundamental role in various body functions, such as conduction in nerves, muscle contraction, and acid-base balance. Electrolyte imbalance can have severe consequences, including cardiac arrhythmias and neuromuscular derangements. Hyperkalemia as well as hypokalemia, for instance, have extensive consequences on cardiac function and must be corrected early. With the evolution of healthcare, the incorporation of the latest technologies and methodologies in fluid and electrolyte management has become more highlighted. For example, new technologies in wearable and implantable devices have shown great potential for continuous monitoring of fluids and electrolytes, which may transform clinicians' treatment of patients (Gao et al., 2021). The infusion of blood products, other than the management of fluid and electrolytes, remains a pillar in the management of critical conditions. Blood transfusion is generally in demand for the essential management of anemia, trauma, or surgery in which there is blood loss. However, transfusion must be guided by a comprehensive understanding of the patient's clinical status, identification of the appropriate blood products, and consideration of potential complications. The current guidelines in blood management emphasize the importance of individualized care plans, with the omission of unnecessary transfusions and the prompt provision of blood products to those who need them. Conceiving a comprehensive framework that incorporates these factors enhances patient outcomes and reflects the complex dynamic of fluid, electrolyte, and blood management in practice (Montero et al., 2022).

8.1. Fluid Balance

Learning Outcome

1. Mechanisms of fluid regulation in the body
2. Assessment of fluid status
3. Consequences of fluid imbalance

Fluid balance is a vital physiological process that maintains homeostasis in the body by controlling the intake and output of fluid. Fluid balance is essential for various functions of the body, such as cellular metabolism, thermoregulation, and the removal of waste substances. A change in fluid balance can lead to disorders like dehydration or fluid overload and can significantly affect health outcomes. For instance, surgical patients or those with chronic illness often present changes in fluid dynamics. Caregivers need to be aware of these changes in order to treat patients effectively. Therefore, regular monitoring and measurement of fluid status should be fundamental components of patient care, linking fluid balance to universal principles of fluid, electrolyte, and blood management in clinical practice. In surgery, precise fluid balance is increasingly critical, and inadequate fluid management contributes to more postoperative complications and prolongs recovery times. Before the guidelines of enhanced recovery after surgery (ERAS), precise fluid management is emphasized to prevent complications and ensure rapid recovery (Gustafsson et al., 2018).

Clinicians utilize evidence-based guidelines to determine appropriate fluid volume and composition, preventing under-resuscitation and fluid overload. Evidence suggests that optimal fluid balance is associated with lower rates of surgical complications, reduced hospital stays, and overall improved patient satisfaction. In addition, taking into account individual patient factors, such as existing disease and current treatment protocols, enables personalized fluid management strategies responding to the diverse clinical needs. Recent evidence has shed light on wide-ranging interactions between fluid balance and immune homeostasis, particularly in infectious disease management, such as COVID-19. The pathophysiologic process of SARS-CoV-2 involves complex immune responses that are regulated by a patient's fluid status, exemplifying the close relationship between fluid balance and immunity (Tay et al., 2020). Fluid-overloaded patients, for example, can develop hyperinflammatory reactions, which might lead to organ dysfunction. Therefore, fluid balance control under such conditions not only meets short-term physiological needs but is also key to modulating immune function and overall disease progression. This integrated approach warrants the application of multi-metric approaches to fluid, electrolyte, and blood management so that clinicians are best placed to enhance patient outcomes in critical care scenarios (Figure 8.3).

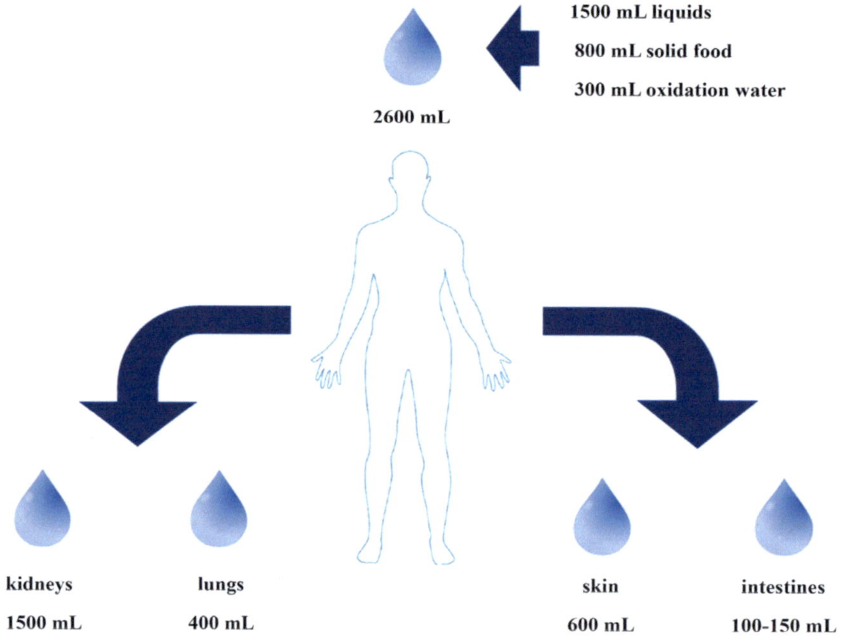

Figure 8.3. Fluid balance is a critical physiological process.

Source: https://www.researchgate.net/publication/337133480/figure/fig3/AS:11431281213118934@1702976900158/Fluid-balance-35-This-figure-shows-the-sites-involved-in-fluid-loss.tif.

8.1.1. Mechanisms of Fluid Regulation in the Body

Regulation of body fluids is a sophisticated process that is primarily managed by the interplay of multiple hormonal and neural mechanisms. The kidneys are the master regulatory organs that regulate water and electrolyte retention or excretion in response to the body's homeostatic needs. This is predominantly mediated by hormones such as antidiuretic hormone (ADH) and aldosterone, which regulate the reabsorption of water and sodium, respectively. As the body changes fluid balance—deprivation or excess—the hypothalamus perceives these changes and triggers the release of ADH to enhance water retention, thereby balancing osmotic levels. It is crucial to understand these processes to be able to manage blood and electrolytes effectively, especially in clinical practice, when fluid imbalance leads to complications that can be harmful. Still another essential aspect of fluid homeostasis is the role of baroreceptors, which are specialized sensory receptors of the cardiovascular system. Baroreceptors respond to changes in arterial pressure and volume and send signals to the central nervous system to adjust fluid balance accordingly. When blood volume decreases, as in hemorrhage, baroreceptors trigger adaptive mechanisms such as increased heart rate, vasoconstriction, and renal sodium retention. This multi-dimensional response complements evidence from Skylab research, which highlights difficulties in atypical fluid-electrolyte regulation under microgravity conditions. These investigations highlight the necessity of considering fluid regulation not only on Earth but also under atypical physiological stressors, thereby validating the relevance of effective fluid management procedures across diverse environments (Leonard, 2025a, b). Besides, the coupling of these regulatory processes with the lymphatic system also points towards the complexity of body fluid management. The lymphatic system plays a pivotal role in interstitial fluid homeostasis and the return of excess fluid into the circulatory system.

Through a network of vessels and nodes, the system facilitates the elimination of pathogens and excess proteins, which are essential in preventing edema and keeping fluid distribution in equilibrium. Involvement between the circulatory and lymphatic systems also becomes highly relevant in disease states, where dysregulation can lead to fluid buildup or dehydration. As explained in recent studies, such as system studies during Skylab flights, a deep understanding of these mechanisms is essential for further refining fluid and electrolyte management protocols, particularly in clinical medicine and spaceflight medicine (Leonard, 2025a, b).

8.1.2. Assessment of Fluid Status

Accurate estimation of fluid status is crucial for managing fluid, electrolyte, and blood balance, especially in at-risk populations such as critically ill neonates. The multifaceted process of managing fluid requires continuous measurement of total fluid intake and output, along with laboratory findings, to avoid errors. Fluid balance documentation is essential, as it directly affects intensive care unit patient outcomes. The issue in clinical practice at this point is the significant quantity of blood required for analysis, which can lead to increased red blood cell transfusion requirement. This question highlights the need for improved assessment methods that cause less harm while preserving precision in fluid status measurements (Milanovic et al., 2013). Such strategies are vital for maximizing fluid management recommendations, thereby improving patient care in high-acuity environments. Fluid status assessment is not limited to neonatal environments but extends to numerous clinical conditions, such as infectious diseases, where fluid imbalance can exacerbate patient conditions. When dealing with infectious enteritis in juvenile and neonatal ruminants, diarrhea leads to significant fluid and electrolyte loss.

Management of such conditions entails careful evaluation of fluid status to guide supportive care, including rehydration of infected animals. Pathogen-targeted interventions are equally important but are complemented by sound fluid management to stabilize the patient's status accordingly. Timeliness and precision in the assessment can minimize the risk of complications such as endotoxemia and sepsis, thereby improving recovery outcomes (Chigerwe et al., 2018). This comprehensive approach identifies the broader consequences of fluid status measurement in various healthcare scenarios. The development of technologies and techniques for fluid status measurement has revolutionized fluid management in clinical practice, improving accuracy. Techniques such as bioelectrical impedance analysis and ultrasound can offer real-time data about the patient's fluid compartments and allow more advanced interventions than earlier. These developments not only provide immediate clinical benefits but also guide subsequent research focusing on optimizing fluid management techniques. As the healthcare industry continues to evolve, the use of technology for fluid status monitoring will be essential in offsetting the dynamics of changing patient states and diverse clinical presentations. The stress on personalized approaches to fluid management goes to validate the importance of accurate measurements in allowing maximum patient advantages in a wide variety of clinical settings, ensuring that electrolyte and fluid balance are at all times preserved (Figure 8.4).

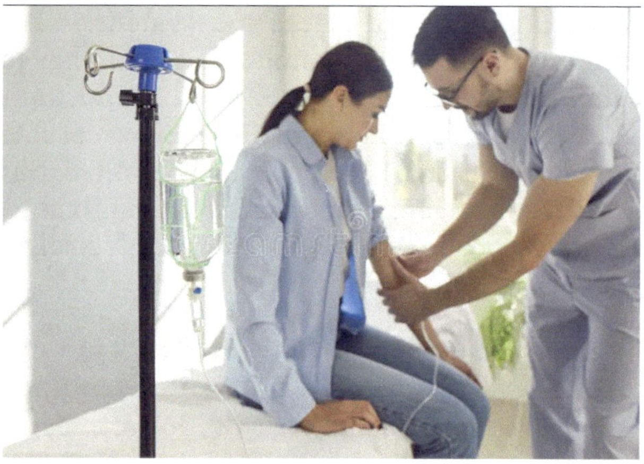

Figure 8.4. Assessment of fluid status in anesthesia.

Source: https://thumbs.dreamstime.com/b/nurse-setting-up-iv-line-patient-close-glass-drip-bottle-stand-hospital-ward-male-doctor-inserting-needle-woman-s-340197607.jpg.

8.1.3. Consequences of Fluid Imbalance

Fluid imbalance can produce profound and multifaceted consequences for various physiological systems in the human body. Excess fluid, or fluid overload, leads to patients developing hypertension, a situation very prevalent among CKD patients. This rise in blood pressure tends to worsen pre-existing conditions, further making treatment and patient management even more challenging. In CKD patients, the utilization of diuretics has frequently been used as a way to manage hypertensive attacks. But evidence regarding how effective these medications are continues to be conflicting, as they have the ability to actually worsen electrolyte imbalance and change kidney function when not closely monitored. Therefore, fluid imbalance and its management in CKD pose a paradox that health practitioners must tread cautiously through (Jo et al., 2023), underscoring why personalized therapy is critical to addressing these complex interactions. Electrolyte imbalances that come with fluid management are another essential domain of patient handling. Fluid imbalance may disrupt the homeostatic control of vital electrolytes such as sodium, potassium, and calcium, leading to lethal complications. For instance, hypernatremia or increased levels of sodium are produced by dehydration. In contrast, hyponatremia or decreased sodium levels are produced by excessive fluid accumulation and may lead to neurological manifestations and cardiovascular stress. Clinical settings need to monitor electrolytes closely because deficiencies and excesses both amplify the effectiveness of fluid management measures. The protocols outlined in evidence-based clinical guidelines point towards a conservative yet assertive approach to fluid and electrolyte balance management, where clinical staff are urged to incorporate best evidence-based practice while applying clinical judgment to assess each patient's case and requirements (Kirchhof et al., 2016).

Furthermore, fluid imbalance and blood management interactions cannot be overlooked, as any alteration in circulating blood volume is directly proportional to hemodynamic stability. Severe fluid shifts, either due to dehydration or fluid overload, in the patient can result in compromised tissue oxygenation, causing numerous effects throughout the system. Such a scenario is commonplace in patients undergoing longer medical procedures or with trauma, in which aggressive fluid resuscitation is important to re-establish hemostasis. Adept blood volume management, combined with close monitoring of electrolytes, becomes imperative to prevent sequelae such as shock or organ failure. For that reason, clinicians are not only tasked with correcting fluid imbalance but also with assessing the degree of its impact on patient outcomes. A sound understanding of these interdependencies is the cornerstone of fluid, electrolyte, and blood management in clinical practice (Jo et al., 2023) (Figure 8.5).

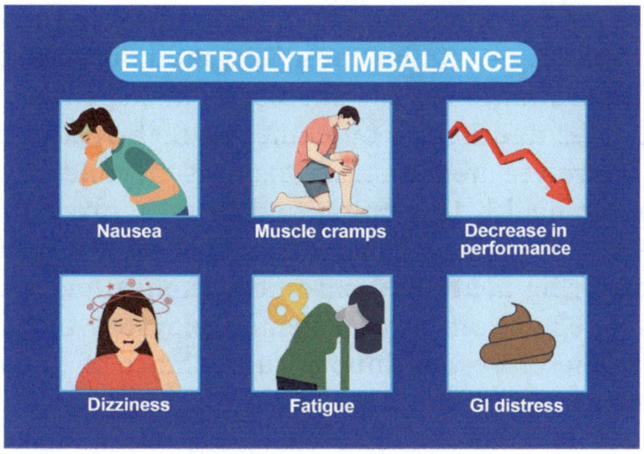

Figure 8.5. Consequences of fluid imbalance.

Source: https://www.sparshdiagnostica.com/wp-content/uploads/2025/02/Electrolyte-Imbalance.jpeg.

Test Your Knowledge

1. What physiological mechanisms, including hormonal and renal processes, help maintain fluid balance in the body?
2. How do the kidneys, cardiovascular system, and osmoreceptors interact to regulate body fluids under normal and stressed conditions?

8.2. Electrolyte Homeostasis

Learning Outcome

1. Key electrolytes and their functions
2. Causes and effects of electrolyte imbalances
3. Monitoring and management strategies

Electrolyte homeostasis is a vital part of physiological balance that supports numerous processes throughout the body, from muscle contraction to neural transmission. Maintenance of appropriate electrolyte levels, such as sodium, potassium, calcium, and chloride, is required for optimal cellular function and overall metabolic processes. Derangements in the maintenance of these levels may occur due to dietary deficiency, endocrine imbalances, or pathologic states involving fluid balance. Proper management of fluid and electrolyte balance is essential in surgeries because inefficient control can lead to severe complications, influencing postoperative recovery and increasing morbidity and mortality. Mechanisms of hormonal regulation, particularly endocrine-mediated pathways, are involved in electrolyte regulation, underscoring the importance of diagnosing and treating endocrine diseases, as documented in the literature, to ensure proper patient outcomes during and following surgery (Rizwan, 2025). In the clinical environment, electrolyte imbalance can occur in numerous ways, particularly among vulnerable groups such as preterm infants. For example, ELBW babies are likely to have an electrolyte imbalance alongside other conditions such as respiratory distress syndrome and anemia. Management of such infants involves addressing their conditions holistically, including observation and intervention procedures to correct electrolyte concentrations, maintain thermoregulation, and restore fluid balance.

Martial arts, like maintenance fluids, nutritional support, and ongoing vital observation, are essential in stabilizing infants and preventing complications. This method provides a rich understanding of the role of interdisciplinary coordination in the successful management of electrolyte homeostasis, thereby improving survival rates and health outcomes in high-risk patient groups (Barawa et al., 2025). The relevance of electrolyte homeostasis extends beyond present-day clinical practice, highlighting its significance for health in general and disease prevention at all stages of the life cycle. Diseases such as heart failure and renal disease in adults have a fundamental effect on electrolyte regulation, endangering acute and chronic complications. For instance, cardiovascular function relies on potassium regulation; hyperkalemia (elevated blood potassium) will result in life-threatening arrhythmias. Therefore, continuous surveillance of electrolytes is imperative across diverse healthcare settings, from emergency departments to routine medical consultations. Bringing advanced monitoring technologies and evidence-based algorithms to the bedside can help ensure the timely identification of imbalances, enhancing patient experience. Maintaining and achieving electrolyte homeostasis is therefore not only imperative for short-term clinical outcomes but also vital to long-term health care management in fluid and blood management systems (Figure 8.6).

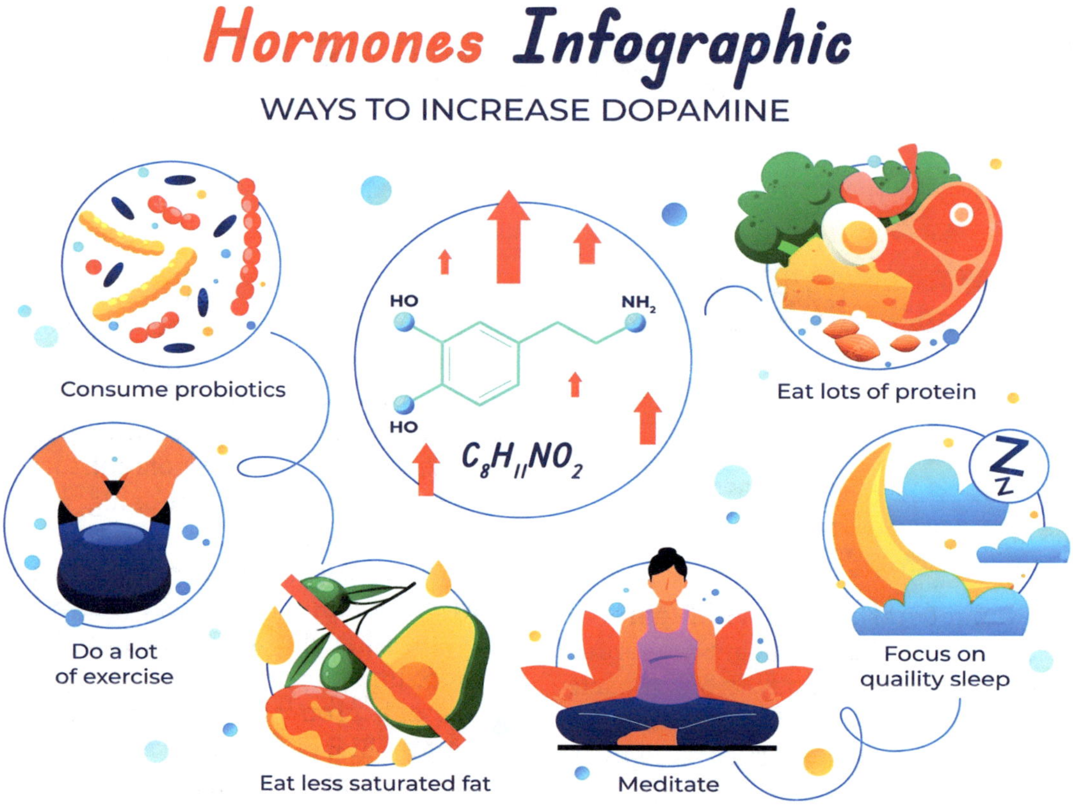

Figure 8.6. Electrolyte homeostasis is a critical aspect of physiological balance.

Source: https://img.freepik.com/free-vector/gradient-hormones-infographic-design_52683-151043.jpg?semt=ais_hybrid&w=740.

8.2.1. Key Electrolytes and Their Functions

Electrolytes play a crucial role in the human body's homeostasis, specifically fluid and blood regulation. Sodium, potassium, calcium, magnesium, and chloride are critical electrolytes involved in various physiological processes, such as nerve transmission, muscle contraction, and fluid balance. Sodium, the most prevalent extracellular cation, plays an essential role in blood volume and pressure maintenance and nerve impulse transmission. In contrast, the chief intracellular cation, potassium, holds a central position in maintaining cardiac function and muscle contraction. The relationship between the two electrolytes underscores the need for efficient monitoring and management, especially in patients with conditions such as ascites and liver disease, where electrolyte balance contributes to the underlying conditions and affects treatment strategies (Scott et al., 2021). Calcium and magnesium have vital but distinct roles in human physiology, both serving significant functions within enzymatic processes and muscle contractions. Calcium is needed for blood clotting and the functioning of numerous cellular processes, as well as serving as a signaling molecule within nerve impulses. Magnesium, on the other hand, is needed for over 300 enzymatic reactions, including those involved in energy generation and protein synthesis. Either of these electrolytes lacking can lead to serious health complications, ranging from muscle cramps, heart troubles, to impaired neurological function. Due to their interconnected roles in multiple biological processes, maintaining optimal levels of calcium and magnesium at any given time is important, particularly in fluid and blood therapy, where the patient's levels may vary depending on the disease or treatment (Gustafsson et al., 2018). Chloride, often not considered among the most crucial electrolytes, plays an equally critical role in fluid balance and acid-base homeostasis. As the principal extracellular anion, chloride maintains osmotic pressure and cell hydration. Chloride is involved in the production of stomach hydrochloric acid, an essential component of digestion, and actively participates in the regulation of pH levels within the body. Disbalances in chloride levels can lead to respiratory alkalosis or metabolic imbalances, potentially complicating management in patients during fluid and electrolyte treatment. Thus, adequate knowledge of significant electrolytes and their functions is required for proper management in clinical practice, particularly in patients with complicated fluid, electrolyte, and blood conditions (Scott et al., 2021).

8.2.2. Causes and Effects of Electrolyte Imbalances

Electrolyte imbalances can be caused by a wide range of factors, significantly impacting people's health. One of the causes is inadequate intake of sodium, potassium, calcium, and magnesium. The conditions are compounded by numerous diseases, including renal disease, in which the kidneys are unable to maintain electrolyte balance. Moreover, acute loss of water through vomiting, diarrhea, or perspiration depletes vital electrolytes, creating a cycle that misrepresents physiological equilibrium. appreciate these root causes, since they struggle to maintain electrolyte levels within baseline limits and consequently prevent complications arising from imbalances. The interaction of these factors underscores the need for an integrated approach to fluid and electrolyte management, particularly in high-risk populations, such as the elderly and those with chronic disease (Alexander et al., 2022). The effects of electrolyte imbalance may be acute or chronic and are likely to manifest in extreme clinical syndromes. For instance, hyponatremia, i.e., low sodium, can result in neurological presentations like confusion, seizures, and even coma in severe cases. Similarly, hyperkalemia with elevated potassium can cause lethal cardiac arrhythmias. Such presentations underscore the central role electrolytes play in cell function and homeostasis, and thus, it is crucial to check their levels in clinical practice. Apart from acute effects on health, long-term electrolyte imbalances can cause chronic conditions, such as osteoporosis due to hypocalcemia. This wide-ranging effect demands a thorough understanding of the physiology of the body regarding electrolyte functions and rigorous monitoring protocols, especially in high-risk patients (Halvorsen et al., 2022). Appropriate treatment of electrolyte imbalances relies on timely detection and intervention. Healthcare providers must undergo thorough assessments to arrive at accurate diagnoses, most often using laboratory tests that measure serum electrolyte levels. Treatment methods can include dietary modification, oral supplementation, or more invasive procedures, such as intravenous electrolyte replacement or hemodialysis in severe cases. In the context of an increasing incidence of electrolyte imbalances based on factors like increased medication use, it is essential that patient and provider education on the need for monitoring electrolytes is highlighted. Furthermore, having established routine protocols in place is necessary to enable timely identification and treatment of such imbalances, especially in the acute care setting. Lastly, an active strategy to fluid and electrolyte balance can minimize the risks of imbalances, resulting in better overall health outcomes (Alexander et al., 2022) (Figure 8.7).

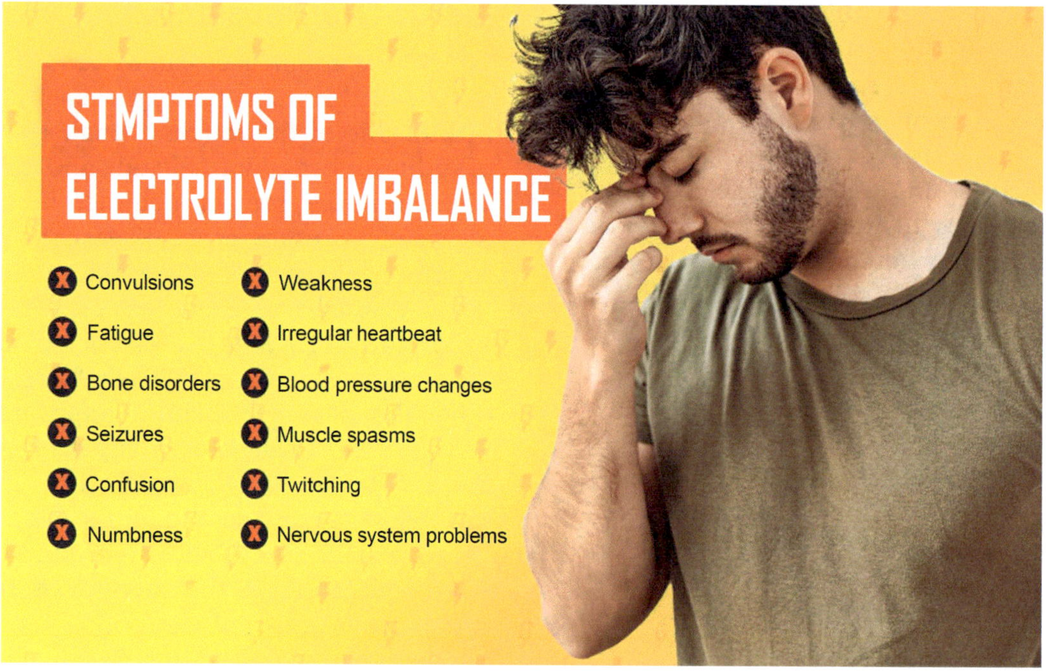

Figure 8.7. Causes and effects of electrolyte imbalances.

Source: https://cdn.shopify.com/s/files/1/0497/3759/7096/files/Symptoms-of-Electrolyte-Imbalance.jpg?v=1665442768.

8.2.3. Monitoring and Management Strategies

Effective monitoring and management strategies are critical building blocks in fluid, electrolyte, and blood management, particularly in patient care. Continuous monitoring of vital signs, fluid intake and output, and laboratory parameters allows physicians to identify departures from the physiological standard that may reflect pathologies. Monitoring is especially vital in patients with acute illness, where timely interventions can have profound effects on outcome. For critically ill patients, technology such as telemetry and intensive laboratory monitoring (e.g., electrolyte levels, blood gases) facilitates rapid identification of complications arising from unbalanced control of fluid and electrolytes. In short, formalized monitoring protocols enhance clinical decision-making, thereby maximizing patient safety and overall quality of care in fluid management. For patients with complex medical issues, individualized management choices become the norm for each case. Individualized options include applying evidence-based practices in the context of patients' clinical status and comorbidities. This includes , determining the optimal type and volume of fluid replacement, and the judicious administration of electrolytes and blood products. The principles of patient-specific therapeutic interventions draw attention to the necessity of thorough comprehension of the pathophysiology in conditions such as diabetes mellitus and COVID-19, where glucose, water, and electrolytes need to be strictly regulated. As indicated in recent studies, optimal management of such patients requires strict monitoring of blood glucose, fluid balance, and electrolytes, stressing the importance of custom-tailored patient care to achieve maximum benefits and eliminate complications (Koliaki et al., 2020; AUTHOR_ID et al., 2020). Finally, integrating newer technology into monitoring processes is transforming fluid, electrolyte, and blood management protocols. Automated monitoring of vital signs and laboratory results provides real-time data, enabling prompt clinical intervention for changes in the patient's condition. The application of decision-support in electronic health records also allows clinicians to easily display historical data and suggestions for fluid and electrolyte therapy. All these technological advances streamline healthcare provision and facilitate the creation of dynamic, adaptive care plans that accommodate changing patient status. The ability to employ innovative monitoring strategies alongside routine assessment procedures is essential for promoting successful management programs and improving patient outcomes in fluid, electrolyte, and blood management practice.

Test Your Knowledge

1. How does the body maintain electrolyte balance, and which organs and hormones are primarily involved in this regulation?
2. What are the consequences of electrolyte imbalances, and how can they affect cellular function and overall health?

8.3. Blood Components

Learning Outcome

1. Overview of blood composition
2. Functions of red blood cells, white blood cells, and platelets
3. Importance of plasma proteins

The intricate composition of blood plays a crucial role in explaining its many roles in the regulation of fluid and electrolytes in the human body. Blood is composed primarily of plasma and cellular components, both of which play crucial physiological roles. Plasma, about 55% of blood composition, is the pale yellowish liquid that carries electrolytes, nutrients, hormones, and waste products. It contains proteins such as albumin, which help maintain oncotic pressure and aid fluid balance between surrounding tissues and blood vessels. The remaining 45% of blood volume is made up of cellular components, including red and white blood cells and platelets. All these cells play important roles in oxygen transport, immunity, and hemostasis, respectively. Knowledge of how these components interact is essential in fluid resuscitation and electrolyte management, particularly in clinical practice, where accurate handling is necessary to achieve homeostasis. Red blood cells (RBCs) cannot be overemphasized in blood components in relation to fluid and electrolyte handling. RBCs are mainly tasked with carrying oxygen from the lungs to the tissues and removing carbon dioxide. This gas exchange is not only crucial in cellular metabolism but also in the body's acid-base balance. An adequate supply of RBCs ensures optimal oxygen delivery, which is critical in surgical procedures involving fluid shifts or volume resuscitation. In hemorrhage or trauma, insufficient RBCs may lead to hypoxia and organ failure.

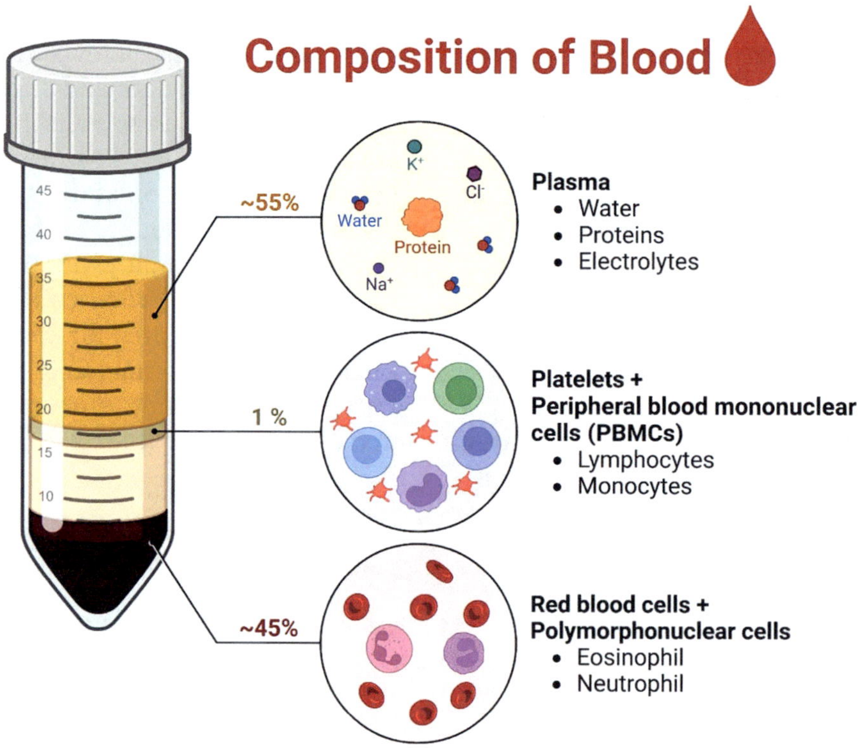

Figure 8.8. The intricate composition of blood.

Source: https://microbenotes.com/wp-content/uploads/2023/04/Composition-of-Blood.jpg.

The monitoring and control of RBC counts, especially in transfusion protocols, represent central aspects of managing both fluid and electrolyte imbalances in patients, highlighting the interrelated nature between blood elements and overall physiological homeostasis. In working with blood elements, the participation of platelets and white cells is also significant, given their roles in hemostasis and immunity. Platelets are responsible for preventing uncontrolled bleeding through clot formation, a process that involves intricate biochemical mechanisms. It is critical to comprehend the process when undertaking procedures that can cause severe blood loss and need immediate regulation of coagulation factors and fluid replacement. On the other hand, white blood cells contribute to immune surveillance and response, defending the organism against invading pathogens and aiding in wound healing. White blood cell count alterations can signal underlying pathology, such as infection or inflammation, which can affect fluid management strategies in general. Recognition of these components' roles allows clinicians to customize interventions—through either blood component transfusions or fluid resuscitation strategies—ultimately enhancing patient outcomes across a range of medical circumstances, thus underlining the importance of holistic knowledge of blood components in fluid, electrolyte, and blood management therapies (Figure 8.8).

8.3.1. Overview of Blood Composition

The structure of human blood is a varied composition necessary for numerous functions of the body, dominated primarily by its cellular and liquid parts. Blood is composed of approximately 45% red blood cells (erythrocytes), white blood cells (leukocytes), and platelets (thrombocytes). Red blood cells have a pivotal role in transporting oxygen, made possible by hemoglobin, while white blood cells are part of the immune system that defends the body against infection. Platelets are also crucial in hemostasis, initiating clot formation to prevent bleeding. The remaining 55% of blood is plasma, a yellowish fluid that serves as the medium for transporting hormones, nutrients, gases, and waste products. Understanding the structure of the blood is a part of managing fluid and electrolyte balance, especially in clinical settings where abnormal blood test results can indicate underlying disease. The significance of blood composition extends beyond simple anatomical information to practical applications in clinical medicine and research, particularly in fields such as space physiology. The findings of study as part of NASAs Life Sciences Research Office, for instance, highlight the importance of blood constituents in physiological response to long-duration space flight. As described in their paper, exercise- and work-related metabolic needs are primarily defined by the composition of the blood, including fluid and electrolyte balance, which is important for maintaining homeostasis under microgravity (Altman et al., 1986). It is thus necessary to measure and regulate blood composition not only for ordinary health needs but also for extraterrestrial conditions in which physical conditions and needs are markedly different from those on Earth. Furthermore, the dynamic nature of blood composition poses challenges and opportunities for fluid and electrolyte regulation. Compensation of adjustments to blood parameters resulting from dehydration or overhydration, for instance, has immediate implications on performance and health outcomes. Studies compiled in NASA's Regulatory Physiology discipline have investigated the interaction between fluid intake, blood volume, and electrolyte levels, providing valuable insight into maximizing physiologic performance (Dickson et al., 2025). This is particularly necessary to ensure control of vulnerable patient groups, such as those with chronic conditions or patients who are having surgery. A sound understanding of blood composition is hence critical for healthcare professionals tasked with creating appropriate treatment regimens that address both immediate and long-term health problems related to fluid balance and blood management.

8.3.2. Functions of Red Blood Cells, White Blood Cells, and Platelets

Red blood cells (RBCs), or erythrocytes, are primarily oxygen carriers in the body, a process that is crucial for cellular and overall body maintenance. Their biconcave shape increases surface area, optimizing oxygen uptake and delivery. One RBC has a cargo of hemoglobin, a protein complex that binds oxygen in the lungs and releases it in tissues to facilitate aerobic respiration. Besides, RBCs transport carbon dioxide to the lungs for exhalation and thus play a role in both modes of gas exchange. Their synthesis, or erythropoiesis, is induced by erythropoietin, which is primarily secreted by the kidneys in response to low oxygen tension. These cells are responsible for maintaining maximum oxygen delivery, particularly under stress conditions such as high altitude or significant blood loss, to emphasize their primary role in fluid, electrolyte, and blood management. In stark contrast, white blood cells (WBCs), or leukocytes, are the body's initial defense mechanisms against infection and other foreign pathogens. They are members of the immune system, and there are several types with distinct functions. For instance, neutrophils immediately mobilize in response to bacterial infections, and lymphocytes, such as B and T cells, play a primary role in adaptive immunity, producing specific antibodies and orchestrating long-term immune responses. The diversified functions of WBCs vary from phagocytosis, in which they engulf pathogens, to the secretion of signal molecules that mobilize other immune cells to the infected site. The constant flow of WBCs through the blood and lymphatic systems enables a rapid response to potential invasion, enhancing the body's ability to maintain homeostasis and defend against disease, thereby integrating their function into the regulation of all fluids and electrolytes in health and during medical interventions (Claassen et al., 2021). Platelets, or thrombocytes, are the most essential components of hemostasis, the physiological body process that prevents unwarranted bleeding when the blood vessels are injured. Small, anucleated cell fragments, platelets are formed from megakaryocytes within the bone marrow and are a critical component of clot development. When there is vascular damage, platelets bind to exposed collagen fibers and aggregate to form a transient plug, a process induced by the release of chemical signals that attract further platelets into the space. The coagulation cascade contributes to this, which eventually converts fibrinogen into fibrin to cement the platelet plug. Therefore, platelet interactions with various clotting factors are essential for modulating bleeding and vascular integrity. By sustaining the delicate coagulation-anticoagulation equilibrium, platelets are important for fluid and electrolyte balance, particularly in the setting of trauma or surgery (Claassen et al., 2021) (Figure 8.9).

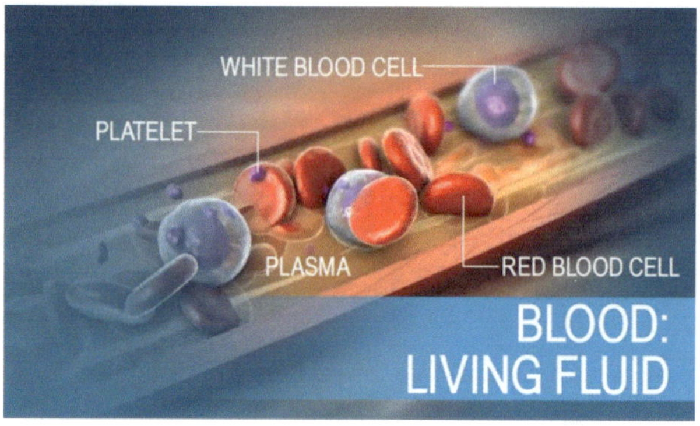

Figure 8.9. Functions of red blood cells, white blood cells, and platelets.

Source: https://www.visiblebody.com/hs-fs/hubfs/Learn_Articles/Circulatory_System/1B-8-Facts-About-Blood.jpg?width=638&height=457&name=1B-8-Facts-About-Blood.jpg.

8.3.3. Importance of Plasma Proteins

The function of plasma proteins in fluid, electrolyte, and blood management cannot be overstated. These proteins, of the vascular space fluid balance. Albumin, the leading plasma protein, is critical in preventing edema by retaining water within the vasculature. This is particularly relevant in the clinical setting, where volume depletion can lead to severe complications. Furthermore, synthesis of plasma proteins is predominantly done in the liver, and this links their levels to liver function as well as overall nutritional status, influencing fluid and electrolyte replacement therapy in patients under treatment for a variety of conditions, such as chronic kidney disease or liver cirrhosis (Alexander et al., 2022). Furthermore, plasma proteins also play a role in the immune system and serve as carriers for other compounds, such as hormones, vitamins, and drugs. Globulins, for instance, play a role in immune reactions, with immunoglobulins having the sole responsibility for defending against infections. In patient fluid management, this is critical because their ability to mobilize immune factors will determine outcomes during recovery. Their drug transport and metabolism cannot be overlooked either; the drug's plasma protein binding will determine the extent and duration of their therapeutic action. The plasma protein concentration thus directly affects a clinician's treatment plan for fluid and electrolyte replacement, as plasma protein-pharmacokinetic interaction becomes more significant during treatment (Percie et al., 2020). Finally, measurement and monitoring of plasma protein levels are essential indicators of health and recovery in fluid and electrolyte management therapy. Hypoproteinemia is an entity that can predispose patients to fluid imbalance and is usually an indicator of latent pathophysiologies, necessitating a multiconstituent intervention strategy. Care professionals should recognize plasma protein levels for the purposes of directing transfusion-related interventions, nutrition management, and fluid therapy. Value for the importance of plasma proteins thus serves the patient ultimately by providing fluid management practice that includes not only hydration but also the biochemical milieu in which these are administered (Alexander et al., 2022; Percie et al., 2020) (Figure 8.10).

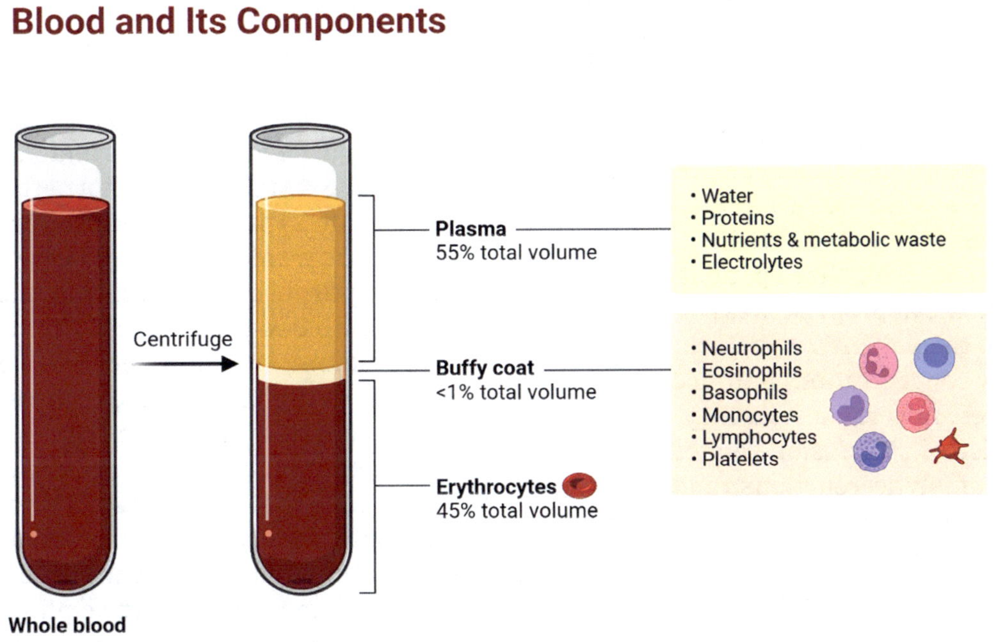

Figure 8.10. The significance of plasma proteins in the context of fluid.

Source: https://endoconsult.b-cdn.net/wp-content/uploads/Components-of-blood.jpg.

Test Your Knowledge

1. What are the major types of plasma proteins, and what are their primary functions in the circulatory system?
2. How do plasma proteins contribute to maintaining blood volume, osmotic pressure, and immune defense?

8.4. Blood Transfusion Practices

Learning Outcome

1. Indications for blood transfusions
2. Types of blood products and their uses
3. Risks and complications associated with transfusions

Blood transfusion is a key aspect of fluid, electrolyte, and blood management in cases of severe hemorrhage or chronic anemia. Blood transfusions can restore hemodynamic stability and reverse coagulopathy, thereby improving tissue oxygenation. However, the decision to transfuse should be wise, weighing risks and benefits. Current guidelines stress the importance of individualized patient assessment to determine the appropriateness of transfusion according to the patient's overall clinical status, hemoglobin concentration, and accompanying comorbidities. Adverse effects may occur, such as in the guise of transfusion-related acute lung injury or hemolytic reactions, and therefore, rigorous screening for blood group and infectious disease must be performed. Transfusion medicine is subject to continuing education on best practices for health professionals to minimize risks and maximize patient outcomes through holistic fluid and blood management practice (Scott et al., 2021). In transfusion practice, the restrictive transfusion strategy has gained favor following evidence that lower transfusion thresholds can benefit certain groups of patients. Research has indicated that maintaining hemoglobin levels between 7 and 8 g/dL in stable, non-cardiac patients may be as effective as, or even better than, more liberal transfusion strategies. This approach not only reduces the risk of transfusion-borne illness but also preserves the availability of blood products for urgently needed patients, such as trauma or surgical patients. In addition, implementing patient blood management strategies, such as optimizing preoperative hemoglobin levels and intraoperative approaches to prevent blood loss, can effectively reduce transfusion needs. These strategies align with the overall principle of not imposing unwarranted intervention and facilitating enhanced patient safety and recovery (Gustafsson et al., 2018). Moreover, the practice of blood transfusion is influenced by technological developments and policy reforms. Innovative transfusion alternatives, such as the use of synthetic blood alternatives and autologous transfusions, are being investigated for the purpose of decreasing the danger of allogeneic blood transfusions. New technological advancements in the processing and storage of blood components have also helped ensure improved safety and efficiency in transfusion practice. Regulatory agencies must enforce strict safety measures, ensure traceability, and monitor adverse events to protect patients. These evolving practices and technologies underscore the importance of a multidisciplinary approach in blood management so that clinicians, transfusion services, and patients are effective in communicating with each other. In recognizing the complexity of transfusion practice in relation to fluid, electrolyte, and blood management, healthcare providers can optimize clinical care and improve patient outcomes (Scott et al., 2021) (Figure 8.11).

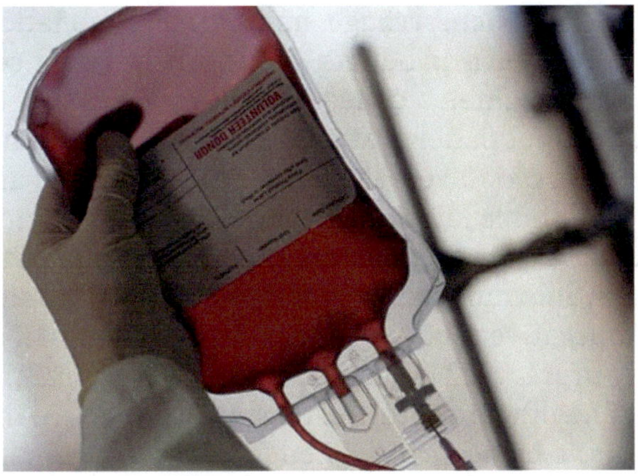

Figure 8.11. The practice of blood transfusion.

Source: https://scx1.b-cdn.net/csz/news/800a/2019/chestbloodtr.jpg.

8.4.1. Indications for Blood Transfusions

The choice to transfuse blood is guided by clearly established clinical indications with consideration of both therapeutic effect and patient safety. In the context of acute medical emergencies, i.e., trauma, hemorrhage, or potentially life-threatening anemia, the urgent correction of blood volume is required in order to stabilize the hemodynamic status of a patient. Transfusions are indicated when hemoglobin levels fall below thresholds, generally 7–8 g/dL in stable patients. This cutoff is not standard, as clinical guidelines recommend that patients with cardiovascular disease require higher levels to prevent complications due to insufficient oxygenation of essential organs (Alexander et al., 2022). The circumstances under which the transfusion is administered tend to determine whether it is needed, especially when immediate intervention can irrevocably affect patient outcomes. Apart from acute conditions, ongoing blood loss, such as that occurring in malignancies or gastrointestinal disease, also necessitates transfusion to improve patients' quality of life and overall functionality. Chronic anemia is typically treated with coordinated care, including transfusion support, with iron supplementation or erythropoiesis-stimulating agents. Blood products, such as packed red blood cells, enhancing oxygen-carrying capacity, thereby alleviating signs of weakness and fatigue, which significantly impact everyday living and quality of life (Halvorsen et al., 2022). Transfusion necessity in such a case transcends mere quantitative considerations; it encompasses a holistic assessment of the patient's clinical condition, underlying disease pathology, and tolerance to prior therapy. In certain groups, such as older patients, transfusion criteria may require particular consideration due to the comorbidities involved and susceptibility to adverse reactions. Transfusions in elderly patients must be carefully decided, remembering that conservatism can often lead to better outcomes without compromising safety. For example, the presence of co-existing underlying diseases, such as chronic cardiac conditions, may require a specialized transfusion strategy to balance the benefits of higher hemoglobin levels against potential risks, including fluid overload or transfusion complications. There must be a proper risk-benefit assessment, so transfusion indications are not just medically indicated but also in agreement with the patients' entire treatment strategies and preferences, thereby fostering the complete care of blood management (Alexander et al., 2022).

8.4.2. Types of Blood Products and Their Uses

In the management of fluids, electrolytes, and blood, understanding various blood products and their applications is necessary for good patient care. Blood products may be categorized into components such as whole blood, red blood cells (RBCs), platelets, plasma, and cryoprecipitate with defined functions in hemostasis, oxygen transport, and volume replacement. Whole blood, though utilized less frequently now, is generally reserved for specific situations such as massive transfusion. Transfusions of red blood cells, however, are central to the treatment of anemia and acute hemorrhage, improving oxygenation and perfusion in hypovolemic individuals. Selective use of such products significantly enhances patient outcomes, particularly in surgery and critical care. Platelet concentrates are required to manage thrombocytopenia and coagulopathy, conditions that put patients at excessive risk of bleeding. Platelets assist in clotting by aggregating at sites of injury in blood vessels. Platelet transfusions are ordered by medical guidelines in platelet counts below acceptable levels, such as before an operation or during chemotherapy. Platelet product use should be a compromise among cost, availability, and clinical need, often requiring close monitoring to prevent transfusion-associated complications. Effective platelet management significantly affects postoperative recovery and minimizes the risk of adverse thrombotic reactions. This targeted use not only preserves hemostasis but also supports the overall objectives of blood management across a range of healthcare settings. Plasma products, in the form of fresh frozen plasma (FFP) and cryoprecipitate, are a critical component of the management of patients with coagulopathy or who require immediate correction of coagulation factors. FFP is applied in instances of massive transfusion, liver disease, or some coagulopathies due to the presence of numerous coagulation factors required for hemostasis. Conversely, cryoprecipitate, a product rich in fibrinogen and factor VIII, is particularly beneficial for the management of conditions such as disseminated intravascular coagulation or hypofibrinogenemia. The prudent use of plasma products is employed to reverse coagulation profiles in critically ill patients, increase survival, and reduce morbidity rates due to bleeding disorders. In the context of the unfolding paradigm in blood management, continuous development of strategies for applying these blood products remains paramount to enhancing clinical outcomes (Daniel et al., 2018; Liang et al., 2020) (Figure 8.12).

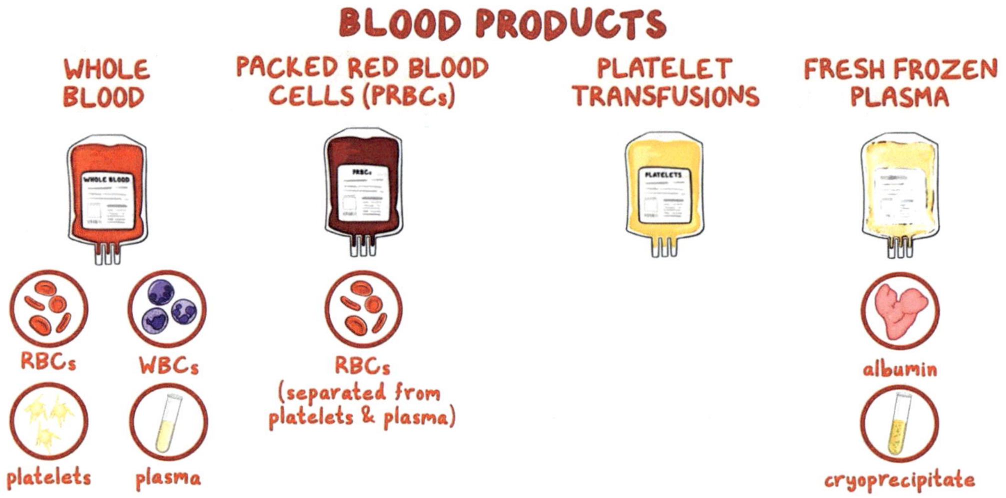

Figure 8.12. Types of blood products and their uses.

Source: https://d16qt3wv6xm098.cloudfront.net/aF4HuG8-Qb_QHZrihh590Bf5QCqTdC4s/_.jpg.

8.4.3. Risks and Complications Associated with Transfusions

The practice of transfusion, while frequently lifesaving, likewise has risks and complications associated with its application, which can have a determinative effect on patient outcomes. Of the numerous complications that can occur, undoubtedly the most immediate is that of transfusion reaction. These may be either mild febrile reactions or acute, life-threatening reactions such as hemolytic reactions and anaphylaxis. Studies have established that specific patient populations, including patients who have received surgical procedures such as total laparoscopic hysterectomy (TLH), experience a higher percentage of blood transfusions, which translates to increased hospital stays and exorbitant healthcare expenses (Cao et al., 2024). Because transfusion patients can develop additional complications from underlying diseases like anemia or coagulopathy, medical professionals must screen for the need for transfusion as well as the risk factors in an orderly fashion. Fluid overload is another important risk of blood transfusions, particularly in groups with existing cardiovascular disease or chronic renal disease. Under such circumstances, blood product transfusion will exacerbate fluid volume disturbances, leading to complications like pulmonary edema or congestive heart failure. Such fluid overload also complicates the treatment of electrolyte imbalances related to the blood transfusion process because increased transfusion of blood products may result in a swift alteration of serum electrolyte levels. Specifically, the threat of hyperkalemia and other electrolyte imbalances necessitates that medical teams scrupulously monitor these values throughout transfusions, thereby promoting maximum patient safety and continuity of care (Sahil et al., 2024). The unification of fluid management and blood transfusion guidelines highlights the imperative need for an integrated approach to preventing such problems. Last but not least, the role of infection in transfusion complications cannot be overlooked. Despite rigorous screening and blood testing before transfusion donation, there is a risk of transmission of infectious agents, including viruses and bacteria. This is particularly true in high-transfusion-volume settings or in immunocompromised patients, who are at increased risk of infection. Infectious complications also lead to , more extended hospital stay, morbidity, and even mortality, and hence proper selection of the patient for transfusion is essential. Identifying safely transfusable patients at minimal risk is important in fluid, electrolyte, and blood care practices (Cao et al., 2024). In conclusion, understanding and managing the risks involved in blood transfusions enables the healthcare provider to prioritize the patient's safety and enhance overall outcomes.

Test Your Knowledge

1. What are the standard practices and protocols for safe blood transfusion, including blood typing and crossmatching?
2. What are the common risks and complications associated with blood transfusions, and how can they be prevented or managed?

8.5. Fluid Therapy

Learning Outcome

1. Types of intravenous fluids
2. Indications for fluid administration
3. Monitoring and adjusting fluid therapy

Fluid management is a primary treatment for the majority of medical illnesses, particularly in the volume-depleted patient with acute or chronic volume depletion. It refers to deliberate administration of fluids to replace or maintain maximal fluid balance to promote maximal organ perfusion and function. Several types of solutions are provided by health workers, e.g., isotonic, hypertonic, and hypotonic fluids, to play a role in the particular clinical setting. For instance, isotonic solutions like normal saline would usually be given to correct hypovolemia, whereas hypertonic solutions could be used in treating specific conditions like cerebral edema. Fluid therapy becomes more effective with the assistance of sophisticated diagnostic instruments, allowing the clinician to individualize interventions without putting the patient at risk of complications, such as fluid overload or electrolyte disturbances. This conservative treatment is advised in individuals with compromised organ systems or undergoing surgeries that place them at risk of developing fluid-related complications. Augmenting traditional methods with technology such as point-of-care ultrasonography (POCUS) has the potential to enhance fluid status assessment and support fluid administration. By enabling hemodynamic bedside evaluation, POCUS allows clinicians to visualize the inferior vena cava and obtain detailed measurements of central venous pressure, providing feedback on a patient's volume status. It is useful because it enables real-time dynamic observation of vascular function, thereby preventing the potential harmful effects of uncontrolled fluid loading. Recent data indicate that the use of such diagnostic tests will stratify patients effectively by volume status and thus maximize the utility of fluid infusion regimens. The evolving strategies in fluid therapy focus on individualizing care, particularly in illnesses such as congestive heart failure, where fluid management remains crucial for preventing renal injury and morbidity in adulthood, according to the literature (Koratala et al., 2022). Secondly, understanding the pathophysiology of fluid management so that an effective treatment strategy can be developed. The interplay between renal perfusion, central venous pressure, and organ congestion exemplifies the responsiveness of fluid therapy. To illustrate, elevated central venous pressure can lead to diminished renal perfusion in the absence of a therapeutic response to fluid therapy. Conditions such as cirrhosis and heart failure illustrate the tightrope that needs to be walked to achieve fluid status without the complications of clinical issues. More recent information on the treatment of related conditions, such as ascites and hepatorenal syndrome, supports the efficacy of customized fluid therapy and underscores the value of focused intervention in achieving major advances in patient outcomes. Thus, clinical evidence integration and new diagnostic approaches enhance the comprehensive system for the treatment of fluid to adapt with the transformation of fluid, electrolyte, and blood management practice (Scott et al., 2021) (Figure 8.13).

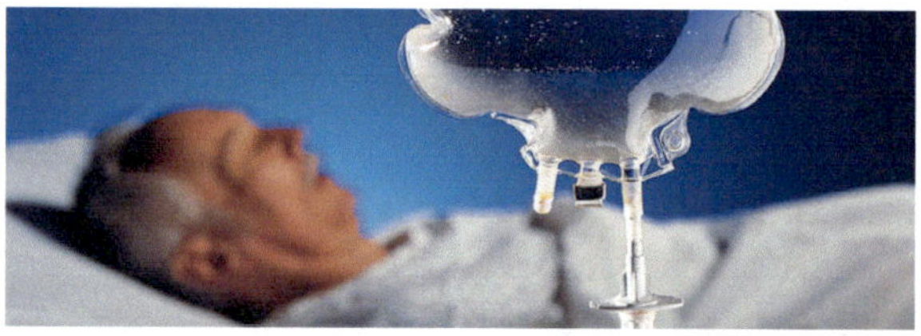

Figure 8.13. Fluid therapy is a critical component of managing various medical conditions.

Source: https://www.baxterprofessional.asia/sites/g/files/ebysai421/files/styles/wide_max/public/IV%20fluids%20landing.png?itok=2Bg1_2JT.

8.5.1. Types of Intravenous Fluids

Fluid and electrolyte management is a critical part of clinical practice, particularly intravenous (IV) fluid therapy. IV fluids are usually categorized into two broad types: crystalloids and colloids. Crystalloids, comprising isotonic solutions like normal saline and lactated Ringer's, are critical in providing hydration and electrolyte balance. They are typically used for daily fluid resuscitation and can quickly shift into the extracellular space. Colloids such as hydroxyethyl starch and albumin, on the other hand, retain bigger molecules within the vascular compartment. This property makes colloids more effective in blood volume expansion, particularly in shock or severe fluid loss. The choice between colloids and crystalloids generally depends on the clinical situation and the patient's specific needs. In addition to crystalloids and colloids, hypertonic solutions constitute a category of intravenous fluids in their own right that are important in some clinical situations. Hypertonic saline is used to correct severe hyponatremia and rapidly normalize sodium levels without jeopardizing osmotic equilibrium. There are hazards involved with the administration of hypertonic solutions, including potential cellular dehydration and the risk of complications such as fluid overload. Therefore, such fluids must be administered cautiously. Additionally, the evidence for many IV fluid categories is still changing, resulting in improved guidelines for their administration. As an example, more recent research highlights the importance of individually oriented administration, whereby fluid types are matched according to the individuals' physiologic needs, thereby maximizing patient outcomes in critical care scenarios. Electrolyte solutions, which form yet another group of intravenous fluids, play a vital role in fluid and electrolyte therapy. Electrolyte solutions, often designed for specific conditions, provide essential ions such as potassium, calcium, and magnesium. Electrolyte solutions are necessary in the treatment of diseases such as hypokalemia or hypocalcemia, where correction is essential to be achieved immediately to re-establish homeostasis. The addition of these fluids into an overall fluid management program underscores the importance of precise electrolyte balance within the clinical environment. Furthermore, the growth in literature describing fluid management underscores evidence-based guidelines as an important consideration for the selection and use of IV fluids. As stressed in the new guidelines of the ERAS Society, proper knowledge of IV fluid types and their use forms the foundation of successful perioperative care and enhanced patient safety in fluid, electrolyte, and blood transfusion management strategies (Gustafsson et al., 2018) (Figure 8.14).

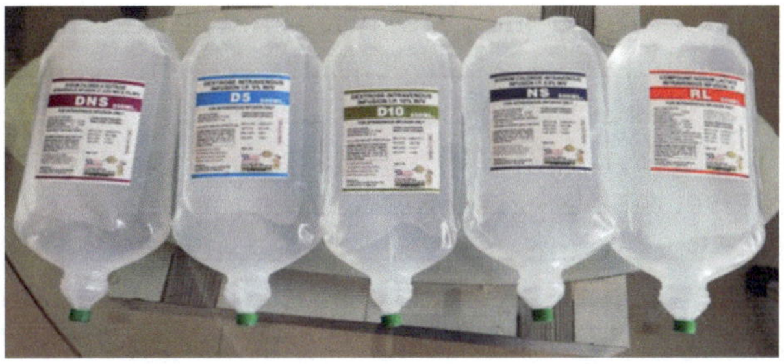

Figure 8.14. Types of intravenous fluids.

Source: https://cpimg.tistatic.com/04553843/b/4/IV-Fluids.jpg.

8.5.2. Indications for Fluid Administration

The contribution of fluid therapy to clinical practice cannot be overstated, as it is fundamental to maintaining homeostasis and supporting patient recovery. The indications for fluid administration largely depend on the clinical situation. For instance, patients with severe fluid loss, say in dehydration or severe hemorrhage, will require immediate fluid resuscitation in a bid to replace vascular volume as well as prevent organ dysfunction. Moreover, disorders with unequal fluid loss, i.e., vomiting, diarrhea, or diuresis, underscore the importance of early fluid replacement. Volumetric response should be carefully monitored through vital signs and urine output, thereby integrating fluid therapy into an overall philosophy of fluid, electrolyte, and blood care in the clinical setting (AUTHOR_ID et al., 2020). Furthermore, fluid management is crucial in surgical procedures and postoperative care. The enhanced recovery after surgery (ERAS) guidelines emphasize the need for physiological fluid management for optimal recovery outcomes. Intraoperative fluid therapy is tailored to prevent hypovolemia, which can occur due to preoperative fasting and intraoperative blood loss. Postoperative fluid management is still crucial in preventing complications such as acute kidney injury and ensuring perfusion. Evidence supporting fluid administration protocols in this case comes from multiple meta-analyses and randomized controlled trials, which establish that meticulous fluid delivery significantly improves recovery trajectories among patients undergoing colorectal surgery (Gustafsson et al., 2018). This once again attests to the critical role fluid management plays in the continuum of patient care. In addition, in critically ill patients, fluid therapy is a vital component of the management of complex clinical syndromes. Sepsis-related shock is a condition that will need aggressive fluid resuscitation to reverse hemodynamic compromise and improve tissue perfusion. In this setting, which type of fluid to administer—colloids or crystalloids—could be determined by clinical parameters such as central venous pressure and serum lactate concentration. The employment of these indicators helps clinicians tailor fluid therapy best, preventing under-resuscitation and fluid overload, which are toxic and lead to inappropriate outcomes such as pulmonary edema. The application of evidence-based guidelines for fluid therapy in critically ill patients is imperative for fluid, electrolyte, and blood management to ensure optimal patient outcomes (AUTHOR_ID et al., 2020) (Figure 8.15).

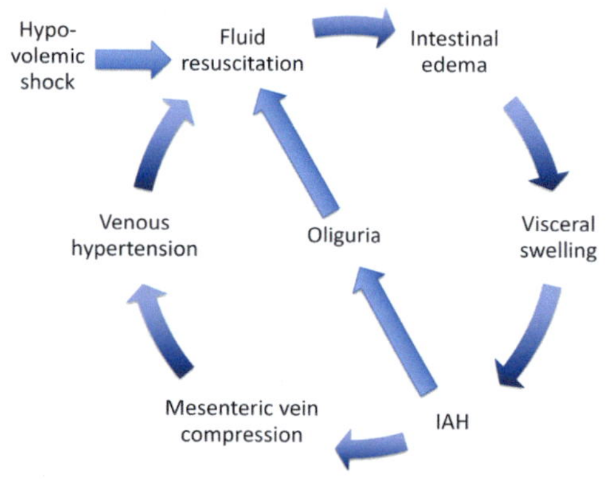

Figure 8.15. Indications for fluid administration.

Source: https://media.springernature.com/lw685/springer-static/image/chp%3A10.1007%2F978-3-031-42205-8_8/MediaObjects/475156_1_En_8_Fig12_HTML.png.

8.5.3. Monitoring and Adjusting Fluid Therapy

Fluid therapy is part of the complete patient care, particularly for surgical and critical care patients. Fluid administration processes are more than mere volume replacement; continuous monitoring of the patient's response to therapy is essential to ensure optimal outcomes. In cases such as pediatric cardiac surgery, methods such as acute normovolemic hemodilution (ANH) are applied to actively manage blood loss without compromising hemodynamic stability. Monitoring indices such as hematocrit, regional cerebral oxygen saturation, and lactate enables clinicians to make immediate fluid therapy interventions. A good example is the use of cerebral oximetry in directing oxygen delivery adequacy decisions when standard transfusion practice is adapted to accommodate patient beliefs or medical requirements (Kang et al., 2013). This situation illustrates the importance of close observation to prevent complications such as impaired tissue perfusion. Fluid therapy approaches should also be modified to address the specific demands arising from electrolyte disturbances or pathologic processes. Pathologic conditions like diabetic ketoacidosis (DKA) illustrate the dynamic interaction between fluid and electrolyte treatment. In treating DKA, it is important to maintain stable glycemic control and prevent sudden electrolyte changes to avert cerebral edema complications. The new two-bag system allows clinicians to address the multi-compartmental needs of children by facilitating rapid isotonic fluid changes, thereby enhancing treatment effectiveness and safety. This system safeguards against the risks of sudden changes in blood glucose levels and reduces the need for acidosis correction to generate better clinical outcomes while ensuring efficient resource use (Patterson et al., 2012). Therefore, an adaptive model of fluid therapy is essential for effectively managing complicated medical conditions. Moreover, the necessity of multidisciplinary collaboration becomes evident in fluid therapy monitoring and control. The integration of nursing, pharmacy, and medical professionals' talents equips each patient's care with a strong foundation, in which all facets of fluid and electrolyte management are harmoniously aligned. With this integration, real-time data such as urine output, vital signs, and laboratory values can be assessed, which are crucial for informing appropriate fluid delivery adjustments. Where blood products are contraindicated by traditional means, as in transfusion-free surgery featured in Kang et al. (2013), multidisciplinary treatments become a forefront in ensuring that patients receive the best possible care without compromising their safety. Such an integrative strategy enhances interhealth team communication and towards patient-centered, high-quality care, ultimately maximizing outcomes in fluid, electrolyte, and blood management.

Test Your Knowledge

1. What are the main indications for fluid therapy, and how do clinicians determine the type and volume of fluids to administer?
2. How does fluid therapy help maintain hemodynamic stability, correct electrolyte imbalances, and support organ function in patients?

8.6. Electrolyte Replacement

Learning Outcome

1. Methods of electrolyte supplementation
2. Guidelines for safe administration
3. Case studies of electrolyte replacement

For electrolyte and blood management as well as fluid in patients, the subtlety of replacing electrolytes is critical to patient management. Electrolytes such as sodium, potassium, calcium, and magnesium are important for several physiological processes, such as cellular function, vascular tone, and neuromuscular impulse transmission. The correct identification of electrolyte abnormalities, such as hyponatremia, is important, especially among patients with pre-existing health conditions such as COVID-19. Recent literature has indicated that hyponatremia in COVID-19 can be caused by various etiologies, and hence, the management strategy for fluid therapy should be tailored. In one such case, hypovolemic hyponatremia required an immediate saline infusion to normalize sodium levels, indicating that appropriate electrolyte repletion methods should be used in acute situations. Ignoring these abnormalities can lead to increased morbidity and mortality, underscoring the importance of prompt, appropriate decision-making in clinical practice (Khan et al., 2020). Correction of electrolyte disorders is more complex than mere correction and requires an in-depth understanding of the pathophysiological background. In difficult situations, during periods of hospital influx during the COVID-19 pandemic, the demand for electrolyte replacement may exceed supply. Medical practitioners are required to use available resources optimally while considering the patient's individual needs. For instance, under emergency conditions, compensatory measures such as reducing the electrolyte dose during supplementation and resorting to conservation techniques become necessary to adequately control the supply of electrolytes and fluids. Such adaptations involve oral replacement therapies or substituting intravenous solutions with oral formulations if feasible. The creation of contingency plans will help ensure that patients receive appropriate care despite impending shortages, ultimately resulting in better patient outcomes and the continuation of effective blood management practices (Burgner et al., 2020). Finally, electrolyte replacement procedures are strongly related to patient monitoring and treatment effectiveness. Ongoing assessment of a patient's clinical status and laboratory results allows for timely modification of electrolyte replacement protocols. Introducing point-of-care testing can enable rapid measurement of electrolyte levels, allowing immediate corrective actions. As an illustration, real-time tracking of potassium levels in patients at risk of hyperkalemia allows clinicians to adjust interventions, such as administering potassium binders or altering diuretic therapy. This shared decision-making process establishes a culture of co-participation between healthcare professionals and patients, making fluid and electrolyte management interventions both effective and efficient. By emphasizing proactive assessment and prompt interventions, patient safety and overall care quality improve, reinforcing the pivotal role of replenishing electrolytes in fluid, electrolyte, and blood management (Khan et al., 2020; Burgner et al., 2020) (Figure 8.16).

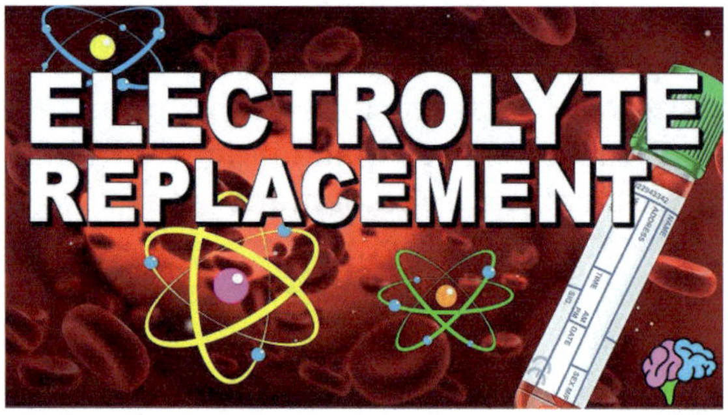

Figure 8.16. The intricacies of electrolyte replacement are critical to patient outcomes.

Source: https://i.ytimg.com/vi/F88DVrHCizQ/hq720.jpg?sqp=-oaymwEhCK4FEIIDSFryq4qpAxMIARUAAAAAGAElAADIQj0AgKJD&rs=AOn4CLDX-0Z5cHs-d3XHdr7pBsWRMOWlbw.

8.6.1. Methods of Electrolyte Supplementation

Electrolyte supplementation is a critical component of fluid, electrolyte, and blood balance regulation, particularly in clinical settings where patients are prone to imbalances. Supplementation can be achieved through numerous methods, ranging from oral rehydration solution to intravenous (IV) therapy. Oral supplementation is typically the first-line treatment, especially for mild-to-moderate deficiency. Supplements that contain sodium, potassium, and glucose can restore intestinal absorption and even replenish depleted electrolytes. Oral supplements may not work for patients with gastrointestinal distress, severe dehydration, or when quick correction of electrolyte imbalance is required, so an IV supplement is a good option too for more serious cases. Intravenous administration of electrolytes provides a quick and controlled method for delivering essential ions directly into the bloodstream. This has some advantages in hospital use, where patients are often monitored for quick shifts in electrolyte balance that may be immediately dangerous to their health. IV fluids may be prepared on an individual patient basis, with the capacity to make fine adjustments to electrolyte composition based on blood test. For instance, hypertonic saline is used to manage hyponatremia, while potassium chloride solutions are used to manage hypokalemia. Physicians need to be careful, however, since wrong concentration or too rapid of infusion may lead to injury, with IV electrolyte administration necessitating a slow and cautious process (Daniel et al., 2018). Beyond more traditional supplementation channels, newer strategies continue to shape best practice in electrolyte management and reassert the importance of staying abreast of current evidence. Enhanced recovery after surgery (ERAS) guidelines, for instance, emphasize multimodal perioperative management and highlight optimizing electrolyte balance as one aspect of recovery (Gustafsson et al., 2018). While traditional methods remain viable, new technologies such as continuous electrolyte monitoring systems are gaining widespread popularity for their ability to predict and correct imbalances before they become difficult to manage. Ultimately, an educated awareness of various supplementation methods enhances the efficacy of fluid and electrolyte management regimens for comprehensive patient care during critical medical interventions and surgeries.

8.6.2. Guidelines for Safe Administration

Administration of fluids, electrolytes, and blood products is a core part of patient care, with strict adherence to established guidelines for safety and efficacy. Safe administration of the components begins with a thorough pre-administration assessment that includes review of the patient's clinical status and past medical history. Clinicians need to establish any endocrine disorders that may interfere with fluid and electrolyte balance, e.g., thyroid disease or adrenal insufficiency. As has been stated in the literature, proper control of these conditions is not only part of metabolic control but also enhances surgical outcomes, especially in anesthetic procedures (Rizwan, 2025). Identification and early management of such comorbidities by clinicians can reduce the risk of complications from fluid overload or electrolyte imbalances. Furthermore, existing guidelines also emphasize the need to monitor patients closely both during and after fluid and blood product transfusions. This includes monitoring of vital signs, fluid responsiveness, and laboratory values such as electrolytes and hematocrit. In trauma treatment, fluid resuscitation must be approached with caution, including interventions like the employment of permissive hypotension for not exacerbating bleeding and coagulopathy. Crystalloid-based resuscitation has been supported by current evidence as the cornerstone. However, it must be in the context of the situation, guided by principles to maintain a minimum blood pressure until hemostasis (Tubert et al., 2024). Continuous re-evaluation of the patient's hemodynamic status is essential, as appropriate compensation of fluid volume and content significantly affects recovery and overall outcomes. Finally, technological advancements in monitoring create new possibilities for the enhancement of secure practice in the administration of fluids and electrolytes. The combination of point-of-care diagnostics and machine learning is able to provide a more precise fluid optimization regimen tailored to the patient's individual needs.

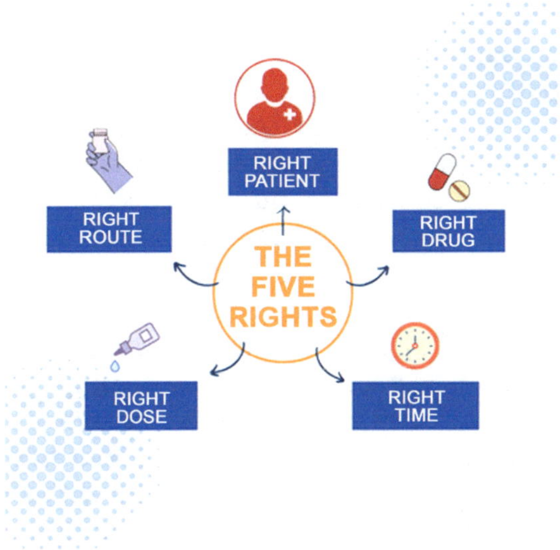

Figure 8.17. Guidelines for safe administration.

Source: https://images.squarespace-cdn.com/content/v1/5d98129f25863e4eb91b5bcd/8f6201dc-ce6e-4f5e-9a1a-18cb8e3c39a7/Five+Rights+of+Medication+Use.png.

These advancements can enable clinicians to address persistent uncertainties through dynamic fluid resuscitation protocols, especially regarding the type and volume of fluids administered. As further studies evolve, there is a need to continue refining guidelines and best practices so fluid management becomes dynamic enough to respond to the evolving paradigm of patient care. By transcending these intricacies, medical practitioners can significantly improve patient safety and outcomes in managing fluid and electrolyte balance (Figure 8.17).

8.6.3. Case Studies of Electrolyte Replacement

The management of diabetic ketoacidosis (DKA) frequently illustrates the central role of electrolyte replacement in optimizing patient outcomes under fluid and blood management treatment. A major component of DKA management is early fluid administration to correct hypovolemia, along with replacement of electrolytes, including potassium. In a study conducted on the management of DKA in patients, potassium phosphate has been found to lead to the quicker resolution of acidosis, which suggests the contribution of electrolyte content to fluid replacement (Loi, 2024). Electrolyte imbalances can further add to the complications, and hence, individualized electrolyte management is critical. The aggressive yet balanced approach to fluid resuscitation not only aids in correcting metabolic derangements but also directly affects patient recovery and clinical outcomes. With analysis of case studies on various fluid regimens in patients with DKA, it becomes clear that the composition of the crystalloid solution can affect recovery pathways. Normal saline (NS) has been the conventional fluid of choice; however, no single fluid type has demonstrated superiority, given the demands of research. The Joint British Diabetes Society and the American Diabetes Association recommend NS with caution for other options, depending on the novelty of clinical outcomes with balanced crystalloids (Loi, 2024). In some cases, the use of balanced solutions seems to improve metabolic parameters more quickly, which calls for careful vigilance to electrolyte composition for effective DKA treatment. Therefore, clinical decisions regarding fluid and electrolyte therapy may substantially impact recovery times and reduce hospitalization. The implications of electrolyte management in DKA extend beyond short-term clinical outcomes to extended patient care. For instance, prolonged hyperchloremia is associated with adverse outcomes such as protracted recovery from acidosis and longer hospital lengths of stay (Müge et al., 2024). This finding underscores the necessity of carefully regulated monitoring of electrolyte levels throughout treatment. By integrating evidence-based electrolyte-replenishment protocols that adjust to individual patients' biochemical markers, providers can enhance patient safety and treatment efficacy. Case series reports of these changes illustrate not only better results but also a greater understanding of the complex interplay between fluid resuscitation and electrolyte replacement. Ultimately, the optimization of DKA patient electrolyte management practices presents a compelling rationale for ongoing research and development of clinical guidelines in fluid, electrolyte, and blood management.

Test Your Knowledge

1. What are the common indications for electrolyte replacement therapy, and how is the choice of electrolyte determined?
2. How can improper electrolyte replacement lead to complications, and what monitoring is necessary to ensure safe correction?

SUMMARY

Adequate fluid, electrolyte, and blood management are the mainstay of clinical practice, particularly among patients with hypovolemic shock. Balanced fluids such as bicarbonated Ringer's solution (BRS) have emerged as an integral part of resuscitation plans. Literature has indicated that BRS not only corrects metabolic acidosis more effectively than standard saline but also provides essential electrolyte replenishment. This improves organ function and tissue perfusion, which is essential in the care of critically injured patients. According to the evidence, BRS should become the priority in clinical practice, especially in emergency and trauma departments, where adequate fluid resuscitation within time will improve patient outcomes and reduce morbidity associated with shock (Wang et al., 2021). Additionally, with advances in healthcare procedures, attention to maintaining acid-base balance through appropriate fluid selection is increasingly important. Evidence has established that BRS infusion leads to significant improvements in base excess and bicarbonate levels and thus demonstrates its superiority compared to the use of normal isotonic fluids. The differential analysis of BRS and other crystalloids calls for health practitioners to evaluate current fluid management practices. Such evidence-based practices are one way to proceed with patient care in critical settings and reflect a step towards administering fluids more in line with physiological states, thereby enhancing recovery outcomes (Wang et al., 2021). Also, the introduction of innovative practices, such as in fluid, electrolyte, and blood management, reflects a broader trend toward personalized medicine. Understanding patient-specific variables, i.e., current health status and resuscitation response, can enable personalized approaches to fluid therapy. Hence, clinical trials and research remain crucial in establishing uniform treatment protocols. With BRS leading the way in novel resuscitation approaches, the healthcare community must also seek novel methods to optimize care while keeping patient safety top of mind. These efforts not only address short-term clinical demands but also provide windows to improved long-term outcomes in the treatment of patients with fluid resuscitation, encouraging an integrative approach in trauma and critical care management.

Knowledge of the physiological principles is required in the management of fluid, electrolyte, and blood parameters. Such processes of management are crucial in avoiding complications of conditions like liver cirrhosis and associated diseases. The subtle balance between fluids and electrolytes is usually disrupted by hepatic decompensation, which typically results in complications in the form of ascites and hepatorenal syndrome (HRS). For instance, ascites formation is associated with declining survival as patients become vulnerable to other infection- and electrolyte imbalance-related hazards. Thus, early identification and management of such complications through appropriate assessments and interventions are necessary in practice (Alexander et al., 2022). These interventions not only alleviate patient distress but also optimize the utilization of resources in healthcare systems. Diuretics and sodium dietary restriction are the most important components of ascites treatment for liver disease. Diuretic therapy should be monitored closely, along with renal function and electrolytes, to prevent complications such as dehydration and electrolyte imbalances. In diuretic use, titration of therapy is done slowly, and dose adjustments are made based on patient response to prevent complications such as muscle cramping and hypotension. Moreover, patient education on sodium intake is important, as adherence to dietary restrictions has a substantial effect on treatment success (Scott et al., 2021). Engagement in the multidisciplinary approach, i.e., consultation with dietitians and frequent follow-up, further enhances patient management, including fluid and electrolyte management. Regular follow-up can facilitate the assurance that treatment regimens of patients are modified according to fluctuating patients' health status. Ultimately, the interchange among fluid management strategies and outcomes in the patient is at the heart of health care. The application of evidence-based recommendations, as established by the American Association for the Study of Liver Diseases, highlights the necessity of comprehensive management guidelines that treat not only pharmacologic management but lifestyle interventions and patient education as well. Adherence to adequate fluid, electrolyte, and blood management may lead to higher survival rates for high-risk patients with chronic diseases. New research and clinical trials will continue to revise these guidelines so that practitioners remain abreast of the latest advancements in the care of disorders related to fluid and electrolyte imbalances (Scott et al., 2021; Alexander et al., 2022). This ongoing evolution underscores the importance of a collaborative, patient-centered approach in improving overall care quality within the field.

KEY TERMS FROM THIS CHAPTER

- Acute kidney injury
- Arrhythmias
- Blood transfusions
- Dysregulation
- Fluid
- Fluid homeostasis
- Antidiuretic hormone (ADH)
- Blood management
- Cytokine release syndrome (CRS)
- Electrolyte
- Fluid balance
- Hepatorenal syndrome (HRS)

CRITICAL THINKING QUESTIONS

1. **Which of the following is a common consequence of hypothermia during the post-operative period?**
   a. Prolonged recovery
   b. Hyperglycemia
   c. Dehydration
   d. Increased appetite
2. **Which complication is characterized by the accumulation of fluid in the chest cavity?**
   a. Pleural effusion
   b. Ascites
   c. Hemothorax
   d. Hydrothorax
3. **What is a potential post-operative complication associated with the administration of excessive intravenous fluids?**
   a. Fluid overload
   b. Dehydration
   c. Electrolyte disturbances
   d. Hyperglycemia
4. **Which condition refers to a decrease in urine output after surgery?**
   a. Oliguria
   b. Polyuria
   c. Hematuria
   d. Dysuria
5. **What is a common post-operative issue that can occur due to poor pain control?**
   a. Immobility
   b. Hyperthermia
   c. Increased appetite
   d. Electrolyte imbalance

Short Answer Questions

1. Discuss the principles of perioperative fluid management.
2. Describe the pathophysiological changes in fluid and electrolyte balance during major surgery.
3. Compare and contrast crystalloids and colloids in the context of intraoperative fluid therapy.
4. Explain the concept of goal-directed fluid therapy (GDFT) and its benefits during anesthesia.
5. Describe the indications for blood transfusion in the operating room.

Answer to Critical Thinking Questions

1. (a); 2. (a); 3. (a); 4. (a); 5. (a)

REFERENCES

1. Altman, P. L., & Fisher, K. D. (1986). Research opportunities in nutrition and metabolism in space. https://core.ac.uk/download/pdf/10458014.pdf (accessed on 28th June 2025).
2. Armstrong, B. (2020). Haematology. *ISBT Science Series, 15*(S1), 46–53. https://doi.org/10.1111/voxs.12588Barawa, W., Lewa, J. D., & Makazi, P. K. (2025). Extremely low birth weight in preterm newborn: A case report. *International Journal of Health, Medicine and Nursing Practice.* https://www.semanticscholar.org/paper/ecf2abd3077af0d7ffe716ac20e5e660aee71515 (accessed on 28th June 2025).
3. Biggins, S. W., Angeli, P., García-Tsao, G., Ginès, P., Ling, S. C., Nadim, M. K., Wong, F., et al. (2021). Diagnosis, evaluation, and management of ascites, spontaneous bacterial peritonitis and hepatorenal syndrome: 2021 practice guidance by the American Association for the Study of Liver Diseases. *Hepatology, 74*, 1014–1048. https://doi.org/10.1002/hep.31884 (accessed on 28th June 2025).
4. Burgner, A., İkizler, T. A., & Dwyer, J. P. (2020). COVID-19 and the inpatient dialysis unit. *Clinical Journal of the American Society of Nephrology, 15*, 720–722. https://doi.org/10.2215/cjn.03750320 (accessed on 28th June 2025).
5. Cao, X., Liu, X., Zhang, X., Zhang, K., Chen, C., Yang, Q., Wang, J., et al. (2024). Risk factors for perioperative blood transfusion in patients undergoing total laparoscopic hysterectomy. *BMC Women's Health, 24.* https://www.semanticscholar.org/paper/9a5235c190931eb6e1f6b31e1b7a564a743984cc (accessed on 28th June 2025).
6. Chigerwe, M., & Heller, M. C. (2018). Diagnosis and treatment of infectious enteritis in neonatal and juvenile ruminants. https://core.ac.uk/download/323068195.pdf (accessed on 28th June 2025).
7. Claassen, J. A. H. R., Thijssen, D. H. J., Panerai, R. B., & Faraci, F. M. (2021). Regulation of cerebral blood flow in humans: Physiology and clinical implications of autoregulation. *Physiological Reviews, 101*, 1487–1559. https://doi.org/10.1152/physrev.00022.2020 (accessed on 28th June 2025).
8. Dickson, K. J., Hess, E., Powers, J. V., & Wallace-Robinson, et al. (2025). Publications of the space physiology and countermeasures program, regulatory physiology discipline: 1980–1990. https://core.ac.uk/download/pdf/42811395.pdf (accessed on 28th June 2025).
9. Ding, X., Cheng, Z., & Qian, Q. (2017). Intravenous fluids and acute kidney injury. *Blood Purification, 43*, 163–172. https://doi.org/10.1159/000452702 (accessed on 28th June 2025).
10. Gao, W., & Yu, C. (2021). Wearable and implantable devices for healthcare. *Advanced Healthcare Materials, 10.* https://doi.org/10.1002/adhm.202101548 (accessed on 28th June 2025).
11. Gustafsson, U., Scott, M. J., Hübner, M., Nygren, J., Demartines, N., Francis, N., Rockall, T., et al. (2018). Guidelines for perioperative care in elective colorectal surgery: Enhanced Recovery After Surgery (ERAS®) Society recommendations: 2018. *World Journal of Surgery, 43*, 659–695. https://doi.org/10.1007/s00268-018-4844-y (accessed on 28th June 2025).
12. Halvorsen, S., Mehilli, J., Cassese, S., Hall, T. S., Abdelhamid, M., Barbato, E., De Hert, S., et al. (2022). 2022 ESC Guidelines on cardiovascular assessment and management of patients undergoing non-cardiac surgery. *European Heart Journal, 43*, 3826–3924. https://doi.org/10.1093/eurheartj/ehac270 (accessed on 28th June 2025).

13. Jo, W., Koh, E. S., & Chung, S. (2023). Therapeutic roles of thiazides and loop diuretics in blood pressure control and renal protection against chronic kidney disease. *Clinical Hypertension, 29.* https://doi.org/10.1186/s40885-023-00238-5 (accessed on 28th June 2025).

14. Kang, S. H., Song, I. K., Kang, J., Lee, J., & Kim, J. T. (2013). Anesthetic management for transfusion-free Rastelli's procedure in a pediatric Jehovah's Witness patient. *Korean Journal of Anesthesiology, 65,* S87–S88. https://www.semanticscholar.org/paper/f8611e5e7f3d00dc50b5003f5d74f91542b9b58a (accessed on 28th June 2025).

15. Khan, A. A., Ata, F., Munir, W., & Yousaf, Z. (2020). Fluid replacement versus fluid restriction in COVID-19 associated hyponatremia. *Cureus.* https://doi.org/10.7759/cureus.9059 (accessed on 28th June 2025).

16. Kirchhof, P., Benussi, S., Kotecha, D., Ahlsson, A., Atar, D., Casadei, B., Castellá, M., et al. (2016). 2016 ESC Guidelines for the management of atrial fibrillation developed in collaboration with EACTS. *European Heart Journal, 37,* 2893–2962. https://doi.org/10.1093/eurheartj/ehw210 (accessed on 28th June 2025).

17. Koliaki, C., Tentolouris, A., Eleftheriadou, I., Melidonis, A., Dimitriadis, G., & Tentolouris, N. (2020). Clinical management of diabetes mellitus in the era of COVID-19: Practical issues, peculiarities and concerns. *Journal of Clinical Medicine, 9,* 2288–2288. https://doi.org/10.3390/jcm9072288 (accessed on 28th June 2025).

18. Koratala, A., & Reisinger, N. (2022). Venous excess Doppler ultrasound for the nephrologist: Pearls and pitfalls. *Kidney Medicine, 4,* 100482–100482. https://doi.org/10.1016/j.xkme.2022.100482 (accessed on 28th June 2025).

19. Lee, D. W., Santomasso, B., Locke, F. L., Ghobadi, A., Turtle, C. J., Brudno, J. N., Maus, M. V., et al. (2018). ASTCT consensus grading for cytokine release syndrome and neurologic toxicity associated with immune effector cells. *Biology of Blood and Marrow Transplantation, 25,* 625–638. https://doi.org/10.1016/j.bbmt.2018.12.758 (accessed on 28th June 2025).

20. Leonard, J. I. (2025a). Description, validation, and modification of the Guyton model for space-flight applications. Part A. Guyton model of circulatory, fluid and electrolyte control. Part B. Modification of the Guyton model for circulatory, fluid and electrolyte control. https://core.ac.uk/download/pdf/42845535.pdf (accessed on 28th June 2025).

21. Leonard, J. I. (2025b). Fluid-electrolyte responses during prolonged space flight: A review and interpretation of significant findings. https://core.ac.uk/download/pdf/42845533.pdf (accessed on 28th June 2025).

22. Liang, H., & Acharya, G. (2020). Novel coronavirus disease (COVID-19) in pregnancy: What clinical recommendations to follow? *Acta Obstetrician Et Gynecological Scandinavica, 99,* 439–442. https://doi.org/10.1111/aogs.13836 (accessed on 28th June 2025).

23. Lyon, A. R., López-Fernández, T., Couch, L. S., Asteggiano, R., Aznar, M. C., Bergler-Klein, J., Boriani, G., et al. (2022). 2022 ESC guidelines on cardio-oncology developed in collaboration with the European Hematology Association (EHA), the European Society for Therapeutic Radiology and Oncology (ESTRO) and the International Cardio-Oncology Society (IC-OS). *European Heart Journal, 43,* 4229–4361. https://doi.org/10.1093/eurheartj/ehac244 (accessed on 28th June 2025).

24. Milanovic, D., & Grošelj-Grenč, M. (2013). Fluid balance in critically ill neonates – ways to improve it. https://core.ac.uk/download/33274565.pdf (accessed on 28th June 2025).

25. Montero-Odasso, M., van der Velde, N., Martin, F. C., Petrović, M., Tan, M. P., Ryg, J., Aguilar-Navarro, S. G., et al. (2022). World guidelines for falls prevention and management for older adults: A global initiative. *Age and Ageing, 51.* https://doi.org/10.1093/ageing/afac205 (accessed on 28th June 2025).

26. Patel, S. M., Venkatesan, V., & Murray, K. J. (2024). Dialysis disequilibrium syndrome with cerebral edema in an adult patient following the initial dialysis session. *Cureus, 16.* https://www.semanticscholar.org/paper/f8d57b0c298d101e542d32affe1d28956dfaaf3e (accessed on 28th June 2025).

27. Patterson, J., Rosenbauer, O., Cinek, A., Neu, A., Schober, E., Parslow, R., Joner, G., et al. (2012). Poster tours. *Pediatric Diabetes, 13.* https://www.semanticscholar.org/paper/e168da338bbc04140a4b77666a5cad897e1beebe (accessed on 28th June 2025).

28. Percie du Sert, N., Ahluwalia, A., Alam, S., Avey, M. T., Baker, M., Browne, W. J., Clark, A., et al. (2020). Reporting animal research: Explanation and elaboration for the ARRIVE guidelines 2.0. *PLOS Biology, 18*, e3000411–e3000411. https://doi.org/10.1371/journal.pbio.3000411 (accessed on 28th June 2025).

29. Rakita, A., Nikolić, N., Mildner, M., Matiasek, J., & Elbe-Bürger, A. (2020). Re-epithelialization and immune cell behavior in an *ex vivo* human skin model. *Scientific Reports, 10.* https://doi.org/10.1038/s41598-019-56847-4 (accessed on 28th June 2025).

30. Rizwan. (2025). Perioperative management of endocrine disorders–practical considerations. *Journal of the Pakistan Medical Association.* https://www.semanticscholar.org/paper/99407d6207cb84d19db2201d1b2b42c7b9117edf (accessed on 28th June 2025).

31. Sam, L. I. (2024). Choice of fluid in the acute management of diabetic ketoacidosis. *Journal of Clinical Review & Case Reports.* https://www.semanticscholar.org/paper/b16011b54d3afea84a6739f5f209b785e146c3a2 (accessed on 28th June 2025).

32. Sezer, M., Karacan, C., Tuygun, N., & Şenel, S. (2024). Evaluation of the effect of fluid and electrolyte therapy on electrolytes and acidosis resolution time in diabetic ketoacidosis. *Turkish Journal of Pediatric Disease.* https://www.semanticscholar.org/paper/580623a7e1062e099da2125e2f3fb09d8b5e428f (accessed on 28th June 2025).

33. Tay, M. Z., Poh, C. M., Rénia, L., MacAry, P. A., & Ng, L. F. P. (2020). The trinity of COVID-19: immunity, inflammation and intervention. *Nature Reviews. Immunology, 20*, 363–374. https://doi.org/10.1038/s41577-020-0311-8 (accessed on 28th June 2025).

34. Tubert, P., Kalimouttou, A., Bouzat, P., David, J. S., & Gauss, T. (2024). Are crystalloid-based fluid expansion strategies still relevant in the first hours of trauma induced hemorrhagic shock? *Critical Care, 28.* https://www.semanticscholar.org/paper/9406dd5bf7728750f917b5679995d230a015753a (accessed on 28th June 2025).

35. Wang, L., Lou, J., Cao, J., Wang, T., Liu, J., & Mi, W. (2021). Bicarbonate Ringer's solution for early resuscitation in hemorrhagic shock rabbits. *Annals of Translational Medicine, 9*, 462–462. https://doi.org/10.21037/atm-21-97 (accessed on 28th June 2025).

36. Wei, P. F. (2020). Diagnosis and treatment protocol for novel coronavirus pneumonia (Trial Version 7). *Chinese Medical Journal, 133*, 1087–1095. https://doi.org/10.1097/cm9.0000000000000819 (accessed on 28th June 2025).

PAIN MANAGEMENT BASICS

9

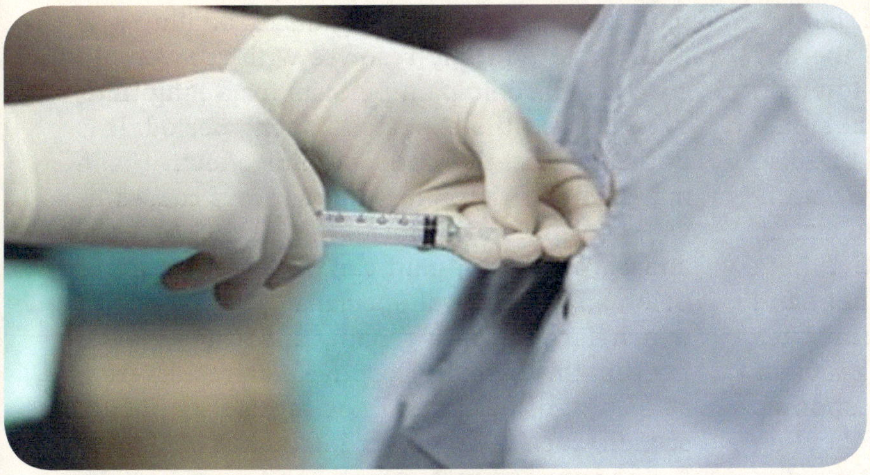

LEARNING OBJECTIVES

After studying this chapter, you will be able to:

1. Understand pain management of anesthesia
2. Focus on pharmacological treatments
3. Discuss the non-pharmacological treatments
4. Focus on role of healthcare professionals
5. Know challenges in pain management
6. Learn about future directions in pain management

Introduction

The first step of pain control is in charge of establishing a successful therapeutic strategy fitted to the patient's individual needs. Pain is a polymorphic phenomenon, both physiological and psychological in nature. It is not just a symptom but a polymorphic experience with emotional, social, and cultural variables. It is thus necessary to have a comprehensive assessment during the initial consultation. Such an assessment may include in-depth patient history, identification of pain description, and evaluation of its impact on activities of daily life. Further, considering pain management options can empower patients, leading to better decisions about their own care. By implementing evidence-based practices, clinicians may design personalized pain management plans that encompass pharmacological, physical, and psychological modalities. Early initiation of collaboration facilitates the establishment of an effective pain management plan, enhancing the patient's quality of life. In the case of pain management, it is imperative to comprehend the different modalities of interventions in order to treat the differing needs of patients appropriately. Pharmacological interventions form the backbone of pain management and include analgesics and adjuvant medications, depending on particular categories of pain, either acute or chronic. For instance, opioids may be employed in the case of severe pain, while NSAIDs may be used in cases of mild to moderate pain. Further, adjuvant therapies like antidepressants or anticonvulsants are helpful in the case of neuropathic pain. Finally, non-pharmacological strategies like physical therapy, acupuncture, and cognitive-behavioral therapy form part of a multifaceted strategy for pain management. An integrative model not only addresses the somatic aspects of pain but also enhances psychological and social function, showing that a mixed bag must be part of the pain management tool kit. Effective pain management requires ongoing assessment and changing treatment plans, which illustrates the importance of patient-healthcare provider communication. Because individual responses to pain treatment can vary, regular follow-up visits are required to monitor progress and modify treatment plans as needed. The use of valid assessment tools can help practitioners evaluate pain severity, functional outcomes, and treatment side effects. Establishing a solid clinician-patient relationship is also important to ensure patient adherence to treatment plans and provide patients with an outlet to express concerns about their pain management. Engaging patients in discussions of their preferences and experiences not only enhances compliance but also leads to a better pain management experience. Overall, an in-depth introduction to pain management is key to a team-based, customized plan that aims to alleviate pain-related distress and improve overall quality of life for patients with pain.

Definition of Pain and Its Types

Pain is a complex and subtle experience usually defined as an unpleasant sensory and affective experience connected with actual or imminent tissue damage. Pain is a key protective function, alerting individuals to harm or the need for medical treatment. The International Association for the Study of Pain (IASP) emphasizes that pain is subjective and varies significantly from person to person, depending on physiological, psychological, and social determinants. Pain categories may be divided into two principal groups: acute and chronic pain, each with distinct characteristics and treatment implications. Acute pain tends to be temporary, due to an illness or injury, and typically resolves with recovery. In contrast, chronic pain persists for a long time, even beyond the expected healing period. It is critical to identify both to tailor effective pain management therapies that address causes as well as relieve symptoms. In addition to acute and chronic pain, pain can also be defined as belonging to several specialized types, one of which is nociceptive pain, and the other is neuropathic pain. Nociceptive pain results from activation of peripheral nociceptors by painful stimuli, such as injury or inflammation, and is further divided into somatic and visceral pain. Somatic pain is focal and characteristically sharp or throbbing, but visceral pain tends to be vague and difficult to localize, owing to the internal organs. In contrast, neuropathic pain occurs as a consequence of injury to the nervous system itself, and its descriptions may involve burning, paresthesia, or numbness. This is critical to clinicians because the pathophysiologic mechanisms of pain will dictate proper treatment modalities. In recent years, the discovery of multidimensional assessment tools has provided easier ways to research such pain and emphasized the need for interdisciplinary approaches in pain therapy (Venkataramu et al., 2022). Moreover, one must also take into account the psychological and emotional aspects of pain, thereby increasing the difficulty of treatment. Chronic pain, in itself, can lead to psychiatric disorders such as depression and anxiety that can significantly worsen a patient's quality of life (Varkey, 2020). The interplay between pain and mental health necessitates an integrative treatment that treats both physical and psychological causes. By embracing both pharmacologic and nonpharmacologic interventions, doctors can design individualized pain management regimens that not only enhance physical symptoms but also promote emotional resilience. This framework for integration enhances the overall effectiveness of pain management interventions, leading to improved patient outcomes. Having a basis in the definition of pain and its different forms enables medical practitioners to develop specific interventions that address the complexity of this multisystem experience, ultimately ensuring higher-quality care for patients with pain (Figure 9.1).

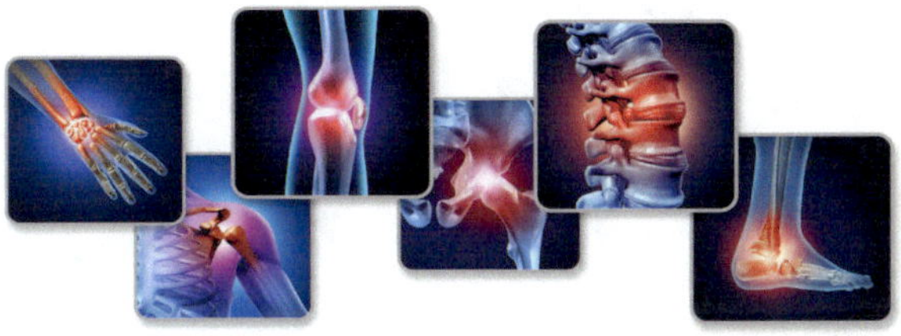

Figure 9.1. Definition of pain and its types.

Source: https://europeanpainfederation.eu/wp-content/uploads/2022/07/pain-body.jpeg.

Importance of Effective Pain Management

Optimal pain management is a pillar of quality healthcare and makes an important contribution to a substantial enhancement of patient outcomes. Recognition of pain as a complex experience necessitates a strategy aimed at its physiological as well as its psychological aspects. Effective management not only alleviates suffering but also enhances general health-related quality of life. Chronic pain, if uncontrolled, will contribute to decreased physical functioning, altered mood, and a domino effect of adverse health consequences that can lead to further dependence on the health care system. Therefore, healthcare providers must comprehend the importance of comprehensive pain management to offer integral care and thereby relieve the socio-economic burden brought about by undertreated pain on patients and society as a whole, as pain tends to indicate a significant reason for which patients seek care at health centers (Umukoro et al., 2025). Moreover, evolving pain management underscores the importance of personalized practice in addressing patients' specific needs. While the opioid epidemic continues to raise alarms regarding the abuse of medications, it is more and more necessary to speak about multidisciplinary strategies involving non-pharmacological and pharmacological interventions. Employing physical therapy, cognitive behavior therapy, and other therapies such as acupuncture or mindfulness-based modalities as adjuncts to pain management regimens can provide significant relief with no risk of more traditional opioid therapy. This delicate handling of the concept of chronic pain and its determinants across multiple dimensions underscores the importance of assessing patients holistically, as effective management can prevent the development of pain problems and promote treatment adherence (Jurayev et al., 2025). Clinicians, therefore, have a responsibility to prioritize effective management in addressing the epidemic of chronic pain to not only provide relief but also empower patients. By providing education and guidance, healthcare professionals empower patients with the knowledge needed to manage their pain proactively. Empowerment enhances patient autonomy, encourages active involvement in their own care, and encourages resilience to the adverse effects of chronic pain. An effective pain management strategy that involves patient involvement not only reduces the incidence of disabling pain disorders but also emphasizes preventive care and potentially lowers the need for hospitalization and more intensive treatments. Lastly, optimal pain control can be the impetus for improved health outcomes and a healthier system, demonstrating the merit of ongoing research and clinical advancement in the field (Umukoro et al., 2025).

Overview of Pain Management Approaches

An effective pain control plan is highly crucial in the management of most forms of pain, particularly in syndromes like chronic low back pain (CLBP), which is highly prevalent and typically resistant to conventional management. As demonstrated in recent studies, lumbar multifidus muscle dysfunction has been recognized as a significant etiology of non-specific CLBP. This dysfunction results from reflex inhibition following an initial injury, which subsequently decreases spinal stability and increases susceptibility to further injury. Pain management for multifidus dysfunction has thus been established, with conservative methods such as patient education, non-steroidal anti-inflammatory medication, and physical therapy.

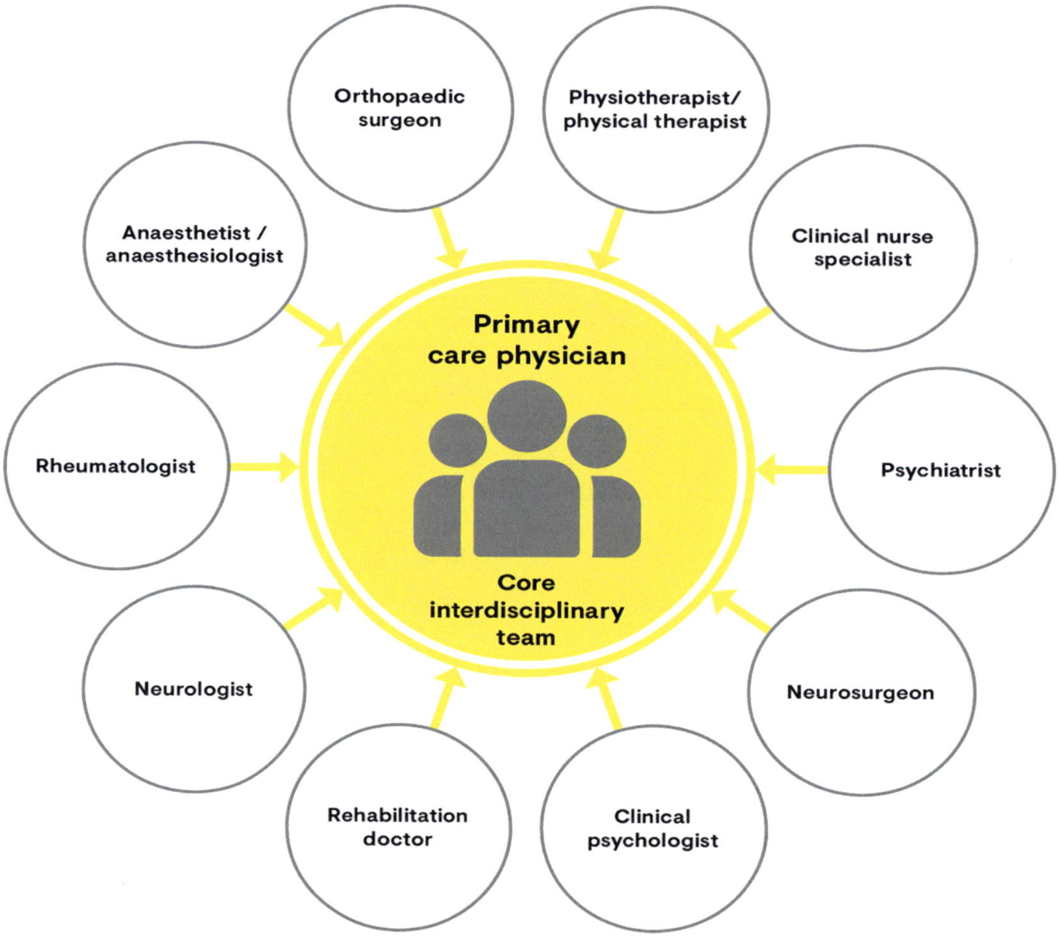

Figure 9.2. An effective pain management approach.

Source: https://www.grunenthal.com/-/media/projects/change-pain/pain-basics/en/p-basics4.png?rev=298f0a5efd7d43619c14681a87869d99&hash=A25EDCF1FBCA61BCE019CA0B8C84C195.

These interventions focus on pain relief but also on rehabilitation of the multifidus' intrinsic function through motor control training and restorative neurostimulation, shifting towards a rehabilitative approach over symptomatic management (Abd-Elsayed et al., 2025). Chronic pain management differs from acute pain, particularly for surgical procedures such as total joint arthroplasties, in that it employs a distinct set of techniques due to its unique physiological mechanisms. Multimodal pain management practices have become increasingly popular in these situations, using a combination of pharmacologic and non-pharmacologic approaches suitable to meet various aspects of postoperative pain. The integration of nerve blocks, analgesics, and adjuvant therapy, like physical rehabilitation, gives the patient a master plan for managing pain. Not only does it set out to maximize pain control and surgical recovery, but it also seeks to decrease opioid dependence, which has been associated with adverse side effects and risk of dependency. The demand for such newer trends reflects the evolving landscape of pain management in clinics (Daniel et al., 2024).

Lastly, the effectiveness of pain management interventions will depend on their adaptability to patients' needs. A one-size-fits-all approach is inadequate in an intervention context that is so intricately linked to subjective experience and clinical presentation. The intersection of evidence-based practice across disciplines—such as psychological interventions for chronic pain management, as well as advanced modalities for postoperative recovery—enables clinicians to construct pain care plans on an individual, case-by-case basis. These individualized plans maximize not only pain results but also overall patient satisfaction, as part of a more cohesive model of care. With more research dedicated to enhancing understanding of pain mechanisms and management, the clinician is better positioned to adapt and modify practice, adding established and new techniques to their portfolio to suit patients' changing needs (Daniel et al., 2024; Abd-Elsayed et al., 2025) (Figure 9.2).

9.1. Understanding Pain

Learning Outcome

1. Physiological mechanisms of pain
2. Psychological aspects of pain perception
3. Impact of chronic pain on quality of life

Pain, as a multifaceted phenomenon, has physiological, psychological, and social components that demand an integrated approach for proper management. Pain is subjective and individual, varying across individuals, with heterogeneity driven by individual thresholds and extrinsic milieu. Pain is also understood by understanding the various forms, such as acute and chronic pain; the latter is a protective response following trauma or surgery, and the former persists beyond the expected healing time, typically causing substantial impairment in quality of life. learn the processes of pain biology, including nociception and neuroplasticity as etiologic factors in chronic pain, as they have direct implications for what is treated and taught in patient education. Clinicians, by enhancing their knowledge of pain, can better craft individualized treatment plans that target not only symptoms but also the patient's well-being and emotional function. Effective management of pain is not confined to pharmacological interventions; it is an approach that takes into consideration the psychological and social elements. The role of caregivers and family members in supporting patients throughout the pain management process is also very important. Of special interest, as stated by He et al. (2005), is the role played by parents in improving a child's postoperative experience by offering emotional support and security. Several parents, however, experience frustration and are not informed about how to properly evaluate and manage pain, as identified in research by Ellerton and Merriam (1994) and O'ConnorVon (2000). Educating parents appropriately and providing them with enough resources on non-pharmacological interventions is critical since these interventions may complement the traditional means of pain relief and enhance patient outcomes. Involvement of caregivers in the pain management process creates a feeling of cooperation that ultimately translates into safer and more effective pain relief. Furthermore, evolving understanding of pain mechanisms and innovative treatment strategies continue to shape paradigms of pain management. For instance, research into biological modifiers of healing illustrates the promise of growth factors in influencing tissue regeneration and pain relief. As noted in the comprehensive review of ligament and tendon injury (Bentley, 2007), new methods, such as gene therapy, are also being explored to enhance healing and reduce pain associated with musculoskeletal disorders. With increased focus on the use of non-pharmacological interventions, evidence is accumulating in support of modalities such as cognitive-behavioral therapy, mindfulness, and physical therapy to enhance quality of life and reduce pain. Despite the complexities of pain perception and control, ongoing research will help close the gap toward greater understanding of pain, ultimately promoting improved patient outcomes and enhanced quality of care across settings.

9.1.1. Physiological Mechanisms of Pain

It is basic to the construction of an effective pain management strategy to comprehend the physiological mechanisms of pain. Pain is fundamentally a defensive reflex mediated by complex neural mechanisms, including nociceptors, spinal cord mechanisms, and supraspinal centers. When tissue is damaged, nociceptors are activated and transmit pain impulses to the spinal cord, where they can be modulated before reaching the brain. The brain then processes this information, which results in the perception of pain. Worth noting is the inclusion of neuroplasticity, allowing for the potential alteration of pain pathways, which is very important in chronic pain conditions. Elucidation of such pathways is vitally important, as it lays the groundwork for interventions guided by the biological mechanism, thereby enhancing patient outcomes in pain management. Psychological processes also play a critical role in the perception and modulation of pain, in that the biopsychosocial model must be adopted in the management of pain. Affect states also influence pain perception, as seen in interactions between the central nervous system (CNS) and various neurotransmitters. For instance, enhanced anxiety and stress can cause enhanced perception of pain through mechanisms such as increased activity of the sympathetic nervous system. By contrast, relaxation methods, such as slow, deep breathing, have been found to stimulate the parasympathetic nervous system, leading to pain reduction and improved overall well-being. These kinds of interventions are particularly relevant to chronic pain patients since they can be utilized to help cure both the physiological and emotional components of pain, complementing an integral pain management program. New studies on pain management procedures are bringing forward the importance of addressing the biological cause of chronic pain. Altius High-Frequency Nerve Block System, for example, offers a new alternative to traditional pain management methods by applying high-frequency alternating current to peripheral nerves. The system establishes a reversible conduction block, decreasing pain without enhancing the patient's reliance on opioids, which are commonly associated with side effects and addiction. Clinical trials have validated remarkable reductions in pain intensity in patients with persistent illnesses, emphasizing the significance of effective treatments capable of addressing the reality of pain. These advances are meant to demonstrate how discovering the physiological underpinnings of pain can potentially unlock therapeutic innovations, ultimately culminating in improved quality of life for sufferers of chronic pain conditions (Figure 9.3).

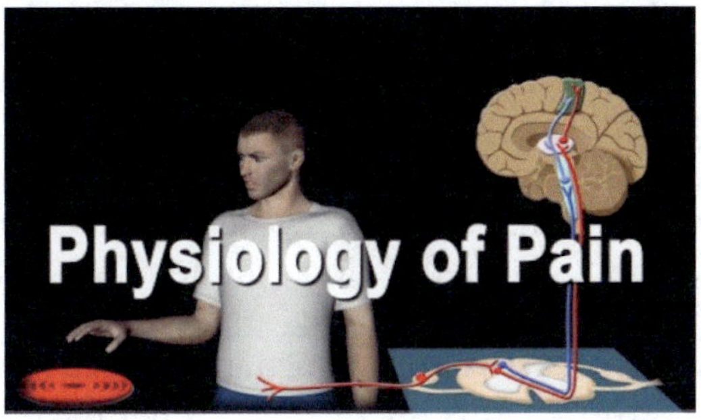

Figure 9.3. The physiological mechanisms of pain.

Source: https://i.ytimg.com/vi/uOaiaYDoUnA/hqdefault.jpg.

9.1.2. Psychological Aspects of Pain Perception

The psychological factors influencing pain perception are highly significant in understanding the way individuals perceive and deal with pain. Pain is not merely a physiological process; it is intertwined with cognitive and affective processes. People's beliefs about pain, prior experiences, and emotional states can significantly influence pain perception. For instance, individuals with fear of pain are found to rate higher pain levels, as fear actually amplifies pain. While biological factors unequivocally contribute to pain transmission, psychological processes can augment or diminish the overall sensation. The interface is designed to draw attention to the need for pain management interventions that address both the physical and psychological dimensions of pain, thereby enhancing patient outcomes and quality of life. Furthermore, contemporary pain management methods recognize the importance of psychological therapy in managing chronic pain. The addition of psychological techniques to treatment programs has been found to improve effectiveness for more traditional pain management treatments. Pain self-management (PSM) programs prioritize group therapy and individual goal-setting, showing that patients can derive internal benefits from sharing stories and peer support.

The affective aspects of pain, such as fear and anxiety, need to be tackled holistically in these frameworks. For instance, (Marom et al., 2025) demonstrates that psychological processes associated with pain perception can be addressed through structured interventions, thereby highlighting the effectiveness of integrating physical and affective strategies to improve pain outcomes. Further, the introduction of a multidisciplinary treatment strategy further emphasizes the importance of psychological factors in chronic pain management. Through the use of multiple therapeutic modalities, such as Pain Neuroscience Education and mindfulness techniques, therapists can equip patients with critical tools to reframe and deal with their pain experiences. Studies have shown that cognitive-behavioral therapy (CBT) and acceptance and commitment therapy (ACT) both significantly decrease pain-related fear and increase coping mechanisms, evidencing their efficacy in changing pain perception. A good example is Venturin et al. (2024), in which a general rehabilitation program considers psychological factors to improve pain relief outcomes. The kind of multidimensional treatment is important because it not only seeks to relieve bodily pain but also seeks to instill an appreciation of the involvement of psychology in the pain perception process, leading to more inclusive treatment of pain management.

9.1.3. Impact of Chronic Pain on Quality of Life

The association between chronic pain and quality of life is of special challenge, affecting individuals' emotional, physical, and social status. Chronic pain is not like acute pain because it does not abate once the body heals. Instead, it persists in time, causing tremendous feelings of hopelessness and frustration to the patients. The ongoing pain may disrupt daily living activities, impair movement, and even impair one's capacity to work or socialize. According to pertinent literature, musculoskeletal pain, which affects nearly half the population of the world, is a classic example of chronic pain being linked to decreased quality of life and increased dependency on healthcare services. Many patients experiencing musculoskeletal pain suffer from chronic problems over extended durations, so there is an absolute need for efficient paradigms of management in a bid to offset these negative consequences (Salah et al., 2021). In addition, the socioeconomic impact of chronic pain cannot be overstated. The constant struggle of coping with pain typically results in increased healthcare costs and lost productivity, entrenching most victims in a cycle of poverty. Chronic pain, in others such as low back pain, remains a significant source of disability throughout the world, with enormous consequences for work attendance and job performance. Such a reality is most acutely felt in the lower socioeconomic classes, where poor access to quality healthcare only exacerbates pain management challenges. As underscored by recent studies, the global burden of low back pain has ballooned in recent decades, necessitating enhanced care interventions aimed at this pervasive condition. Closing the gap between optimal pain management practice and actual patient care is crucial in reclaiming quality of life for patients with chronic pain (Buchbinder et al., 2020). In managing the multifaceted disability caused by chronic pain, a comprehensive and multidisciplinary pain management strategy becomes necessary. These actions should encompass pharmacologic treatment, physical therapy, and behavioral interventions to improve physical and psychological well-being. Present-day practice tends to support the utilization of multimodal analgesia, whereby multiple healing approaches are used in concert in an effort to reap maximum benefits without being overly dependent on medications alone. This tailor-made approach not only promotes greater activation of active control of pain but also results in a better quality of life for individuals with chronic pain syndromes. Lastly, a commitment to greater awareness and improved treatment routes is significant in countering the adverse impacts of chronic pain on quality of life (Salah et al., 2021) (Figure 9.4).

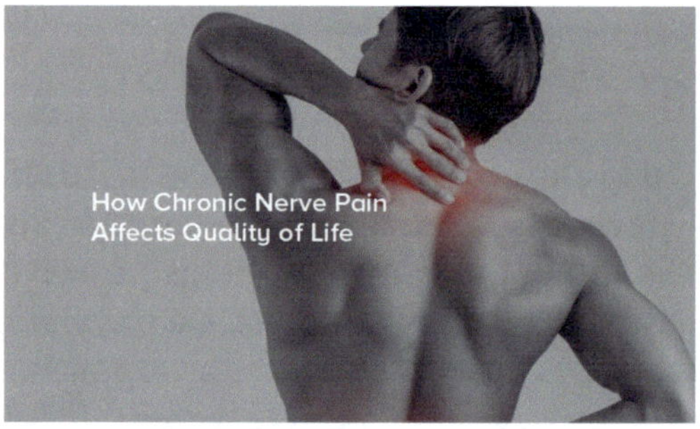

Figure 9.4. The interplay between chronic pain and quality of life presents significant challenges.

Source: https://www.citizenshospitals.com/static/uploads/9312319c-253f-4028-899a-536b03c122a6-1737368086937.jpg.

Test Your Knowledge

1. What are the main physiological pathways involved in the perception and transmission of pain from the site of injury to the brain?
2. How do nociceptors, neurotransmitters, and the central nervous system interact to modulate pain signals?

9.2. Pharmacological Treatments

Learning Outcome

1. Non-opioid analgesics
2. Opioid medications
3. Adjuvant therapies (e.g., antidepressants, anticonvulsants)

Treatment of pain often involves the use of pharmacological therapy, which can be grouped into several classes based on their mode of action and the types of pain to be alleviated. The principal drugs in clinical use are non-steroidal anti-inflammatory drugs (NSAIDs), acetaminophen, and opioids. The NSAIDs work by inhibiting cyclooxygenase enzymes, which are central to the inflammatory response and therefore abate pain. Acetaminophen, which is useful for pain management, does not have the anti-inflammatory action of NSAIDs. Opioids like morphine and oxycodone are usually reserved for severe or moderately severe pain since they are likely to cause dependence and produce side effects. Despite common use, opioid use has now become controversial, warranting a reconsideration of pharmacologic means of pain control that are both effective and safe. In certain conditions, the efficacy of pharmacological treatment can vary significantly. In patients with rheumatoid arthritis (RA), for instance, chronic pain represents a frequent manifestation, which can complicate their management in general. Current guidelines prefer the use of disease-modifying anti-rheumatic drugs (DMARDs) to manage the activity of the disease and, concomitantly, pain relief. Empirical evidence shows that synthetic and biologic DMARDs are highly effective in relieving pain associated with RA, as systematic reviews have concluded that they are superior to placebo (Cox et al., 2025). As a result, studying the broader scope of pharmacotherapy and its application to specific patient populations becomes important for optimizing pain management practice. Neuropathic pain is a unique challenge to pharmacologic interventions, and unique therapeutic strategies are required. Anticonvulsants and antidepressants are the first-line therapies and exert their actions by modifying neurotransmitter concentration and altering pain pathways. Gabapentin and pregabalin are efficient in the treatment of neuropathic pain, although in practice their action is typically temporary, and there is vast patient heterogeneity (Andreji et al., 2025). Recent research into newer, more sophisticated therapies such as monoclonal antibodies and N-methyl-D-aspartate (NMDA) receptor antagonists holds the potential to revolutionize the pharmacological management of neuropathic pain. With ongoing progress in research, cross-disciplinary collaboration and serial clinical trials will be key to refining treatment therapies and improving the welfare of patients with complex pain syndromes.

9.2.1. Non-Opioid Analgesics

In the management of pain, non-opioid analgesics are of utmost importance in order to manage various types of pain without the risk associated with their application. They are commonly employed since they are effective and also entail less dependence risk. Some examples of these include NSAIDs and acetaminophen. These medications inhibit the cyclooxygenase enzymes and therefore block inflammation and pain. For example, ibuprofen and naproxen are typically prescribed for conditions that range from arthritis to acute trauma. Acetaminophen's antipyretic and analgesic effect, meanwhile, makes it an ideal drug in fever management and milder pain, particularly among patients who may be susceptible to the gastrointestinal adverse effects of NSAIDs. This complex mechanism puts non-opioid analgesics as key pieces of the puzzle in coordinated pain treatment models. While having their own merits, the non-opioid analgesics also have their own limitations and side effects. For instance, repeated administration of NSAIDs has adverse gastrointestinal effects, like ulcers and bleeding, along with renal damage. Further, while acetaminophen is quite safe at doses prescribed for its application, it possesses catastrophic risks when administered in overdose doses, which mainly affect liver function. Doctors must strictly analyze patient profiles on a case-by-case basis and consider the comorbidities involved and concomitant medications used. The education of the patient cannot be overstated since most patients will unconsciously misuse these medications. Medical professionals favor the use of the minimum dose for the shortest duration to avoid adverse effects.

This active approach is vital in guaranteeing that non-opioid analgesics are responsible for pain management without unnecessarily inducing health problems. Continued studies enlighten us further on non-opioid analgesics and their potential in pain management. Recent studies have examined novel delivery methods, such as the use of lipid-based nanoparticles, in improving analgesic bioavailability. Remarkably, this route has been highly promising for achieving targeted relief, especially for centrally acting drugs that require penetration of the blood-brain barrier to be effective. The intranasal route, particularly when combined with new drug formulations such as in situ gel systems, has opened new avenues in pain relief pharmacology. This approach not only enhances drug absorption but also may reduce systemic side effects, enabling patients to undergo effective treatment with reduced risk. As the area continues to evolve, ongoing clinical trials will be at the forefront of determining the efficacy and safety of such novel delivery systems in comparison to non-opioid analgesics, leading to better patient outcomes in pain management (Ivan et al., 2024; Koo et al., 2024) (Figure 9.5).

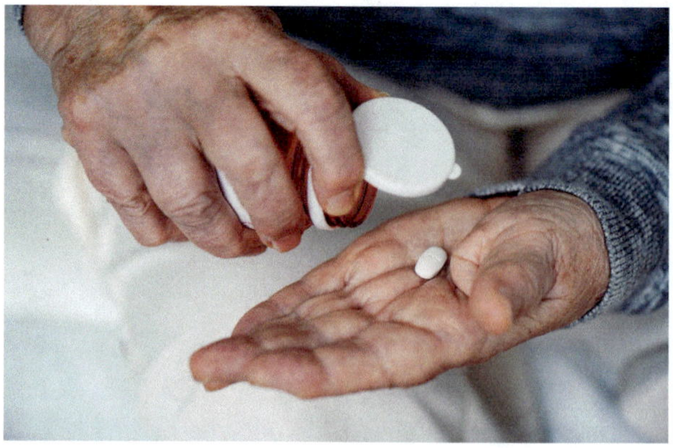

Figure 9.5. The non-opioid analgesics.

Source: https://paininjuryrelief.com/wp-content/uploads/2019/01/rawpixel-973106-unsplash-3.jpg.

9.2.2. Opioid Medications

The challenge of complexity with opioid medicines is significant, particularly in the case of pain management. These medicines, including morphine, oxycodone, and the controversial fentanyl, are potent analgesics commonly utilized to deal with severe pain, particularly following surgery or cancer. Their benefit must be weighed against potential risks like addiction and overdose. Opioid drugs produce their effect by binding to specific receptors of the brain and spinal cord, modifying pain transmission mechanisms. Although the effect can be effective in analgesia, tolerance formation and dependence are also risks, requiring careful prescribing practice. Physicians have a key role to play in educating patients on these medications, clearing misconceptions regarding their usage and explaining the risks involved, thus setting proper pain-relief strategies while curtailing their abuse and addictiveness potential (Mary et al., 2023). The opioid crisis has brought attention to how medical professionals should balance pain relief with risks from opioid medications. Education of patients, particularly regarding the role and function of opioids, is paramount in effective pain management and the removal of opioid use stigma. Patients will come with medication misinformation, imagining that opioid treatment is an irreversible treatment for pain and not part of a big, multimodal management plan. This is the wrong line of thinking that leads to unnecessary assessments and interventions, which waste valuable healthcare resources. Evidence shows that educating patients to be cognizant of the pathophysiologic mechanisms of pain can improve patient perception and outcomes (Mary et al., 2023). Efforts to counteract this misperception through targeted education can improve functional status and quality of life in patients with chronic pain. Opioid medication, as much as it has been found to work for disabling pain, still lags behind maximum use due to addiction and abuse fears.

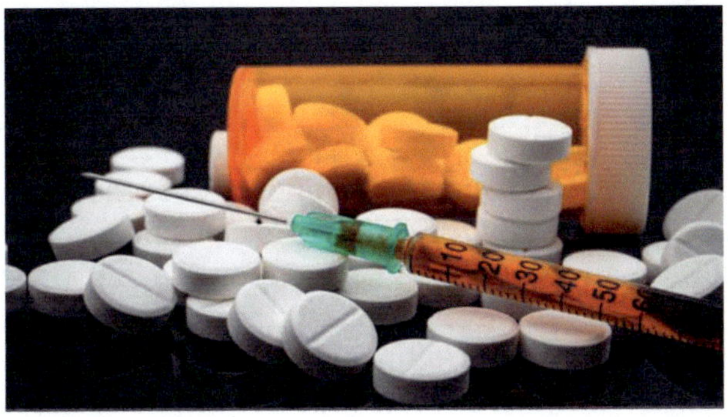

Figure 9.6. The complexity surrounding opioid medications.

Source: https://www.hopkinsmedicine.org/-/media/feature/nested/opioid-teaser-v1.jpg.

There is an ample knowledge deficit in physician training when it comes to opioid use disorder (OUD) treatment, driving ongoing mortality due to opioid overdose. Opioid use disorder medications have been shown to decrease mortality significantly and are critical in the management of this public health crisis, but are often underprescribed due to discomfort on the part of providers and education deficits. Educational courses directed towards medical students discussing the pharmacology of opioids, principles of pain management, and principles of addiction treatment are crucial. The more confident medical professionals become that they can prescribe and treat opioid drugs without risk, the better they will be able to manage the intricacy of pain care while working proactively to combat the opioid crisis (Figure 9.6).

9.2.3. Adjuvant Therapies (E.g., Antidepressants, Anticonvulsants)

Adjuvants play crucial roles as adjuncts to the general pain management, particularly in chronic pain syndromes when the use of routine analgesics is unsatisfactory. With the inclusion of drugs such as antidepressants and anticonvulsants, clinicians can modulate pain by non-analgesic means. Antidepressants, specifically the tricyclics and the serotonin-norepinephrine reuptake inhibitors, have been found to modify the mechanisms of pain, enhancing analgesia in neuropathic pain. Anticonvulsants like gabapentin and pregabalin have similarly been found to be effective in alleviating nerve pain by inhibiting the release of excitatory neurotransmitters and stabilizing neuronal membranes. These treatments illustrate the value of a multimodal pain management strategy, where the clinician can tailor treatment regimens to maximize efficacy while minimizing the use of opioids and other conventional analgesics. Moreover, the use of adjuvant treatments in pain management also indicates that multimodal analgesia has evolved as a useful method for managing postoperative pain. From a literature review, the coordination of therapeutic modalities is found to enhance analgesia as well as reduce opioid consumption, thereby avoiding opioid side effects and chronic pain development. Adjuvant treatments may prove especially useful in the postoperative period, where analgesia is crucial to maximize recovery. The application of adjuvant drugs together with conventional analgesics, though, encourages an integrative treatment approach that manages acute pain and discourages chronic pain development. Embracing such a multi-modal approach not only improves patient results but also harmonizes with current healthcare methods, prioritizing holistic pain treatment protocols. Additionally, as healthcare professionals continue to research the efficacy of adjuvant treatments, it is vitally essential to establish a sound foundation of knowledge in pharmacology and its influence on pain management. Educational content, as used here in Epicore et al. (2023), can be invaluable in teaching practitioners about the pharmacodynamics and pharmacokinetics of such drugs. Understanding how adjuvant treatments act on pain pathways is critical in optimizing treatment regimens. In addition, research on the application of such therapeutic medications, as emphasized by multimodal analgesia studies (Martins et al., 2023), is critical in the formulation of pain management guidelines. By leveraging the potential of adjuvant therapies, professionals can significantly enhance the quality of treatment provided to individuals with acute and chronic pain, thereby improving health outcomes and quality of life.

Test Your Knowledge

1. What are the common classes of non-opioid analgesics, and how do they relieve pain at the molecular and cellular levels?
2. What are the advantages and limitations of non-opioid analgesics compared to opioid medications in pain management?

9.3. Non-Pharmacological Treatments

Learning Outcome

1. Physical therapy and rehabilitation
2. Cognitive-behavioral therapy
3. Alternative therapies (e.g., acupuncture, massage)

The introduction of non-pharmacological interventions into models of pain management is a significant development in clinical practice. These interventions include cognitive-behavioral therapy, physical therapy, and complementary therapies such as acupuncture and mindfulness. Conversely, pharmacological interventions provide immediate relief. Non-pharmacological interventions are, however, commendable for addressing psychological and emotional dimensions of pain, leading to coping mechanisms in the long run. For instance, cognitive-behavioral therapy teaches patients to shift their perception of pain, enhancing their resilience and self-efficacy. Integrating these practices enables clinicians to design a more holistic treatment plan that not only alleviates pain but also improves patients' overall health, as evidenced by research demonstrating the effectiveness of combining these approaches with standard practices (Raja et al., 2025). Music therapy, another non-drug method of treatment, has also been seen throughout many fields of medicine for its ability to relieve pain and anxiety. Studies have shown that listening to or playing music enhances the release of endorphins, resulting in reduced self-reported pain. This method is particularly beneficial to use within settings such as children's hospitals and dental work, where anxiety serves to exacerbate pain experience. By reducing anxiety, music therapy makes the treatment atmosphere more patient-centered, promoting patient compliance and satisfaction. The non-invasive nature of the intervention makes it appealing, especially for patients who do not wish to subject themselves to the side effects of pharmacological interventions. Cumulative evidence supports that non-pharmacological interventions, such as music therapy, can optimize pain management outcomes across diverse patient populations (Sahu et al., 2025). Also, the potential of non-medication interventions extends beyond reducing short-term pain to creating resilience and long-term improvements in health. Interventions involving physical activity, like exercise therapy, not only reduce pain but also assist in the recovery of strength and function in patients undergoing surgery or suffering from an injury. Of special note is that these interventions have been successful in the rehabilitation of long-standing chronic pain conditions like arthritis and fibromyalgia, where medication for long periods of time can be hazardous. The combination of physical therapy and cognitive-behavioral methods constitutes a multimodal treatment that addresses both the physical and psychological aspects of pain. With advances in research, there is more than ever an awareness of the importance of integrating these diverse modalities into everyday practice, reemphasizing that effective pain management should be pharmacologic as well as non-pharmacologic (Raja et al., 2025).

9.3.1. Physical Therapy and Rehabilitation

Physical therapy and rehabilitation are also vital in the management of pain through care of physical and functional recovery aspects. The interventions aim to restore function and enhance quality of life for patients with pain resulting from injury, surgery, or chronic disease. By ensuring active engagement in the process, physical therapy enables patients to be actively involved in their rehabilitation. An intensive exercise regimen, led by a physically licensed therapist, can alleviate pain, build strength, and introduce flexibility. In addition, the use of manual therapy techniques and modalities, such as heat or ultrasound, can contribute to increased pain reduction and healing. Physical therapy is thus an integral component of pain management strategies, in that it not only alleviates the symptom of pain but also the causative mechanisms producing pain. Aside from physical therapy, rehabilitation interventions usually include interdisciplinarity with healthcare practitioners from different disciplines. This integrative approach provides a holistic care program for patients since pain may have diverse sources, which include physical, psychological, and external causes. By integrating mental health care, dietary counseling, and education on pain management measures, rehabilitation practitioners can significantly enhance patient outcomes. This approach aligns with evidence-based practice recommendations, which call for the multidimensionality of pain and the personalization of treatment regimens. Furthermore, such interprofessional clusters encourage frequent communication among practitioners, therefore enhancing continuity of care throughout the healing process. This collusion eventually yields an intensified pain management plan that is holistic and adaptive to the patient's unique needs. The effectiveness of rehabilitation and physiotherapy in pain management is further supported by ongoing research, highlighting the necessity of evidence-based practice. Various studies have established the benefits of personalized exercise therapy in reducing pain and improving overall function in patients with musculoskeletal diseases and post-surgery patients (François et al., 2019). These findings establish that some physical therapy techniques not only relieve pain but also lead to long-term improvements in the individual's physical state. Moreover, new rehabilitative trends, such as aquatic therapy or virtual reality, are constantly emerging, offering alternative methods for pain relief. As rehabilitation practice continues to evolve, it is more critical than ever for rehabilitation practitioners to stay informed about emerging therapies and studies so that patients receive optimal treatment and pain management (Arthur et al., 2018) (Figure 9.7).

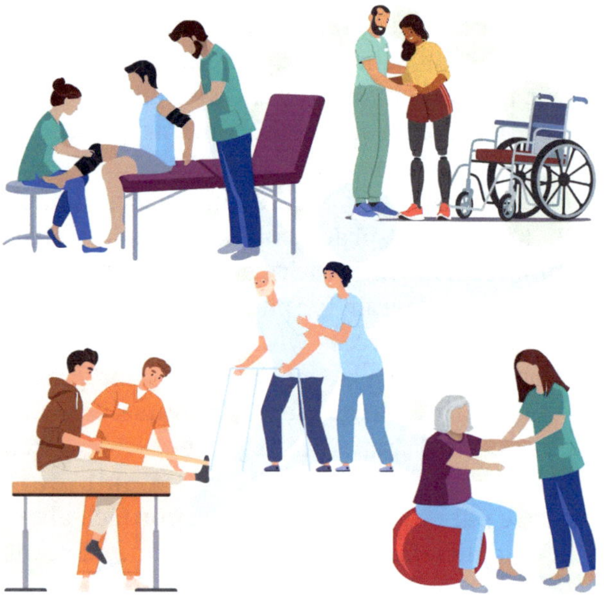

Figure 9.7. Physical therapy and rehabilitation.

Source: https://neemtreehealthcare.com/wp-content/uploads/2024/12/What-is-Physiotherapy-Rehabilitation.webp.

9.3.2. Cognitive-Behavioral Therapy

Cognitive-behavioral therapy (CBT) has become more frequently utilized as a mainstay in the treatment of chronic pain, equipping patients with skills to relearn how they perceive and respond to pain. CBT targets the interaction between thought, feeling, and action, allowing an individual to develop coping skills capable of diminishing the emotional and psychological effects of pain. Studies have demonstrated that CBT can lead to significant reductions in pain interference, which is particularly important in those suffering from CLBP. For instance, a recent trial indicated medium-to-large reductions in pain interference among patients undergoing videoconference-delivered CBT, demonstrating its efficacy irrespective of modality. Hence, introducing CBT in pain management therapies can provide patients with the necessary tools to improve their quality of life and help them engage in activities of daily life, thus facilitating a more integrative pain management strategy (Day et al., 2024). The explanation for CBT's success in pain management lies in cognitive restructuring and activation. By helping the patients to identify and reverse distorted thought patterns, CBT encourages a shift toward healthier accounts of pain, resulting in a reduction of distress emotions associated with chronic illness.

Further, the therapy may involve behavioral strategies such as activity scheduling or exposure exercises, which can enable people to re-engage with life despite persistent pain. Evidence supporting the proposition that patients using CBT interventions report decreased pain and improved functioning in the long term derives from various clinical trials. Therefore, the practicability of CBT—whether delivered face-to-face or via telehealth platforms—indicates its relevance in pain management today, particularly given access issues to healthcare (Abdullah et al., 2024). Integrating CBT into multimodal pain treatment programs emphasizes the need for an integrated approach to addressing chronic pain. Clinicians, such as physiotherapists and nurses, can work cooperatively to apply CBT methods and improve the patient's therapeutic experience. This cooperation has the potential to close the gap between psychological and bodily pain treatment options, such that patients gain access to integrated care that addresses their specific circumstances. While evidence continues to establish the effectiveness of CBT, clinical practice also increasingly needs to place such interventions at the center of pain management models. By promoting psychological resilience and empowering patients with coping strategies, CBT not only reduces the burden of chronic pain but also promotes a sense of control among sufferers, allowing them to manage the experience of pain more effectively (Day et al., 2024).

9.3.3. Alternative Therapies (E.g., Acupuncture, Massage)

The increasing popularity of complementary therapies such as acupuncture and massage highlights the evolving context of pain relief. They provide holistic approaches that accommodate not only the medical models of symptom relief but also patients' notions of health and well-being. Acupuncture, a treatment founded on traditional Chinese medicine, employs extremely thin needles inserted at targeted points to stimulate the body's mechanisms with significant benefit to conditions of osteoarthritis and migraines. Massage therapy, on the other hand, is reported to enhance blood circulation, ease muscle tension, and calm the mind, which ultimately leads to improved functional gains among patients suffering from various types of pain. As discussed in the literature, the concurrent application of these therapies amplifies conventional treatment and establishes an integrated pain management model, improving subjective well-being and symptomatic relief. The effectiveness of acupuncture and massage is evidenced by accumulating evidence-based research, revealing their potential as evidence-based alternatives or adjuncts to pharmaceutical interventions. Research indicates that acupuncture may modulate pain perception by initiating the release of endorphins and activating the body's own pain-relieving mechanisms. Similarly, research indicates that massage can also significantly reduce inflammation and relieve musculoskeletal pain. These points clearly suggest that the incorporation of alternative therapies in pain management programs will enhance patient outcomes, particularly in patients with drug intolerance to conventional medicines. For instance, osteoporotic pain patients can perhaps derive improved quality of life from such non-invasive therapies since pharmacological intervention is likely to have high side effects. It is therefore increasingly critical for doctors to consider these other therapeutic approaches in their treatment programs. Promoting alternative therapies in mainstream medical practice requires educating patients and applying personalized treatment that considers individual preferences. As the medical community is aware of the limitations of traditional therapeutics, the potential of benefits from acupuncture and massage therapeutics presents a path towards more holistic pain management approaches. Acknowledging the physiological and psychological underpinnings of pain can help patients make better decisions about their treatments. Given the available evidence on their effectiveness, practitioners should advise patients on incorporating these therapies as part of their management plan. Further, research can assess their long-term outcomes and impacts across various populations. By advocating a holistic approach that incorporates complementary therapies, health practitioners are best placed to address the multi-dimensional nature of pain and enhance patients' satisfaction in general, especially for conditions with chronic pain etiology and care, as highlighted in the rising literature on these therapies (Seppi et al., 2019; Meryl et al., 2022) (Figure 9.8).

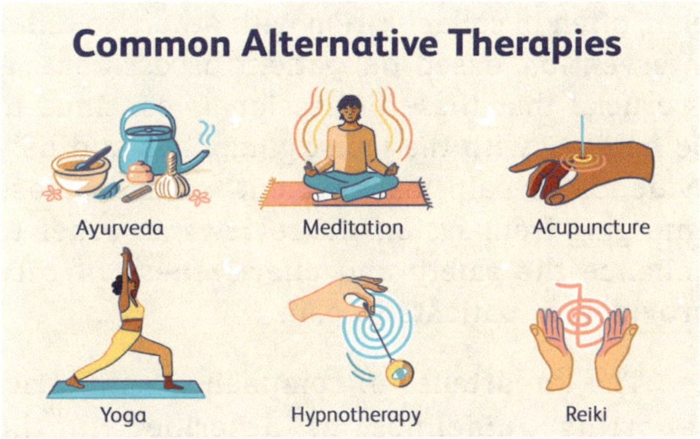

Figure 9.8. The increasing acknowledgment of alternative therapies.

Source: https://www.verywellmind.com/thmb/puRzNEXvSspRLcSSf5sXgVTWEgU=/1500x0/filters:no_upscale():max_bytes(150000):strip_icc()/alternative-therapies-types-and-uses-5207962_final-406a673fa76e41d9add8ce4771222dd0.png.

Test Your Knowledge

1. What are the common classes of non-opioid analgesics, and how do they relieve pain at the molecular and cellular levels?
2. What are the advantages and limitations of non-opioid analgesics compared to opioid medications in pain management?

9.4. Role of Healthcare Professionals

Learning Outcome

1. Pain specialists and their functions
2. Importance of interdisciplinary teams
3. Patient education and self-management strategies

The role of healthcare professionals in effective pain management is multifaceted and vital to patient comfort and quality of life. Practitioners such as physicians, nurses, and pharmacists require a broad knowledge base of pain mechanisms and the many treatment modalities. Each professional has a unique role in developing an integrated pain management plan, often in collaboration with others to tailor intervention based on patient assessment. It is crucial that these professionals continue to be familiar with the latest guidelines and best evidence in pain management, such as those emerging from systematic reviews, in order to enhance the safety and effectiveness of care provided to patients in pain.

The importance of compliance with strict reporting guidelines, as described in the PRISMA 2020 statement, cannot be overstated, as they provide transparency and replicability in clinical practice, which is important for pain management (Matthew et al., 2021). For complex patients, such as those with advanced dementia, healthcare professionals have some issues to address, particularly when assessing pain efficiently. Evidence suggests that advanced dementia patients are more likely to have pain poorly managed due to difficulties of communication and the inability to measure their level of pain accurately. The registered nurses, who are primarily responsible for controlling the pain in such patients, report various difficulties, including distinguishing between pain symptoms and emotional distress, and controlling medication. Additionally, involvement of family members in this challenge is equally important since they can have an instrumental role in explaining patients' pain behavior and implementing appropriate interventions. Therefore, enhancing communication skills and relational rapport among patients' families and the healthcare team is essential to improving overall pain management practice (Lundin et al., 2021). Additionally, the incorporation of specialized education for health professionals is essential for addressing the nuances of pain care, especially among high-risk populations. As the paradigm for pain care continues to shift, it becomes for all patients. In response, health organizations need to invest in ongoing education and the integration of best practices in palliative and geriatric care. Specifically, increasing nurses' competence in pain assessment and intervention can lead to better patient outcomes, especially when complex dementia is a concern, such as in nursing homes. With healthcare systems working to increase quality care, ensuring health professionals receive the latest recent studies and training will be instrumental in increasing their role as trained patient advocates for individuals in pain (Lundin et al., 2021).

9.4.1. Pain Specialists and Their Functions

One of the core components of quality pain care, pain specialists are medical doctors who diagnose and treat various pain disorders. Pain specialists are a team of medical doctors who consist mainly of anesthesiologists, physiatrists, neurologists, and rheumatologists, each with their own set of skills and areas of expertise in pain management. This multidisciplinary approach enables pain clinicians to develop comprehensive treatment plans that may involve medication, physical therapy, psychological therapy, and more complicated interventional techniques. The interprofessional practice ensures greater holistic care of patients with chronic and acute pain, taking into consideration the significance of an advanced understanding of the biopsychosocial determinants causing pain experiences. One of the functions of pain specialists is to conduct thorough pain evaluations in order to diagnose the underlying causes properly. Using standardized evaluation protocols and patient histories, specialists can determine the underlying cause of pain, thereby enabling them to tailor treatment. For instance, a prescriptive intervention involving customized foot orthoses (CFOs) to control foot pain can be a significant intervention (Leach et al., 2024). Furthermore, pain specialists must consider patients' specific circumstances, i.e., psychological state and lifestyle, when developing treatment plans. The integrative assessment process is a significant function of pain specialists in maximizing patient outcomes and minimizing the risk of treatment-related complications. The other significant function of pain specialists is the implementation of new strategies for the management of pain, including integrating complementary strategy. For example, evidence has shown that combining physiotherapy with modalities such as transcutaneous electrical nerve stimulation (TENS) significantly reduces postoperative pain, underscoring the value of interdisciplinary pain management (Pilch et al., 2024). Pain specialists can use such data to further evidence-based practice and enhance patient education regarding the latest treatment modalities. Their pain management abilities not only address bodily pain but also provide a platform where patients are engaged in their recovery process, eventually helping them manage their pain effectively (Figure 9.9).

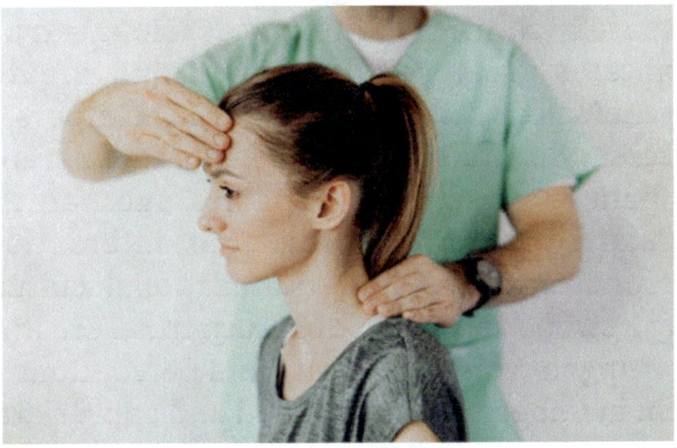

Figure 9.9. Pain specialists and their functions.

Source: https://irp.cdn-website.com/afe9686a/dms3rep/multi/Capture-16c49c19.PNG.

9.4.2. Importance of Interdisciplinary Teams

Pain management, particularly chronic pain management, can be effectively enhanced by interdisciplinary teams comprising a multidisciplinary range of health professionals. Pain management is multifaceted and requires consultation with various disciplines, such as doctors, nurses, psychologists, and physiotherapists. Interdisciplinary teams leverage each team member's multidisciplinary expertise to address patients' multi-dimensional needs and integrate medical, psychological, and social interventions to achieve the best possible results. Within a decentralized care environment, in which chronic pain often involves emotional and psychological components, synclinality among different perspectives fosters an integrated patient-centered approach. By emphasizing collaboration, interprofessional teams can create tailored treatment plans that address all facets of a patient's life, thereby improving the overall quality of care and patient satisfaction. Interprofessional trust is essential for effective interdisciplinary team practice in pain management. Trust is the basis of collaboration, on which healthcare professionals feel secure enough to share information, knowledge, and resources. As research confirms, interprofessional trust facilitates greater collaboration and greater psychological safety among team members, a necessary characteristic in a field as vulnerable as pain management. Variables such as the regularity of interprofessional interaction, personal attitude, and organizational culture play a strong role in building such trust. Creating a setting in which the values and perceptions of team members are understood and appreciated not only raises job satisfaction but also improves teamwork effectiveness, ultimately resulting in better patient welfare and safety in pain management practices (Corbaz-Kurth et al., 2025). Interdisciplinary pain management education programs are essential for the evolution of strong collaborative healthcare practice. These programs offer the prospects of knowledge exchange and skill development between disciplines and allow members to address the complex biopsychosocial aspects of chronic pain. Research highlighted the process of formulating such training programs with input from multidisciplinary expert groups that can identify barriers and the individual skills necessary for integrated pain management approaches (Munneke et al., 2024). Joint development of these training programs results in a more capable workforce for delivering integrated care. Through interdisciplinary training, healthcare systems can establish a multidisciplinary culture that ultimately enhances the quality of care and brings professionals together for a common patient-centered goal under the banner of pain management.

9.4.3. Patient Education and Self-Management Strategies

Proper patient education is paramount in maximizing pain control through self-manageable techniques. Awareness of the character of their pain allows patients to become active participants in the management plans. Education allows patients to recognize pain precipitants, utilize coping mechanisms, and adhere to treatments as prescribed. In addition, by delivering concise and informative information and communication on pain management options, patients are more likely to be included in their care. This interaction encourages autonomy over their condition, which has been demonstrated to enhance overall well-being and satisfaction with treatment. Including learning activities enables healthcare providers to ensure that patients are well-informed regarding their condition and therapy options, consequently eliminating fear of the unknown and encouraging adherence to management plans. Self-management behaviors, like developing individualized pain management plans, are the key to empowering patients. These plans may incorporate the utilization of a number of approaches, such as physical therapy, management of a medication regimen, and alternative approaches, such as yoga or mindfulness. If patients understand how these approaches work separately and in combination, they are most likely to use them appropriately. The incorporation of technology, such as mobile apps for pain monitoring, can further enhance self-management by allowing patients to track their symptoms and identify patterns that inform treatment adjustments. These proactive strategies enable patients to observe their improvement and to reshape their management plans as necessary, learn how to cope with chronic pain, and promote long-term adherence to self-management practices. Additionally, regular monitoring of patient improvement is critical in maximizing self-management practices. Healthcare professionals must provide regular communication with patients, emphasizing the benefit of frequent follow-ups to measure the effectiveness of pain management practices. This cooperative approach not only strengthens the pedagogic aspects of treatment but also allows for much-needed specification of evolving pain experiences. Additionally, addressing such a problem as workplace stress, which affects quality of life and care behavior negatively, is of paramount significance in a health care setting (Babapour et al., 2022). By recognizing these dynamics and incorporating patient feedback, health care providers can create a more comprehensive, user-oriented model for managing pain, ultimately leading to improved patient outcomes and satisfaction.

Test Your Knowledge

1. How do healthcare professionals educate patients to promote self-management of chronic conditions, and why is this important for improving health outcomes?
2. What strategies and tools can patients use to effectively manage their health, and how do healthcare providers support their implementation?

9.5. Challenges in Pain Management

Learning Outcome

1. Opioid crisis and its implications
2. Variability in patient responses to treatment
3. Barriers to effective pain management

The pain management industry is plagued by a variety of challenges that can render possible positive treatment results moot. Included among these is the multifaceted nature of pain, which can be acute or chronic and varies significantly from person to person. Those variables of the character of the injury, psychological status, and pre-existing medical conditions contribute to the subjective experience of the pain and complicate the creation of a single treatment approach for all by medical professionals. The challenge is exacerbated by the differences in the experience of pain based on demographic variation, including age and culture. Besides, the increasing chronic pain burden in older individuals magnifies the need for customized interventions that take into account diverse patient needs because muscle function is lost during aging. Physical inactivity prevail (Míkel et al., 2021). As such, clinicians must contend with a multifaceted backdrop as they strive to implement successful pain management strategies. The second fundamental challenge of pain management occurs in the realm of pharmacological treatment, namely, the risk of opioid use. As potent as they have been in managing acute pain, opioids have proven to be a factor in an increase in addiction and overdose rates, prompting a sober reappraisal of their role in treatment protocols. The opioid epidemic has led to the adoption of other ways of pain control, including the use of non-opioid analgesics, regional blocks, and multimodal regimens that include more than one therapeutic modality (Chin et al., 2021). It is not without its challenges, however. Physicians must balance the need for pain control against the risk of addiction and side effects, requiring ongoing research and education to establish long-term and safe alternatives for pain relief that do not involve opioids. Additionally, the adoption of innovative pain management techniques is frequently constrained by organizational barriers, including limited access to care and variation in healthcare providers' training. For instance, regional anesthesia has been demonstrated to be an effective technique in reducing systemic use of opioids and improving postoperative recovery, but has not been utilized adequately in the majority of clinical practices due to variations in practitioner skill and insufficiency in exposure to novel techniques (Chin et al., 2021). The increasing complexity of pain management necessitates that healthcare systems innovate to address these deficiencies, providing practitioners with training in novel pain-relief techniques and encouraging patient access to comprehensive pain management services. These systemic challenges must be addressed to improve patients' health outcomes and to develop a humane, effective strategy for pain management (Figure 9.10).

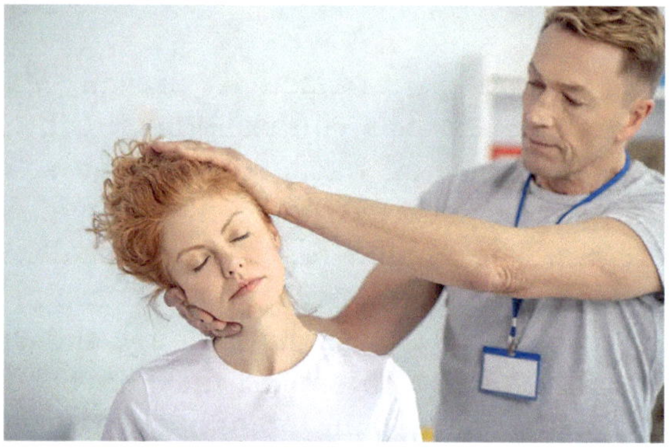

Figure 9.10. The field of pain management is fraught with a multitude of challenges.

Source: https://www.outsourcestrategies.com/wp-content/uploads/2024/10/navigating-pain-management-billing-coding.webp.

9.5.1. Opioid Crisis and Its Implications

The United States opioid epidemic is a complex public health problem characterized by an unprecedented increase in prescription and misuse of opioid medications. Initially being touted for their efficacy in pain relief, opioids have brought about extensive addiction and overdose mortality, transforming practices in pain management in medical institutions. It requires an integrative vision to grasp the consequences of this crisis, one that not only considers the biological origins of addiction but also the socioeconomic factors underlying its dissemination. Patients with chronic pain, once relying on opioids for succor, are now being subjected to harsh regulation and a shift toward non-opioid treatment. As medical professionals navigate this landscape, they are forced to weigh the need for effective pain relief against the necessity of minimizing the harms of opioid therapy, moving pain management into an increasingly cautious and informed profession. The effect of the opioid epidemic is not limited to personal health but extends into public health infrastructure and economic systems. Increased healthcare spending is derived from the treatment of addiction to opioids, complication management, and mental health interventions for individuals who have been impacted. Opioid overdose patients inundate emergency departments with intensive use of resources in acute states that could have been avoided had intervention occurred sooner and education been offered. In addition, stigma associated with dependence on opioids also discourages individuals from seeking help, hence perpetuating the disease and addiction process. This health crisis calls for the full extent of policy interventions, including the roll-out of public health campaigns among healthcare practitioners and patients alike. Additional training in pain management and prescribing practices is crucial, so that future generations of doctors can effectively treat pain at minimal risk of opioid treatment. As the healthcare setting evolves to the opioid crisis, attention turns to developing alternative pain management practices. Non-opioid drugs, including NSAIDs, antidepressants, and analgesics, represent possible options for pain control without risking the vices of opioid dependence. Alongside this, integrative therapies, including physical therapy, acupuncture, and cognitive-behavioral therapy, are proving useful components of an integrated pain management protocol. Assessment of such alternatives is central to addressing the needs of chronically painful patients while reducing opioid dependency. Research into new therapies and the role of multidisciplinary care teams are central to creating holistic pain management programs that prioritize patient safety and long-term well-being. Through these combined efforts, the health implications of the opioid epidemic can be appropriately addressed, paving the way to a more sustainable approach to pain management (Figure 9.11).

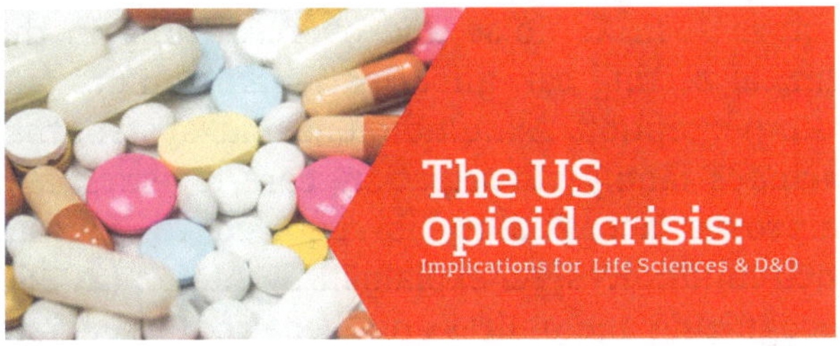

Figure 9.11. The opioid crisis in the United States represents a complex public health challenge.

Source: https://media.licdn.com/dms/image/v2/C4D12AQGsQb8YM1KVVA/article-cover_image-shrink_720_1280/article-cover_image-shrink_720_1280/0/1593090439715?e=2147483647&v=beta&t=cvW2UPymTnlkDIlZodm_FbtoFwNMEzeVnBxa_KGh2Q0.

9.5.2. Variability in Patient Responses to Treatment

Variability in patient response to treatment is a core aspect of pain management that health practitioners must address if maximum therapeutic results are to be realized. Patients may react variably to pain management therapy as a function of an infinite number of factors, such as gene pool, environmental factors, and comorbidities. A case in point is pharmacogenomics— the study of how genes affect an individual's response to drugs—whose role is crucial in tailoring pain management treatments. Metabolic pathway differences can lead to varied responses to a single drug, underscoring the need for patient-specific treatment approaches that account for individual characteristics. The necessity of this patient-specific treatment method is emphasized in recent guidelines, which suggest individualized approaches based on patient-specific features to improve intervention efficiency in pain management and patient satisfaction (Williams et al., 2018). In addition to biological factors, psychological factors also contribute importantly to the impact of pain management treatment efficacy. Patients' beliefs and attitudes toward pain, treatment, and their contributions to healing can modulate their response to various therapies. Cognitive-behavioral approaches can be used to counteract unpleasant thoughts and behaviors, ultimately enhancing compliance and outcomes. Also, affective states such as depression and anxiety can be responsible for pain intensification as well as undermining the success of treatment. This necessitates comprehensive evaluations that involve both the psychological and the physical. The combination of mental health care with medication, healthcare professionals may observe heightened sensitivity to pain management interventions, resulting in improved quality of life in patients (Keith et al., 2018). Lastly, my social determinants of health cause variation in patients' responses to treatment. Socioeconomic status, access, and beliefs about pain and treatment can hinder or advance successful pain management. As an example, individuals of lower socioeconomic status may have even greater obstacles to contend with, such as poor insurance or lack of ability to see a specialist, that add to their pain problems and hinder successful pain management. Moreover, the effect of cultural beliefs on the experience of pain is a significant consideration in treatment adherence and long-term prognosis. Understanding these social contexts is essential for healthcare workers, as integrating knowledge of patients' backgrounds can lead to more equitable and effective pain management interventions. Coordination of these different factors not only enhances clinical effectiveness but also enables patient-centered care in pain management (Williams et al., 2018).

9.5.3. Barriers to Effective Pain Management

Breaking through the barriers to effective pain treatment is significant in the broader context of patient care, given the multi-dimensional aspects of pain experience and response. One of the most significant barriers may be the absence of adequate provider knowledge and education, which can lead to the misapplication of pain measurement and inadequate treatment regimens. Nurses and healthcare professionals are critical advocates of pain control, but most are not fully trained to use pain management methods. This disparity not only affects patient outcomes but also underscores the need for recurrent education programs focused on an integrative understanding of pain. As Salameh et al. (2025) have argued, more knowledge about pain management is essential to facilitating an empathic care approach, which can ultimately improve patient satisfaction and recovery trajectories. Organizational and structural obstacles in the healthcare environment also further complicate efforts at pain management. Most clinical environments are likely to lack policy or resources to implement comprehensive pain management protocols. Such shortcomings can take many forms, including inappropriate medications for pain relief, suboptimal staff-to-patient ratios, and insufficient availability of interdisciplinary teams of care providers. Moreover, communication deficits and hierarchical barriers typically impede the sharing of information about significant patients' pain experiences, thereby limiting effective management strategies. Correction of these organizational limitations is imperative to enable healthcare professionals to deliver effective pain relief and develop a setting conducive to active pain management programs, according to Atefeh (2025). Besides, personal and contextual variables are of paramount importance for the barriers against effective pain management. Parents' concerns and myths regarding pain medication among children may result in treatment avoidance, thereby exacerbating the pain process. Technical problems, including difficulties accessing appropriate equipment for pain control or communication aids, can hinder prompt pain relief. In addition, environmental factors such as noise and overcrowding in the clinical setting can affect patients' comfort and pain perception. A multidimensional system that includes family participation, care logistics, and improved accessibility is required to address such hindrances. As explained by Atefeh (2025), recognizing and addressing these contextual and personal factors can enhance the performance of pain management tactics, leading to better patient outcomes and quality of care (Figure 9.12).

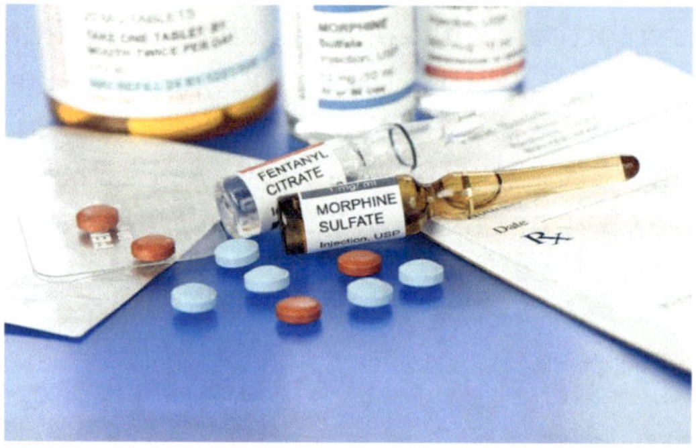

Figure 9.12. The barriers to effective pain management.

Source: https://www.drjimcollins.com/wp-content/uploads/2020/02/2020-03-30-Barriers-to-Effective-Pain-Management-in-Senior-Care-770x500.jpg.

Test Your Knowledge

1. What are the main challenges in managing pain effectively while minimizing the risks associated with opioid use?
2. How has the opioid crisis affected clinical pain management practices, and what strategies are being implemented to address its public health implications?

9.6. Future Directions in Pain Management

Learning Outcome

1. Advances in pain research
2. Emerging technologies (e.g., neuromodulation)
3. Personalized medicine approaches

The evolving pain management landscape is increasingly technology- and data-analytics-driven. Among the most important aspects of future pain management are the use of big data and the Internet of Things (IoT). With wearable technology and smart devices tracking patients' vitals and pain intensity in real-time, medical professionals can offer personalized treatment plans that adjust based on patients' responses. This technology not only optimizes greater effective pain relief but also enhances patient activation by allowing patients to participate in their care process actively. As clinicians embrace evidence-based practices, they can recognize trends and patterns that facilitate easier and better chronic pain management and overall patient safety, thereby revolutionizing traditional care models. Moreover, advances in cloud computing are creating new opportunities for collaborative care in pain management. The ability to store and process large amounts of patient data in the cloud safely enables healthcare providers to access integrated health records, including prior pain management history. Having a unified perspective on data is essential for medical professionals determined to deliver interventions tailored to the uniqueness of individual patients, according to recent studies emphasizing the need for precision medicine. In this regard, the Global Burden of Diseases, Injuries, and Risk Factors Study (GBD) has an important role in providing evidence-based data that can inform public health programs and ultimately help practitioners make more informed decisions regarding pain management practices (Alize et al., 2024). In the near future, pain management will also prioritize multidisciplinary care that incorporates mental health and integrative therapies. Knowledge of the biopsychosocial model of pain will be essential, recognizing that pain management extends beyond pharmacological treatment. Incorporating psychological counseling and alternative therapies, such as mindfulness and cognitive-behavioral therapy, will help identify the emotional and cognitive components of pain and foster multidisciplinary healing. Future research will need to examine the potential benefits of such interventions in an IoT-enabled context, where real-time monitoring and feedback systems enhance adherence to therapy. With new strategies coming forward, concerns such as ensuring patient privacy and security in digital healthcare solutions also need to be addressed so that patients develop trust in new health technologies and applications (Dang et al., 2019).

9.6.1. Advances in Pain Research

Research in pain management has made significant advances, changing the approaches to pain relief at its very foundation. The reliance on opioids has traditionally marked conventional management of pain. In contrast, modern pain management strategies emphasize an interdisciplinary approach involving the amalgamation of pharmacological and non-pharmacological practices. Existing evidence identifies several alternatives to the traditional opioid treatments such as tramadol and buprenorphine, which ensure effective relief of pain with decreased potential for opioid dependency. This evolution of pain treatment not only seeks to diminish pain but also to optimize patients' global quality of life, testifying to the value of holistic paradigms of care that resonate with the multicultural essence of pain itself, highlighted in recent literature (Bashir, 2023). Also, advancing knowledge of the neurobiological mechanisms that drive pain has fueled new paradigms of treatment.

For instance, improvements in interventional therapies, such as nerve blocks and spinal cord stimulation, represent an outstanding step towards more targeted and effective pain relief treatments. Such improvements allow doctors to tailor treatments to specific patients based on their pain profiles, thereby enhancing effectiveness and safety. Moreover, the use of cognitive-behavioral therapy and physical rehabilitation in pain treatment protocols demonstrates an integrated stance towards pain management, recognizing the psychological and social dimensions of pain. This multidimensional model is supported by ongoing research into these dynamic approaches, with an emphasis on patient-focused pain management (Bashir, 2023).

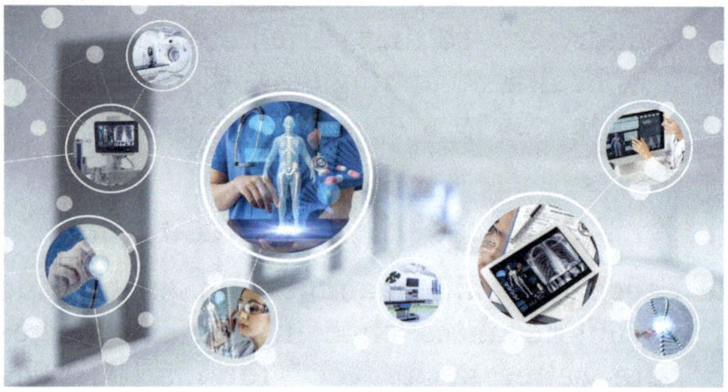

Figure 9.13. Research in the field of pain management has witnessed significant advancements.

Source: https://i0.wp.com/pswordpress-production.s3.amazonaws.com/2020/08/AdobeStock_230968424-smaller.jpg?fit=1800%2C961&ssl=1.

The use of anesthesia in perioperative pain management reflects advances in pain relief approaches over recent years. With advances in more potent anesthetic medications and techniques, the specialty has improved the surgical experience for patients. Improvements in perioperative analgesia emphasize pain relief not only during surgery but also during postoperative recovery. Both analgesia and anesthesia have therefore been emphasized, leading to improved patient outcomes and satisfaction by relieving pain shortly after surgical procedures. Research in the area continues to yield valuable insights into the effectiveness of modern anesthetic approaches and their role in facilitating pain control in therapeutic settings. Ultimately, such improvements welcome a new era for tailored pain management treatments, where not only is pain treated rightfully, but it is also effectively done, in order to improve overall perioperative management of the patient (Figure 9.13).

9.6.2. Emerging Technologies (E.g., Neuromodulation)

With advances in the field of pain management, new technologies such as neuromodulation are gaining importance for enhancing therapeutic outcomes. Neuromodulation refers to the controlled application of stimuli that alter nerve function, thereby modulating pain mechanisms in the nervous system. The technology encompasses a number of techniques, including spinal cord stimulation and peripheral nerve stimulation, which have shown promise in alleviating chronic pain conditions. These treatments, in providing a more focused approach to pain modulation, can significantly reduce reliance on opioids and other pain medications, frequently followed by catastrophic side effects. The integration of neuromodulation into treatment planning is a significant step toward individualized pain management strategies that improve patients' quality of life. In addition to neuromodulation, advances in biomarker discovery promise to revolutionize the definition and treatment of pain. The National Institutes of Health (NIH) has emphasized the importance of establishing objective biomarkers to enable the development of non-addictive therapeutics for pain treatment. Such biomarkers promise to enable different pain states to be classified by their individual pathophysiologic profiles, ultimately yielding more targeted and effective therapeutic strategies. NIH's Helping to End Addiction Long-term (HEAL) Initiative will support this discovery process by collaborating with industry leaders and academics. By focusing on rigorous validation, the initiative aims to accelerate research toward developing neurotherapeutics with the capacity to bring relief without the addictive liability of current pain medications, thus ending the escalating opioid crisis (Karen et al., 2020). Moreover, the synergy between neuromodulation and emerging technologies such as triboelectric nanogenerators (TENGs) offers promising avenues for pain management. The TENG technology has shown potential not only for energy harvesting but also for designing self-powered devices and sensors that can be integrated into wearable pain management systems. This can facilitate the development of smart systems that provide real-time monitoring and modulation of pain pathways. By harnessing the capabilities of TENG to make wearable, energy-efficient devices, clinicians can improve treatment adherence and patient engagement. As such technologies advance, how they will complement existing pain management processes will be critical in advancing towards an ever-more dynamic and responsive approach to managing chronic pain conditions in the future (Zhu et al., 2020) (Figure 9.14).

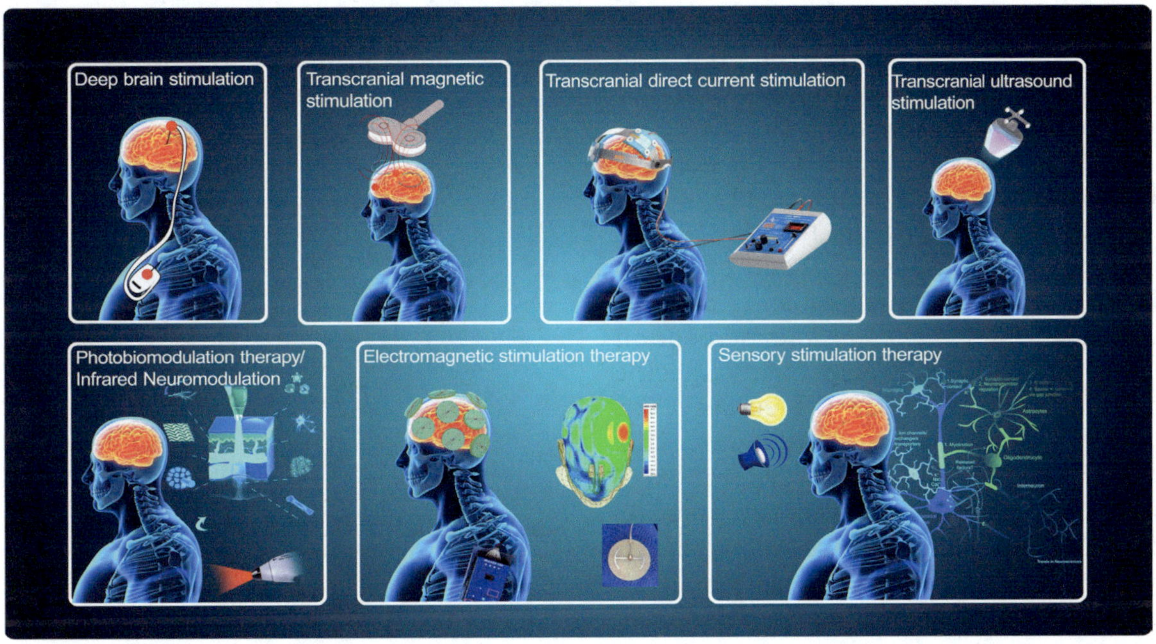

Figure 9.14. The landscape of pain management continues to evolve, emerging technologies.

Source: https://www.mdpi.com/cells/cells-14-00122/article_deploy/html/images/cells-14-00122-g002.png.

9.6.3. Personalized Medicine Approaches

The integration of personalized medicine strategies into pain treatment represents a significant paradigm shift in healthcare. To date, pain treatment methods have relied on a one-size-fits-all model, which often produces less-than-ideal outcomes in patients with heterogeneous response patterns to therapies. Personalized medicine seeks to address this issue by tailoring treatment plans to patient-specific attributes, including genetic profiles, environmental factors, and disease phenotypes.

In the management of pain, this approach can optimize the performance of interventions and minimize side effects, thereby enhancing overall patient quality of life. By applying data analysis and molecular stratification, medical practitioners can establish adaptive treatment regimens that closely fit the individual needs of each patient and set the stage for enhanced efficacy in treating chronic pain disorders and improving adherence to therapeutic measures. Moreover, personalized medicine embeds numerous new approaches with the potential to revolutionize pain therapy. For instance, pharmacogenomics, the investigation of how genes affect an individual's response to drugs, has proved invaluable in understanding how a patient metabolizes a medicine. This helps health practitioners provide the best painkillers for a patient according to his/her genetic predisposition, reducing the incidence of harsh side effects of conventional therapy. In addition, approaches such as biomarker discovery are establishing the foundations for personalized pain treatment that addresses the condition's underlying mechanisms. Specific biomarkers of pain response and perception are being targeted to develop highly specific therapies that can optimize the efficacy and safety of pain management regimens. This evolution foretells a possible incorporation of personalized therapies into everyday practice, thus making pain management as individualized as possible. The application of personalized medicine in pain management is particularly relevant to multimodal therapy involving multiple therapeutic modalities. Such a modality recognizes that pain relief is often achieved through a combination of pharmacologic and non-pharmacologic interventions, tailored to the patient's needs. For instance, the use of digital health technologies, such as wearable devices and mobile applications, can facilitate continuous monitoring of pain severity and treatment response, enabling timely dosage adjustments. Similarly, as with the management of diseases such as irritable bowel syndrome (IBS) and lung cancer pain, personalized medicine can entail the incorporation of genomic study insights to inform treatment. These advancements create an integrated system for pain management that not only alleviates suffering but also addresses the complexity of patient profile diversity, paving the way for further innovation in pain management principles (Figure 9.15).

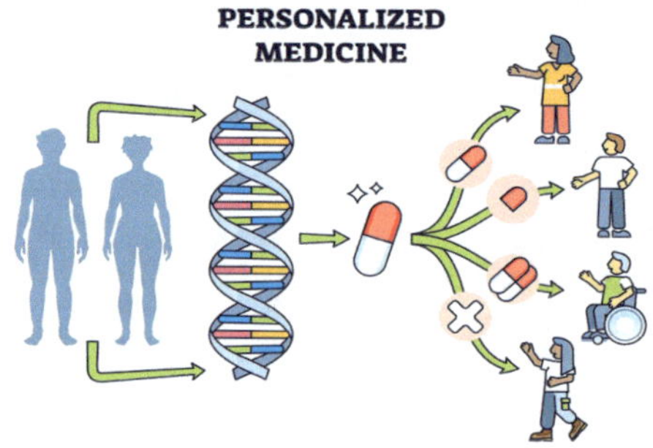

Figure 9.15. The integration of personalized medicine approaches.

Source: https://www.medznat.ru/uploads/images/post_content/7182/image_3/1690458980image_3.webp.

Test Your Knowledge

1. How can personalized medicine approaches improve the effectiveness and safety of pain management for individual patients?
2. What role do genetic, molecular, and patient-specific factors play in guiding future pain management strategies?

SUMMARY

Effective management of pain is a multifaceted process that requires an extensive understanding of various strategies and tools employed by medical professionals and patients. Effective management of pain begins with recognizing individualized patient needs and the various types of pain they may be exposed to. Individualized planning of pain management is important in maximizing patient outcomes and improving health. New technologies, such as smartphone apps, have been shown to have potential to increase self-management capacity among people with chronic pain, but further evidence is essential to ensure their effectiveness. The reality that limited apps present at the moment meet the needed quality indices demonstrates the necessity for continued investigation and development in the field (Devan et al., 2019). Furthermore, collective effort by patients, clinicians, and application developers can lead to more advanced tools tailored to address particular populations, cultural, and contextual factors in pain control. For instance, the lack of cultural competence in pain management applications today indicates a vital gap that must be addressed to enhance user interaction and performance. The capacity of smartphone apps to serve as interventions with scalability enables greater accessibility, but medical practitioners and users must be mindful of the boundaries of such devices. Thus, improving the quality of pain management apps can make a monumental contribution to the healthcare field as a whole if the apps are scientifically tested for clinical effectiveness (Joseph et al., 2017). It is, in the end, a conclusion that refers to complete and evidence-based practice fused with innovations by means of technology. Formulated on an individual basis and towards the evolving facets of treatment in research undertakings and self-management assistance, clinicians must develop strategies for pain management. By encouraging an integrative method of pain management grounded in knowledge built through clinical guidelines and patient experience, healthcare workers are better able to meet patients' needs and support healing. Combining these efforts will improve the overall face of pain management, ensuring that people in pain receive optimal quality of care and support tailored to their unique needs.

A good pain management strategy is critical in addressing the issues faced by patients with various kinds of pain, particularly in today's environment influenced by external drivers such as the COVID-19 pandemic. An appreciation for the complexity of pain—whether acute or chronic—requires a comprehensive approach that includes both pharmacological and non-pharmacological measures. Key components of pain management include assessment of pain intensity, emotional status, and the patient's overall health. Moreover, compliance of the patient with tailored treatment plans is important because patients arrive in unique combinations of pain, comorbid conditions, and lifestyle variables that drive their disease. With appropriate pain relief, patients can improve quality of life, and the integration of this component into health system management is thus emphasized (Appoh et al., 2025). The availability to apply nonsteroidal anti-inflammatory drugs (NSAIDs), including Nimesulide, indicates a pharmacological approach for managing musculoskeletal pain syndrome conditions, such as low back pain (LBP). Recent research shows a high prevalence of LBP, especially in patients with post-COVID-19, whose pain may be precipitated by various factors, including systemic. Nimesulide, which was also found to be effective in alleviating pain, has an acceptable safety and tolerability profile relative to other NSAIDs. However, its administration should be balanced against the risk of drug interaction with the presence of other concomitant drugs and comorbid medical illnesses. Hence, careful consideration of patients' histories is necessary to minimize risks and enhance treatment outcomes (Kamchatnov et al., 2022). Beyond pharmaceutical interventions, the adoption of innovative human resource technologies in practice in pain management can improve the quality of the patient experience. Certain technologies, such as data analytics for predictive modeling and AI-based platforms, can help personalize interventions to better cater to the unique needs of individual patients. By applying these advances, practitioners can facilitate medication management, improve patient education, and facilitate increased compliance with treatment regimens. Virtual reality simulations can also serve as adjunct therapy for pain management by providing immersive experiences that distract and inform patients about their pain conditions. Lastly, adopting a holistic, tech-inclined approach to managing pain will enable better outcomes and enhanced patient satisfaction, again highlighting the necessary imperative to treat both the biological and psychosocial aspects of pain (Appoh et al., 2025).

KEY TERMS FROM THIS CHAPTER

- Acceptance and commitment therapy (ACT)
- Chronic low back pain (CLBP)
- Communication
- Holistic approach
- Non-steroidal anti-inflammatory drugs (NSAIDs)
- Pain self-management (PSM)
- Central nervous system (CNS)
- Cognitive-behavioral therapy (CBT)
- Disability
- Musculoskeletal disorders
- Pain management
- Pharmacological landscape

CRITICAL THINKING QUESTIONS

1. Which of the following drugs is most commonly used for Patient-Controlled Analgesia (PCA)?

a. Midazolam

b. Fentanyl

c. Ketorolac

d. Morphine

2. What is the primary advantage of multimodal analgesia?

a. Reduced surgery time

b. Elimination of opioid use

c. Improved renal function

d. Enhanced pain control with fewer side effects

3. Which receptor is primarily responsible for the analgesic effect of opioids?

a. GABA-A

b. NMDA

c. Mu (μ) opioid receptor

d. Alpha-2 adrenergic receptor

4. Which of the following is an advantage of using regional anesthesia for postoperative pain?

a. Increased risk of systemic side effects

b. Delayed ambulation

c. Reduced need for systemic opioids

d. Increased sedation

5. Ketamine produces analgesia primarily through antagonism of which receptor?

a. AMPA

b. Mu opioid

c. GABA

d. NMDA

Short Answer Questions

1. Describe the physiological mechanisms of pain perception and modulation. How do anesthetic agents interfere with pain pathways at different levels of the nervous system?
2. Compare and contrast the pharmacology, indications, and side effects of opioids and non-opioid analgesics used in anesthesia.
3. Discuss the principles of multimodal analgesia in perioperative care.
4. Explain the role of regional anesthesia techniques (e.g., spinal, epidural, nerve blocks) in perioperative pain management.
5. Evaluate the risks and benefits of Patient-Controlled Analgesia (PCA).

Answer to Critical Thinking Questions

1. (d); 2. (d); 3. (c); 4. (c); 5. (d)

REFERENCES

1. Abd-Elsayed, A., Kurt, E., Kollenburg, L., Hasoon, J., Wahezi, S. E., & Storlie, N. R. (2025). Lumbar multifidus dysfunction and Chronic low back pain: overview, therapies, and an update on the evidence. *Pain Practice, 25*(5), e70044. https://doi.org/10.1111/papr.70044
2. Copy to clipboardAbdullah, S., Al Saloum, A., Qadim, K., Alshammari, Z., Farhan, F., Albanaqi, R., Tawfiq, N., et al. (2024). Pain management beyond pills: The physiotherapist-nurse dynamic in non-pharmacological interventions. *Power System Technology.* https://www.semanticscholar.org/paper/22e68307fcddff071076bd66bfcd53fe228a7cbf (accessed on 28th June 2025).
3. AL Zahrani, A. S. (2023). The role of anesthesia in pain management: Advancements in perioperative analgesia. *Journal of Medical Science and Clinical Research.* https://www.semanticscholar.org/paper/0cc94f9f605d4b2b8b0c625efcbba3ab1fec63ea (accessed on 28th June 2025).
4. Andrejić, N., Božović, I., Moradi, H., Tataei, R., & Knezevic, N. (2025). Neuropathic pain management: A focused review of current treatments and novel data from main ongoing clinical trials. *Expert Opinion on Investigational Drugs, 34*, 287–299. https://www.semanticscholar.org/paper/4733ba8ffedc3900e72f45fb5a293702ce87d974 (accessed on 28th June 2025).
5. Appoh, M., Gobile, S., Alabi, O. A., & Oboyi, N. (2025). Innovative HR technologies: Transforming expatriate management and immigration services for the 21st century. *International Journal of Multidisciplinary Research and Growth Evaluation.* https://www.semanticscholar.org/paper/9b560ec032b8575c5fdba4dafb81a01b564be4a3 (accessed on 28th June 2025).
6. Atefeh, S. (2025). Barriers and facilitators of pain management in children: A scoping review. *BMC Anesthesiology, 25.* https://www.semanticscholar.org/paper/abd94a664f89130307ae4ed05fc5a4360d3b1bed (accessed on 28th June 2025).
7. Babapour, A. R., Gahassab-Mozaffari, N., & Fathnezhad-Kazemi, A. (2022). Nurses' job stress and its impact on quality of life and caring behaviors: A cross-sectional study. *BMC Nursing, 21.* https://doi.org/10.1186/s12912-022-00852-y (accessed on 28th June 2025).
8. Bashir, M. K. (2023). Recent advances in pain management. *medtigo Journal of Medicine.* https://www.semanticscholar.org/paper/1ca33b64af62ec655113b205717e035358696739 (accessed on 28th June 2025).
9. Bentley, G. (2007). Repair and regeneration of ligaments, tendons and joint capsule. *Annals of The Royal College of Surgeons of England, 89*, 329–330. https://www.semanticscholar.org/paper/3fe21e5a329697eee2fa08132bd9e1e33d9e5745 (accessed on 28th June 2025).
10. Buchbinder, R., Underwood, M., Hartvigsen, J., & Maher, C. G. (2020). The Lancet Series call to action to reduce low value care for low back pain: An update. *Pain, 161*, S57–S64. https://doi.org/10.1097/j.pain.0000000000001869 (accessed on 28th June 2025).
11. Burnett, A. L., Nehra, A., Breau, R. H., Culkin, D. J., Faraday, M. M., Hakim, L., Heidelbaugh, J. J., et al. (2018). Erectile dysfunction: AUA guideline. *The Journal of Urology, 200*, 633–641. https://doi.org/10.1016/j.juro.2018.05.004 (accessed on 28th June 2025).
12. Carmichael, J. C., Keller, D. S., Baldini, G., Bordeianou, L., Weiss, E. G., Lee, L., Boutros, M., et al. (2017). Clinical practice guidelines for enhanced recovery after colon and rectal surgery from the American Society of Colon and Rectal Surgeons and Society of American

Gastrointestinal and Endoscopic Surgeons. *Diseases of the Colon & Rectum, 60*, 761–784. https://doi.org/10.1097/dcr.0000000000000883 (accessed on 28th June 2025).

13. Chin, K. J., Mariano, E. R., & El-Boghdadly, K. (2021). Advancing towards the next frontier in regional anesthesia. *Anesthesia, 76*, 3–7. https://doi.org/10.1111/anae.15321 (accessed on 28th June 2025).

14. Corbaz-Kurth, S., Weissbrodt, R., Juvet, T., Hannart, S., Krsmanovic, B., Salamin Plaschy, I., & Terrier, P. (2025). How does trust emerge in interprofessional collaboration? A qualitative study of the significance, importance, and dynamics of trust in healthcare teams and networks. *Journal of Interprofessional Care.* https://www.semanticscholar.org/paper/5717fdcba767130fabe5a7cc214ee192dd5477cd (accessed on 28th June 2025).

15. Cox, N., Mallen, C. D., & Scott, I. C. (2025). Pharmacological pain management in patients with rheumatoid arthritis: A narrative literature review. *BMC Medicine, 23.* https://www.semanticscholar.org/paper/c0895a91516ff64477e2f68f443bf2f5196b0a20 (accessed on 28th June 2025).

16. Dang, L. M., Piran, M. J., Han, D., Min, K., & Moon, H. (2019). A survey on Internet of Things and cloud computing for healthcare. *Electronics, 8*, 768. https://doi.org/10.3390/electronics8070768 (accessed on 28th June 2025).

17. Davis, K. D., Aghaeepour, N., Ahn, A. H., Angst, M. S., Borsook, D., Brenton, A., Burczynski, M. E., et al. (2020). Discovery and validation of biomarkers to aid the development of safe and effective pain therapeutics: Challenges and opportunities. *Nature Reviews Neurology, 16*, 381–400. https://doi.org/10.1038/s41582-020-0362-2 (accessed on 28th June 2025).

18. Day, M., Ciol, M. A., Mendoza, M. E., Borckardt, J., Ehde, D., Newman, A. K., Chan, J., et al. (2024). The effects of telehealth-delivered mindfulness meditation, cognitive therapy, and behavioral activation for chronic low back pain: A randomized clinical trial. *BMC Medicine, 22.* https://www.semanticscholar.org/paper/01e183c4876bc8b44117df3f39ac82e56fe448e2 (accessed on 28th June 2025).

19. de Souza, D. N., Lorentz, N. A., Charalambous, L. T., Galetta, M., Petrilli, C. A., & Rozell, J. (2024). Comprehensive pain management in total joint arthroplasty: A review of contemporary approaches. *Journal of Clinical Medicine, 13.* https://www.semanticscholar.org/paper/e23d3d2c9fac9a9aa1ac32c3f525ecda60c914d0 (accessed on 28th June 2025).

20. Devan, H., Farmery, D., Peebles, L., & Grainger, R. (2019). Evaluation of self-management support functions in apps for people with persistent pain: Systematic review. *JMIR mHealth and uHealth, 7*, e13080–e13080. https://doi.org/10.2196/13080 (accessed on 28th June 2025).

21. El-Tallawy, S. N., Nalamasu, R., Salem, G. I., LeQuang, J. A., Pergolizzi, J. V., & Christo, P. J. (2021). Management of musculoskeletal pain: An update with emphasis on chronic musculoskeletal pain. *Pain and Therapy, 10*, 181–209. https://doi.org/10.1007/s40122-021-00235-2 (accessed on 28th June 2025).

22. Erickson, S., & Sturdy, L. (2023). The language of medical terminology II. https://doi.org/10.29173/oer43 (accessed on 28th June 2025).

23. Ferrari, A. J., Santomauro, D., Aali, A., Abate, Y. H., Abbafati, C., Abbastabar, H., Abd ElHafeez, S., et al. (2024). Global incidence, prevalence, years lived with disability (YLDs), disability-adjusted life-years (DALYs), and healthy life expectancy (HALE) for 371 diseases and injuries in 204 countries and territories and 811 subnational locations, 1990–2021: A systematic

analysis for the Global Burden of Disease Study 2021. *The Lancet, 403*, 2133–2161. https://doi.org/10.1016/s0140-6736(24)00757-8 (accessed on 28th June 2025).

24. Hwang, W. (2025). Evolution of pain management in lung cancer surgery: From opioid-based to personalized analgesia. *Anesthesia and Pain Medicine, 20*, 109–120. https://www.semanticscholar.org/paper/d9584d4ee8bb52ff9ce2a87d2a00876460254e71 (accessed on 28th June 2025).
25. Izquierdo, M., Merchant, R. A., Morley, J. E., Anker, S. D., Aprahamian, I., Arai, H., Aubertin-Leheudre, M., et al. (2021). International exercise recommendations in older adults (ICFSR): Expert consensus guidelines. *The Journal of Nutrition Health & Aging, 25*, 824–853. https://doi.org/10.1007/s12603-021-1665-8 (accessed on 28th June 2025).
26. Jurayev, K., & Akhmadjonov, U. (2025). Treatment and prevention of acute suppurative otitis media. *The American Journal of Medical Sciences and Pharmaceutical Research.* https://www.semanticscholar.org/paper/f5462c0daf0caea00f9e67d6d4bae9800c72e9a0 (accessed on 28th June 2025).
27. Kamchatnov, P., & Chugunov, A. V. (2022). Management of patients with musculoskeletal pain syndrome during COVID-19 pandemic. *Doctor.Ru.* https://www.semanticscholar.org/paper/54a68ec65792e4657a861aef02d890c2cbf8548c (accessed on 28th June 2025).
28. Khalid, S. I., Veludandi, N., Agwu, C., & Slavin, K. V. (2025). Altius electrical nerve stimulation for post-amputation pain treatment: A comprehensive review. *Pain Management.* https://www.semanticscholar.org/paper/6c4bdc80000e62e260e8ddde8ab7f7d16a43c9c4 (accessed on 28th June 2025).
29. Kharb, D., Kharb, P., Jawaid, S., & Singh, A. (2025). Innovative approaches in managing irritable bowel syndrome: From personalized medicine to gut microbiome therapies. *International Journal of Health Sciences and Research.* https://www.semanticscholar.org/paper/6cc0e3248a32f69e8f00be334f3ed5d739b5b36c (accessed on 28th June 2025).
30. Koo, J., Lim, C., & Oh, K. T. (2024). Recent advances in intranasal administration for brain-targeting delivery: A comprehensive review of lipid-based nanoparticles and stimuli-responsive gel formulations. *International Journal of Nanomedicine, 19*, 1767–1807. https://doi.org/10.2147/ijn.s439181 (accessed on 28th June 2025).
31. Leach, E., Cowley, E., & Bowen, C. (2024). The experiences of podiatrists prescribing custom foot orthoses and patients using custom foot orthoses for foot pain management in the United Kingdom: A focus group study. *Journal of Foot and Ankle Research, 17.* https://www.semanticscholar.org/paper/11df17e65e13f0ec8bed1bf02a34d26d40e3337f (accessed on 28th June 2025).
32. LeBoff, M. S., Greenspan, S. L., Insogna, K., Lewiecki, E. M., Saag, K. G., Singer, A., & Siris, E. S. (2022). The clinician's guide to prevention and treatment of osteoporosis. *Osteoporosis International, 33*, 2049–2102. https://doi.org/10.1007/s00198-021-05900-y (accessed on 28th June 2025).
33. Lindor, K. D., Bowlus, C. L., Boyer, J. L., Levy, C., & Mayo, M. J. (2018). Primary biliary cholangitis: 2018 practice guidance from the American Association for the Study of Liver Diseases. *Hepatology, 69*, 394–419. https://doi.org/10.1002/hep.30145 (accessed on 28th June 2025).

34. Lundin, E., & Godskesen, T. (2021). End-of-life care for people with advanced dementia and pain: A qualitative study in Swedish nursing homes. *BMC Nursing, 20.* https://doi.org/10.1186/s12912-021-00566-7 (accessed on 28th June 2025).

35. Mach, F., Baigent, C., Catapano, A. L., Koskinas, K. C., Casula, M., Badimón, L., Chapman, M. J., et al. (2019). 2019 ESC/EAS guidelines for the management of dyslipidemias: Lipid modification to reduce cardiovascular risk. *European Heart Journal, 41,* 111–188. https://doi.org/10.1093/eurheartj/ehz455 (accessed on 28th June 2025).

36. Marom, P., Novak, A., Heruti, R. J., & Lev-Ari, S. (2025). Enablers, barriers and practical applications of a group-based pain self-management program for patients receiving medical cannabis: A qualitative study of patients and clinicians. *Pain Practice, 25.* https://www.semanticscholar.org/paper/b0985e523f51a3268aef82b106427fa74eb130de (accessed on 28th June 2025).

37. Martins, T. M., Souza, D. M., & Souza, D. M. (2023). Use of multimodal anesthesia in the treatment of postoperative pain. *Brazilian Journal of Pain, 6.* https://doi.org/10.5935/2595-0118.20230075-en (accessed on 28th June 2025).

38. Munneke, W., Demoulin, C., Nijs, J., Morin, C., Kool, E., Berquin, A., Meeus, M., et al. (2024). Development of an interdisciplinary training program about chronic pain management with a cognitive behavioral approach for healthcare professionals: Part of a hybrid effectiveness-implementation study. *BMC Medical Education, 24.* https://www.semanticscholar.org/paper/d9c703fd19777dc3bc8b9d958ab0fe986afc6bf8 (accessed on 28th June 2025).

39. Ooi, K. B., Tan, G. W. H., Al-Emran, M., Al-Sharafi, M. A., Căpăţînă, A., Chakraborty, A., Dwivedi, Y. K., et al. (2023). The potential of generative artificial intelligence across disciplines: Perspectives and future directions. *Journal of Computer Information Systems.* https://doi.org/10.1080/08874417.2023.2261010 (accessed on 28th June 2025).

40. Page, M. J., Moher, D., Bossuyt, P. M., Boutron, I., Hoffmann, T., Mulrow, C. D., Shamseer, L., et al. (2021). PRISMA 2020 explanation and elaboration: Updated guidance and exemplars for reporting systematic reviews. *BMJ.* https://doi.org/10.1136/bmj.n160 (accessed on 28th June 2025).

41. Pilch, A., Jekiełek, M., Stach, B., Zyznawska, J., & Klimek, M. (2024). Impact of obstetric physiotherapy and transcutaneous electrical nerve stimulation (TENS) on pain management and gastrointestinal function following cesarean birth: A randomized controlled trial. *European Journal of Midwifery, 8.* https://www.semanticscholar.org/paper/e1e312fa3ae731d9556c6cf59b70f9e56ae92491 (accessed on 28th June 2025).

42. Raja, J., Parmar, D., Subramaniam, S. D., Nagella, S. P., Pappulwar, S. M., Mehlawat, R., & Maini, A. (2025). Anxiety and pain management in dental patients: A systematic review of pharmacological and non-pharmacological approaches. *Journal of Pharmacy and Bioallied Sciences.* https://www.semanticscholar.org/paper/7bd514d588d36e550c4118f5129b16d9e1f9e236 (accessed on 28th June 2025).

43. Sahu, P., & Patel, R. (2025). Improving pediatric pain management: A comparative analysis of pharmacologic vs. non-pharmacologic treatments. *Journal of Neonatal Surgery.* https://www.semanticscholar.org/paper/b5c01879adc9191a251629f3f8e171a84baa8511 (accessed on 28th June 2025).

44. Salameh, B., Nawajah, I., Al-Nawaja'a, I. A., Alkubati, S., Khatatbeh, H., ALbashtawy, M., Rababa, M. J., et al. (2025). Determinants of effective pain management in pediatric patients: An assessment of attitudes and barriers. *Journal of Pain & Palliative Care Pharmacotherapy.* https://www.semanticscholar.org/paper/2fc1b5ea818452e9fcdfd2f258dfa515617a0d92 (accessed on 28th June 2025).

45. Schneider, B. J., Naidoo, J., Santomasso, B., Lacchetti, C., Adkins, S., Anadkat, M. J., Atkins, M. B., et al. (2021). Management of immune-related adverse events in patients treated with immune checkpoint inhibitor therapy: ASCO guideline update. *Journal of Clinical Oncology, 39*, 4073–4126. https://doi.org/10.1200/jco.21.01440 (accessed on 28th June 2025).

46. Semernik, I. V., & Samonova, C. V. (2024). Investigation of noise immunity of a multichannel underwater wireless optical communication system. https://doi.org/10.34660/inf.2023.53.92.429 (accessed on 28th June 2025).

47. Seppi, K., Chaudhuri, K. R., Coelho, M., Fox, S. H., Katzenschlager, R., Pérez-Lloret, S., Weintraub, D., et al. (2019). Update on treatments for nonmotor symptoms of Parkinson's disease—An evidence-based medicine review. *Movement Disorders, 34*, 180–198. https://doi.org/10.1002/mds.27602 (accessed on 28th June 2025).

48. Taldone, S., Lemmon, S. K., Bianco, S. D. C., St. Onge, J. E., Ford, H. R., Cox, L., Serota, D. P., et al. (2022). Opioid use disorder curriculum: Preclerkship pharmacology case-based learning session. *MedEdPORTAL.* https://doi.org/10.15766/mep_2374-8265.11255 (accessed on 28th June 2025).

49. Umukoro, E., Elijah, O., Igben, V., & Moke, E. G. (2025). The pharmacological profile, therapeutic importance and limitations with the use of oxycodone: A review. *African Journal of Tropical Medicine and Biomedical Research.* https://www.semanticscholar.org/paper/2d7ed59602e02c28165a52b826bc9d326341ed42 (accessed on 28th June 2025).

50. Varkey, B. (2020). Principles of clinical ethics and their application to practice. *Medical Principles and Practice, 30*, 17–28. https://doi.org/10.1159/000509119 (accessed on 28th June 2025).

51. Venkataramu, V. N., Ghotra, H. K., & Chaturvedi, S. K. (2022). Management of psychiatric disorders in patients with cancer. *Indian Journal of Psychiatry, 64*, S458–S472. https://doi.org/10.4103/indianjpsychiatry.indianjpsychiatry_15_22 (accessed on 28th June 2025).

52. Venturin, D., Battimelli, A., di Cara, G., & Poser, A. (2024). The multidisciplinary team in the management of chronic pain and pain-related fear: An evidence-based approach in a clinical case. *Physiotherapy Theory and Practice, 41*, 447–464. https://www.semanticscholar.org/paper/4645c86b0e55bce592257fd0dd8ab01019630af7 (accessed on 28th June 2025).

53. Volcheck, M. M., Graham, S. M., Fleming, K. C., Mohabbat, A. B., & Luedtke, C. A. (2023). Central sensitization, chronic pain, and other symptoms: Better understanding, better management. *Cleveland Clinic Journal of Medicine, 90*, 245–254. https://doi.org/10.3949/ccjm.90a.22019 (accessed on 28th June 2025).

54. William, L. (2006). Commentary on He H-G, Pölkki T, Pietilä A-M and Vehviläinen-Julkunen K (2005). A survey of Chinese nurses' guidance to parents in children's postoperative pain relief. *Journal of Clinical Nursing, 15*, 1585–1586. https://www.semanticscholar.org/paper/ba626b5bc310e18eaa10b35988da2a52e324633c (accessed on 28th June 2025).

55. Williams, B., Mancia, G., Spiering, W., Rosei, E. A., Azizi, M., Burnier, M., Clement, D. L., et al. (2018). 2018 ESC/ESH guidelines for the management of arterial hypertension. *European Heart Journal, 39*, 3021–3104. https://doi.org/10.1093/eurheartj/ehy339 (accessed on 28th June 2025).

56. Wydro, M., Grotowska, M., Łukasiewicz, M., & Strawińska, A. (2025). The role of controlled breathing in pain management. *Quality in Sport.* https://www.semanticscholar.org/paper/b4af662e6304fe1abf6a64cac229ec2c7c07f8ae (accessed on 28th June 2025).

57. Xu, P., Ji, X., Li, M., & Lu, W. (2023). Small data machine learning in materials science. *npj Computational Materials, 9.* https://doi.org/10.1038/s41524-023-01000-z (accessed on 28th June 2025).

58. Zhu, J., Zhu, M., Shi, Q., Wen, F., Liu, L., Dong, B., Haroun, A., et al. (2020). Progress in TENG technology—A journey from energy harvesting to nano energy and Nano system. *EcoMat, 2.* https://doi.org/10.1002/eom2.12058 (accessed on 28th June 2025).

POSTPARTUM PAIN MANAGEMENT AND RECOVERY IN ANESTHESIA

10

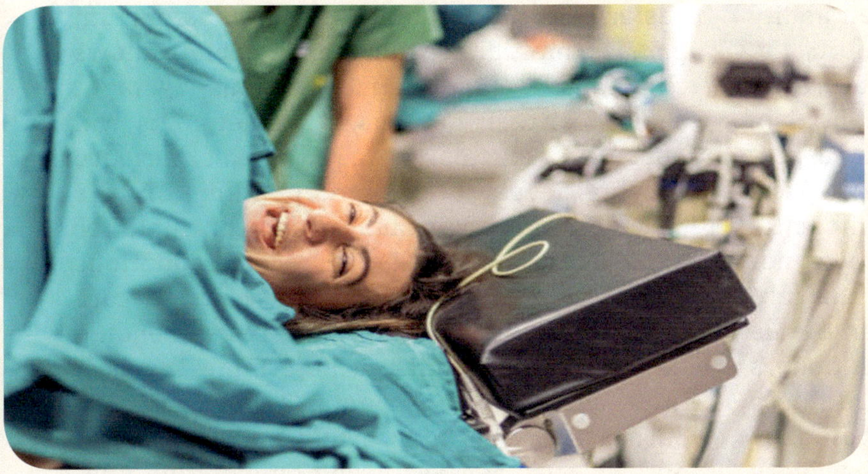

LEARNING OBJECTIVES

After studying this chapter, you will be able to:

1. Explain the types of postpartum pain
2. Understand pain management strategies
3. Discuss the role of healthcare providers
4. Discuss the impact of postpartum pain on recovery
5. Focus on cultural considerations in pain management
6. Know long-term effects of postpartum pain

Introduction

The transition to motherhood, while wonderfully delightful, is a phase that is traditionally marred by tremendous physical and emotional trials, particularly in coping with postpartum discomfort. Effective coping strategies are key not only to upgrading maternal recovery but also to achieving maximum health of the infant. Anesthesia is also at the focal point here, since it renders pain mitigation at the time of and after parturition feasible, impacting recovery periods and the potential for caregiving. Familiarity with the various modalities of pain mitigation, along with the physiological complexities of recovery in the postpartum context, is necessary for healthcare personnel who are to provide care for new mothers. Besides, altering practice in anesthesiology has revealed new paradigms that orient toward patient-centered care, thereby establishing the distinctiveness of personal experiences throughout the postpartum progression. Equally critical is the management of maternal physiological responses during labor, which, if poorly regulated, may lead to complications in both the mother and the fetus. Emerging research indicates the adverse effects associated with traditional practices, such as the sustained Valsalva bearing down efforts, and how they can be quite harmful even as they raise questions about the efficacy of such practices towards guaranteeing safe delivery. Anesthesia practice should be evidence-based and embrace these findings. Through adjusting pain management practices to address the unique obstacles of labor and postpartum recovery, practitioners can enhance maternal confidence in their ability and reduce the risk of injury. Therefore, the inclusion of evidence from the literature on maternal care and anesthesia is essential in informing effective methodologies that respect both the physiological and psychological aspects of birth. Finally, the importance of hospital discharge readiness measurement should not be overlooked in the effective postpartum care model. The readiness for hospital discharge scale (RHDS) is useful, allowing health practitioners to quantify a patient's perceived readiness following childbirth. Strong psychometric underpinnings established through confirmatory factor analysis make it possible for clinicians using the RHDS to determine intervention areas pre-discharge, enabling more informed, individualized care planning. These tools are not only critical to the optimization of post-anesthetic pain control, but also to overall recovery. By incorporating instruments such as the RHDS, medical professionals can ensure smoother hospital-to-home transitions for patients, thereby supporting sustained recovery processes in postpartum patients and ultimately improving their motherhood experience.

Definition of Postpartum Pain

Postpartum pain is a multifaceted phenomenon that affects women after giving birth and is a significant component of the recovery process. Postpartum pain results from various causes, including physical trauma associated with vaginal delivery or cesarean section, uterine involution, and perineal trauma. These physiological causes often contribute to feelings of mild to severe pain and hence deserve close consideration of their impact on women's health following childbirth. The postpartum pain experience stems not only from physiological transformation but also emotional and psychological ones, which can increase pain perceptions and hinder recovery. Proper management of postpartum pain, in turn, is crucial to maximizing maternal well-being and making the motherhood transition easier. The understanding that postpartum pain is a multidimensional phenomenon allows clinicians to personalize pain management choices for their patients. A blanket policy will not suffice, considering that women experience varying levels of pain depending on the specific birth circumstances and threshold for pain. Additionally, existing recommendations emphasize significantly patient-centered care in managing postpartum pain, recommending in-depth assessments to determine the best interventions for a woman's best interest. Such approaches may include pharmacologic options, such as NSAIDs and opioids, and non-pharmacologic methods, including physical therapy and counseling support. With various management options, health care practitioners can reduce the risks of intractable postoperative pain, enhancing recovery and quality of life for new mothers. In particular, the interaction between postpartum pain management and anesthesia affects women's recovery experience. Effective anesthesia not only reduces postpartum pain but can also prevent the establishment of chronic pain in the long term. Providers are encouraged to consider how postoperative care relates to pain control protocols, as uncontrolled pain may have such complications as postpartum depression or disability. To normalize care practice, current recommendations emphasize the necessity of monitoring pain intensity and, if necessary, adjusting management plans based on patient reports. Additionally, consideration of the impact of anesthetic choice is important, especially in the context of latent bleeding disorders that can affect recovery, as illustrated by the presentation of von Willebrand disease in postpartum management (Nathan et al., 2021). Thus, postpartum pain management must have a multidisciplinary view of the patient's past and history to achieve the optimal outcomes (Figure 10.1).

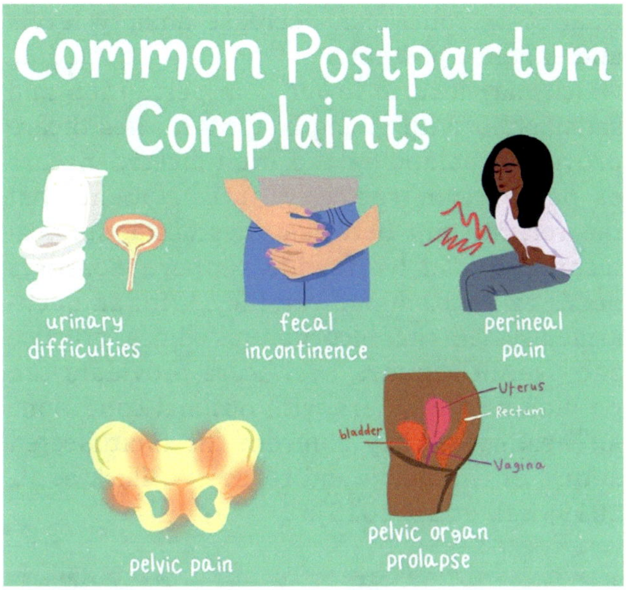

Figure 10.1. Postpartum pain is a multifaceted phenomenon experienced by women following childbirth.

Source: https://pelvicpainrehab.com/wp-content/uploads/2024/10/image1-1-1024x1024.jpg.

Importance of Effective Pain Management

Proper management of pain is also necessary in the postpartum stage, which plays a significant role in a woman's recovery process following delivery. Uncontrolled pain can hinder movement, interfere with the initiation of breastfeeding, and negatively affect maternal-infant bonding. Postpartum pain is diverse, depending on the type of delivery and individual levels of pain tolerance. Current practices favor a multimodal approach for pain control, using both pharmacological and non-pharmacological methods. By managing pain through various modalities, health care professionals can tailor interventions to individual needs, thereby increasing overall patient satisfaction. Individualized treatment, beyond ensuring enhanced physical rehabilitation, contributes to psychological well-being that is critical for new mothers as they adjust to the challenges of motherhood. Adequate pain control therefore forms an essential aspect for the facilitation of not just physical rehabilitation but emotional stability among postpartum women. Postpartum pain mechanisms are complex and need an integrated management approach. Research finds that unnoticed acute pain experienced in labor and delivery can lead to chronic pain states many years after hospital discharge. Some predictors of chronic pain, such as a history of pain and the type of anesthesia used in delivery, imply hidden risk factors that need individualized pain management. For instance, while epidural analgesia can alleviate pain during labor, the reverse may not always be the case with post-delivery pain, and adjunct therapies can be applied to prevent the development of chronic pain. According to recent literature, there is a need to target effective interventions that are capable of addressing acute pain and preventing its long-term consequences, thus emphasizing the importance of active pain management strategies in the post-delivery period (Fabris, 2011). Furthermore, poor pain management has wider consequences for healthcare outcomes among new mothers than mere short-term physical pain; it extends to other healthcare usage. Improperly managed pain will add to greater healthcare utilization through complications from poor healing and over-stress. It will also hurt the mental well-being of mothers, causing conditions like post-partum depression. Therefore, healthcare professionals owe a responsibility other than clinical intervention; they must support new mothers emotionally and psychologically. Strategies, such as explicit communication about pain experience and incorporating women's own choices into treatment decisions, are essential to effective pain management. Lastly, postpartum pain management is crucial not only to alleviate pain but also to improve long-term health outcomes in infants and mothers (American College of Obstetricians and Gynecologists et al., 2007).

Overview of Anesthesia in Postpartum Care

Management of anesthesia in the postpartum period is a critical component of recovery support in post-childbirth women, particularly those who experience pain following surgery such as cesarean sections. Anesthesia techniques such as epidurals and spinal anesthesia are not just for the alleviation of postoperative pain but are also designed to enhance the recovery process of patients. By effectively managing pain relief, these methods can enable mothers to be more involved in their postpartum care and in bonding with their newborns. On top of that, effective administration of anesthesia can minimize the psychological effect of delivery, improving maternal experience and facilitating a smooth transition into motherhood. With recent controversy regarding anesthesia management, it is well worth noting how differences in maternal health, such as prior disabilities, might influence anesthetic techniques and results. Pregnant women with disabilities may have unique needs during and following delivery that necessitate customized anesthetic strategies for satisfying their physical and psychosocial needs. Anesthesia providers need to be equipped with knowledge regarding such challenges so that they can offer personalized care that celebrates the individuality of every patient. Understanding the experiences of disabled mothers allows the healthcare system to develop an inclusive setting and support system that ensures higher satisfaction and recovery. Engrafting such thinking into anesthesia practice is essential in order to enable all women, regardless of the health context in which they find themselves, to receive optimal care during the postpartum period. Also, the role of support systems, such as doulas, in postoperative care can significantly affect the effectiveness of anesthesia management. Doulas provide emotional and physical support, adding a layer of care that complements medical procedures. Doulas' presence can decrease anxiety levels and enhance postpartum women's satisfaction, which may lead to lower pain perception and satisfaction with giving birth. With healthcare providers balancing the multifaceted nature of postpartum recovery, it is evident that the relationship between anesthesia, surgical technique, and worldwide support measures needs to be examined carefully. With an open-armed system that incorporates clinical practice and overall support, healthcare providers can provide new mothers with optimal conditions for healing as they confront the multifaceted nature of childbirth and recovery (Clark et al., 2019; Bell et al., 2015).

10.1. Types of Postpartum Pain

Learning Outcome

1. Physical pain from childbirth
2. Emotional and psychological pain
3. Pain related to breastfeeding

The postpartum period is typically characterized by a variety of pain modes, which consequently can have serious impacts on healing and overall maternal health. One of the principal sources of discomfort is the physical trauma incurred during the delivery process. This includes perineal pain from vaginal lacerations or episiotomies, which can be chronic and influence a woman's ability to perform normal activities or bond with her infant. Additionally, cesarean section also has its own complications, such as surgical wound incisional pain that may require further intervention. It is important to know the variation in types of pain following both vaginal and cesarean delivery since mismanagement will lead to prolonged recovery time and dissatisfaction among women (Dowell et al., 2022). Lower gastrointestinal symptoms are also a big category of postpartum pain that is frequently overlooked. Constipation, hemorrhoids, or anal fissures are widespread among most women and are intensified by the physiological impact of pregnancy and the stresses of new motherhood. For instance, the prevalence of hemorrhoids has been reported to be as high as 86% during pregnancy and extends to the postpartum period. The discomfort caused by these conditions may be significant and reduce quality of life during an already challenging transition period. The professionals need to be cautious of these complications and provide the appropriate treatment options. Adequate management not only alleviates immediate distress but also supports the overall maternal health profile during recovery (Rao et al., 2022). Secondly, psychosomatic pain due to emotional and psychological change cannot be ruled out. Postpartum anxiety and depression can manifest physically, hence contributing to hypersensitivity to pain. New mothers can become more tense in muscles, develop headaches, and basically do not manage pain well due to their psychological state. This bond between psychological well-being and bodily suffering points towards the requirement of comprehensive postpartum care covering both aspects. By encouraging open communication about mental health and revisiting healthcare strategies for pain management, medical professionals can better support new mothers in their recovery, with bodily and emotional needs met simultaneously (Dowell et al., 2022; Rao et al., 2022) (Figure 10.2).

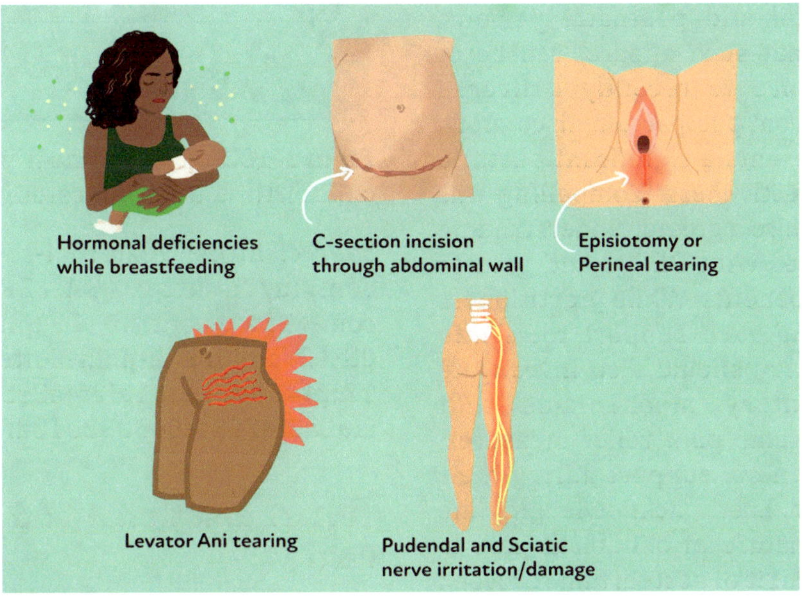

Figure 10.2. Postpartum pain occur.

Source: https://pelvicpainrehab.com/blog/recovering-postpartum-pain-and-perineal-tears/.

10.1.1. Physical Pain from Childbirth

The physical pain resulting from childbirth is a multifaceted experience that can significantly impact a woman's postpartum recovery. During labor, women often endure intense contractions and pressure, leading to a range of physical discomforts that can persist long after the birth experience.

It is not confined to the immediate postpartum stage alone but also to various phases of the recovery process because women experience complications such as perineal trauma, incisional pain due to a cesarean section, and uterine involution. Adequate management of pain is required to facilitate recovery so that new mothers can engage in caregiving and acquire knowledge about their new roles free from the suppressive effect of uncontrolled pain. Health care providers must be aware of the continuum of pain experiences and offer one-on-one interventions that take into account the physical and psychological aspects of postpartum recovery from childbearing. New findings are pointing towards the potential of new support systems for managing postpartum pain. One of these is the use of dynamic elastomeric fabric orthoses (DEFO), which has proven useful in alleviating pain and enhancing functional ability during the prenatal and postnatal periods. Evidence reveals that such apparel can be of significant assistance to recently delivered mothers suffering from postpartum discomfort, but compliance presents a significant obstacle to their overall effectiveness. Compelling this compliance will require a greater understanding of users' experiences with DEFOs and greater education on their benefits. While practitioners consider integrating such support tools into postpartum care, they should also investigate other complementary mechanisms that would enhance regular pain relief measures, offering mothers general support during their recuperation period. Lastly, acknowledging the psycho-emotional nature of childbirth pain is critical within the ambit of postpartum recovery. Many women experience various degrees of traumatic stress response following childbirth, which may manifest in the form of severe physical and emotional distress. Research indicates that between 10% of women may experience high levels of postnatal traumatic stress, affecting their overall well-being and healing process. The interface of physical trauma associated with childbirth, such as cesarean section or labor distress, and vulnerability to postnatal PTSD underlines the intracommunicativity of pain management. Effective screening procedures and therapeutic strategies, such as cognitive-behavioral therapy (CBT), can become instrumental in managing this psychological aspect of postpartum recovery. By providing an integrated approach that encompasses physical and mental health measures, health professionals are better able to help women control the problems of postpartum pain and emotional distress, thus creating a less stressful recovery experience (Figure 10.3).

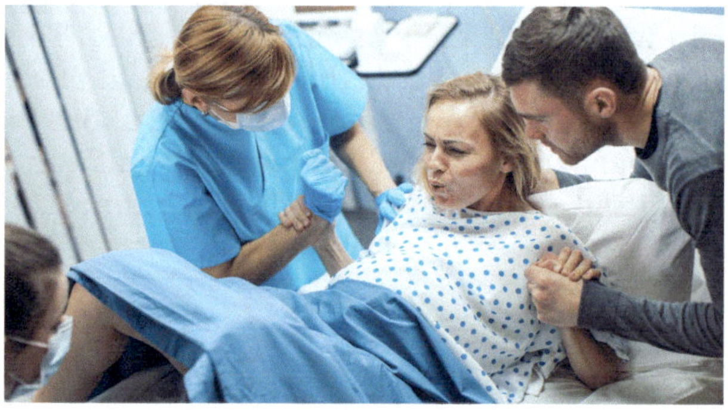

Figure 10.3. The physical pain resulting from childbirth is a multifaceted experience.

Source: https://external-content.duckduckgo.com/iu/?u=https%3A%2F%2Fparentology.com%2Fwp-content%2Fuploads%2F2023%2F03%2Fchildbirth-pain-Edited.png&f=1&nofb=1&ipt=06c448dd1f52f4a3eed58de15d8eafdb3fa92a2f47931f545832018df7b2db2f.

10.1.2. Emotional and Psychological Pain

The emotional and psychological pain of postpartum women is a significant aspect of their recovery process. Following delivery, many women go through varying degrees of feelings ranging from joy to profound sorrow, accompanied by hormonal shifts and lifestyle changes. This emotional upheaval can lead to postpartum depression (PPD), a condition that is described in roughly 15% of new mothers.

The PPD experience is usually characterized by feelings of insufficiency, despair, and worry that may disrupt both recovery from physical pain and bonding with the infant. Identification and stabilization of these psychological difficulties are critical in the provision of holistic postpartum care, as they will influence a mother's adherence to self-care and her capacity for self-control of the physical pain. Thus multifaceted postpartum pain management is necessary. Non-pharmacological treatments have been discovered to provide relief not only from bodily pain but also from distress related to emotions in women postpartum. Treatments such as mindfulness, cognitive behavioral treatment (CBT), and peer support interventions can significantly improve anxiety and depression. Studies have shown that engaging in structured physical exercise can improve mood and emotional well-being by stimulating the release of endorphins, natural mood elevators. Specifically, research indicates that exercise lowers emotional pain and enhances overall recovery. All these approaches agree with findings that advise on the management of emotional pain being the key to effective postpartum recovery, particularly when integrated with the use of non-pharmacological intervention (Acharya et al., 2024). Furthermore, the management of emotional as well as physical pain in an overarching way is now universally accepted as best practice in postpartum care. For instance, structured physical activity interventions have been linked to cardiovascular health benefits, reduction of blood pressure, and enhanced mental health outcomes, demonstrating the interdependence of physical and psychological well-being (Chawrylak et al., 2024). Additionally, innovative interventions such as online counseling for health and mobile phone reminders have also shown promise to get postpartum women involved in recovery behavior. By offering personalized assistance and resources, such strategies promote resilience and help women cope with the complexities of postpartum emotions. As emotional suffering comes to be understood differently, it becomes vital to give top priority to holistic care models that acknowledge and respond to the complex nature of postpartum recovery (Figure 10.4).

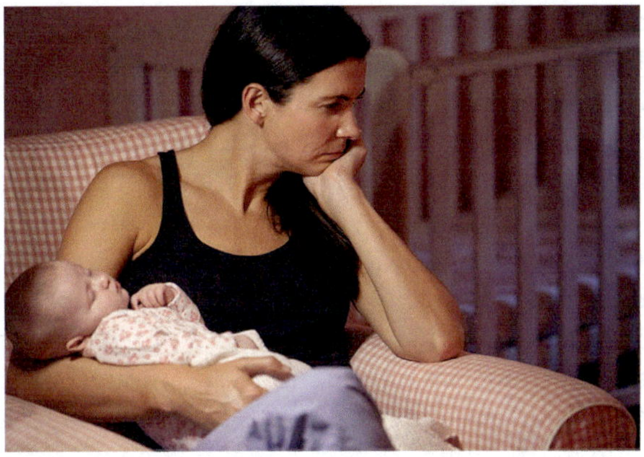

Figure 10.4. Postpartum depression.

Source: https://owh-wh-d9-prod.s3.amazonaws.com/s3fs-public/images/blog-postpartum-depression.jpg.

10.1.3. Pain Related to Breastfeeding

The pain of breastfeeding is a universal problem for the majority of postpartum women, having an impact on their overall recovery and well-being. The breastfeeding pains can occur in the form of sore nipples, engorgement, and even more severe ones like mastitis. These pains not only discourage the act of breastfeeding, but they also interfere with the mother's mental health, thereby triggering the feeling of inadequacy and stress. Determining the cause of this pain is essential to manage it effectively; causes such as faulty latch, inadequate positioning, and pre-existing medical conditions can become the causes of distress. By early intervention through counseling and support of these conditions, pain can be reduced, encouraging mothers to continue breastfeeding, which is a well-documented intervention with beneficial effects on both mother and infant. Pain management for lactating mothers must be multi-faceted in its approach, addressing physical as well as emotional factors. These include , techniques such as proper positioning for breastfeeding, the use of breast pads, and gentle compressions of the breasts, which can ease pain. The use of drugs that are safe when breastfeeding can also be contemplated, guided by recommendations that prioritize the healing of the mother without risk to the baby. Non-pharmacologic interventions such as warm compresses or ice packs can also yield considerable relief. By applying a multidisciplinary approach that includes emotional support and education on breastfeeding expectations, health care professionals can help mothers navigate the often challenging experience of breastfeeding while minimizing pain and maximizing maternal confidence. Furthermore, stigma surrounding pain from breastfeeding can complicate new mothers' experiences. New mothers are self-conscious about reporting difficulties, fearing they will be judged or found wanting, which can leave them more isolated and exacerbate pain management issues. This discrimination may deny mothers access to assistance or advice on the right care practices, which are essential for successful postpartum recovery. Encouraging open discussions of breastfeeding issues may empower mothers to seek help and make their experiences 'normal.' There is a need for health professionals to use a trauma-informed model that allows mothers, developing an environment of trust and empathy. By challenging such social stigmas and emphasizing the role of compassionate care, we can reinforce the success of breastfeeding and overall maternal health in the postpartum period (Dowell et al., 2022; Andrea et al., 2021).

Test Your Knowledge

1. What are the different types of postpartum pain experienced by women after childbirth, and what are their common causes?
3. How do the intensity and duration of various postpartum pains differ between vaginal delivery and cesarean section?

10.2. Pain Management Strategies

Learning Outcome

1. Pharmacological options
2. Non-pharmacological methods
3. Alternative therapies

Effective pain management treatments are significant in postpartum care as they can reliably affect a mother's ability to care for her newborn and improve overall health. Among many different interventions, the use of dynamic elastomeric fabric orthoses (DEFO), specifically compression garments, has been yielding increased research evidence. The clothes are designed to alleviate pain resulting from obstetric conditions by improving abdominal support. Evidence shows that DEFOs may help manage pain and enhance functional capacity during the postpartum period. Although compliance with wearing these support garments is generally poor, research into novel designs may improve wearability and facilitate compliance in postpartum women (Hing et al., 2019). With such technologies, healthcare providers can offer more targeted pain management strategies tailored to the individualized needs of postpartum women. In addition to clothing for physical support, psychological well-being is also a significant factor in managing pain after childbirth. A growing evidence base indicates that some women do experience severe traumatic stress reactions associated with childbirth, and these have the potential to make recovery more complicated and increase pain perception. Studies indicate that as much as 10% of women experience severe traumatic stress responses, but only a few develop chronic postnatal posttraumatic stress disorder (PTSD) (Ayers et al., 2004). Psychological interventions like cognitive-behavioral therapy (CBT) have been suggested to treat these distress responses. By incorporating psychological support in pain management methods, healthcare providers can reverse the multifaceted quality of postpartum pain, leading to a more comprehensive method of healing.

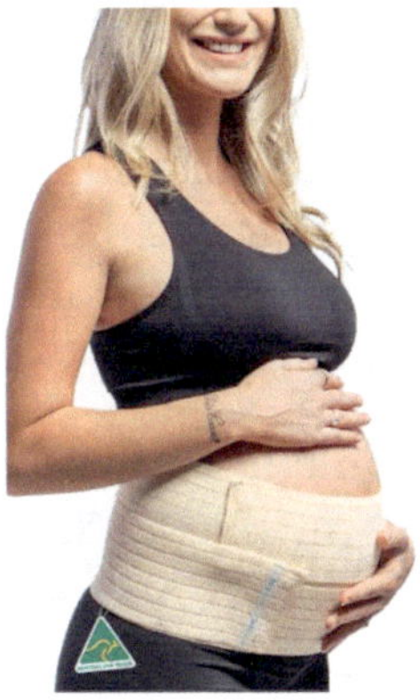

Figure 10.5. Dynamic elastomeric fabric orthoses (DEFOs).

Source: https://www.parents.com/thmb/CxNoKGichyVjrUFEsTSW-M62qu8=/fit-in/1500x1001/filters:no_upscale():max_bytes(150000):strip_icc()/bellybands-3-in-1-belly-band-for-pregnancy-postpartum-c-section-b53c682adf344f0facefb6f5373e8751.jpg.

A multidisciplinary model that integrates both physical and psychological interventions can yield the best outcomes in postpartum pain management. By combining the application of DEFOs with psychotherapy methods such as CBT, healthcare professionals are able to enable women to explore the physical and emotional problems of the postpartum process. This integrative model acknowledges that pain is a multifaceted experience that is not only physical but is also closely linked to emotional well-being. Areas of research for the future must continue to examine the effectiveness of combining these interventions and to expand understanding of barriers to compliance. By offering solid guidelines and easy access to appropriate support, women can enjoy a healthy quality of life during the vulnerable postpartum period, enabling them to integrate into motherhood (Ayers et al., 2004; Hing et al., 2019) (Figure 10.5).

10.2.1. Pharmacological Options

Appropriate management of postpartum pain is paramount in optimizing recovery and enhancing the general quality of life for newly delivered women. A key role in this is played by pharmacological intervention, for which a wide range of analgesics exists that can be matched to each patient's needs. Opioids remain a daily choice due to their potent analgesic efficacy, particularly for the pain of acute type following cesarean section or severe perineal laceration. However, their use comes at the cost of potential side effects like sedation and respiratory depression that complicate recovery. This is why healthcare providers should weigh the utility of opioid use against these complications and also factor in adjunctive therapies. This is pivotal in allowing women to participate maximally in their postpartum care, including bonding with their newborns and meeting everyday responsibilities. In addition to opioids, nonsteroidal anti-inflammatory drugs (NSAIDs) are another drug option in pain relief postpartum. These drugs are useful in the management of mild to moderate pain and are convenient in relieving pain as well as inflammation that accompanies perineal pain and uterine contraction. The bimodal action of NSAIDs on pain and inflammation, rendering them a viable, safer alternative, is normally advised before escalating to more potent analgesics. As confirmed by recent studies, multimodal analgesic protocols combining both opioids and NSAIDs have been proven to optimize pain relief and limit opioid dependence. The combination approach not only optimizes pain relief but also minimizes potential side effects with higher doses of opioids, thereby making the entire postpartum recovery experience safer. Beyond conventional oral medications, emerging pharmacological options are expanding the range of postpartum pain management. Novel interventions with regional anesthesia techniques or adjuvant therapy, such as nerve blocks, can provide improved pain relief with fewer systemic effects. Regional anesthesia, for instance, can alleviate pain from specific sources without the wide-ranging effects of systemic opioids, fulfilling short-term recovery needs and long-term management. Besides, new techniques, such as the application of autologous platelet-rich plasma to promote healing in certain conditions, have shown promise for pain relief while enabling quick recovery. However, as Wang et al. (2024) observe, the efficacy and safety of such novel interventions must be evaluated comprehensively to ensure they are indeed helpful. Last but not least, enhancing postpartum pain management will involve continued reevaluation of pharmacologic agents to offer comprehensive care for recovering mothers.

10.2.2. Non-Pharmacological Methods

Non-pharmacologic interventions are a must in alleviating pain during the postpartum period as well as recovery, of great benefit to the overall well-being of new mothers. Modalities such as physical therapy, relaxation, and support devices all help alleviate discomfort without side effects such as those seen with pharmacologic relief. For instance, physical interventions, such as pelvic floor exercises and stretches, have been shown to enhance recovery by increasing muscle tone and reducing tension. Furthermore, cognitive-behavioral interventions can empower women to manage pain well, which results in greater control during the period of recovery. These methods, while often adjunctive to traditional analgesia, emphasize taking a total postpartum approach to combining physical and mental health. The inclusion of non-pharmacologic measures also addresses the demand for safer pain-relief medication, particularly in institutions where the use of opioids is an issue. In addition to the high opioid dependence rates and risk of unwanted side effects, there is greater awareness of measures that minimize opioid dependency throughout the recovery period. For example, integrating mindfulness and breathing into therapy can help regulate levels of anxiety and stress, which can exacerbate pain syndromes. Furthermore, support groups as well as peer-to-peer programs provide emotional and social support that significantly influences pain perception and coping.

This emphasis on creating a caring environment is in line with the general goals of maximizing recovery results for mothers, encouraging evidence-based and compassionate practice like that described in Pilkington et al. (2024). There is still room to explore new non-pharmacological interventions, including technology, to enhance postpartum care. Patient-controlled analgesia devices and interventions that allow for dialogue with healthcare professionals are a paradigm shift in pain management. These technologies allow for real-time modification of care plans, but also allow patients to be actively engaged with the recovery process. Such incorporation enables a multimodal approach to pain management that can produce better results without the side effects of pharmaceutical interventions. In addition, having guidelines that focus on non-opioid approaches facilitates a culture that is conducive to holistic care. Postpartum pain management directions in the future should prioritize such new, evidence-based practices to optimize the recovery experience for mothers, as encouraged by the recent review of pain management practices by Almottowa et al. (2025) (Figure 10.6).

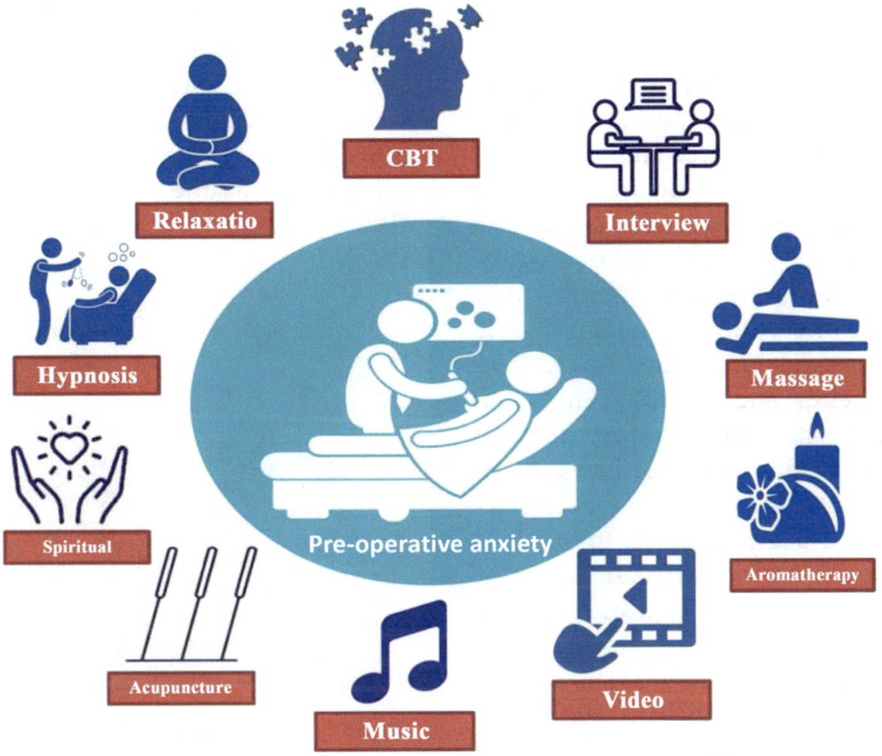

Figure 10.6. Non-pharmacological methods play a crucial role in postpartum pain management and recovery.

Source: https://www.researchgate.net/publication/359874670/figure/fig1/AS:11431281242160893@1715412829002/Non-pharmacologic-approaches-in-preoperative-anxiety.tif.

10.2.3. Alternative Therapies

Complementary therapy has become increasingly prominent over the past few years as an adjunct to conventional pain relief measures in postpartum women. The majority of new mothers experience a range of aches and pains, including perineal discomfort and backache, which hinder recovery and affect overall well-being. Holistic treatments like acupuncture, massage, and yoga are becoming increasingly popular for general benefit, to counter physical and mental health aspects of postpartum recovery. It has been established in research that alternative therapies to enhance emotional support and reduce anxiety, crucial during postnatal periods. By assisting in potentially alleviating pain and improving mobility, alternative therapies are capable of providing a multidimensional care that touches on the many-sided requirements of postpartum women on the road to recovery. The incorporation of alternative therapies into traditional medical care can lead to better treatment outcomes in postpartum pain care. The evidence would suggest that if nonpharmacologic modalities are combined with usual analgesics, there is greater relief from pain and less drug consumption, which carries a heavy side effect burden. That is of particular interest in that there is inadequate relief of pain by the current standard therapy for some women. Moreover, research into new therapies based upon a better understanding of pain, such as targeted drug treatments, may be directed by results of various methodologies. In this context, clinicians are increasingly recommending the integration of pharmacologic and nonpharmacologic modalities to achieve maximum pain relief and overall functional benefit, consistent with contemporary medical practice that promotes individualized treatment. Central to the efficacy of alternative interventions is the need for large-scale research to validate their benefits, especially in postpartum settings. As the health climate continues to transform, the deployment of alternative interventions must be supported by robust evidence bases and an empirical understanding of how they work. For instance, while studies have established that there are possible benefits of interventions like acupuncture in pain relief for diseases such as osteoarthritis, their identification as relevant to postpartum healing remains vital. Also, the role of medical marijuana as a pain relief option, most extensively researched in cancer pain, presents avenues for its investigation in postpartum application (Kopczy et al., 2024). Thus, advancing the scientific literature on complementary treatments might contribute to the arsenal of options available for postpartum treatment, alleviating the physical pain and psychological ailments that a new mother experiences as she progresses through this life-altering stage (Farinelli et al., 2024) (Figure 10.7).

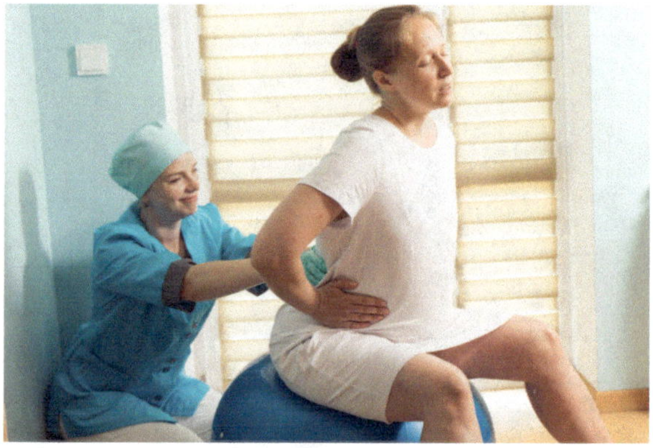

Figure 10.7. Alternative therapies.

Source: https://images.saymedia-content.com/.image/t_share/MTk5MjkzMjEyMjExMjkxNTUw/pain-relief-options-during-labor.png.

Test Your Knowledge

1. What are the main pharmacological options available for pain management, and how do they differ in terms of mechanism of action and side effects?
2. How can alternative therapies such as acupuncture, physiotherapy, relaxation techniques, and herbal treatments complement conventional pharmacological pain management?

10.3. Role of Healthcare Providers

Learning Outcome

1. Assessment of Pain Levels
2. Development of Personalized Pain Management Plans
3. Education and support for new mothers

In the complex landscape of postpartum pain, the role of healthcare professionals becomes pivotal in the provision of effective recovery for new mothers. Professionals must conduct thorough pain assessments that account for the physiological and psychological determinants of each patient's pain. Knowledge of unique postpartum recovery needs enables healthcare professionals to tailor pain management strategies that significantly impact the mother's health. Empathic communication empowers providers to encourage mothers to report pain severity and concerns, thereby facilitating collaborative care. This individualized approach not only addresses acute pain but also considers long-term recovery patterns, resulting in improved outcomes. Emphasizing patient-centered care through prioritization of it empowers healthcare providers to support mothers, with a favorable impact on postpartum outcomes. The application of mixed modalities in postpartum care also reflects the role of healthcare providers in pain management. From the literature, complementary and traditional treatments like acupuncture and herbal medicine have proven to be effective in alleviating postpartum pain. However, evidence favoring these treatments remains mixed and inconclusive to a certain extent, and hence more studies need to be conducted to confirm their effectiveness (Smith et al., 2020). Health professionals are in a position to help patients make well-informed decisions consistent with their values and health needs, and urge them to decide accordingly. This renders interdisciplinary care by health professionals even more important in enabling an integrated approach to pain management in postpartum women. Together through such alliances, care strategies are better positioned to be refined and tailored to meet the diverse needs of new mothers. When complex health conditions such as opioid use disorder (OUD) are involved in complicating postpartum recovery, the roles of healthcare practitioners include advocacy as well as specialized services. Research shows that recovering mothers employ specific strategies to obtain their own needs met as well as their infants' needs met despite experiencing systemic stigma and judgment from society (Mattson et al., 2021). Providers have the opportunity to demystify these mothers' experiences by fostering an open, supportive environment. By actively providing social support, promoting self-care behaviors, and distributing educational materials, providers can enhance health for both the infant and the mother. Understanding the complexity of OUD in postpartum care underscores the need for healthcare workers to remain informed and compassionate, ultimately improving recovery rates among vulnerable populations.

10.3.1. Assessment of Pain Levels

Accurate assessment of pain severity in postpartum women is crucial to effective pain management and recovery. Following delivery, women are likely to experience various degrees of physical distress, possibly significantly affecting their overall health and ability to care for their newborns. Systematic assessment of pain is needed, using standardized tools such as the Numeric Rating Scale or Visual Analog Scale, which allow healthcare providers to measure pain intensity objectively. Pain level quantification not only allows for individualized treatment but also identifies women who may become at risk for developing chronic pain syndromes. Further, newer studies also indicate measuring both the psychological and physiological aspects of pain, since emotional triggers such as anticipation and previous trauma have been shown to increase pain sensations during the postpartum phase. Appropriate pain monitoring ensures timely, evidence-based interventions that ultimately optimize recovery outcomes. Pain relief is not merely physically significant; it also contributes to mental well-being and overall quality of life for new mothers. Pain postpartum can lead to severe emotional distress, including postpartum depression and anxiety. Knowledge of the psychophysical relationship between pain and mental status is essential so that caregivers can manage these related illnesses. Research has shown that effective pain management techniques can reduce the susceptibility to develop postpartum post-traumatic stress disorder (PTSD), especially in women who face elevated pain severity during delivery (Sghaier et al., 2024). By acknowledging the multidimensional character of pain, health care providers can adopt holistic pain management strategies that involve psychosocial support in conjunction with drug therapies. These integrative approaches can improve both maternal and infant health outcomes, providing a comprehensive picture of postpartum care. In addition, the importance of regular pain assessment is underscored by the need for plan individualization. Postpartum women are likely to have unique experiences of pain that can be related to multiple factors, such as mode of delivery and individual tolerance of pain. For instance, a significant percentage of women suffer from moderate to extreme levels of pain following cesarean deliveries, underscoring the significance of successful pain relief strategies (Matthew et al., 2025). Poor pain assessment and management lead to prolonged suffering and are detrimental to the recovery process, affecting the ability of a mother to engage in bonding with her baby. As new evidence emerges daily about pain management, guidelines and classification systems for pain intensity will be essential. It is ultimately through a thoughtful evaluation process that suffering may be alleviated and the quality of life enhanced for postpartum women, facilitating easier transitions to motherhood (Figure 10.8).

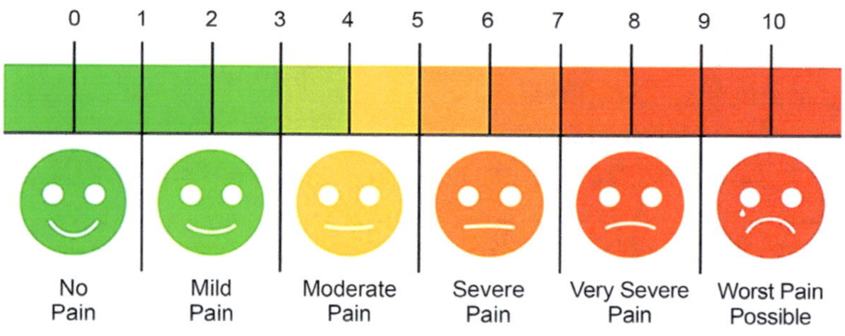

Figure 10.8. Pain scale.

Source: https://d1zxene68j3keg.cloudfront.net/sites/default/files/Resouces/images/Manage%20Pain.jpg.

10.3.2. Development of Personalized Pain Management Plans

Individualized pain management programs are an essential factor in the process of caring for postpartum pain, which can significantly influence mothers' recovery and general well-being. Postpartum women's individual needs and experiences ensure that a tailored approach must consider a range of issues, from the subjective experience of pain to variations in individuals' threshold of pain and individual circumstances of childbirth. Research indicates that psychological and emotional factors, including stress and anxiety levels during pregnancy, are factors influencing what pain is like after giving birth. Therefore, individualized programs must incorporate measures that target not only the physical aspect of pain but also its emotional and psychological causes. The synergistic integration of these elements can lead to enhanced maternal satisfaction and shorter post-delivery recoveries, as evidenced by the increasing use of holistic approaches, e.g., music and mindfulness therapies, which have been found to minimize stress and, as a result, pain perception (Dixon et al., 2024). In addition to psychological considerations, though, effective individualized pain management programs must also be responsive, acknowledging variability in medical, social, and cultural determinants of maternal care. To confirm, variability in the types of health facilities—ranging from urban birth centers to safety-net clinics—underscores the need for individualized approaches that align with the specific needs and resources of different populations (Cook et al., 2009). Incorporating patient experience into the care model enables providers to design interventions grounded in personal experience and choice. It is a methodology that not only empowers women but also improves the understanding of pain management. Prioritizing women's engagement in design by allowing their voices to be heard throughout the development process helps providers ensure care is responsive and sensitive to the diverse experiences of new mothers during recovery. Besides, ongoing assessment and adaptation of patient pain plans are essential in ensuring maximum outcomes. Pain management is not supposed to be a fixed procedure but something flexible as patients' healing continues. Ongoing monitoring enables health workers to detect varying pain levels, drug side effects, and the efficacy of other interventions. Such malleability is significant in that postpartum recovery can vary significantly depending on a variety of external variables such as hormonal shifts, home care complications, and individual health status. By maintaining open lines of communication among clients and health care providers, the effectiveness of personalized pain relief strategies can be maximized, leading to a more attentive and supportive health environment that prioritizes the needs of postpartum women and enhances their recovery (Dixon et al., 2024).

10.3.3. Education and Support for New Mothers

New mother support and education are key ingredients in creating effective postpartum pain control and facilitating overall postpartum recovery. As the new mom navigates the complexities of her new role, access to holistic education programs can significantly enhance her sensitivity to the physical and emotional health needs of the postpartum stage. Such awareness allows mothers to make educated decisions regarding pain control techniques, which can include self-control practices, drug selections, and life alteration. Moreover, understanding normal complications and signs during this period can help determine when specialist services might be needed, allowing timely intervention that could prevent complications or worsening of pain. Introducing maternal health-specific educational resources can ultimately increase outcomes of recovery and overall mother and infant health. Along with education, there needs to be support systems in place for new mothers who are not recovering from postpartum recovery. Family, friends, or even medical care providers can help a lot in alleviating the psychological distress that is typically associated with postpartum problems. Research has shown that newly delivered mothers who are well supported feel less lonely, anxious, or depressed, which tends to worsen pain and impede recovery. Peer support groups are also useful venues for exchanging experiences, offering encouragement, and providing advice on pain management. In addition, healthcare providers can help mothers by actively treating postpartum pain and preparing them with necessary resources and referrals to mental health services, as appropriate. Thus, the interaction between education and social support is important in enabling new mothers to navigate postpartum life. The importance of culturally competent education and support systems cannot be overstated, particularly in minority and underprivileged populations. Multicultural populations of new mothers may face unique barriers to postpartum care, producing disparities in recovery outcomes and pain management outcomes. Culturally responsive programs can help close these gaps by honoring and respecting the special needs and beliefs of mothers, thereby establishing an environment in which they are valued and appreciated. For instance, some groups of people will value some dietary recommendations or other methods of pain relief that are consistent with their cultural practices. Additionally, education programs that incorporate family members into the learning process can ensure more positive home environments for new mothers. To this end, consideration of cultural issues is essential to improving support for all mothers, enhancing their postpartum experience and health outcomes (Figure 10.9).

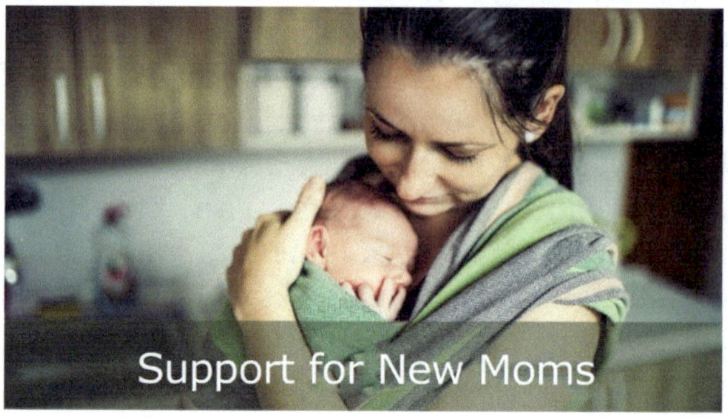

Figure 10.9. Education and support for new mothers are critical components in fostering effective postpartum pain management and facilitating overall recovery.

Source: https://external-content.duckduckgo.com/iu/?u=https%3A%2F%2Fwww.motherrisingbirth.com%2Fwp-content%2Fuploads%2F2014%2F08%2FSupport-for-New-Moms.jpg&f=1&nofb=1&ipt=d99837ca04e07e20226b45b44a2ff7c12d0e3384dc5ce10ac6f5cd7ec7a4c4c1.

Test Your Knowledge

1. How do healthcare providers assess individual patient needs to develop personalized pain management plans?
2. What is the role of multidisciplinary healthcare teams in implementing, monitoring, and adjusting personalized pain management strategies?

10.4. Impact of Postpartum Pain on Recovery

Learning Outcome

1. Physical recovery and mobility
2. Emotional well-being and mental health
3. Effects on bonding with the newborn

Postpartum pain management is important to the healing of recently delivered mothers, as it affects physical recovery as well as psychological status. Pain after delivery can be due to several causes, including perineal trauma, surgical interventions such as cesarean delivery, and organic disorders such as constipation, which are specifically prevalent in the postpartum period. Understanding the complexity of postpartum pain allows healthcare providers to tailor pain management strategies that not only manage acute pain but also allow for a more optimal recovery trajectory. Ideal pain management can significantly benefit a mother's ability to care for her infant, support her emotional health, and maintain overall health in the early postpartum period. The ramifications of poor pain control extend past the early post-childbirth period and result in long-term consequences. Studies have demonstrated that women who experience unrelieved postpartum pain are at increased risk of a long-term chronic pain state, both physically and mentally. For instance, persistent pain can disrupt a mother's ability to engage in bonding activities with her baby and can lead to feelings of incompetence or postpartum depression. At times, pain diminishes a woman's enthusiasm for performing essential rehabilitation activities, thereby prolonging recovery. Such issues of pain have to be addressed to facilitate women's adjustment to motherhood and also enhance their standard of living during the transitional period. The implementation of evidence-based processes in postpartum care remains paramount, especially when considering existing recommendations for pain management. Healthcare providers are encouraged to utilize multimodal therapy employing pharmacological and non-pharmacological interventions, sufficient to relieve pain without threatening possible side effects, such as opioid medication. Current guidelines lay great stress on accurate assessment and individualized management to achieve optimal outcomes in women with postpartum pain. Through their application, clinicians are able to aid in the mitigation of pain's adverse effects on healing, ultimately ensuring maternal health during the postpartum period. Proper management in alignment with best-practice standards can readily redefine the postpartum experience for new mothers, resulting in healthier families and communities (Rao et al., 2022; Dowell et al., 2022) (Figure 10.10).

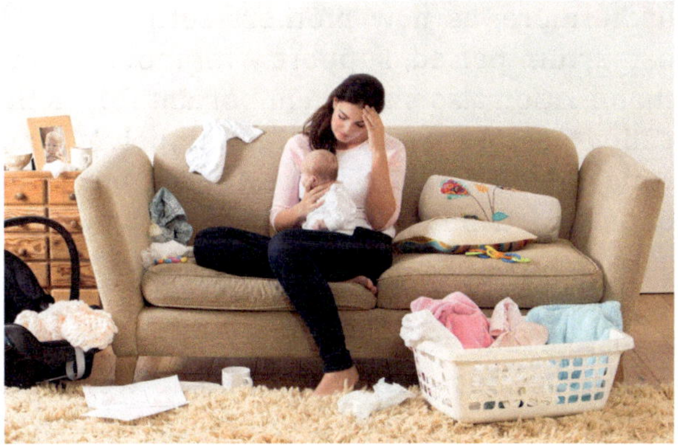

Figure 10.10. The management of postpartum pain is critical for the recovery of new mothers.

Source: https://external-content.duckduckgo.com/iu/?u=https%3A%2F%2Famericanpregnancy.org%2Fwp-content%2Fuploads%2F2020%2F09%2Fpostpartum-depression-1024x683.jpg&f=1&nofb=1&ipt=b7eb8481b0fe31d79dad0bf245814782282500c716908170d2e83ee7dd51d813.

10.4.1. Physical Recovery and Mobility

In postpartum recovery, there are important roles played by physical recovery and mobility in the return to well-being and function. Most women, having given birth, experience numerous physical problems, such as pain and limited mobility, caused by hormone changes, labor, and physical stressors of giving birth. Engaging in regular, moderate exercise is important because it aids both in physical healing and alleviating symptoms of postpartum depression and anxiety. According to existing studies, improving physical fitness plays a significant role in general health, for example, by reducing the risk of non-communicable diseases and improving cognitive health (N/A, 2023). With such outstanding advantages in increased mobility, postpartum treatment planning ought to encourage new mothers to incorporate safe, effective exercise practices into their recovery regimen, with an emphasis on both short- and long-term benefits of increased physical fitness. Furthermore, as new mothers settle into the postpartum period, support with mobility and rehabilitation also plays an important role in the healing process. Exercises for the pelvic floor, gentle stretching, and progressive strengthening not only contribute to physical recovery but also enable women to develop mastery and autonomy over their bodies. Technological advancements in postpartum exercise programs may enable virtual workout sessions and home workouts, which have gained additional importance during the COVID-19 pandemic (Bansal et al., 2022). These resources may make exercise more accessible to postpartum patients, enabling them to rehabilitate at their own pace and enhance mental well-being. An individualized model of physical rehabilitation enables mothers to navigate their unique physical landscapes after successful childbirth, facilitating mobility and mental well-being. Lastly, the symbiotic relationship between physical recovery and mental well-being is particularly important in the postpartum period. While physical mobility is an appropriate indicator of recovery, psychological gains resulting from increased mobility must also be recognized. Engagement in physical rehabilitation exercises can enhance social interaction and societal support, which are vital against feelings of loneliness that some new mothers experience. Increased physical activity can markedly improve mood and well-being and inhibit the onset of chronic diseases in the long run (N/A, 2023). Therefore, postpartum care needs to include organized support measures for both physical and psychological well-being, so that new mothers have not merely been taught how to manage pain but also empowered to gain a full recovery that propels them towards future health and mobility (Figure 10.11).

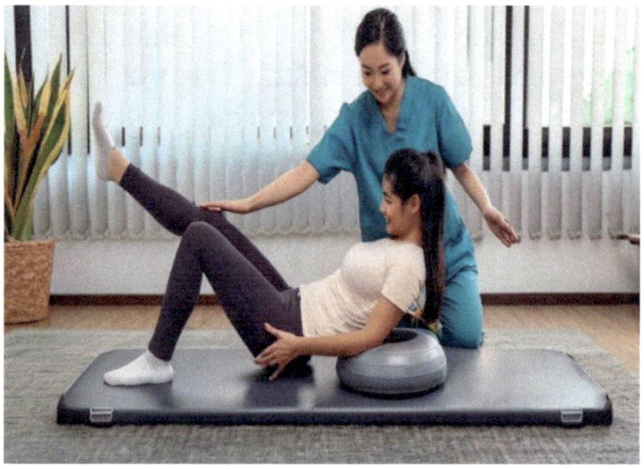

Figure 10.11. Physical recovery and mobility.

Source: https://www.thehealthsite.com/pregnancy/postpartum-recovery-tips-new-mothers-physiotherapy-support-back-pain-breastfeeding-posture-health-post-pregnancy-1127190/.

10.4.2. Emotional Well-Being and Mental Health

Postpartum is afflicted by emotional challenges that can significantly affect a new mother's emotional and overall health, as well as her frame of mind. It's a delicate balancing act between physical recovery from giving birth and emotional well-being, as unchecked pain can have adverse psychological effects. Research has shown that social support is absent among those who are at risk for postpartum depression (PPD), with significant consequences both for the mother and for the growth and development of her child. In this sense, PPD can be a biological signal, alerting mothers to the greater expense of coping with poor support and the potential evolutionary costs of investing in a troubled offspring. Understanding this connection allows clinicians to intervene in ways that not only facilitate physical healing but also improve emotional health, underscoring the need for an integrated approach to postpartum care that addresses both pain management and mental health (Hagen et al., 1999). On top of this, emotional distress during the postpartum period can manifest in various ways, one of which is postnatal posttraumatic stress disorder (PTSD). Research has shown that 10% of women are able to experience extreme traumatic stress responses following childbirth, creating a volatile intersection of emotional wellness and labor and delivery outcomes. Previous psychiatric history, type of delivery, and level of labor support have been named primary predictors of symptomatology of postnatal PTSD. Since these stress responses can compromise maternal functioning and disrupt infant bonding, identification of at-risk individuals within routine assessment becomes crucial. Postpartum care that includes screening tools for emotional disorders enables practitioners to better respond to the psychological dimensions of recovery, such that mothers are given timely and appropriate intervention (Ayers et al., 2004). Encouraging postpartum emotional health involves an interdisciplinary pain management process that also attends to the psychological impact of childbirth. Interventions such as cognitive-behavioral therapy (CBT) have been effective in alleviating extreme traumatic stress reactions and PTSD symptoms, enabling women to incorporate their birth experiences positively. In combining these treatment techniques, practitioners must also take steps to ensure that pain management does not have the unintended consequence of reinforcing feelings of helplessness or emotional tension. Providing women with comprehensive strategies addressing both physical pain and emotional distress can enable a better overall recovery process. This integrated process is required to maximize short-term outcomes, such as alleviating pain, and long-term emotional health, thereby providing a nurturing environment conducive to effective maternal-infant attachment and care (Ayers et al., 2004).

10.4.3. Effects on Bonding with the Newborn

The early postpartum period is also when a close bond between a mother and newborn can be established, as early bonding deeply affects the infant's future social and emotional maturity. However, bonding can be interfered with by uncontrollable pain that results from childbirth. Physical pain may get in the way of a mother connecting with their newborn intimately, depriving them of the intimate interaction essential for attachment. Severely postpartum painful mothers might find it difficult to initiate contact between their skin and the baby's or respond promptly to the demands of the baby, which might undermine the success of breastfeeding as well as overall infant care. According to the referrals by research, emotional suffering that accompanies physical pain may be a limiting factor in caring interactions, therefore supporting the use of adequate pain management methods shortly after delivery to facilitate bonding with the infant. Oxytocin, or the bonding hormone, is central to maternal-infant attachment development. During childbirth and lactation, the hormone is secreted, stimulating feelings of attachment and caregiving behavior. Adequate postpartum pain relief can maximize oxytocin secretion, therefore creating a caregiving environment essential for bonding. At a state of physical comfort, mothers are more likely to have positive social interactions with their newborns that are able to further stimulate oxytocin. Furthermore, oxytocin's anti-stress activity and capacity to enhance resilience could provide mothers with the emotional stability needed during the postpartum period. Hence, postpartum pain management not only ensures physical recovery but also optimizes the hormonal context that promotes the development of safe attachment to infants, thereby improving infant and maternal health outcomes (Carter et al., 2020). Moreover, the bonding processes are integrated with the psychological implications of postpartum recovery. Managing pain effectively, mothers also experience greater satisfaction with their birthing and postpartum experience, which can translate into more emotional bonding with their baby. Conversely, when they are having chronic pain, they may become withdrawn and depressed, having less interaction with their baby. The same can also be a cause-and-effect scenario, in which less bonding further worsens the mother's feelings of inadequacy or distress. A pain management strategy that includes physical and emotional support is thus central to healthy mother-infant relations. Offering comfort and emotional well-being, health care professionals can foster an environment conducive to the formation of maternal bonds, with implications for mother and child in their early interactions and future development (Wolters et al., 2021) (Figure 10.12).

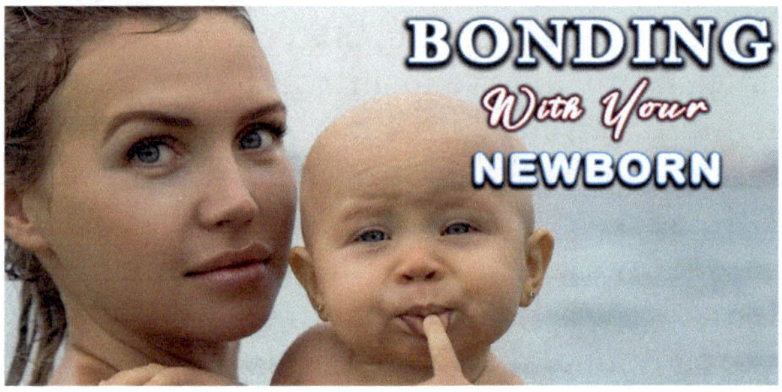

Figure 10.12. The early postpartum period is critical for establishing a strong bond between a mother and her newborn.

Source: https://external-content.duckduckgo.com/iu/?u=https%3A%2F%2Fi.ytimg.com%2Fvi%2FRv56muLG5vk%2Fmaxresdefault.jpg&f=1&nofb=1&ipt=3be90719c707a732cbe66b1ceaa571e93b4d73b9da39794fb1eb121e92904803.

Test Your Knowledge

1. How does postpartum pain affect a mother's physical recovery, emotional well-being, and ability to care for her newborn?
2. What strategies can be used to effectively manage postpartum pain and promote faster recovery?

10.5. Cultural Considerations in Pain Management

Learning Outcome

1. Variations in pain perception
2. Cultural practices and beliefs about postpartum care
3. Access to resources and support

Cultural knowledge of pain control is essential to healthcare providers when delivering care to postpartum women with special needs. Culture influences what patients feel pain to be and how they anticipate care. For instance, collectivist postpartum women may appreciate family involvement in decisions about their care because they are cared for through shared communal practices rather than individualized medical care. By comparison, patients who have come from more collectivist cultures might appreciate autonomy and direct communication with healthcare providers regarding their options for managing pain. It is this variation that indicates a call for culturally competent care that integrates cultural norms, beliefs, and values into practice. By conforming pain management practices to culturally specific expectations, healthcare providers can enhance patient outcomes, satisfaction, and even trust within the healthcare system. Language differences and modes of communication also significantly contribute to pain management in postpartum care. Healthcare providers should recognize that language differences may affect patients' ability to express their pain and needs effectively. Mistranslation may be possible when the patients are not fluent in the dominant language, and may lead to inappropriate pain relief or wrong treatment choices. Having professional interpreters and culturally sensitive educational information can help patients express their concerns effectively. Healthcare providers should also recognize and because they acknowledge differences in nonverbal communication, as body language and distress behavior, may vary. By opening channels of communication and actively seeking patient feedback, clinicians may improve pain assessment and treatment, ultimately benefiting a more equitable postpartum stay. Additionally, socioeconomic factors entangled in culture pose other hurdles to the practice of pain management. Income, education, and access to care inequities affect the way postpartum women perceive and react to pain. For lower socioeconomic individuals, delayed access to prolonged postpartum care may increase distress and a sense of failure in controlling pain. This situation can be further aggravated by cultural values that discourage the expression of pain or a lack of knowledge about treatment options. Eradicating such disparities requires a strategy that targets both the cultural construction of pain and the institutionally located barriers faced by postpartum women. Initiatives aimed at facilitating greater access to culturally responsive care can bear great fruit, reinforcing the importance of promoting health equity in the context of postpartum recovery and pain control (Joseph et al., 2021; Gavin et al., 2021).

10.5.1. Variations in Pain Perception

The postpartum pain experience is heterogeneous across women due to numerous biological, psychological, and social determinants. Variability in individual psychological status, the cultural background of the woman, and the experience of previous pain all ensure variability of experience. Psychological determinants such as depression and anxiety are well-documented to worsen pain and hamper recovery. Furthermore, research is indicative of the fact that cultural environments also influence women to perceive and report their pain, and this directly can affect whether or not they can seek treatment or employ coping strategies. For example, women from stoic cultures tend to underestimate their pain, and hence their postpartum pain relief and therapy are compromised. An understanding of such differences is necessary for health care providers to tailor pain management approaches that are effective and culturally appropriate to achieve better outcomes for all postpartum women (Brodbeck et al., 2022). Neurobiological mechanisms also play a significant role in modulating pain perception in the postpartum period. Research has proven that post-delivery hormonal fluctuations—primarily estrogen and progesterone level fluctuations—are capable of influencing a woman's pain tolerance directly. The hormones also communicate with the nervous system, controlling the way pain messages are received and interpreted. The pain of childbirth itself also usually has a central role to play in pain perception; for instance, some women may become pain-sensitive following an abusive delivery. This becomes important in documenting the imperative of holistic pain assessments based on individualized biological responses and psychosocial markers to counter postpartum pain adequately. Further, increased understanding of such neurobiological differences will inform the design of individualized interventions that address the specific pain experiences of postpartum women (Craft-Blacksheare, 2012). Multimodal pain treatment also must take these differences in pain experience into account to achieve maximum recovery. The interventional modalities may include pharmacological interventions, such as nonsteroidal anti-inflammatory agents or opioids, and non-pharmacological interventions, such as cognitive-behavioral therapy and mindfulness practices. Healthcare providers must engage in open conversations with patients to identify the individual experiences of their pain and affect states, thus enabling personalized pain treatment programs. Educating healthcare providers about the multidimensional array of factors influencing pain perception not only optimizes their care for postpartum women but also advances patient-centered care within healthcare settings. Lastly, obtaining solutions to the complexities of pain sensation is integral to effective interventions on postpartum pain control and recovery strategies that yield favorable health outcomes (Brodbeck et al., 2022) (Figure 10.13).

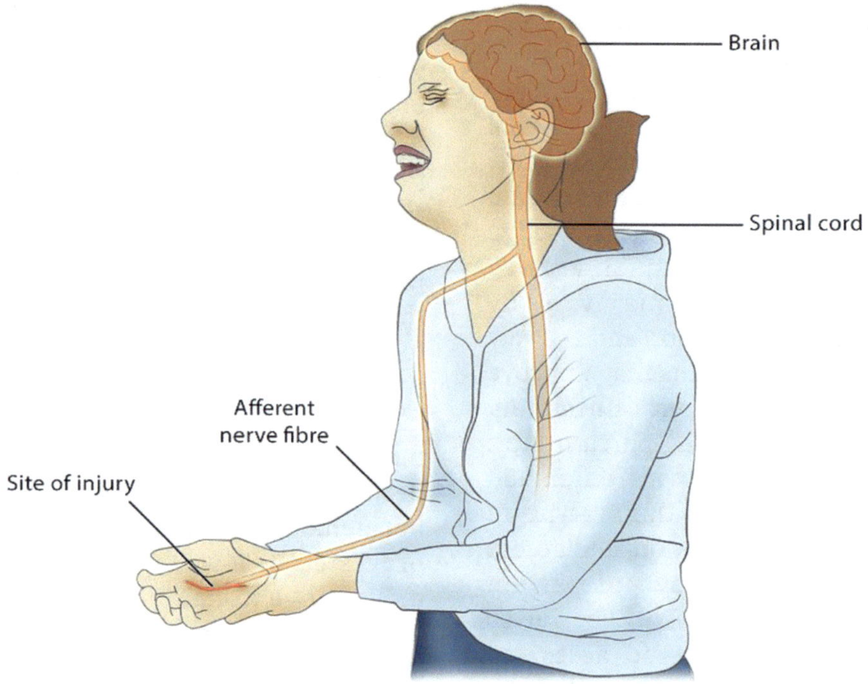

Figure 10.13. The experience of pain during the postpartum period varies significantly among women due to multiple biopsychosocial factors.

Source: https://external-content.duckduckgo.com/iu/?u=https%3A%2F%2Fimages.fineartamerica.com%2Fimages%2Fartworkimages%2Fmediumlarge%2F2%2Fpain-perception-maurizio-de-angelisscience-photo-library.jpg&f=1&nofb=1&ipt=f82a8fed2056e7e3cc67ef0fe8dec7906dc425db b2da784601465be0ae0deda4.

10.5.2. Cultural Practices and Beliefs About Postpartum Care

The postpartum care practice and cultural beliefs are deeply rooted in the culture and tradition of specific communities, identifying how new mothers perceive pain relief and recuperation. Postpartum, by and large, remains a time of vulnerability for both newborns and mothers across cultures, therefore eliciting healing practices and customs. For example, in India, the TBAs prefer to take a leading role in helping mothers adhere to these practices. Despite efforts towards promoting skilled birth attendants, research indicates that TBAs still play a dominant role in providing postpartum care, including adhering to local traditions, including some dietary practices and bathing rituals. Such practices strike a balance between biomedical advice and traditional knowledge, suggesting that culturally informed care can optimize women's recovery experiences and pain relief outcomes (Adamson et al., 2010). Additionally, postpartum care is also closely linked with the mental well-being of recently given birth mothers, suggesting the utmost importance of considering cultural beliefs in pain management interventions. Perinatal mental health, such as the emotional and psychological problems for women before, during, and after childbirth, is an essential factor in the recovery process. For instance, racial and ethnic minority women frequently experience obstacles that impede their access to mental health care. Asian American women, for example, have been underresearched when it comes to postpartum care, despite experiencing unique challenges such as acculturative stress and discrimination. It is essential to recognize these cultural determinants in the development of effective postpartum care programs addressing the special needs of various population groups. Mental health interventions for these women should integrate traditional values and adopt a collaborative approach to empower mothers in their recovery (Yuen et al., 2022). The interface of cultural beliefs and postpartum care practices also includes community support networks, which unite around new mothers. Collective childcare has been a characteristic of postpartum life in most cultures, in which mothers receive active care from members of their community and family. Collective childcare has the added advantage of supporting physical recuperation and developing emotional resilience through a sense of shared experience and resourcefulness. Some of these collective practices can entail the mutual sharing of postpartum care knowledge that is traditionally passed down and the provision of emotional care. By embracing such culture-embedded practices, healthcare practitioners can establish an environment that not only addresses physical pain relief but also sustains the mental well-being of mothers. : Appreciating and embracing these cultural elements within postpartum care interventions are important for improving maternal outcomes in pain management and overall recovery (Adamson et al., 2010).

10.5.3. Access to Resources and Support

Access to resources and support is a central tenet of effective postpartum care and recuperation. New mothers are likely to experience a cluster of physical and emotional problems following birth, which demand individualized care beyond standard healthcare settings. The contemporary world witnesses digital health platforms, in this instance, mobile apps for postpartum care, becoming significant assets. These apps can provide immediate access to mental health care, guided exercises, and pain management techniques. With the latest technology, new mothers can leverage customized support that empowers them during the healing process. Since these platforms are more accessible, their ability to shape postpartum care and address complications such as postpartum depression becomes highly relevant, which is why it is important to systematize incorporating these resources into everyday healthcare practices (Almalki et al., 2025). Additionally, access to healthcare centers is also crucial for postpartum recovery. In the majority of low- and middle-income countries, issues with healthcare infrastructure can compromise access to prompt medical care and support, aggravating maternal health disorders. Availability of postpartum care facilities, for instance, including pain management protocols and psychological counseling, may be limited by the unavailability of necessary resources and training within available health facilities. From the recent studies, the implementation of standard guidelines and protocols can enhance the quality of postpartum women's care, but does this with high levels of investment in training healthcare providers and the supply of appropriate resources (Aimagambetova et al., 2024). With a focus on comprehensive strategies that cater to both physical and psychological health needs in mothers, the healthcare systems are better positioned to enhance postpartum pain relief as well as recovery results. Also worth noting in the consideration of access to resources in postpartum care is the social support role. Friends, family, and community networks all offer critical emotional and practical support that can significantly alleviate distress for new mothers. These support systems are not only valuable for the physical aspect of the recovery process, such as managing pain and stressful infant tasks, but also play a general role in mental health. Incorporating community-based initiatives that not only teach families but also reinforce support networks can create an environment conducive to healthier postpartum experiences. When mothers receive appropriate emotional and physical support from their inner circles, they are in the strongest position possible to navigate recovery processes more effectively. Relying on the full spectrum of resources available—everything from technological aids to family support—will ultimately maximize postpartum pain management techniques and promote overall recovery practice (Figure 10.14).

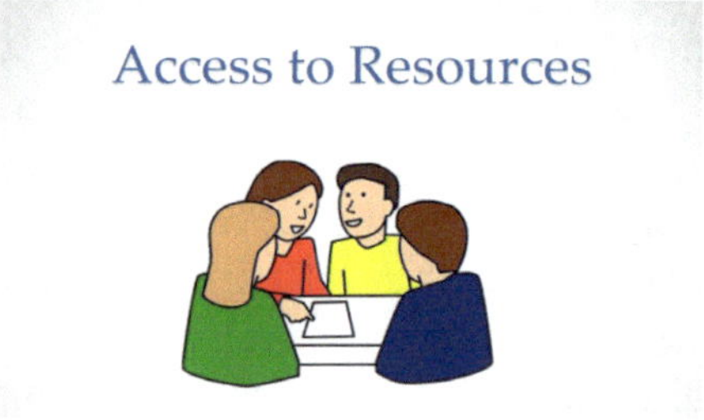

Figure 10.14. Access to resources and support.

Source: https://external-content.duckduckgo.com/iu/?u=https%3A%2F%2Fimage5.slideserve.com%2F9457071%2Faccess-to-resources-l.jpg&f=1&nofb=1&ipt=6e8d79110d9c36dbf36fdac494e1f49800546f8f8359972198dcb55ab58caf6c.

Test Your Knowledge

1. How do cultural beliefs and practices influence the perception, expression, and management of postpartum pain?
2. Why is cultural sensitivity important in developing effective and acceptable pain management strategies for postpartum women?

10.6. Long-term Effects of Postpartum Pain

Learning Outcome

1. Chronic pain conditions
2. Impact on future pregnancies
3. Influence on maternal mental health

The long-term effects of postpartum pain extend beyond brief physical discomfort, significantly affecting a woman's overall health and quality of life. After giving birth, many women experience various forms of pain, such as musculoskeletal pain and lumbopelvic pain, lasting for months or years. This chronic pain can impede normal function and limit physical mobility, making a sequence of unwanted consequences such as decreased social engagement and lower physical fitness more likely. As suggested by recent studies, participation in organized physical exercise may be crucial for reducing such symptoms. Specifically, regular moderate-intensity exercise has been shown to enhance cardiovascular fitness, muscle strength, and postpartum depression and hence treat both the physical and emotional effects of postpartum pain (Chawrylak et al., 2024). Furthermore, the psychological effects of having postpartum pain can be severe, resulting in the development of long-term mental health disorders like postpartum depression (PPD) and anxiety disorders. The connection between PPD and chronic pain is established, with studies showing that women who have chronic pain are most likely to develop depressive symptoms. Adequate postpartum pain management techniques, therefore, become vital not only for physical recovery but also for psychological well-being in new mothers. Innovative interventions, such as progressive muscle relaxation training and structured parenting programs, have shown beneficial effects on maternal attachment and reduced feelings of isolation, underscoring the importance of integrated care in the management of the mental and physical health consequences of postpartum pain (Chawrylak et al., 2024). The use of maternity support belts and dynamic elastomeric fabric orthoses (DEFOs) has been a notable intervention in the management of postpartum pain. Studies have shown that such orthotic devices can significantly reduce pain and improve functional ability in the postpartum period. Nonetheless, adherence to conventional support mechanisms has been poor, necessitating the introduction of more comfortable and attractive alternatives. Research has shown that if women wear these supportive garments regularly, they better manage pain and have better quality of life. These, however, are additional efforts that need to be made to discover consumer-friendly designs and educational strategies to motivate acceptance of these interventions. By prioritizing an interdisciplinary strategy that includes not only physical interventions but mental health care as well, healthcare providers can lay the groundwork for optimal management and recovery from postpartum pain as a whole and for attending to mothers in the long term.

10.6.1. Chronic Pain Conditions

Chronic pain conditions impact postpartum recovery quite significantly, tending to complicate the process of healing after delivery. Chronic pain in new mothers may lead to more difficulties in their physical well-being and in caregiving too. The interplay between pain and emotional well-being is particularly critical; unresolved bodily pain can exacerbate issues such as depression or anxiety, making it even harder to recover. When mothers experience the ordeal of dealing with babies, the long-term burden of suffering can lead to an experience of powerlessness and unhappiness. As the root cause of major unipolar depression is adverse life events, postpartum can serve as an initiator to the onset of such symptoms, thereby ensuring that pain management should be multidimensional and address physical and psychological needs to provide the best possible recovery in new mothers (Hagen et al., 2002). Effective treatment of chronic pain is paramount in allowing postpartum recovery and maximizing the overall quality of life of postpartum women. Treatment modalities commonly involve a multidisciplinary regimen of physical therapy, medication, and psychological counseling. Health care providers with experience in the dynamics of postpartum pain are available to allow individuals to receive customized interventions based on individual needs. Furthermore, improved access to resources can guarantee better health outcomes for mothers who are not covered by certain services or insurance schemes. Integrated support systems can assist the healthcare system in addressing the specific challenges of chronic pain conditions among the postpartum population. Thus, strategies that consider both the physical suffering and the psychological dimensions of chronic pain are essential in facilitating resilience and recovery during this vulnerable phase of life (Fortuny et al., 2011). Identification of chronic pain disorders in postpartum treatment not only impacts mothers but also guarantees healthier development processes in children. Psychological distress associated with chronic pain can have catastrophic effects on maternal-infant bonding and overall family interactions. Painful mothers are less likely to be completely present with their children, which may lead to behavioral or developmental difficulties in their children. In addition to the challenges of child-rearing and pain management, healthcare services must intervene in the broader implications of maternal health on childhood development. Using two-generational service delivery models, it is feasible to bridge the gap between maternal health service interventions and the needs of expected children, positioning postpartum pain management as an important aspect of integrated family healthcare (Fortuny et al., 2011) (Figure 10.15).

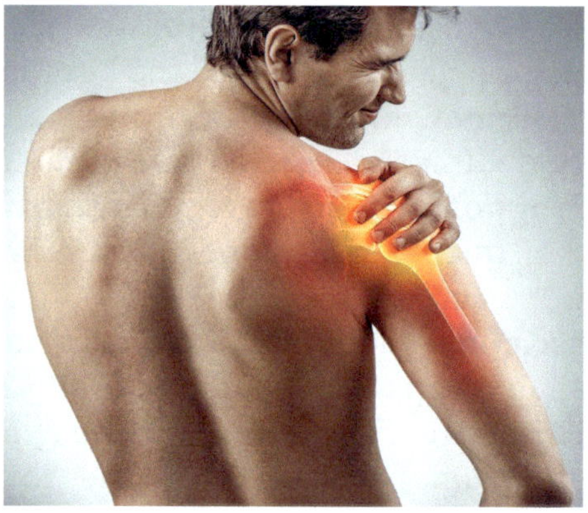

Figure 10.15. Chronic pain conditions significantly impact postpartum recovery.

Source: https://external-content.duckduckgo.com/iu/?u=https%3A%2F%2Fi0.wp.com%2Fnew.completemedicalwellness.com%2Fnew%2Fwp-content%2Fuploads%2F2021%2F06%2FBanner-2.webp%3Ffit%3D1920%252C1080%26ssl%3D1&f=1&nofb=1&ipt=6a2e23f9a7ce4453e05923e1a970073c71e8162ac37adb329e3694d36f56abb9.

10.6.2. Impact on Future Pregnancies

The implications of postpartum pain management extend far beyond the immediate recovery period and have the potential to leave a lasting legacy on subsequent pregnancy. Women who experience uncontrolled or undertreated pain following childbirth may be at heightened risk for a range of complications in subsequent pregnancies. Some complications, such as CS, may result in permanent effects that induce anxiety and fear in terms of modes of delivery during subsequent pregnancies. Research indicates that women with a history of CS have higher risks of complications in subsequent pregnancies, like uterine rupture and placental pathology, necessitating careful planning for future delivery operations (Nedopekina et al., 2021). Hence, adequate pain control during the postpartum period can result in better maternal health and outcomes in subsequent pregnancies, making it necessary to have effective pain control methods following delivery. In addition, the physiological consequences of the previous pregnancies, combined with inadequate postpartum care, yield chronic outcomes such as lumbosacral dysfunction. According to one research study, a high percentage of women with multiple pregnancies reported suffering from dysfunction of the lumbosacral region, which previous pelvic and lower back pains can explain suffered after delivery (Aranake et al., 2024). These musculoskeletal disorders, if left untreated, can limit a woman's physical activity, her ability to care for her newborn, and her overall health. Furthermore, postpartum pain on a chronic basis may create a pattern of avoidance behavior, which may affect the decision to have a second child. Hence, understanding and managing the physical implications of postpartum pain is crucial towards guaranteeing not only recovery but also well-being in future pregnancies. Finally, the psychological effects of postpartum pain cannot be ignored since they are likely to have long-lasting impact on subsequent pregnancy outcomes. Women who go through chronic pain following childbirth may end up with heightened anxiety regarding future pregnancies. It is assumed that this fear can have an impact on maternal decision-making and behavior for subsequent pregnancies, e.g., deciding on attempting a vaginal delivery after cesarean (VBAC) or preparing for subsequent cesarean delivery (Nedopekina et al., 2021). Furthermore, the emotional cost of managing postpartum pain may create fear of childbearing or feelings of inadequacy, perhaps deterring women from subsequent pregnancies. Therefore, integrated postpartum pain care with psychological counseling plays a crucial role in nurturing the self-esteem of women who are expecting future pregnancies and ultimately realizes healthier results for the mothers and their children.

10.6.3. Influence on Maternal Mental Health

The intersection between postpartum pain management and maternal mental health has increasingly been understood as being central to comprehending the delicate process of recovery after giving birth. Proper education imparted to mothers regarding their recovery process carries a significant influence on maternal mental health. Through studies, it is seen that inadequate knowledge about postpartum wellbeing negatively impacts mental health, leading to health factors such as postpartum depression (PPD). By providing mothers with what they need and an understanding of their recovery, healthcare systems can create an environment that supports healthy mental well-being. Programs such as Exploring Postpartum Care: A Guide for Mothers are exemplary of this endeavor because they address important aspects of the postpartum process, such as self-care, pain management, and mental health education, ultimately contributing to better maternal outcomes (Matlock et al., 2024). Post-delivery exercise is also a significant consideration with profound effects on maternal psychological health. A minimum of 150 minutes of moderate intensity aerobic exercise weekly is recommended according to guidelines, which has been found to lower postpartum depression symptomatology and overall well-being. Studies indicate that regular exercise not only enhances cardiovascular health and muscle strength but also promotes mental well-being by building emotional resilience and reducing anxiety (Chawrylak et al., 2024).

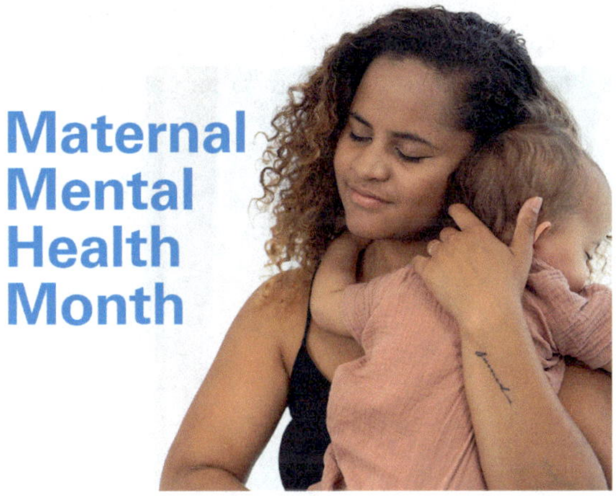

Figure 10.16. Influence on maternal mental health.

Source: https://external-content.duckduckgo.com/iu/?u=https%3A%2F%2Fwww.ahealthierupstate.org%2Fwp-content%2Fuploads%2F2024%2F05%2FMaternal-Mental-Health-Month-Social-Media-Image-EX-FINAL-copy.jpg&f=1&nofb=1&ipt=f6c9656f96db45cec8386d32e177695513690ffae207a5571e874b989c84bc25.

Addition of organized physical activity to postpartum recovery regimens can serve as a crucial component for mothers, allowing them to optimize mental well-being while simultaneously addressing pain alleviation and post-childbirth recovery. Also important is the role of integrated caregiving interventions, such as occupational therapy, in supporting maternal mental health during the postpartum period. Occupational therapists can provide personalized interventions that respond to day-to-day strategies to improve everyday functioning and mental health. The incorporation of new practices, such as online health counseling and progressive muscle relaxation, has been shown to offer significant benefits for reducing PPD and promoting maternal attachment (Chawrylak et al., 2024). Through integrating exercise with psychological assistance and education, there exists a complete model of recovery that addresses not just pain control but also the mental health of mothers, thereby improving their postpartum experience and long-term status (Figure 10.16).

Test Your Knowledge

1. What are the potential long-term physical and psychological effects of unresolved postpartum pain on maternal health?
2. How can persistent postpartum pain contribute to mental health conditions such as postpartum depression and anxiety?

SUMMARY

It is critical to highlight the significance of personalized methods that value maternal and fetal health. Standard practice is frequently found to advocate for directed pushing maneuvers in labor, even though there is evidence to support potential harm in the form of reduced fetal oxygenation and damage to maternal structures. It is through these observations that traditional practices related to the second stage of labor need reassessment. Implementation of evidence-based practices, such as facilitating spontaneous bearing down rather than forced efforts, has the potential to improve outcomes for both mother and infant. Improved pain management guidelines that incorporate these physiological approaches enable healthcare professionals to contribute to safer, more streamlined childbirth outcomes for women, culminating in better postpartum recovery pathways. Besides, emphasis on the contribution of spontaneous maternal bearing down, as supported by overwhelming scientific proof, must be a key pillar in managing labor. It not only adheres to the natural physiological pathway but also builds greater confidence among laboring mothers. The potential adverse effects associated with Valsalva pushing call for a relook at traditional approaches to managing the second stage of labor. As practitioners incorporate alternative methods—such as open-knee-chest position or altered breathing routines—into practice, they can mitigate the risks associated with forceful pushing. By doing this, healthcare providers are in a stronger position to help women in their unique birthing processes, striving toward less traumatic and healthier births following giving birth, including alleviating pain and enhancing emotional and physical well-being. Lastly, the commitment to adjusting guidelines for labor management based on growing evidence will not only improve maternal care but also demonstrate the wider implications for anesthesia practice in the postpartum period. The findings highlight the need for continuous professional development and clinical education among practitioners to maintain the latest evidence-based practice. Nursing and medical personnel will face challenges in applying these physiologic approaches, but the potential for improved outcomes is well worth it. Through the active support and promotion of women's spontaneous bearing down during labor, healthcare professionals can promote recovery from anesthesia, creating a holistic plan for postpartum care that is supportive of maternal autonomy and security, opening the door to healthier families.

Effective pain management during the postpartum period is of paramount importance in the convalescence of new mothers, particularly those who have undergone a cesarean section (CS). Pain has been the chief obstacle to early mobilization and optimal rehabilitation, both physical and emotional. Literature indicates that inadequate pain control leads to hospital delay in discharge and interferes with the mother-baby bonding process. Anesthesia techniques, including multimodal analgesia, enable improved outcomes by delivering a constellation of drugs that address multiple pain mechanisms. Along with alleviating pain, such a technique results in fewer side effects of single-drug administration. The implementation of individualized pain management protocols has the potential to significantly enhance recovery, allowing mothers to become more engaged in their postpartum care and nurturing. While the medical community continues to see the importance of effective pain management, evidence-based guidelines should now be the norm everywhere to improve maternal outcomes. The rising rate of cesarean sections throughout the world raised the issue of more scrutiny of the factors that determine women's options for delivering. The motivations behind wanting CS are more often than not fear-based, in the form of fear of pain (and possibly injury) due to the labor process, as highlighted in recent qualitative research (Colomar et al., 2021).

Women are usually apprehensive about the dangers of vaginal delivery and believe that CS is the safer route. Second, more women report feeling in control of the birth process with a planned cesarean, and this finding further attests to their preference. These findings point toward a timely alignment of psychological factors and clinical practices in the decision of maternal preference. Medical professionals must have serious discussions on birth options, ensuring that women are well-informed regarding the implications of vaginal and cesarean delivery. This promotes informed decision-making and fosters a culture of support and trust. Furthermore, an appreciation of the different perceptions women have towards pain relief and recovery is needed. Evidence indicates that anxiety regarding pain during labor significantly influences women's requests for cesarean section, typically resulting in calls for surgical intervention in the lack of medical necessity (Colomar et al., 2021). Consequently, healthcare workers are responsible for allaying such phobias by developing a system that prioritizes adequate pain management and awareness of the process of labor. Interventions must transcend alleviating bodily pain to relieving anxiety regarding delivery choices. Healthcare systems can also be improved through policies that facilitate patient-centered care, allowing mothers to express their needs and actively engage in their care plans. In acknowledging and acting on the complex factors involved in pain control and healing, medical care providers can establish a better postpartum experience for women across varying settings.

KEY TERMS FROM THIS CHAPTER

- Dynamic elastomeric fabric orthoses (DEFO)
- Endorphins
- Maternal health
- Patient feedback
- Postnatal posttraumatic stress disorder (PTSD)
- Postpartum pain management
- Empathetic communication
- Healthcare professionals
- Newborn
- Personalized care
- Postpartum
- Postpartum period

CRITICAL THINKING QUESTIONS

1. **Which of the following is considered first-line pharmacologic treatment for postpartum uterine cramping pain?**
    a. Ibuprofen
    b. Morphine
    c. Acetaminophen
    d. Ketamine
2. **What is the preferred regional anesthesia technique for cesarean section recovery?**
    a. Epidural anesthesia with opioids
    b. Spinal anesthesia with intrathecal morphine
    c. General anesthesia followed by IV PCA
    d. Local wound infiltration only
3. **What is the most common side effect of intrathecal morphine in postpartum patients?**
    a. Hypotension
    b. Respiratory depression
    c. Itching (pruritus)
    d. Nausea and vomiting
4. **Which of the following analgesic medications is safe for breastfeeding mothers?**
    a. Codeine
    b. Oxycodone
    c. Morphine
    d. Meperidine
5. **Enhanced Recovery After Cesarean (ERAC) protocols typically include:**
    a. Routine use of PCA morphine
    b. Delayed ambulation and minimal oral intake
    c. Multimodal analgesia and early mobilization
    d. Exclusive use of general anesthesia

Short Answer Questions

1. Discuss the principles and benefits of multimodal analgesia in postpartum pain management.
2. Explain the role of intrathecal morphine in cesarean section anesthesia.
3. Describe the Enhanced Recovery After Cesarean (ERAC) protocols.
4. Evaluate the role of regional anesthesia techniques such as TAP blocks and epidurals in managing postpartum pain. Include indications, mechanisms, and benefits.
5. What are the considerations for postpartum pain management in special populations, such as opioid-tolerant patients or those with a history of substance use disorder?

Answer to Critical Thinking Questions

1. (a); 2. (b); 3. (c); 4. (c); 5. (c)

REFERENCES

1. Acharya, D., & Regmi Khadka, N. (2024). Patient perspectives on post-surgical pain management after C-section using non-pharmacological methods. https://core.ac.uk/download/638725899.pdf (accessed on 28th June 2025).
2. Saravanan, S., Turrell, G., Johnson, H., & Fraser, J. (2010). Birthing practices of traditional birth attendants in South Asia in the context of training programmes. *Journal of Health Management, 12*(2), 93–121. https://doi.org/10.1177/097206341001200201Aimagambetova, G., Bapayeva, G., Sakhipova, G., & Terzic, M. (2024). Management of postpartum hemorrhage in low- and middle-income countries: Emergency need for updated approach due to specific circumstances, resources, and availabilities. *Journal of Clinical Medicine, 13.* https://www.semanticscholar.org/paper/831af730f43429e920382c0175f049bc051e1faf (accessed on 28th June 2025).
3. Almalki, M., & Mehmood, A. (2025). Assessing the features of mobile apps for self-management of postpartum depression. *African Journal of Reproductive Health, 29*(3), 132–142. https://www.semanticscholar.org/paper/0b50ded8a0626b07a083775ad4aa3828ad3f89d5 (accessed on 28th June 2025).
4. Almottowa, H. A., Seraj, A. S., Darwish, H. J., Khubyah, S. Y., Jan, R. H., Hanbashi, A. I., Almutair, R. K., et al. (2025). Patient-centric innovations in pain management for postoperative care. *International Journal of Community Medicine and Public Health.* https://www.semanticscholar.org/paper/55f3792df5e9c5ae0e46734efbf65113a6197619 (accessed on 28th June 2025).
5. American College of Obstetricians and Gynecologists, Roberts, J., Hanson, L., Lothian, J., Ponkey, S. E., Rothman, B. K., Simkin, P., et al. (2007). Best practices in second stage labor care: Maternal bearing down and positioning. https://core.ac.uk/download/213087164.pdf (accessed on 28th June 2025).
6. Ancona, J., Archer, J., Baird, S., Holmes, G., et al. (2007). Perceived readiness for hospital discharge in adult medical-surgical patients. https://core.ac.uk/download/213076329.pdf (accessed on 28th June 2025).
7. Aranake, A. P., Gaikwad, D. V., & Kanase, S. B. (2024). Prevalence of lumbo-sacral dysfunction in multiparous women. https://core.ac.uk/download/622174134.pdf (accessed on 28th June 2025).
8. Atefeh, S. (2025). Barriers and facilitators of pain management in children: A scoping review. *BMC Anesthesiology, 25.* https://www.semanticscholar.org/paper/abd94a664f89130307ae4ed05fc5a4360d3b1bed (accessed on 28th June 2025).
9. Ateya, A. A., EL-Kholy, G. A., Hassan, A. A., et al. (2020). Breast engorgement among women with Caesarean section: Impact of nursing intervention. https://core.ac.uk/download/327125352.pdf (accessed on 28th June 2025).
10. Ayers, S. (2004). Delivery as a traumatic event: Prevalence, risk factors, screening & treatment. https://core.ac.uk/download/9982834.pdf (accessed on 28th June 2025).
11. Bansal, G., Rajgopal, K., Chamola, V., Xiong, Z., & Niyato, D. (2022). Healthcare in metaverse: A survey on current metaverse applications in healthcare. *IEEE Access, 10*, 119914–119946. https://doi.org/10.1109/access.2022.3219845 (accessed on 28th June 2025).

12. Brodbeck, A., Helminak, G., Jacobson, E., Islas, D., Esser, M. S., Phelps, E. M., Streeton, A. C., et al. (2022). NANN Research Summit 2022. *Advances in Neonatal Care, 22*, E78–E85. https://www.semanticscholar.org/paper/067cac7462808f5dbbac8715ea18c595b53c6b18 (accessed on 28th June 2025).

13. Buley, A. (2019). A quality improvement study of the implementation of the Vermont Newborn Plan of Safe Care among nursing staff at Vermont hospitals. https://core.ac.uk/download/223071442.pdf (accessed on 28th June 2025).

14. Carter, C. S., Kenkel, W. M., MacLean, E. L., Wilson, S. R., Perkeybile, A. M., Yee, J. R., Ferris, C. F., et al. (2020). Is oxytocin "nature's medicine"? *Pharmacological Reviews, 72*, 829–861. https://doi.org/10.1124/pr.120.019398 (accessed on 28th June 2025).

15. Chawrylak, K., Krzemińska, K., Kubas, M., et al. (2024). Physical activity during postpartum period–An analysis of the latest studies and guidelines. https://core.ac.uk/download/620863064.pdf (accessed on 28th June 2025).

16. Cook, A., & Palmer, L. (2009). Providing maternity care to the underserved: A comparative case study of three maternity care models serving women in Washington, D.C. https://core.ac.uk/download/71348405.pdf (accessed on 28th June 2025).

17. Craft-Blacksheare, M. (2012). Self-reported explanations of recurrent chlamydia infections and urban females. *Journal of Obstetric, Gynecologic, & Neonatal Nursing, 41*. https://www.semanticscholar.org/paper/eb4be672da8561a06fc583e57e73f3114248ef27 (accessed on 28th June 2025).

18. Dixon, D. E. (2024). A holistic approach to music for stress management during pregnancy. https://core.ac.uk/download/621476222.pdf (accessed on 28th June 2025).

19. Dowell, D., Ragan, K., Jones, C. M., Baldwin, G., & Chou, R. (2022). CDC clinical practice guideline for prescribing opioids for pain—United States, 2022. *MMWR Recommendations and Reports, 71*, 1–95. https://doi.org/10.15585/mmwr.rr7103a1 (accessed on 28th June 2025).

20. Farinelli, L., Riccio, M., Gigante, A., & De Francesco, F. (2024). Pain management strategies in osteoarthritis. *Biomedicines, 12*. https://www.semanticscholar.org/paper/9a155ac2b3cb12840869cfe2e70b28a88ebdfe74 (accessed on 28th June 2025).

21. Fine, J. S., Ambrose, A. F., Didehbani, N., Fleming, T. K., Glashan, L., Longo, M., Merlino, A., et al. (2021). Multi-disciplinary collaborative consensus guidance statement on the assessment and treatment of cognitive symptoms in patients with post-acute sequelae of SARS-CoV-2 infection (PASC). *PM&R, 14*, 96–111. https://doi.org/10.1002/pmrj.12745 (accessed on 28th June 2025).

22. Fortuny, K., & Golden, O. (2011). Improving the lives of young children: Meeting parents' health and mental health needs through Medicaid and CHIP so children can thrive. https://core.ac.uk/download/71357294.pdf (accessed on 28th June 2025).

23. Goodwin, M. L., Loomans, J. I., Barzilai, O., Dea, N., Gasbarrini, A., Lazáry, Á., Netzer, C., et al. (2025). Frontline voice: AO Spine member survey regarding spine oncology knowledge generation and translation needs. *Global Spine Journal*. https://www.semanticscholar.org/paper/cc008ea7db550aa9c83f5ec711e23a563e54b1f1 (accessed on 28th June 2025).

24. Hagen, E. H. (2002). The bargaining model of depression. https://core.ac.uk/download/pdf/85221.pdf (accessed on 28th June 2025).

25. Herrera, J. E., Niehaus, W., Whiteson, J., Azola, A., Baratta, J. M., Fleming, T. K., Kim, S. Y., et al. (2021). Multidisciplinary collaborative consensus guidance statement on the assessment and treatment of fatigue in post-acute sequelae of SARS-CoV-2 infection (PASC) patients. *PM&R, 13*, 1027–1043. https://doi.org/10.1002/pmrj.12684 (accessed on 28th June 2025).

26. Hing, W. A., Milne, N., Pope, R. R., et al. (2019). Effectiveness, feasibility, and acceptability of dynamic elastomeric fabric orthoses (DEFO) for managing pain, functional capacity, and quality of life during prenatal and postnatal care: A systematic review. https://core.ac.uk/download/225011383.pdf (accessed on 28th June 2025).

27. Kim, Y. D. (2025). Association between postoperative pain management and long-term patient outcomes. *Journal of the Korean Medical Association.* https://www.semanticscholar.org/paper/bb46f1c64120a483ad1dcee92e42e1a36acdd0fe (accessed on 28th June 2025).

28. Kopczyński, C., Kopczyńska, U., Malinowski, P., Sikorski, P., Gurdak, K., Dydyk, M., Dyrek, M., et al. (2024). Harnessing cannabis: Pain management strategies for oncology patients–A narrative review. *Journal of Education, Health and Sport.* https://www.semanticscholar.org/paper/af8de1d2090d7af5eb3adb66e8bc4169ce651ccf (accessed on 28th June 2025).

29. Matlock, A. J. (2024). Exploring postpartum care: A guide for mothers. https://core.ac.uk/download/622190549.pdf (accessed on 28th June 2025).

30. Mattson, N. M. (2021). Processes used by mothers in opioid recovery to manage the needs of the maternal-infant dyad: A grounded theory study. https://core.ac.uk/download/516098702.pdf (accessed on 28th June 2025).

31. Nedopekina, E. (2021). Cesarean section. Impact on postpartum recovery, subsequent pregnancy and delivery. https://core.ac.uk/download/388619946.pdf (accessed on 28th June 2025).

32. Niyonkuru, E., Iqbal, M. A., Zhang, X., & Ma, P. (2024). Complementary approaches to postoperative pain management: A review of non-pharmacological interventions. *Pain and Therapy, 14*, 121–144. https://www.semanticscholar.org/paper/7e73de5526954cd7f5a26210457020457b40dd49 (accessed on 28th June 2025).

33. Patil, V. R., & Sharma, R. K. (2025). Effectiveness of modified sacroiliac belt on pelvic girdle pain in postnatal. https://core.ac.uk/download/640070535.pdf (accessed on 28th June 2025).

34. Pavord, S., Daru, J., Prasannan, N., Robinson, S., Stanworth, S., & Girling, J. (2019). UK guidelines on the management of iron deficiency in pregnancy. *British Journal of Hematology, 188*, 819–830. https://doi.org/10.1111/bjh.16221 (accessed on 28th June 2025).

35. Perkins, G. D., Gräsner, J. T., Semeraro, F., Olasveengen, T. M., Soar, J., Lott, C., Van de Voorde, P., et al. (2021). European Resuscitation Council Guidelines 2021: Executive summary. *Resuscitation, 161*, 1–60. https://doi.org/10.1016/j.resuscitation.2021.02.003 (accessed on 28th June 2025).

36. Petersen, E. E., Davis, N. L., Goodman, D. A., Cox, S., Mayes, N., Johnston, E., Syverson, C., et al. (2019). Vital signs: Pregnancy-related deaths, United States, 2011–2015, and strategies for prevention, 13 states, 2013–2017. *MMWR Morbidity and Mortality Weekly Report, 68.* https://doi.org/10.15585/mmwr.mm6818e1 (accessed on 28th June 2025).

37. Piacentine, L., & Weiss, M. (2006). Psychometric properties of the readiness for hospital discharge scale. https://core.ac.uk/download/213077027.pdf (accessed on 28th June 2025).

38. Pilkington, M., Pentz, B., Short, K., Marchand, T., Aziz, S., Lam, J. Y., Spencer, A., et al.

(2024). Enhanced recovery after surgery (ERAS) consensus recommendations for opioid-minimizing pharmacological neonatal pain management. *BMJ Pediatrics Open, 8.* https://www.semanticscholar.org/paper/6e0f23a68e1f6e89120a4e7f32ef600c6fe8b9c5 (accessed on 28th June 2025).

39. Prastyo, W. A., & Nugraheni, A. I. (2025). Management strategies and surgical outcomes for pediatric appendicitis: A literature review. *The Indonesian Journal of General Medicine.* https://www.semanticscholar.org/paper/c374d2637d025348d46ce4a7e0264de8ff56e249 (accessed on 28th June 2025).

40. Rao, S. S. C., Qureshi, W., Yan, Y., & Johnson, D. A. (2022). Constipation, hemorrhoids, and anorectal disorders in pregnancy. *The American Journal of Gastroenterology, 117,* 16–25. https://doi.org/10.14309/ajg.0000000000001962 (accessed on 28th June 2025).

41. Sghaier, N., Ben Soussia, R., Bouchahda, H., Belhadj, I., Ben Garouia, H., & Khiari, H. (2024). Post-traumatic stress disorder after childbirth: A Tunisian study. *European Psychiatry, 67,* S664. https://www.semanticscholar.org/paper/f825eddfb6f561866c7e8c73ad7b28d9e94fbfbc (accessed on 28th June 2025).

42. Silow-Carroll, S. (2008). Brigham and Women's Hospital: "Moving the needle" takes people, processes, and leadership. https://core.ac.uk/download/71349641.pdf (accessed on 28th June 2025).

43. Smith, E. (2020). Traditional Chinese medicine and its role in women's health. https://core.ac.uk/download/322850890.pdf (accessed on 28th June 2025).

44. Wang, Y., Shen, Y., Guo, H., You, D., Jia, S., Song, G., & You, X. (2024). Non-oral pharmacological interventions in the management of herpes zoster-related pain: A review of current research. *Frontiers in Pain Research, 5.* https://www.semanticscholar.org/paper/c6682009dd1543b590a7dab905f36fd5872fd8a9 (accessed on 28th June 2025).

45. Weber, A. N., Miskle, B., Lynch, A., Arndt, S., & Ación, L. (2021). Substance use in pregnancy: Identifying stigma and improving care. *Substance Abuse and Rehabilitation, 12,* 105–121. https://doi.org/10.2147/sar.s319180 (accessed on 28th June 2025).

46. Wolters, V., Heimovaara, J. H., Maggen, C., Cardonick, E., Boere, I., Lenaerts, L., & Amant, F. (2021). Management of pregnancy in women with cancer. *International Journal of Gynecological Cancer, 31,* 314–322. https://doi.org/10.1136/ijgc-2020-001776 (accessed on 28th June 2025).

47. Yu, R., & Lin, X. (2024). Different doses of epidural morphine combined with multimodal analgesia strategies for postpartum pain management: Study protocol for a single-center, double-blind randomized, pragmatic clinical trial. *BMJ Open, 14.* https://www.semanticscholar.org/paper/0da1291d59404b4e86f4989356ba190f948c0f05 (accessed on 28th June 2025).

48. Yuen, J. (2022). Filling the GAAAPPS: Generating affirming Asian American perinatal psychological services. https://core.ac.uk/download/552888487.pdf (accessed on 28th June 2025).

COMPLICATIONS AND EMERGENCIES IN ANESTHESIA

11

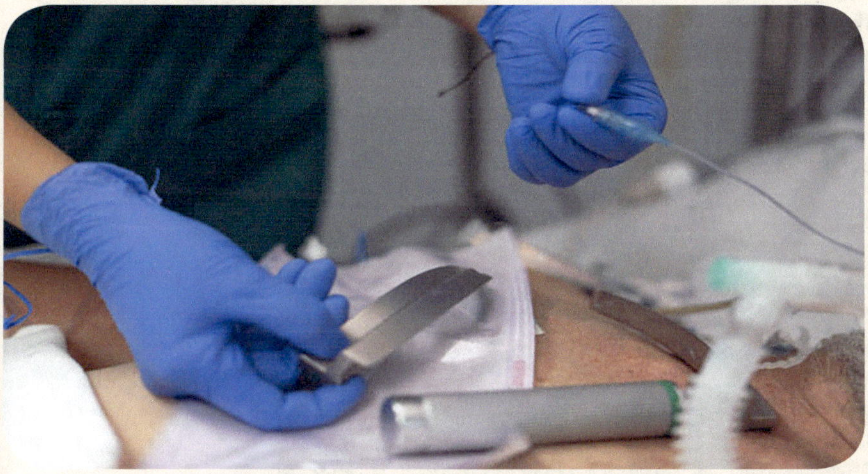

LEARNING OBJECTIVES

After studying this chapter, you will be able to:

1. Discuss the types of anesthesia
2. Explain the common complications in anesthesia
3. Focus on risk factors for anesthesia complications
4. Understand emergencies in anesthesia
5. How to implement effective prevention strategies
6. Focus on management of anesthesia emergencies

Introduction

Anesthesia is an integral component of modern-day surgical practice, often at the leading edge of surgical accidents and catastrophes. The role of anesthesia extends beyond inducing unconsciousness; it encompasses a range of management strategies that critically influence patient outcomes. Poor anesthesia and resultant development of complications can contribute not only to prolonged recovery but also to morbidity and mortality. For instance, among older patients undergoing hip fracture operations, postoperative delirium (POD) has been reported to occur at varying rates, pointing to a pressing requirement for efficient preoperative assessment and treatment methods to prevent such an aftermath (Anita et al., 2022). The incidence of various secondary medical complications from anesthesia cannot be overstated with the growth of elective and emergency procedures against the backdrop of an aging population with multiple comorbidities. In emergency settings, complexity is compounded by the emergent nature of the operations and the often unstable physical status of the patients. Research has shown that post-emergency laparotomy mortality is up to 18%, emphasizing the need for precise anesthetic management (Oumer et al., 2021). Emergency surgeries often present with complexities that require prompt assessment and decision-making by the surgical and anesthetic teams, further complicating perioperative care. Preventive strategies and the early identification of complications should be at the forefront of anesthesia practice, particularly among high-risk patients. The combination of multidisciplinary interventions, such as educating healthcare professionals, advanced pain management practices, and comprehensive preoperative evaluations, can significantly improve patients' outcomes. By focusing on risk factors associated with complications like POD among elderly patients or the catastrophic results involving high mortality with emergency surgeries, health practitioners can enhance generic institutional protocols with regard to anesthesia (Anita et al., 2022; Oumer et al., 2021). Hence, the function of well-educated and intelligent interventions is key to providing security to patients and optimizing recovery within the dynamic field of anesthesia (Figure 11.1).

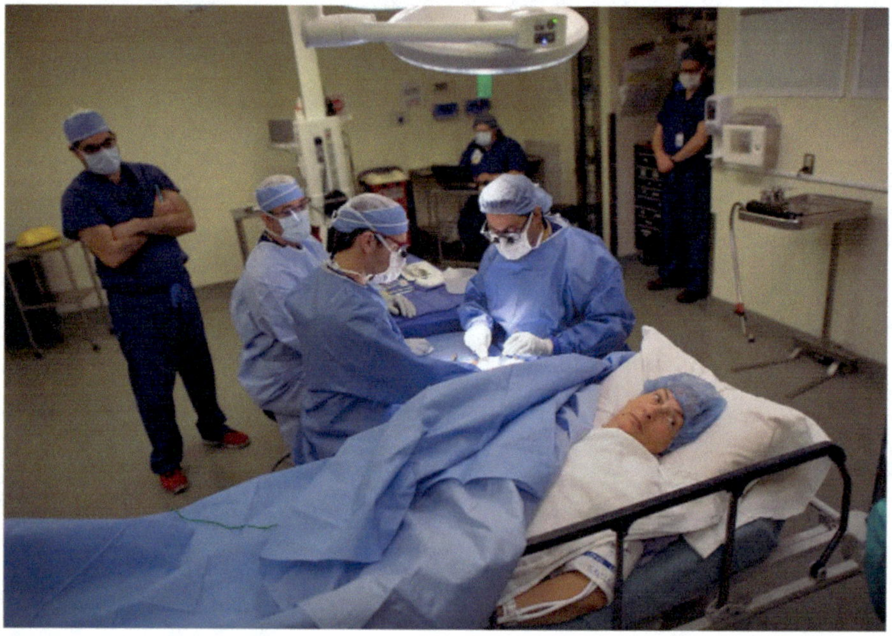

Figure 11.1. The practice of anesthesia is a critical component of modern surgical procedures.

Source: https://static01.nyt.com/images/2017/03/25/science/26AWAKE4/26AWAKE4-jumbo.jpg?quality=75&auto=webp.

Definition of Anesthesia

Anesthesia is a medical technique that causes temporary loss of consciousness or sensation, allowing surgery and diagnosis to be carried out. It comprises multiple techniques depending on the patient's condition and the type of procedure. The major forms of anesthesia include general anesthesia, which makes the patient fully unconscious; regional anesthesia, administered to a specific area of the body; and local anesthesia, which numbs a particular area. All three methods utilize different protocols and medications that act on the body's nervous system to cause intended effects, with the goal of facilitating improved patient comfort and procedural success. A complete understanding of the subtleties of anesthesia is essential because complications and disasters under anesthesia can arise from a myriad of factors, such as patient physiology, drug interactions, and procedural delivery technicalities. Administration of anesthesia requires a complete understanding of pharmacokinetics and pharmacodynamics, as well as accurate planning and monitoring during the perioperative period. Every anesthetic drug has individual properties that determine its use, effect, and potential hazards. For instance, while general anesthesia is beneficial in that it provides unconsciousness, it is also associated with conditions such as respiratory depression and cardiovascular instability. Regional anesthesia can minimize systemic complications by impacting pre-planned nerve pathways, but it might not apply to all procedures or patients. The safety of the patient must always be the priority, facilitated by meticulous preoperative examinations that consider the patient's medical history and the type of surgical intervention. A sound skillset and deep knowledge base, therefore, must be owned by an anesthesiologist in a position to foresee and manage potential complications effectively (Charles et al., 2019). In addition, anesthesiology practice has evolved to incorporate newer technologies and techniques, such as ultrasound to guide regional anesthesia. Perioperative ultrasound enhances the precision of interventions, minimizes complications, and overall maximizes patient outcomes by facilitating real-time imaging of anatomical structures. This advancement is due to the requirement for continuous education and development of the anesthesiology profession for minimizing risks associated with anesthetic practice. With procedural complexity, acquiring knowledge to integrate emerging technologies, such as ultrasound, into anesthesia practice and training will be the order of the day. Notably, considerable attention has been paid to standardizing and enhancing ultrasonic education in anesthesiology, highlighting the possibility of reducing anesthesia-related emergencies (Mahmood et al., 2016). This reflects a shift towards a centering nucleus of skills all practitioners must achieve to ensure high-quality care and optimal patient safety in surgical care.

Importance of Understanding Complications

The subtlety of anesthesia is a complex landscape in which to practice, where the expertise of complications can exert a significant influence on patient outcomes. Anesthetists must be well-grounded in knowledge and in a position to anticipate and deal with complications that can arise during procedures. Such complications, ranging from airway obstruction to cardiovascular instability, are capricious and can occur at any moment, requiring immediate and expert decision-making. This cannot be overstressed; anesthesiologists are typically the initial point of contact with intraoperative crises. By fostering a thorough appreciation of the potential complications associated with different anesthesia methods, practitioners can refine their response plan and reduce risks effectively. Moreover, existing research indicates that a systematic sedation practice, including the evaluation of underlying medical conditions and potential drug interactions, enhances safety in high-risk populations, such as children receiving procedures (Charles et al., 2019). This emphasizes the importance of proper training and ongoing education regarding complications that arise during a medical practitioner's professional life. Also, the inclusion of newer methods, such as perioperative US, in anesthesiology practice underscores the evolving nature of clinical training. An understanding of how to properly use US can significantly reduce the occurrence of complications by providing improved visualization during procedures, particularly in acute settings. Society of Cardiovascular Anesthesiologists has encouraged a formal US education as an integral component of training in anesthesia with a strong focus on the use of ultrasound for improving patient safety and outcomes (Mahmood et al., 2016). Because anesthesiologists use US in practice, the ability to identify and address potential complications in real time is significantly enhanced. Thus, the educational curriculum needs to incorporate specialized training in the use of US for the correction of catheter placement issues or for the assessment of hemodynamic stability in critically ill patients.

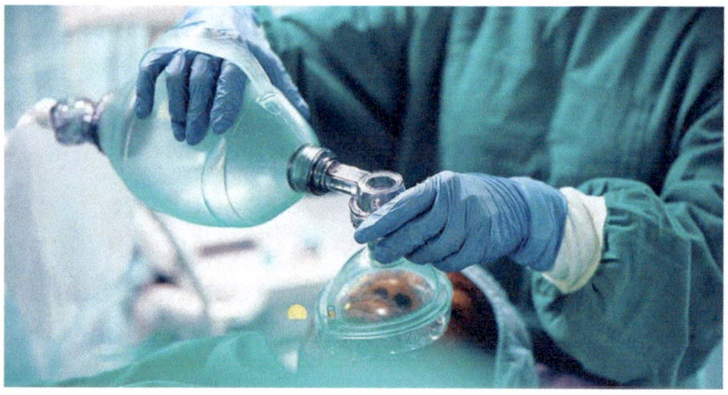

Figure 11.2. The intricacies of anesthesia present a complex landscape where understanding complications.

Source: https://medicalbuyer.co.in/wp-content/uploads/2024/01/Anesthesia-workstations-%E2%80%93-Relentless-technological-transformation.jpg.

This modification not only complies with best practices but also equips anesthesiologists with expertise they can use to manage evolving issues in a rapidly developing specialty. Lastly, ongoing education for anesthesiologists on complications ensures that practitioners can handle emergencies effectively. Owing to the dynamic nature of the medical field, the development of training standards is necessary to facilitate optimal levels of care. Emphasis on understanding complications in anesthesia fosters a safety culture among anesthesiologists, challenging them to remain vigilant and proactive in practice. In the process, they not only maintain their proficiency but also ensure they are prepared for the unforeseen nature of operating room work. In addition, with the increasing use of technology such as point-of-care ultrasound, a thorough understanding of its importance for patient safety is becoming increasingly important (Mahmood et al., 2016). This ongoing commitment to education and awareness will ultimately result in improved patient care and decreased incidence of anesthesia complications, with resulting benefits to the healthcare system as a whole (Figure 11.2).

11.1. Types of Anesthesia

Learning Outcome

1. General anesthesia
2. Regional anesthesia
3. Local anesthesia

Anesthesia comprises different types, all designed to meet the demands of specific surgeries and patients. General anesthesia, for instance, induces a reversible condition of unconsciousness and pain alleviation so that primary operations can be conducted in the absence of pain. Used primarily in extensive procedures such as open heart or brain surgery, general anesthesia contains inherent risks that must be managed, including respiratory depression, cardiovascular instability, and postoperative issues such as nausea and vomiting. All of these risks are important to know in anticipation of complications that may arise during or after administration, because patient safety is always the number one consideration in anesthesia procedures. Regional anesthesia is yet another common type of anesthesia comprising techniques such as spinal and epidural anesthesia. The process involves administering anesthetic medication near a cluster of nerves to eliminate sensory perception in a specific region of the body. Regional anesthesia would typically be ideal for pelvis or lower limb surgeries because it keeps the patient awake and typically allows a faster recovery with fewer systemic side effects compared to general anesthesia. Regional anesthesia is not, however, complication-free, and complications such as inadvertent dural puncture, infection at the injection site, or hematoma may arise, leading to neurological compromise if treated late. The significance of such risks demonstrates the need for strict observation during and after the procedure with regional anesthesia techniques. Local anesthesia is also a significant category, typically used for minor surgery in which only one isolated area of tissue needs anesthetic.

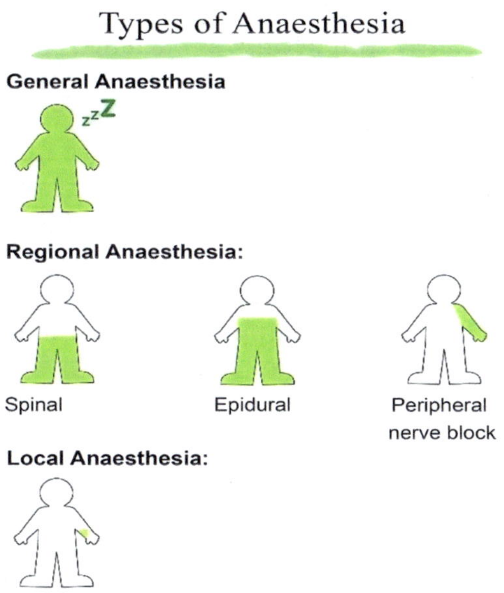

Figure 11.3. The landscape of anesthesia encompasses.

Source: https://cdn.medizzy.com/BJcrAzHLknwiLQCm_IihLA6wmlU=/680x711/img/posts/76bc973e-831e-4adc-bc97-3e831e4adc78.

For this use, local anesthetic medication such as lidocaine or bupivacaine is administered or applied locally to the tissue to block pain. At the same time, the patient remains fully conscious. While local anesthesia is effective and safe, there may be complications arising from it, for instance, allergic reactions, systemic toxicity, or inadequate anesthesia leading to distress in the patient. With value-based care at the center of healthcare, strict adherence to evidence-based approaches, including those recommended by ERAS guidelines, can optimize outcomes while minimizing complications related to anesthesia. Timely performance of these protocols plays a critical role in addressing the challenges of varied types of anesthesia and improvement of overall care of patients, as seen from studies conducted by the ERAS Society, showing significant decreases in complications and hospital stay with well-organized approaches (Joseph et al., 2017; Ljungqvist et al., 2017) (Figure 11.3).

11.1.1. General Anesthesia

In anesthesia, general anesthesia offers distinct benefits and associated risks that warrant critical consideration in operating rooms. The method is characterized by the use of pharmacological agents to induce unconsciousness and insensitivity to pain. While it keeps such a state effectively manageable for a variety of operations, it is also characterized by heightened complications, particularly among susceptible populations. For instance, existing studies highlight the need to follow up on patients who may be affected by other diseases, such as COVID-19. In a recent review, patients diagnosed with SARS-CoV-2 received cesarean sections, and the anesthetic method employed demonstrated efficiency as well as challenge, particularly in terms of hypotension during epidural anesthesia that requires special consideration during the administration of general anesthesia (Chen et al., 2020). The intricacies of general anesthesia necessitate a comprehensive knowledge of its potential complications. Research indicates that the patient population and underlying health conditions influence the risk of anesthetic complications. A 17.5% rate of complications was observed in horses that were subjected to general anesthesia during a retrospective analysis, with the suggestion that complications tend to crest in recovery phases. Variables such as increased weight, advanced age, and longer anesthesia time significantly increased risk, indicating the need for individualized anesthetic management (Laurenza et al., 2020). These findings underscore the importance of an anticipatory model of risk assessment for human patients, in which explicit determination of these variables can inform anesthesia protocols and improve patient outcomes. Ultimately, the complexity of general anesthesia demands a more thorough examination by medical experts. Continuing advances in anesthetic technique and monitoring practices aim to minimize risks, but the necessity for emergency occurrences remains a problem. The necessity of highly coordinated intervention by operating room staff, anesthesiologists, and nurses is imperative for the patient's maximum safety. With clear knowledge of potential complications and a sequential policy for their resolution, the risk for adverse events can be reduced. Amid the growing incidence of complications in routine and emergency cases, there is a need for education and training to recognize and manage general anesthesia-related complications among clinicians (Chen et al., 2020; Laurenza et al., 2020).

11.1.2. Regional Anesthesia

In anesthesiology, regional anesthesia has also gained considerable prominence due to its specific concern for pain relief with minimal systemic effect. Regional anesthesia encompasses the administration of anesthetic agents in a specific, i.e., sensation-blocking, manner in the surgical region. The primary benefit of regional anesthesia is its lower risk of postoperative complications than general anesthesia. For instance, studies indicate that while patients undergoing regional anesthesia for surgeries such as hip arthroplasties have lower postoperative complication rates, such as pneumonia and deep vein thrombosis, which are common among elderly patients (Desai et al., 2018). Additionally, the technique can lead to fewer emergency department visits and readmissions, which indicate why regional anesthesia plays a vital role in improving patient safety and satisfaction in ambulatory surgery and inpatient treatment. Although it has advantages, regional anesthesia is not without complications or emergency situations. One of its primary risks is the potential for nerve injury due to the deposition of local anesthetics near vulnerable neural elements. Although such occurrences are relatively rare, they can lead to permanent sensory or motor deficits, significantly impacting a patient's lifestyle. Also, the formation of a hematoma, particularly after a spinal or epidural block, is highly risky, particularly in patients with coagulation disorders. They suggest meticulous patient assessment and awareness of an individual's risk factors before regional anesthesia. Application of protocols for monitoring and controlling these complications is essential in the perioperative setting to ensure patient safety and to avoid risks associated with this type of anesthesia. Regional anesthesia emergencies can also be caused by inappropriate response to the block, such as incomplete analgesia or systemic toxicity. Incomplete analgesia may necessitate supplemental analgesics, potentially compromising patient care and recovery times. In addition, systemic anesthetic toxicity due to local anesthetics, being rare as it is, can induce severe cardiovascular and neurological complications, thus requiring immediate action. Anesthesia practitioners require identification and management guidelines for such complications. For example, institutions encourage protocols for the management of local anesthetic systemic toxicity, with a need to be prepared to provide resuscitative treatment. Overall, while regional anesthesia offers significant benefits for surgical pain management, the risks necessitate careful observation and prompt response to any complications, underscoring the value of expert training and preparedness for anesthesia professionals (Bryan et al., 2018) (Figure 11.4).

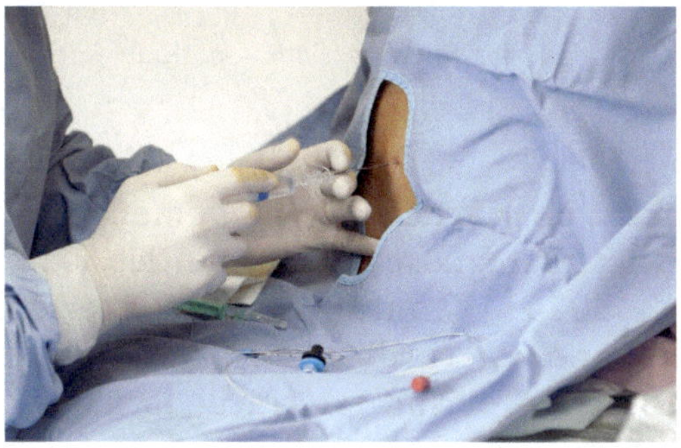

Figure 11.4. The regional anesthesia.

Source: https://www.verywellhealth.com/thmb/YwoG7Rb7TaAEUUS1pxNEMCUEcvQ=/1500x0/filters:no_upscale():max_bytes(150000):strip_icc()/GettyImages-154725435-59a034a50d327a001006171b.jpg.

11.1.3. Local Anesthesia

Local anesthesia is a vital component of modern medical practice, enabling procedures to be performed with minimal distress for patients without putting patients to sleep. The procedure involves delivering anesthetic chemicals to specific areas of the body, effectively blocking nerve impulses to prevent pain. Although local anesthesia is safe in most instances, complications can arise, and proper monitoring and care must be exercised to address them. Of interest, local anesthetics are capable of inducing systemic toxicity, especially when they are accidentally injected into the vascular space, leading to serious outcomes such as cardiovascular collapse or central nervous system toxicity. Moreover, side effects such as site infection, nerve injury, and allergy may affect the efficacy of local anesthesia, delaying recovery or necessitating additional interventions, underscoring the importance of proper administration techniques and thorough patient history-taking before treatment. Complications with local anesthesia must be handled at a subtle level, drawing on both the pharmacological properties of the anesthetic agents and the physiological effects they may induce. For instance, cardiovascular toxicity may generally be attributed with the application of the agents in excess dosage or improperly directed injections. Therefore careful vigilance should be exercised when injecting them. Clinical practice guidelines suggest the implementation of safety practices that include pre-procedure assessment and weight-based dosing calculations to prevent possible overdose situations. Training healthcare professionals to recognize early warning signs of systemic toxicity, such as tinnitus or seizure, is essential for timely intervention. In addition, adequate post-procedure pain management modalities can minimize systemic opioids, thus reducing the risk of opioid-related complications as reported in recent literature (Jennifer et al., 2016). Continuous education and practice of current clinical practice guidelines are essential for maintaining patient safety and effective pain management. Despite its advantages, local anesthesia is not devoid of potential emergencies. Risk for complications necessitates an overall approach to patient evaluation, including potential pre-existing medical conditions and drug interactions that would impact outcomes. For instance, individuals with allergies or specific cardiac conditions might be at increased risk from local anesthetic administration. Additionally, infection in the injection site is a source of potential complications, such as abscess formation, which necessitates sensitive assessment prior to the procedure. Generally, the integration of enhanced recovery protocols taking into account the modes and timing of local anesthesia delivery has been theorized to increase postoperative outcomes, especially with procedures like colorectal surgery, where postoperative recovery protocols have become standard practice in today's practice (Joseph et al., 2017). Ongoing dedication to safety protocols and education will be paramount as anesthetic practice continues to evolve to meet the needs of diverse surgical patients.

Test Your Knowledge

1. Differentiate between general, regional, and local anesthesia in terms of mechanism, administration, and clinical applications.
2. What factors influence the selection of general, regional, or local anesthesia for a particular patient and surgical procedure?

11.2. Common Complications in Anesthesia

Learning Outcome

1. Allergic reactions
2. Respiratory complications
3. Cardiovascular complications

Anesthesia is a part and parcel of modern surgical practice; however, it is not devoid of complications that arise in the perioperative period. The most commonly encountered complications are respiratory, typically due to airway obstruction or inadequate ventilation. Inadequate preoperative assessment, anatomical airway abnormalities, and suboptimal monitoring are some of the causes that can enhance these risks, particularly in high-risk groups, e.g., pediatric patients and obese patients. The need for a proper preanesthetic evaluation, including identification of potential airway complications, has become more evident for improving patient safety under sedation and anesthesia (Charles et al., 2019). Correct airway management, with appropriate equipment and personnel, is essential to avoid such complications and to guarantee patient safety during surgery. Apart from respiratory problems, cardiovascular complications are at high risk of anesthesia. Anesthetics induce hemodynamic alterations, which can lead to hypotension, arrhythmias, or even cardiac arrest in individuals with pre-existing cardiovascular disease. The increase in maternal death due to anesthesia administration serves as a grim reminder of this potential complication, particularly in women who may be hiding undiagnosed comorbidities (Carvalho et al., 2019). Monitoring and meticulous maintenance of cardiovascular status during the operative period is critical to avoid such complications. Furthermore, preoperative patient optimization through selective screening and implementation of anesthetic care practice guidelines significantly reduces cardiac-related events, enhancing the general safety and outcomes of patients. Complications from anesthesia also involve neurologic events, which, although rare, come with profound implications for patients.

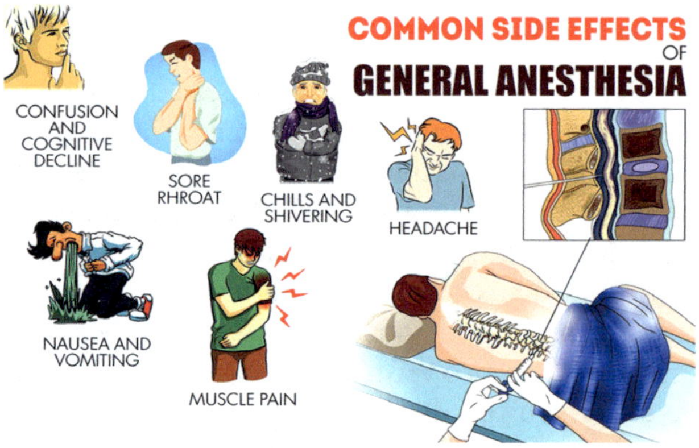

Figure 11.5. Common complications in anesthesia.

Source: https://i.pinimg.com/736x/cc/16/6e/cc166ed3b11071daf36075a767cd1a67.jpg.

Neurologic complications may manifest as postoperative cognitive dysfunction or, in sporadic cases, as cerebrovascular accidents. Those who are more vulnerable, like the elderly and individuals with cerebrovascular disease, need careful evaluation before surgery. The interaction among anesthetic drugs and their neurotoxic potential supports careful usage and continuous monitoring during sedation (Charles et al., 2019). Additionally, increasing awareness among anesthesiologists of individual patient risk factors will provide a platform to optimize anesthesia techniques and reduce neurologic complications, thereby enhancing patient care in operating rooms (Figure 11.5).

11.2.1. Allergic Reactions

Allergic responses are a serious problem in anesthesia practice, as they have the potential to cause serious complications during anesthesia. Administration of anesthetic and adjuvant drugs has the potential to induce hypersensitivity reactions in patients. Such allergic reactions can range from mild cutaneous manifestations, i.e., urticaria, to potentially life-threatening situations like anaphylaxis, and hence prompt identification and treatment are the necessities of the hour. Complications from anesthesia under the World Health Organization typically stem from unforeseen allergic reactions, further emphasizing the need for proper preoperative testing that identifies patients who are at risk for such occurrences. Having anesthesiologists properly sensitized to potential allergens and having emergency kits on hand are simple measures that can help limit the risks of allergic reactions under anesthesia (Jain et al., 2025). Planning and prudence in the identification and management of allergic reactions are crucial to anesthesiologists and operating room personnel. A striking example involved a patient who developed anaphylaxis following the administration of oxytocin during an emergency cesarean section. The patient had signs of acute respiratory distress and hypotension following intravenous oxytocin, followed by emergency intubation and intense resuscitation. This incident underscores the importance of keeping drug reserves on hand and the need for specialized training in the management of allergy-related emergencies in the operating room. Anesthesiologists must be proficient not only in the pharmacological profiles of the drugs being administered but also in identifying allergic responses and implementing rapid intervention procedures to ensure patient safety (Aithal et al., 2024). In addition, the importance of taking careful patient histories cannot be emphasized enough in preventing unintended anesthetic-related allergic reactions. In the pre-anesthetic interview, it would be appropriate to elicit information about past allergic reactions to drugs, foods, or latex, as this information would be useful in choosing anesthetic agents. Knowledge of a patient's past helps anesthesiologists tailor their practice to individual needs and apply appropriate precautions when administering anesthetics and adjunct medications. Secondarily, intraoperative monitoring should be increased in patients with a history of allergy because anticipatory caution helps early recognition of any allergic phenomenon. By promoting a safety and readiness culture, operating teams can minimize the risk of allergic complications, ultimately enhancing patient outcomes in anesthesia practice (Jain et al., 2025).

11.2.2. Respiratory Complications

Respiratory complications during anesthesia can have significant implications for patient safety and outcome and are thus of paramount importance to anesthesiologists. Respiratory complications range from minor, e.g., hypoxemia, to severe, e.g., ARDS and pneumonia. Among the factors most likely to lead to respiratory complications are the patient's underlying condition, e.g., COPD or obesity, which can complicate the anesthetic management. In addition, the intraoperative environment, such as mechanical ventilation methods and anesthesia duration, can also augment the risk of respiratory events. Understanding such factors in anesthetic preparation is important, as careful consideration can reduce risk and improve outcomes, thereby lowering the incidence of respiratory complications in the operating room. In a retrospective analysis of anesthesia-related complications, a staggering 22.6% of complications were respiratory complications, highlighting the prevalence of this complication in practice (Laurenza et al., 2020). These finding highlights that observing respiratory parameters is paramount in anesthesia, particularly in patients with known risk factors. Effective management protocols should include early detection strategies and timely interventions for respiratory failure. Choice of anesthetic technique and effective use of adjunctive drugs will also affect respiratory function. Anesthesiologists must be proficient in assessing and providing ventilation throughout surgery to reduce the risk of adverse respiratory outcomes. Further, practice modifications in anesthetic care during the COVID-19 pandemic have highlighted respiratory complications in vulnerable populations, such as pregnant SARS-CoV-2 infected women (Chen et al., 2020).

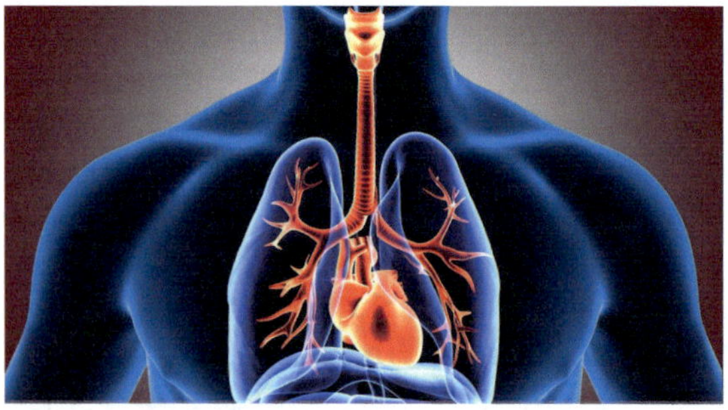

Figure 11.6. Illustration of the human respiratory system, highlighting the lungs, trachea, and heart.

Source: https://www.drugdiscoverytrends.com/wp-content/uploads/2019/10/ddd1703_respiratory.jpg.

An increased incidence of complications, such as significant intraoperative hypotension has fueled anesthesia provision for cesarean delivery in these patients. Standardized regulations ensure that general and epidural anesthesia were employed safely; however, the documented cases of hypotension indicate the delicate balance attained in anesthesia management in respiratory infections. The adoption of such lessons in anesthesia practice can enhance safety precautions and preparedness, ultimately improving patient outcomes for routine and emergency cases, particularly those involving respiratory complications (Figure 11.6).

11.2.3. Cardiovascular Complications

Cardiovascular complications during anesthesia are a serious concern as they may have a specific impact on the patient's outcome. The interaction of anesthetic agents with existing cardiovascular diseases requires careful observation and management throughout surgery. Anesthesia can cause several cardiovascular effects, such as altered heart rate, alteration in blood pressure, and even cardiac arrest in susceptible patients. Such factors as advanced age, pre-existing cardiac disease, and the surgical invasiveness pose greater risks of unwanted cardiovascular complications. For instance, complications can be reduced by methods tailored to fit individual patient groups. One needs to appreciate the physiological effects of anesthetics, such as vasodilation and changes in myocardial contractility, in maintaining hemodynamic stability in the perioperative period, and the importance of vigilance among practitioners in the anesthetic disciplines. Management of cardiac complications must be multifactorial, including preoperative assessment and continued intraoperative monitoring. Guidelines and protocols, such as those provided by the American Society of Colon and Rectal Surgeons, are critical to maximizing the safety and efficacy of anesthesia in the patient at risk for cardiovascular disease. These recommendations encourage optimization of patients' condition prior to surgery, including optimization of comorbidities and risk factors that may contribute to cardiac adverse effects. Accordingly, with the introduction of enhanced recovery programs, the significance of multidisciplinary strategy in the identification of at-risk patients is yet again emphasized, thus enabling individualized anesthetic techniques and interventions to be applied. This method not only raises the level of patient safety but also aims to enhance recovery outcomes, highlighting the necessity for anesthetists to be vigilant and proactive in their work (Joseph et al., 2017). In addition to preoperative and intraoperative concerns, post-anesthesia care must also focus on ongoing cardiovascular monitoring to detect and treat any developing complications.

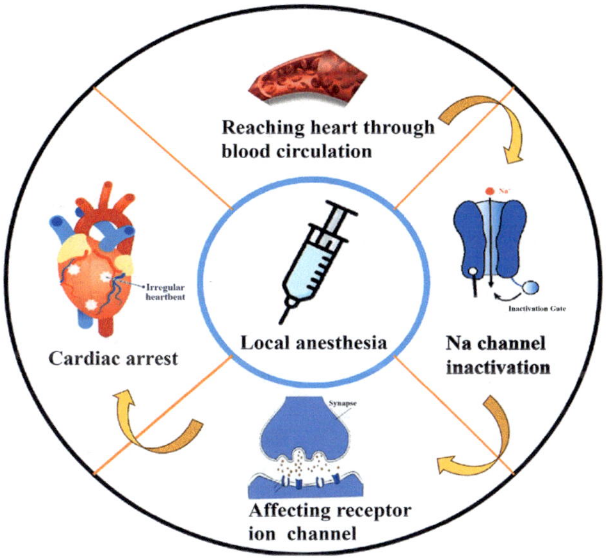

Figure 11.7. Cardiovascular complications during anesthesia.

Source: https://ars.els-cdn.com/content/image/1-s2.0-S0890850824000173-ga1_lrg.jpg.

The early recovery phase is especially important because cardiovascular events usually occur at this time. Heart rhythm, blood pressure, and observation for signs of compromised perfusion should be monitored to alert clinicians to potential postoperative problems. Early detection and intervention are the keys to preventing the risks of complications such as myocardial infarction or cardiac arrest. Further, postoperative follow-up and patient education are crucial steps that ensure patient preparation for potential cardiovascular complications after discharge. By facilitating an inclusive approach that spans the entire care continuum—from preoperative assessment to postoperative recovery—caregivers of anesthesia can significantly enhance patient safety and minimize the incidence of cardiovascular complications during procedures (Laurenza et al., 2020) (Figure 11.7).

Test Your Knowledge

1. What are the most common respiratory complications associated with anesthesia, and what mechanisms lead to their development?
2. How can perioperative monitoring and management strategies reduce the risk of respiratory complications during and after anesthesia?

11.3. Risk Factors for Anesthesia Complications

Learning Outcome

1. Patient-related factors
2. Surgical factors
3. Anesthesia provider factors

In determining the risk factors for anesthetic complications, the medical and physiological history of the patient is critical. Pre-existing medical illnesses such as obesity, diabetes, and cardiovascular disease can significantly increase the chances of complications due to anesthesia. For instance, obese individuals can be predisposed to obstructive sleep apnea, increasing airway complications and hypoxemia during procedures under anesthesia. Furthermore, conditions like undiagnosed or inadequately controlled diabetes can lead to metabolic instability, an additional risk factor for surgery. Adequate preoperative workups must be performed to properly assess these risks and to arrange appropriate anesthetics for each patient's unique case. Beyond patient-specific factors, the type of surgical procedure and the method of anesthesia employed can also influence the incidence of complications. Certain operations, such as those within the thoracic cavity or major vascular surgery, are inherently higher risk due to their inherent complexity and the physiological stresses they incur. Similarly, decision-making for the administration of general vs. regional anesthesia is not risk-free. General anesthesia, although effective in most cases, is associated with several possible complications, including airway obstruction or laryngospasm, particularly in those with preexisting recognized airway problems. In contrast, however, regional anesthesia, even if typically associated with fewer complications at a systemic level, may also induce complications such as nerve damage or hematoma formation. As a result, both the surgical site and the anesthetic approach must be well chosen to prevent risks. Last but not least, the anesthesia professional's expertise and ability are strongly associated with the development of complications. Anesthesia is a highly specialized area of medicine that requires long-term training and experience to manage its risks successfully. Less competent specialists are more prone to misestimate at critical points, such as during intubation or the administration of anesthetic medications. Furthermore, intraoperative monitoring skills, essential for the early identification of subsequent complications, may vary among individuals. More recent evidence indicates that greater levels of competence among caregivers are associated with fewer complications. Continuous education and simulation training here are essential for anesthesia personnel to keep up with emerging techniques and technologies, thereby maintaining patient outcomes during surgery (Сметанин, 2024; Fomina et al., 2024) (Figure 11.8).

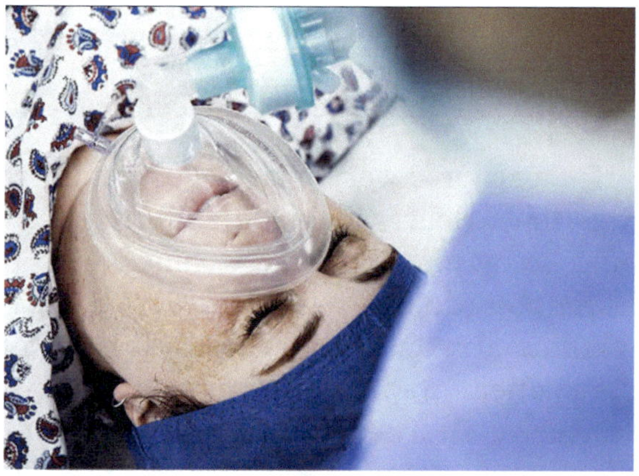

Figure 11.8. The risk factors for anesthesia complications.

Source: https://media.post.rvohealth.io/wp-content/uploads/sites/3/2021/11/general_anesthesia_GettyImages910493382_Thumb.jpg.

11.3.1. Patient-Related Factors

In anesthetics, patient issues are crucial in determining the success of surgery and the risk of complications. Patient issues include a variety of individual health parameters like age, comorbidities, and psychological status, all of which can significantly impact anesthesiology care and perioperative management. For instance, older patients often present with several comorbid diseases, such as cardiovascular and respiratory diseases, which can complicate perioperative risks and necessitate modifications to standard anesthesia regimens. Mental status, such as anxiety and depressive disorders, has also been demonstrated further to add complexity to pain perception and impact recovery, revealing the necessity for comprehensive evaluation prior to administration of anesthesia. These patient-specific factors are at the forefront of optimizing outcomes and minimizing postoperative complications, evidence of the ultimate importance of personalized care in anesthetic practice. The second most important patient-related factor is the role of prior conditions in the efficacy and safety of anesthesia. Obesity, diabetes, and obstructive sleep apnea are conditions that need to be intensively examined since they can lead to intra- and post-operative complications. Obesity, for instance, may complicate airway management and enhance the risk of respiratory complications in the postoperative period, requiring careful preoperative assessment and customized anesthetic practice. Similarly, diabetes can affect wound healing and render patients more susceptible to infection after surgery and, thus, compound the complexity of anesthetic management. The team of anesthesiologists should take such variables into account while crafting a perioperative plan, which entails evaluating the appropriateness of the anesthetic agents used as well as the monitoring strategy. The intricate interplay between patient-related factors and anesthesia outcomes underscores the need for close collaboration in patient management to identify and treat risks appropriately. The patient's psychosocial and cultural history also warrants examination when dealing with anesthesia and surgical complications. Awareness of a patient's emotional status, socioeconomic status, and culture may have a significant influence on their response to anesthesia and recovery. For example, patients from different cultures may have different beliefs about medication and pain management and therefore will react differently to postoperative treatment protocols. Also, greater levels of anxiety, which in certain instances can be observed in patients with traumatic past or pain catastrophizing, may lead to greater medication demands and latency of recovery. Comprehensive preoperative education and customized education measures are most critical to account for these variables and to improve communication and patient confidence. By making these psychosocial considerations a priority, health care professionals can develop more effective anesthetic services, ultimately leading to better patient experiences and fewer anesthetic complications (Jennifer et al., 2016; Joseph et al., 2017).

11.3.2. Surgical Factors

The operating room setting is plagued by many factors that can potentially play a significant role in patient outcomes and complication possibilities in anesthesia. A prime example of one of these important factors is the operation's emergency status. Emergency operations, such as those performed for a strangulated hernia or trauma, are prone to having unique considerations that can exacerbate complications. For instance, those requiring emergent surgery tend to be of higher comorbidity rates and may present with more advanced stages of disease than their elective counterparts. This added complexity may translate into longer operating times and increased anesthetic risk, as evidenced by findings that longer operating times are associated with higher complication rates. Therefore, anesthesiologists must familiarize themselves with the surgical environment to devise the appropriate strategies that mitigate such risks without affecting patient safety or effective care (Ayd et al., 2021). Another crucial surgical element to consider is the technique used during surgery. Different surgical approaches, such as laparoscopic versus open surgery, carry differing risk profiles that can affect anesthetic management. During procedures such as inguinal herniotomy, the Transabdominal Preperitoneal (TAPP) and Lichtenstein approaches have different effects on postoperative outcomes and anesthesia time. Literature indicates that procedures that consume more operating time not only increase expenses but also postoperative complications. For example, anesthesia time for inguinal herniotomies had a mean of 155 minutes, which shows the relationship between applied surgical technique and potential complications.

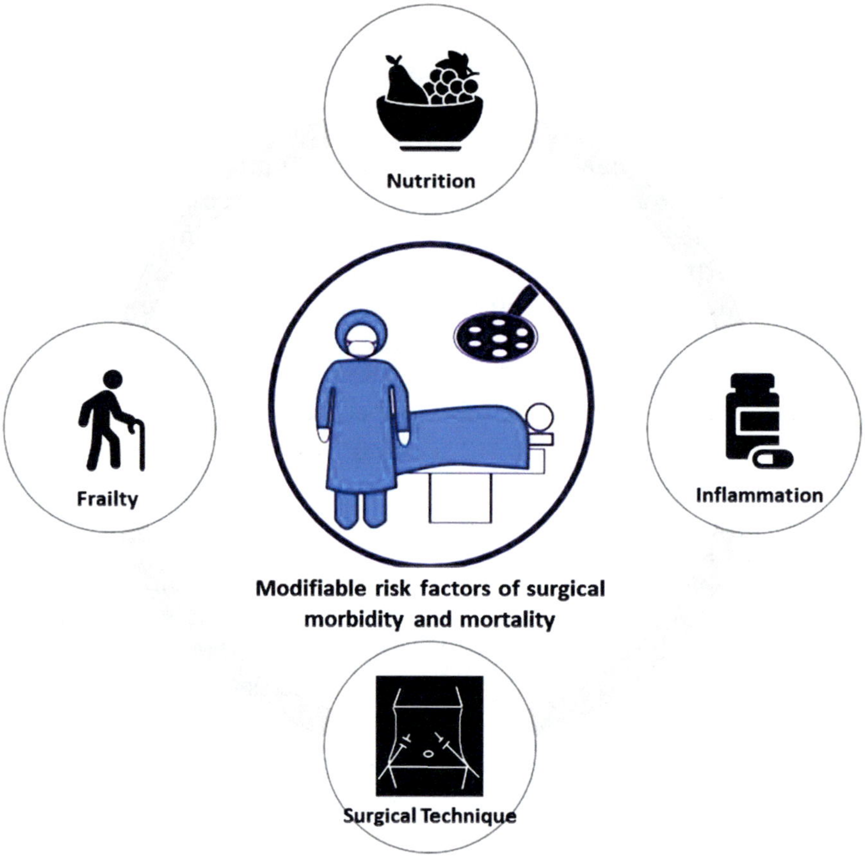

Figure 11.9. The surgical landscape is fraught with various factors.

Source: https://www.mdpi.com/nutrients/nutrients-14-03107/article_deploy/html/images/nutrients-14-03107-g001.png.

This information is paramount to anesthesiologists, who must adjust their anesthetic plan accordingly to optimize patient safety based on surgical complexity (Ayd Mın et al., 2021). Further, where the surgery is being conducted is integral to the risk of anesthetic complications. Environmental factors, whether the surgery occurs in a clean operating room or an emergency department, can have a profound impact. For instance, emergency tracheostomies performed outside of controlled environments were seen to increase significantly the rate of complications and risk of mortality. Out of 402 patients in one study on the context of surgery as a predictor of poor outcomes, those who had neck pathology were discovered to be at greater risk. These findings prepare anesthesiologists to encounter unexpected challenges in non-traditional environments and highlight the importance of proactive risk reduction efforts for immediate surgical procedures (Figure 11.9).

11.3.3. Anesthesia Provider Factors

Anesthesia care professionals' skill and experience have a strong influence on patient outcomes during procedures. Anesthesia professionals, either anesthesiologists or nurse anesthetists, must possess not only technical skill but also significant knowledge of patient physiology, pharmacology, and complications. According to studies, the provider's experience and knowledge of specific procedures have been shown to significantly reduce the risk of complications arising from anesthetic administration, thereby ensuring patient safety during the procedure. Additionally, an adequately prepared anesthesia team is equally critical in managing emergencies that may arise during surgical procedures, such as general allergic reactions or cardiovascular instability, thereby reducing morbidity rates during and after surgery. Decision-making by anesthesia providers is important during the perioperative period as well. Reliable preoperative assessment identifies patients at higher risk of complications. For example, the presence of comorbid conditions such as heart disease or obesity might necessitate a special anesthetic approach or maneuvers. The anesthesia providers must inform the surgical team of these risks and adjust their approach accordingly. The postoperative recovery-anesthetic management relationship merely reinforces the importance of such preoperative evaluations, as seen in cases where caregivers must anticipate ahead of time complications like postoperative delirium. Recognition of such risk factors allows caregivers to implement measures that can prevent negative outcomes in and after surgery, for example, the complex relationship between provider-related factors and patient safety. Emergency situations call on anesthesia providers to act quickly, an action that can ultimately determine patients' survival and recovery. In high-stress scenarios such as cardiac arrest or anaphylaxis, an agile and experienced provider can effectively stabilize a patient and deliver the complexities of advanced airway management and medication administration. Prompt settlement of the situation, along with appropriate decision-making, hinges significantly on the provider's training and experience. Emergent situations are often exacerbated by inappropriate anesthetic management, particularly in those with vulnerabilities. Curiously, appropriateness and timing remain essential because deviations result in grave complications or deaths. Consequently, the work of anesthesia professionals in the management of emergencies is directly linked to patient outcomes, further emphasizing the necessity of ongoing training and simulation exercises in anesthesia practice (Choi et al., 2020; Lee et al., 2023).

Test Your Knowledge

1. What patient-related and procedure-related factors increase the risk of complications during anesthesia?
2. How does preoperative assessment of risk factors help in preventing and managing anesthetic complications?

11.4. Emergency Situations in Anesthesia

Learning Outcome

1. Anaphylaxis
2. Malignant hyperthermia
3. Cardiac arrest

Emergency anesthesia cases pose a range of challenges that require immediate action and professional skills from healthcare providers. The complexity of such cases is generally heightened by patients' heterogeneous medical histories, particularly in an emergency operating room, where predisposing conditions may complicate anesthetic management. For instance, anesthesiologists need to be prepared to treat poorly controlled or uncontrolled acute postoperative pain, which, if not treated, can lead to severe complications, as per recent guidelines on pain management for emergency procedures. These recommendations for a multidisciplinary approach to pain management, based on patient needs and varying by procedure and disease, highlight the importance of timely evaluation and appropriate intervention in these high-risk environments (Coccolini et al., 2022). Complexity is added to the anesthesia crisis in pediatric patients by the unique physiological and anatomical characteristics of younger patients. Safe sedation of children requires thorough pre-sedation evaluation to establish potential risks due to anesthetic agents. It entails evaluation for underlying disease states that predispose the child to side effects and screening for satisfactory fasting before drug administration. Adequate, age-specific equipment and well-trained personnel are also critical in case of airway emergencies, especially in light of the likelihood of airway obstruction with children bearing anatomical variations such as enormous tonsils. Improved knowledge of pharmacokinetics and drug interaction risks enables anesthesiologists to manage such emergency complications more safely and effectively (Charles et al., 2019). The importance of close monitoring under anesthesia cannot be overstressed, especially in emergencies where complications can arise at any moment. Anesthesiologists are required to implement rigorous monitoring protocols to detect real-time changes in a patient's vital signs because such changes can indicate life-threatening conditions such as hypoxia or arrhythmias. The integration of advanced monitoring technology enables immediate data collection, informing clinical interventions to stabilize the patient effectively. Coupled with well-delineated post-procedure recovery procedures, such protocols would allow patients to be kept under observation in proximity until they reach their baseline state of consciousness. Through disciplined practice that focuses on preparedness and timely response, the safety of individuals with anesthesia complications can be significantly enhanced (Charles et al., 2019; Coccolini et al., 2022) (Figure 11.10).

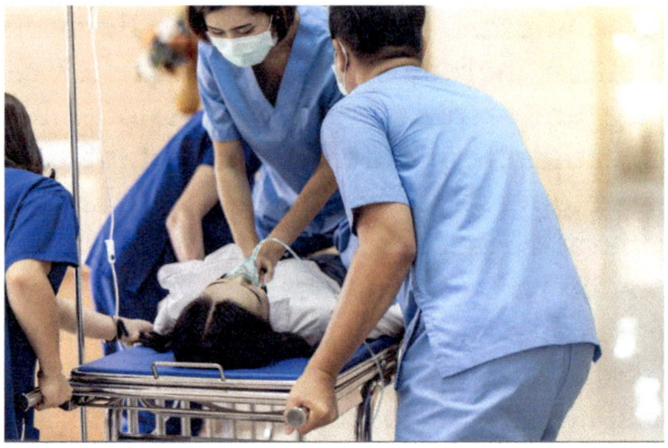

Figure 11.10. Emergency situations during anesthesia.

Source: https://esaic.org/wp-content/uploads/2024/02/bigstock-medical-team-do-cpr-cardiopulm-383305994-scaled-1.jpg.

11.4.1. Anaphylaxis

Anaphylaxis, or acute, severe allergic reaction, is a grave emergency that can be difficult to manage under anesthesia. Since exposure to several allergens during the perioperative period, such as drugs, latex, or specific foods, is feasible, anesthetic personnel must be adequately trained in identifying the symptoms of anaphylactic shock. Physicians primarily rely on a wide range of clinical presentations, including urticaria, angioedema, bronchospasm, and hypotension, to detect this deadly condition early. Anaphylaxis must be recognized early, as symptoms rapidly evolve to impair respiration and precipitate cardiovascular collapse, necessitating rapid intervention (Busse et al., 2020). Anaphylactic management of anesthesia emphasizes the rapid administration of epinephrine as the first-line treatment. This potent vasoconstrictor not only alleviates hypotension but also reduces bronchospasm and improves pulmonary ventilation, correcting critical aspects of the reaction. In addition to epinephrine, follow-up intramuscular administration of antihistamines and corticosteroids can help reduce the inflammatory response. The anesthesiology service must also be prepared to provide supplemental oxygen, intravenous fluids, and advanced airway management if respiratory compromise or cardiovascular instability occurs during the attack (Kheterpal et al., 2020). Successful management thus hinges upon both early recognition and collaborative response. Preventive interventions are necessary to limit the risk of anaphylaxis in patients undergoing anesthesia. Anesthesiologists are required to conduct thorough preoperative examinations, such as eliciting complete medical histories of allergies and a history of reaction to anesthetics and other drugs. Also, the use of allergen-specific testing, when available, may be helpful in determining possible sensitization before anesthesia induction. In environments where anaphylaxis is common, implementing protocols and training staff can increase preparedness, equipping teams to recognize the signs of anaphylaxis and administer appropriate emergency care. Emphasizing prevention and preparedness can go a long way in minimizing the dangers of anaphylaxis in the operating room (Busse et al., 2020).

11.4.2. Malignant Hyperthermia

Malignant hyperthermia (MH) is a severe but rare complication of the anesthetic practice, particularly an acute hypermetabolic state in susceptible individuals, typically triggered by certain types of anesthetic drugs. It occurs primarily as a result of a genetic predisposition, which manifests as a skeletal muscle and which leads to a life-threatening release of sarcoplasmic reticulum calcium when exposed to depolarizing muscle relaxants such as succinylcholine and inhalational anesthetics such as halothane. Understanding of this condition is especially crucial in resource-constrained settings, as evidenced by accounts from sub-Saharan Africa, where early diagnosis and management were vital in averting surgical mortality (Ndikontar et al., 2020). The rarity of MH incidents may lead to underdiagnosis and inadequate preparedness, making proper education and training of anesthesiology personnel in the identification of its signs and symptoms all the more important. Prompt identification of malignant hyperthermia is of utmost relevance in clinical practice since the condition may advance rapidly into a life-threatening crisis if not addressed in due course of time. Early presentations often feature a sudden increase in end-tidal carbon dioxide, muscle stiffness, and tachycardia—a presentation that might be misattributed to other intraoperative events. A case of a 9-year-old child experiencing masseter rigidity following succinylcholine and sevoflurane underscores the urgency of the situation; the anesthetic team diagnosed MH and administered dantrolene—its drug of choice as an antidote—within minutes, resulting in a favorable patient outcome (Lapisatepun et al., 2020). This case demonstrates the value of expectant watchfulness on the part of the operating room surgical care team and emphasizes the value of having dantrolene immediately available in every operating room since early treatment can turn a potentially fatal condition into a treatable one. The significance of malignant hyperthermia for anesthesia extends beyond immediate clinical challenges; it also encompasses aspects of anesthetic planning and patient safeguards. Of particular note, patients with a history of known MH or risk factors, which may include family history, must be appropriately screened prior to any surgical operations. Preoperative assessment should include thorough counseling on potential anesthetic agents and backup plans to mitigate MH risks. In addition, health facilities must implement comprehensive emergency plans that not only identify MH recognition and treatment but also training simulations for anesthesiology staff. In the treatment of malignant hyperthermia, anesthesia providers play a central role in fostering a safety culture that prioritizes close observation and immediate intervention to guarantee that patients are protected from this rare but serious complication (Ndikontar et al., 2020) (Figure 11.11).

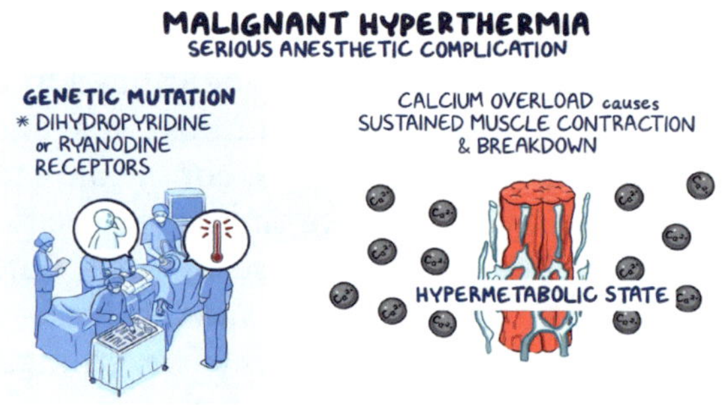

Figure 11.11. Malignant hyperthermia (MH).

Source: https://d16qt3wv6xm098.cloudfront.net/VQ4ghCc9Qz6cTHDSBBb0eK_qToyDZixe/_.jpg.

11.4.3. Cardiac Arrest

Cardiac arrest is an urgent, life-threatening condition that could happen acutely in patients undergoing anesthesia. When the heart ceases to beat, blood flow to the vital organs ceases, triggering a cascade of physiological derangements. Anesthesiologists must keep in mind that cardiac arrest is highly likely to occur with some procedures, especially those involving sedation and airway management. For instance, sedation with the use of drugs like dexmedetomidine has been shown to result in a non-zero rate of severe side effects, including cardiac arrest, although at relatively low rates relative to other methods of sedation. In assessing the risk of cardiac arrest, the anesthesiologist must consider patient-specific factors such as a history of pre-existing cardiovascular disease, age, and the surgery being performed (Sulton et al., 2016). Effective management of anesthesia-induced cardiac arrest needs the anesthesiology team to respond promptly and in a well-coordinated manner. The American Heart Association emphasizes that early detection and intervention, i.e., provision of cardiopulmonary resuscitation (CPR) and defibrillation as may be necessary, needs to be done to improve outcomes. The complexity of managing a cardiac arrest situation is compounded in the operating room, where equipment availability and team readiness directly influence resuscitation success. Anesthesiologists need first to guarantee attainment of advanced airway management because deficits in this regard complicate resuscitation as well as increase the risk of secondary complications. Studies have indicated that each failed attempt at intubation can effectively add significantly to the risk of complications, including hypoxia risk and aspiration, further complicating the patient's status during an incident of cardiac arrest (Bernhard et al., 2015). Training and preparation are key determinants of lowered risks of anesthesia-related cardiac arrest. Continuing education and simulation training in emergency airway management, along with exposure to the entire operating room staff to resuscitation guidelines, can enhance the rates of successful first-pass intubation attempts. Enhancing performance skills and stress decision-making allows anesthesiologists to handle complex airway cases more effectively, thereby reducing the number of events leading to cardiac arrest. Besides, there should be constant review and practice of emergency protocols as institutional standards with an environment that prioritizes patient safety. By encouraging rigorous training programs and emphasizing the importance of team-based approaches to crisis management, anesthesia professionals can significantly curb occurrences of cardiac arrest in high-risk situations (Bernhard et al., 2015; Sulton et al., 2016).

Test Your Knowledge

1. What are the most common emergency situations encountered during anesthesia, and how should they be managed promptly and effectively?
2. How does preparation, monitoring, and teamwork contribute to the successful handling of anesthetic emergencies?

11.5. Prevention Strategies

Learning Outcome

1. Preoperative assessment
2. Monitoring during anesthesia
3. Postoperative care

While under anesthesia, prophylactic treatment is most vital for minimizing complications and emergencies. Maternal hypotension is a standard risk of spinal anesthesia that can occur in a high percentage of patients unless actively prevented. Studies have indicated that the implementation of prophylactic interventions, such as phenylephrine administration, can significantly minimize spinal anesthesia-related hypotension. In a clinical trial, patients who received a phenylephrine infusion experienced hypotensive events at a much lower frequency than those who received colloid infusions, further substantiating the relevance of strategic pharmacological intervention in emergency situations. By practicing such targeted prevention, medical professionals can ensure optimal patient safety and outcomes, particularly with high-risk procedures such as cesarean sections, where rapid hemodynamic stability is required (Subhani et al., 2025). Another central element of anesthesia prevention practice is the evaluation and treatment of risk factors for surgical complications that endanger patients. The increasing prevalence of multimorbidity among surgical patients demands a high level of awareness of these factors, as has been extensively studied in several studies examining their association with anesthesia complications. For instance, age, comorbidities, and the nature of the surgical procedure significantly influence the risk of complications. Consequently, anesthesiologists must perform a detailed preoperative assessment to formulate individualized anesthetic plans, keeping in view patient-specific risks. This proactive approach not only minimizes the risk of complications but also establishes a safety culture in which patients and healthcare practitioners can work together to overcome the challenges in anesthesia care (Ziganshin et al., 2024). Finally, enhancing communication and collaboration among surgical and anesthetic teams is essential to effective prevention strategies. Complications in examples can often be traced to breakdowns in communication at critical junctures of patient care. Using systematic communication tools, such as checklists and transparent protocols, can significantly reduce the risk of errors and ensure that each team member has a clear understanding of the patient's requirements and the planned anesthetic. Moreover, repeated simulation training has the ability to cultivate not only technical competency but also teamwork skills, with teams being more adept at responding to emergencies. By fostering open communication and collaborative training, healthcare teams can develop a cohesive approach that focuses on patient safety and effectively addresses potential complications in the administration of anesthesia (Figure 11.12).

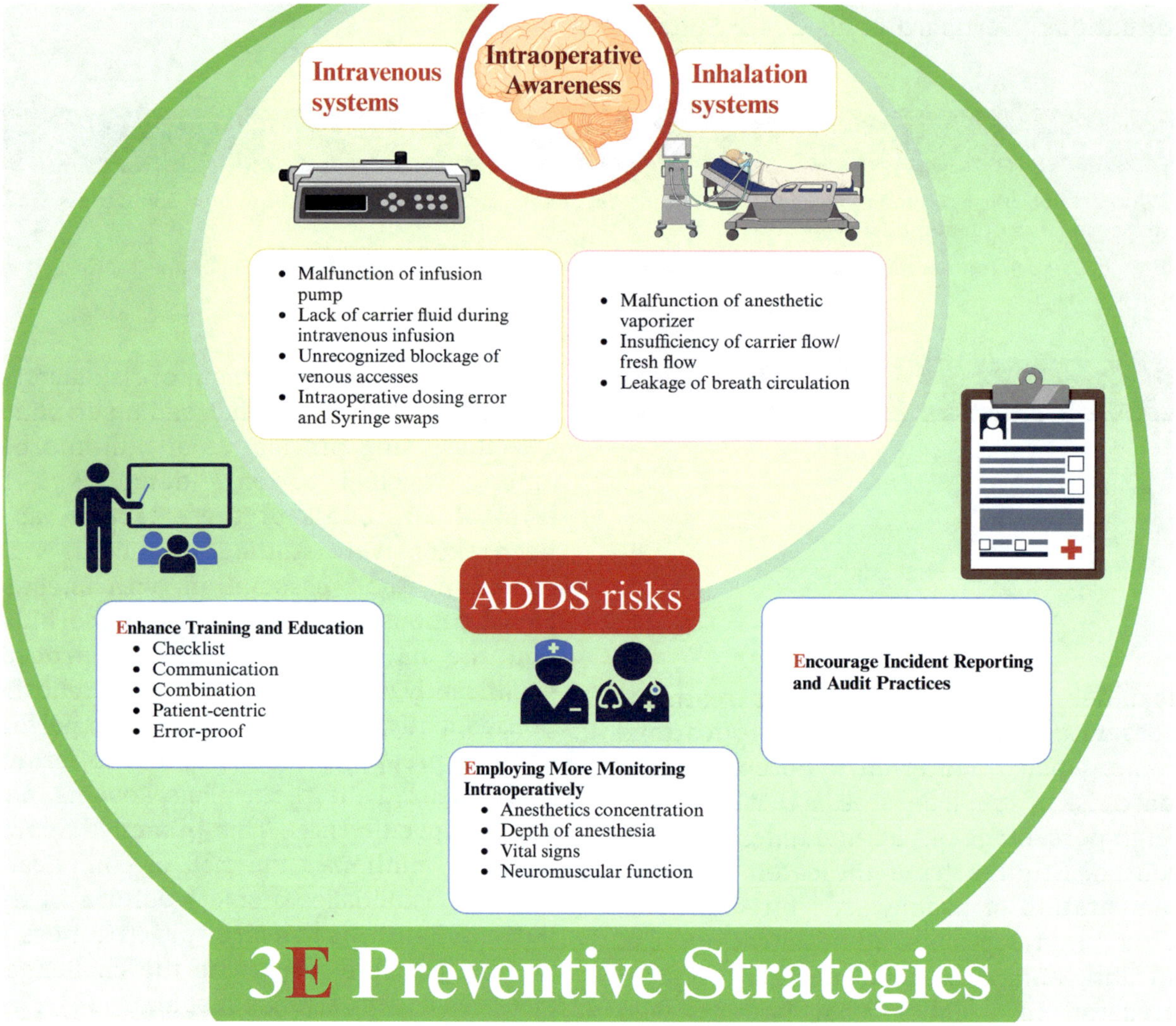

Figure 11.12. The implementation of effective prevention strategies.

Source: https://www.frontiersin.org/files/Articles/1566185/fphar-16-1566185-HTML-r1/image_m/fphar-16-1566185-g001.jpg.

11.5.1. Preoperative Assessment

Preoperative evaluation is an essential aspect of anesthesiology practice on which the foundation of patient safety and the minimization of complications in the operating room is built. Thorough examination before anesthesia not only facilitates the identification of concealed anesthesia-related hazards but also enables the anesthetist to create an individualized anesthetic plan. The significance of adequate preoperative assessment is attested to by statistics showing that the incidence of difficult tracheal intubation ranges from 1.5% to 8% in cases of general anesthesia. Failure of intubation complications can lead to severe outcomes, including brain damage and death. To prevent these outcomes, the anesthetist must assess a number of factors, including the patient's anatomy of the airway and relevant medical history, which can influence the risk of postoperative complications. Better preoperative evaluation is a key determinant of improved anesthesia-related outcomes and reduced patient morbidity and mortality (Tamire et al., 2019). Several preoperative assessment tools have been standardized to anticipate possible intubation difficulty and enhance patient safety. Mallampati classification, interincisor distance, and thyromental distance are basic tests that can help anesthetists anticipate difficult airway conditions. These assessment methods have worked well in clinical settings, with evidence demonstrating that effective implementation can minimize the number of patients who develop intubation complications. In addition, incorporating these tests into routine practice not only streamlines the preoperative process but also enables better use of resources, allowing surgical and anesthetic personnel to be assigned more easily. Education programs aimed at improving anesthesia providers' knowledge and use of these tools are essential for promoting best practices (Tamire et al., 2019). In addition, guidelines published by organizations such as the American Society of Colon and Rectal Surgeons (ASCRS) and the Society of American Gastrointestinal and Endoscopic Surgeons (SAGES) emphasize the importance of comprehensive preoperative counseling as part of preassessment. This policy encourages a culture of communication between patients and healthcare professionals, facilitating patient education regarding the operation and the risks involved. Preoperative counseling has been shown to improve patient outcomes after surgery by reducing uncertainty about discharge criteria and postoperative expectations and fostering a more informed, active patient. Those protocols have been linked to reduced hospital stay lengths and complication rates, affirming the substantial impact that meticulous preoperative assessment can have on patient quality care.

11.5.2. Monitoring During Anesthesia

Field monitoring in anesthesia is a critical part that has a significant influence on patient outcomes and safety. Continuous monitoring of life-sign vital parameters, such as blood pressure, heart rate, and oxygen saturation, allows anesthesiologists to identify deviations from baseline levels that may signal complications. In particular, the use of perioperative US techniques has transformed the traditional monitoring protocols by offering enhanced visualization of anatomical structures and physiology during surgery. The application of US for vascular access or cardiac assessment has thus becoming central to anesthesia practice; thus, there is a necessity for a teaching curriculum that acclimates anesthesiologists to the level of competence required for these advanced modalities. By incorporating these technologies into routine practice, the risk of harm from unrecognized hemodynamic changes can be markedly reduced, resulting in improved surgical outcomes and increased patient safety (Mahmood et al., 2016). Moreover, unexpected complications such as hypotension, hypoxia, and arrhythmias can occur in the perioperative period, which demand careful and vigilant monitoring protocols. Anesthesiologists use a variety of devices to monitor vital parameters, including end-tidal carbon dioxide, electrocardiography, and temperature, with the aim of ensuring optimal patient management throughout the surgical procedure. Specifically, oxygenation monitoring in close detail is of the highest priority since hypoxemia is potentially devastating to neurological function if not resolved quickly. The capacity of the anesthesiologist to read these figures in real time and interpret them accordingly is therefore crucial so that immediate intervention may be undertaken to stem potential crises. In furtherance, a comprehensive understanding of the physiological implications of aberrant values enhances decision-making in high-risk situations, emphasizing the importance of ongoing education and training in monitoring techniques and technologies (Mónica et al., 2015). Finally, cooperation between the anesthesiology team and operating room staff is an essential aspect of effective monitoring under anesthesia.

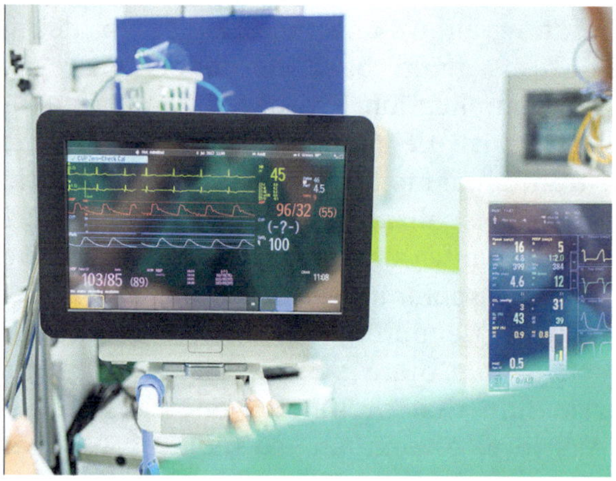

Figure 11.13. Monitoring during anesthesia.

Source: https://www.apsf.org/wp-content/uploads/newsletters/2019/3402/or-monitoring-featured.jpg.

Transfer of information regarding the patient's status, especially in patients with established risk factors, allows immediate adjustment of anesthetic care to prevent intraoperative difficulties. Notably, incorporating high-fidelity simulation training can enhance team performance and refine communication strategies in the operating room. As the era of anesthetic practice evolves with technological development, so must training paradigms encompass monitoring techniques. Future anesthesia specialists ought to develop a firm set of skills that combines traditional and innovative monitoring techniques to address patient care challenges effectively. Through such stern training, anesthesiologists will be more effective in managing emergencies and anesthesia-related complications, thereby promoting patient welfare (Mahmood et al., 2016) (Figure 11.13).

11.5.3. Postoperative Care

Effective postoperative care is essential in avoiding complications following surgery, particularly anesthetic procedures. The postoperative recovery period after surgery demands vigilance over patients as they emerge from general anesthesia. Major factors considered at this stage include assessment of respiratory function, observation for vital signs, and identification of any symptoms of complications such as suboptimal ventilation or aspiration. Because of the risks associated with anesthesia, medical practitioners must be prepared to act quickly in the event of complications. Foreign object aspiration, for instance, objects such as dental objects utilized in surgical procedures, can be very hazardous to patient safety. Prompt action, for instance, bronchoscopy to evacuate, can be essential in such a case. This emphasizes the need for structured postoperative care pathways that focus on timely observations and interventions, maintaining patient safety, and minimizing the risk of complications (Gandagule et al., 2025). An additional essential component of postoperative care is the management of potential complications related to underlying conditions, especially in the setting of perioperative COVID-19 infection. Studies have shown that patients who have undergone surgery and have developed COVID-19 have higher mortality and respiratory complications than their healthy counterparts. In this context, individualized postoperative care has been seen to improve outcomes. Clinicians are required to take the patient's age, comorbid conditions, and the nature of the surgery into consideration. Individualization of care protocols based on these determinants can have a real impact on recovery trends and reduce the risk of severe complications. This makes it essential to include a complete evaluation of each patient's personal risk profile in postoperative care plans to ensure optimal patient outcomes in today's complex medical landscape (Kim et al., 2025). Moreover, the use of the multidisciplinary team in postoperative care is important for managing the wide variety of potential complications that may arise. Coordination among anesthesiologists, surgeons, nurses, and other medical staff ensures responsiveness in postoperative care and a holistic approach. A team-based approach can ensure close monitoring and open communication, allowing early detection and correction of complications and thus assuring patient safety. Education and training of medical professionals in recognizing emergent situations, coupled with rigorously established intervention strategies, can further enhance practices of postoperative care. Encouraging a culture of shared responsibility and active management, healthcare teams can significantly improve recovery experiences among surgical patients and limit the incidence of complications that have adverse effects on long-term results in anesthesia and surgical care (Gandagule et al., 2025) (Figure 11.14).

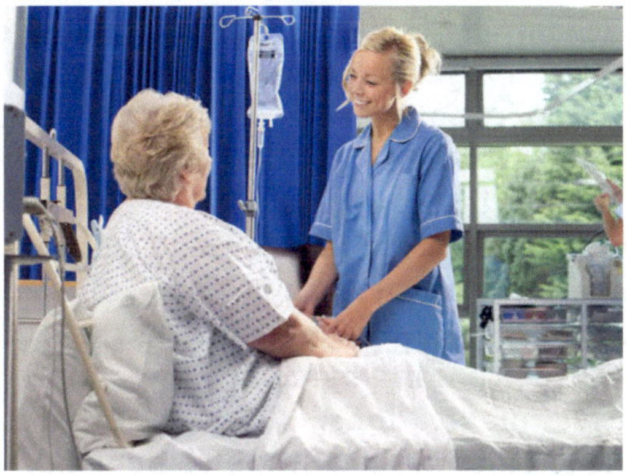

Figure 11.14. The postoperative care.

Source: https://media.post.rvohealth.io/wp-content/uploads/2020/08/postoperative-care_thumb.jpg.

Test Your Knowledge

1. How does thorough preoperative assessment help identify risks and guide safe anesthetic planning?
2. Why is continuous monitoring during anesthesia essential, and which vital parameters must be closely observed?

11.6. Management of Anesthesia Emergencies

Learning Outcome

1. Immediate response protocols
2. Use of emergency medications
3. Role of the anesthesia team

Management of anesthesia emergencies is a critical component in ensuring patient safety during surgical operations. Anesthesia crises may range from airway obstruction and cardiovascular instability to drug reaction and equipment failure. Treatment of these crises begins with early detection of symptoms and application of appropriate interventions. For instance, crises such as hypoxia or hypoventilation necessitate urgent management of the airway and oxygenation. The interdisciplinarity of risk identification and the effective handling of acute emergencies limits their effects. Subsequent monitoring of vital signs can enable early detection of deterioration, prompting interventions that can prevent serious complications or even death. Hence, high levels of preparedness, as reflected in intensive training and protocol compliance, are essential in anesthesia management. Within specialty environments such as hyperbaric oxygen treatment, the trajectory of managing anesthesia crises presents new challenges. One study examined the requirement for anesthesia in mechanically ventilated patients undergoing hyperbaric oxygen treatment. It determined that significant requirement for sedation caused significant patient-ventilator asynchrony in 88.2% of the instances. Almost 29.4% of patients had bradycardia, hypertension, and desaturation develop as treatment complications, emphasizing the emergency need for personalized anesthesia management. Employment of a variety of sedative medications, such as midazolam, dexmedetomidine, and propofol, demands care to maximize sedation and avoid side effects. The case calls special emphasis not just to clinical competency needed for anesthesia emergencies, but also to having these strategies modified to special environments. The collaborative effort of anesthesiologists and other healthcare professionals is essential to achieving favorable outcomes in such challenging cases (Furkan et al., 2025). Current advancements in neuroanesthesia emphasize the necessity of having adequate knowledge and rigorous management protocols in intraoperative emergencies. Literature focuses on intracranial pressure (ICP) management and cerebral perfusion optimization to effectively manage traumatic brain injury. Innovative approaches, such as multimodal monitoring, may provide a more comprehensive profile of the patient's status than monospecific therapy. Further, studies compare general anesthetics with sedation techniques and conclude that both are effective, but the choice may influence rates of recanalization during endovascular therapy. Continuing education and multidisciplinary collaboration remain key to optimizing these approaches to neuroanesthesia. In doing so, anesthetists must be attentive and reactive, integrating new evidence into practice to ensure the highest level of patient safety and minimize the frequency and severity of anesthesia-associated emergencies (Sleiman et al., 2025) (Figure 11.15).

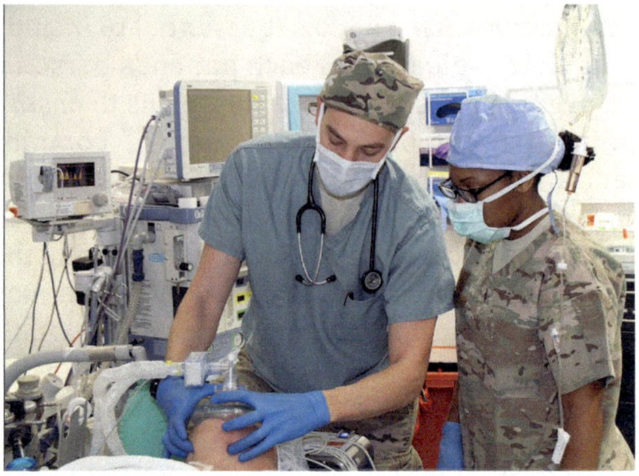

Figure 11.15. Management of anesthesia emergencies.

Source: https://upload.wikimedia.org/wikipedia/commons/thumb/7/74/Physician_anesthesiologist.jpg/1200px-Physician_anesthesiologist.jpg.

11.6.1. Immediate Response Protocols

In the context of anesthetics, immediate response protocols are critical in managing complications that could arise during surgical procedures. Such protocols involve a series of predefined steps designed to stabilize the patient and address specific adverse events promptly. For instance, when unexpected hemorrhagic complications occur, as in procedures such as orthognathic surgery, maintaining hemodynamic stability becomes paramount. Utilizing hypotension protocols can effectively control bleeding and enhance the visualization of the surgical site, thereby mitigating potential risks associated with blood loss. Notably, although numerous variations of these protocols have been proposed, their impact on systemic changes remains under-researched, underscoring the need for ongoing evaluation in clinical practice (Monnazzi et al., 2024). Furthermore, the effectiveness of immediate response protocols extends beyond the operating room into recovery phases, particularly in the post-anesthesia care unit (PACU). Immediate mobilization, mandated by enhanced recovery after surgery (ERAS) guidelines, serves as a case study in optimizing postoperative recovery. Investigations demonstrate that initiating mobilization within 30 minutes of arrival in the PACU may significantly affect physical activity levels, thus enhancing overall recovery. However, recent findings indicate that this immediate intervention does not necessarily translate into increased physical activity compared to traditional mobilization practices, suggesting that immediate responsiveness must be tailored to specific patient needs to achieve desired outcomes (Th Wörn et al., 2024).

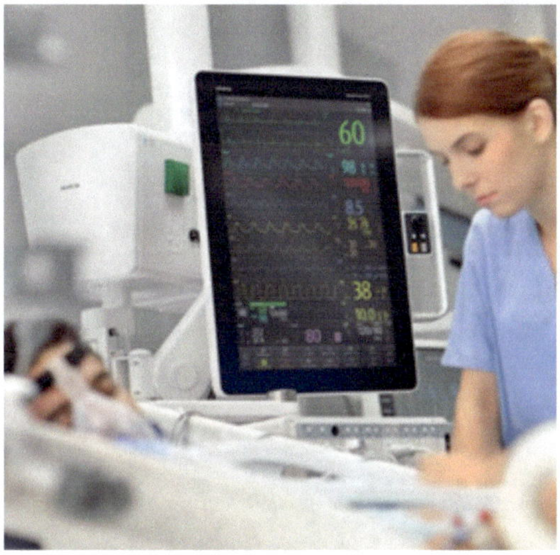

Figure 11.16. Healthcare professional monitoring vital signs in the post-anesthesia care unit.

Source: https://www.mindray.com/content/xpace/en_us/news-and-events/blog/the-importance-of-patient-monitoring-in-the-post-anesthesia-care-unit.thumb.319.319.png.

The implementation of immediate response protocols requires education and training for healthcare teams to ensure efficacy and safety in emergencies. Staff competence in recognizing signs of complications, such as hypoxia or cardiovascular instability, can lead to a more efficient application of the established protocols. Continuous training and simulations can prepare teams to respond cohesively, ultimately minimizing the risks associated with anesthesia-related emergencies. Moreover, the evaluation and refinement of these protocols based on real-time feedback are essential for adapting to evolving clinical environments, reinforcing the notion that immediate response protocols are dynamic processes aimed at improving surgical safety and patient outcomes in anesthesia practices (Figure 11.16).

11.6.2. Use of Emergency Medications

In anesthesia practice, the proper use of emergency drugs is vital for managing unforeseen issues during surgical procedures. Anesthesiologists are trained to act promptly in solving crises such as severe hypotension, aspiration, or anaphylaxis, which all demand immediate pharmacologic interventions. In fact, medications such as epinephrine to reverse rapid anaphylaxis or atropine for treating bradycardia underscore the value of preparedness in critical situations. Furthermore, the current opioid crisis complicates pain management after surgery, as physicians must balance the benefits of analgesia against the dangers of overdose and addiction. The complexities involved in managing opioids intraoperatively and postoperatively illuminate the entire dilemma that anesthesiologists face when balancing pain management with patient safety, thus outlining the importance of emergency drugs in the practice of anesthetics (Jennifer et al., 2016). Effective postoperative complications management does not end with surgical procedures but also encompasses the appropriate use of emergency drugs. For instance, in UK, after ureteral stenting following renal procedures, studies indicate that medications such as alpha blockers and antimuscarinics can complement each other to ameliorate stent symptoms. In case of an emergency, the anesthesiologist will need to be prepared to administer these medications, as well as others, to alleviate pain and prevent unscheduled emergency visits. Recent advances in pharmacology and biomaterials enhance this field of care, as stents that are biodegradable and nonsteroidal anti-inflammatories exist as new means of reducing pain and complications. The capabilities for deploying these drugs and treatment strategies emphasize multidisciplinary practice to manage complications, ensuring high-quality patient care in and out of the operating room (Ben et al., 2015). As well, the context of emergency use of drugs in anesthesia is constantly evolving through ongoing research and clinical practice guidelines aimed at further optimizing patient outcomes. Anesthesiologists are increasingly being asked to embrace emerging standards around opioid prescriptions, particularly given the unprecedented rates of opioid misuse pre- and post-op. Emergency drugs are not only a means of action to respond to acute emergencies but also for avoiding iatrogenic opioid dependence-related complications. The overall aim in employing such drugs is not only to guard against immediate risk but to encourage a general system that steers clear of long-term complication risks resulting from inappropriate use. As the specialty progresses, responsible use of emergency drugs will play an increasingly crucial role in both preoperative planning and intraoperative care, necessitating ongoing education and retraining from anesthesia providers (Jennifer et al., 2016) (Figure 11.17).

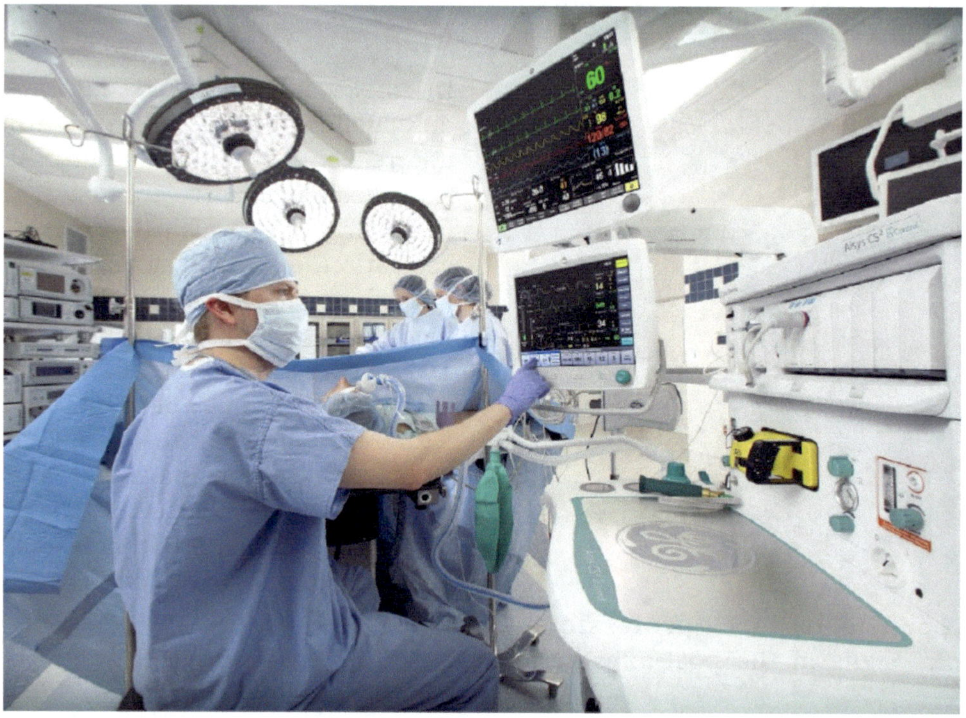

Figure 11.17. The judicious use of emergency medications.

Source: https://images-cdn.welcomesoftware.com/Zz01MjRkMGFkOGI2ODMxMWVjODhkZDFhZmYzM2ZiN2NhNg==/Aisys%202%201200_900.jpg.

11.6.3. Role of the Anesthesia Team

The role of the anesthesia team is a critical component in assuring the safety and efficacy of anesthetic care, particularly in situations of potential complications and emergencies. The team of anesthesiologists, anesthetists, and nurses has the duty to perform a thorough preoperative assessment to identify all factors that can increase the risk of adverse events during procedures. At this point, the team considers the patient's history, medications, and related anesthesia issues. All this planning allows the team to implement tailored anesthetic protocols while anticipating possible critical events. As unpredictable complications such as respiratory failure or allergic reactions can arise, an effective anesthesia team helps manage them and thereby reduce risks during anesthesia administration. Within the operating room, the work of the anesthesia teams is not limited to administering anesthetic drugs; they ought also to be vigilant observers of physiological parameters during surgery. Monitoring vital signs such as heart rate, blood pressure, and oxygen saturation can be utilized to provide real-time feedback on the status of the patient. Any abnormality that might be identified can be the start of a complication that must be treated in a timely manner. For safety, for example, in a respiratory emergency, the anesthesia team is trained to perform airway management maneuvers that are fundamental to patient protection. Additionally, their ability to introduce sophisticated resuscitation methods under unforeseen circumstances helps ensure the patient's safety and the environment, thereby cementing the anesthesia team's place as frontline guardians against toxic outcomes in anesthesia. Effective intercommunication between anesthesia staff members and with the remainder of the surgical team is central to the management of possible complications and emergencies. All team members must be knowledgeable about the procedures and expectations that guide anesthetic care so they can respond predictably in changing situations. Moreover, the establishment of proper infection-control guidelines, especially in the context of contemporary global health issues, underscores the need for teamwork to reduce risks. For instance, during outbreaks like the 2019-nCoV pandemic, the anesthesia team must ensure greater safety standards and be trained in the use of personal protective gear to prevent viral transmission, which underscores their contribution not only to procedural safety but also to ensuring the health of patients and healthcare workers (Randy et al., 2020). Eventually, continuous learning and simulation training can equip the team to be better prepared for emergencies, enabling them to sustain their responsiveness and effectiveness when facing adversity, thereby validating their essential role in anesthetic practice (Charles et al., 2019).

Test Your Knowledge

1. What are the key steps in the immediate management of common anesthesia-related emergencies such as airway obstruction, hypotension, and cardiac arrest?
2. How do standardized emergency protocols and team communication improve outcomes during anesthetic crises?

SUMMARY

The complexities involved in anesthesia highlight the necessity of proper preoperative assessment and meticulous management strategies to minimize complications to a bare minimum. The information from several studies indicates that while profound adverse events are rare in standard procedures, certain risk factors significantly increase the rate of complications. For instance, a pediatric study of patients who underwent bone marrow aspirations and lumbar punctures had a serious event incidence of 1.7%, with prematurity and emergency states found to be major predictors of respiratory complications (Dagher et al., 2024). This indicates the necessity of an individualized approach in patients with identifiable risk factors to make appropriate adjustments to anesthesia practices to avoid potential adverse effects. Besides, the data also show that anesthetic management has changed, and some surgeries are nowadays performed successfully without direct action by anesthesiologists. This shift, in particular observed with hand surgeries where surgeons administer regional or local anesthetic themselves, has resulted in satisfactory efficacy rates greater than 98% and with fewer cases of adverse effects (Andrzej, 2024). However, despite data indicating that most complications are treatable, the capacity to implement emergency intervention remains primary. These results require a reevaluation of traditional anesthetic practices and prompt reassessment of roles within the surgical team to maximize overall patient safety and procedural success. Lastly, as anesthesia science continues to evolve, ongoing education and training for surgeons and anesthesiologists are mandatory. The evolving environment demands careful examination of the latest developments in anesthetic techniques and the management of complications to achieve optimal patient outcomes. In this type of environment that promotes coordination between anesthesiologists and surgeons to communicate and share information effectively, the risk of adverse events can be further reduced. In offering safe anesthesia care, the healthcare sector must concentrate on evidence-based practices with keenness to adapt to the evolving challenges in the practice of anesthesia, thereby providing safety and health to all surgical patients.

Anesthesia complications and emergencies are multifaceted issues that require a thorough understanding of the pharmacological and physiological mechanisms involved in anesthesia. Of most significant importance is perioperative anticoagulant management, which has become increasingly relevant with the growing number of patients treated with anticoagulants. Particularly, recommendations specify the necessity of cautious preparation in terms of when to stop these drugs, particularly direct oral anticoagulants (DOACs) and antiplatelet medications, before surgery. Use of the Grading of Recommendations Assessment, Development and Evaluation (GRADE) lexicon allows clinicians to evaluate the strength of the recommendation for managing anticoagulation in the perioperative setting, thereby facilitating decision-making in surgical interventions with a higher risk of bleeding (Keeling et al., 2016). An awareness of these nuances can affect patient safety and outcomes, underscoring the importance of individualized risk assessment during surgical intervention planning. In emergency situations, certain complications can necessitate appropriate management plans. For anticoagulated patients, early surgical intervention may be necessary, prompting guidelines that determine when surgery is safe to perform and whether it involves pharmacologic reversal agents or other treatments, such as tranexamic acid, to support hemostasis. Pre-operative parenteral tranexamic acid administration has been shown in research to reduce blood loss without increasing thrombotic risk, an important consideration in the patient population. With evolving guidelines, the need for bridging with low-molecular-weight heparin

(LMWH) is also being questioned. Though bridging is intended to mitigate thromboembolic risk during gaps in anticoagulant therapy, it carries a potential for increased bleeding. It should thus have its risks versus benefits weighed carefully in cases of emergency (John et al., 2016). Finally, anesthesia practitioners must also factor in the potential for drug allergy reactions to drugs used in surgery. An adverse event can cause innumerable complications, from trivial to lethal, underscoring the importance of vigilance and preparedness. Knowing common anesthetic drugs and their side effects, along with good monitoring practices, allows clinicians to respond in a timely fashion to signs of complications such as allergic reactions, anaphylaxis, or airway compromise. Furthermore, the application of findings from emerging research to anesthetic practice can lead to improved patient outcomes and minimize anesthesia-related risks. With health increasingly prioritizing evidence-based medicine, continuing professional education on evolving anesthesia practices is essential for clinicians to refresh their strategies for the prevention and management of anesthesia-related emergencies, thereby making surgical environments safer overall (Keeling et al., 2016).

KEY TERMS FROM THIS CHAPTER

- Arthroplasties experience
- Central nervous system
- Local anesthesia
- Optimal patient safety
- Patient discomfort
- Postoperative delirium (POD)
- Cardiovascular
- Healthcare system
- Neurological events
- Pain management
- Patient safety
- Potential complications

CRITICAL THINKING QUESTIONS

1. **Which of the following is the most common cause of intraoperative anaphylaxis?**
   a. Midazolam
   b. Neuromuscular blocking agents
   c. Inhalational agents
   d. Opioids
2. **A patient under general anesthesia suddenly develops hypotension, bronchospasm, and rash. What is the most likely diagnosis?**
   a. Pulmonary embolism
   b. Myocardial infarction
   c. Anaphylaxis
   d. Tension pneumothorax
3. **Which of the following is the first-line treatment for malignant hyperthermia?**
   a. Naloxone
   b. Flumazenil
   c. Dantrolene
   d. Atropine
4. **What is the most reliable early sign of malignant hyperthermia?**
   a. Hyperthermia
   b. Bradycardia
   c. Increased end-tidal CO_2
   d. Cyanosis
5. **Which complication is most likely with spinal anesthesia?**
   a. Malignant hyperthermia
   b. High spinal block
   c. Bronchospasm
   d. Aspiration pneumonia

Short Answer Questions

1. Discuss the causes, clinical presentation, and management of malignant hyperthermia during general anesthesia.
2. Describe the pathophysiology, risk factors, and perioperative management of aspiration pneumonitis in anesthetized patients.
3. Explain local anesthetic systemic toxicity (LAST): causes, clinical features, treatment options, and prevention.
4. Describe the emergency management of difficult or failed intubation.
5. Explain the causes and emergency treatment of tension pneumothorax during positive pressure ventilation under anesthesia.

Answer to Critical Thinking Questions

1. (b); 2. (c); 3. (c); 4. (c); 5. (b)

REFERENCES

1. Aithal, N. S., & B, N. P. D. (2024). A case of anaphylactic reaction to oxytocin in a parturient undergoing emergency caesarean section. *World Journal of Biology Pharmacy and Health Sciences, 20*(1), 151–152. https://doi.org/10.30574/wjbphs.2024.20.1.0726Albanese, A. M., Ramazani, N., Greene, N., & Bruse, L. (2022). Review of postoperative delirium in geriatric patients after hip fracture treatment. *Geriatric Orthopedic Surgery & Rehabilitation, 13.* https://doi.org/10.1177/21514593211058947 (accessed on 28th June 2025).
2. Aydın, M., Fikatas, P., Denecke, C., Pratschke, J., & Raakow, J. (2021). Cost analysis of inguinal hernia repair: The influence of clinical and hernia-specific factors. *Hernia, 25*, 1129–1135. https://doi.org/10.1007/s10029-021-02372-1 (accessed on 28th June 2025).
3. Bean, B. A., Connor, P. M., Schiffern, S. C., & Hamid, N. (2018). Outpatient shoulder arthroplasty at an ambulatory surgery center using a multimodal pain management approach. *JAAOS Global Research and Reviews, 2*, e064. https://doi.org/10.5435/jaaosglobal-d-18-00064 (accessed on 28th June 2025).
4. Bernhard, M., Becker, T. K., Gries, A., Knapp, J., & Wenzel, V. (2015). The first shot is often the best shot. *Anesthesia & Analgesia, 121*, 1389–1393. https://doi.org/10.1213/ane.0000000000000891 (accessed on 28th June 2025).
5. Bou Sleiman, V., Benson, B., & Gumbert, S. (2025). Anesthetic management of neurosurgical emergencies. *Current Opinion in Anesthesiology.* https://www.semanticscholar.org/paper/cb91dfc99a6245bb350c5e0950290123642166e4 (accessed on 28th June 2025).
6. Busse, P., Christiansen, S. C., Riedl, M. A., Banerji, A., Bernstein, J. A., Castaldo, A. J., Craig, T., et al. (2020). US HAEA Medical Advisory Board 2020 guidelines for the management of hereditary angioedema. *The Journal of Allergy and Clinical Immunology: In Practice, 9*, 132–150.e3. https://doi.org/10.1016/j.jaip.2020.08.046 (accessed on 28th June 2025).
7. Carmichael, J. C., Keller, D. S., Baldini, G., Bordeianou, L., Weiss, E. G., Lee, L., Boutros, M., et al. (2017). Clinical practice guidelines for enhanced recovery after colon and rectal surgery from the American Society of Colon and Rectal Surgeons and Society of American Gastrointestinal and Endoscopic Surgeons. *Diseases of the Colon & Rectum, 60*, 761–784. https://doi.org/10.1097/dcr.0000000000000883 (accessed on 28th June 2025).
8. Carvalho, B., & Mhyre, J. M. (2019). Centers of excellence for anesthesia care of obstetric patients. *Anesthesia & Analgesia, 128*, 844–846. https://doi.org/10.1213/ane.0000000000004027 (accessed on 28th June 2025).
9. Chen, R., Zhang, Y., Huang, L., Cheng, B., Xia, Z., & Meng, Q. (2020). Safety and efficacy of different anesthetic regimens for parturients with COVID-19 undergoing cesarean delivery: A case series of 17 patients. *Canadian Journal of Anesthesia/Journal Canadine Anesthesia, 67*, 655–663. https://doi.org/10.1007/s12630-020-01630-7 (accessed on 28th June 2025).
10. Chew, B. H., & Seitz, C. (2015). Impact of ureteral stenting in ureteroscopy. *Current Opinion in Urology, 26*, 76–80. https://doi.org/10.1097/mou.0000000000000234 (accessed on 28th June 2025).
11. Choi, S., Jung, I., Yoo, B., Lee, S., & Kim, M. C. (2020). Risk factors for postoperative delirium in elderly patients after spinal fusion surgery. *Anesthesia and Pain Medicine, 15*, 275–282. https://www.semanticscholar.org/paper/71afff84833cd8ddba75665b7fd7c78eb0b7fcff (accessed on 28th June 2025).

12. Coccolini, F., Corradi, F., Sartelli, M., Coimbra, R., Kryvoruchko, I. A., Leppäniemi, A., Doklestić, K., et al. (2022). Postoperative pain management in non-traumatic emergency general surgery: WSES-GAIS-SIAARTI-AAST guidelines. *World Journal of Emergency Surgery, 17.* https://doi.org/10.1186/s13017-022-00455-7 (accessed on 28th June 2025).

13. Coté, C. J., & Wilson, S. (2019). Guidelines for monitoring and management of pediatric patients before, during, and after sedation for diagnostic and therapeutic procedures. *Pediatrics, 143.* https://doi.org/10.1542/peds.2019-1000 (accessed on 28th June 2025).

14. Dagher, K., Benvenuti, C., Virag, K., & Habre, W. (2024). The incidence of postoperative complications following lumbar and bone marrow punctures in pediatric anesthesia: Insights from APRICOT. *Journal of Pediatric Hematology/Oncology, 46*, 165–171. https://www.semanticscholar.org/paper/a190bf0bf9253dfd6387187af799ca3b7d0a711c (accessed on 28th June 2025).

15. del-Río-Vellosillo, M., & García-Medina, J. J. (2015). Anesthetic considerations in *HELLP* syndrome. *Acta Anesthesiologic Scandinavica, 60*, 144–157. https://doi.org/10.1111/aas.12639 (accessed on 28th June 2025).

16. Desai, V., Chan, P. H., Prentice, H. A., Zohman, G. L., Diekmann, G. R., Maletis, G. B., Fasig, B. H., et al. (2018). Is anesthesia technique associated with a higher risk of mortality or complications within 90 days of surgery for geriatric patients with hip fractures? *Clinical Orthopedics and Related Research, 476*, 1178–1188. https://doi.org/10.1007/s11999.0000000000000147 (accessed on 28th June 2025).

17. Fomina, E., Pochinok, E. M., Bedash, K. I., & Ponomareva, M. N. (2024). Disorders of binocular balance and accommodation as myopia progression criteria. https://doi.org/10.34660/inf.2020.26.65.009 (accessed on 28th June 2025).

18. Gandagule, R., Korde, S., Masih, A., & Saini, N. (2025). Accidental aspiration of an implant driver into the right bronchus during implant surgery. *Cureus, 17.* https://www.semanticscholar.org/paper/490d60424f3916b2fc864aaa6b035d9ea96f5e28 (accessed on 28th June 2025).

19. Jain, M., Sakale, H., & Shyam, A. (2025). Safe surgery is everyone's responsibility. *Journal of Orthopedic Case Reports, 15*, 1–3. https://www.semanticscholar.org/paper/ca300531416f19249d095f79c8d508ed0b2ff3b7 (accessed on 28th June 2025).

20. Keeling, D., Tait, R. C., & Watson, H. G. (2016). Peri-operative management of anticoagulation and antiplatelet therapy. *British Journal of Hematology, 175*, 602–613. https://doi.org/10.1111/bjh.14344 (accessed on 28th June 2025).

21. Kheterpal, S., Vaughn, M. T., Dubovoy, T., Shah, N., Bash, L. D., Colquhoun, D. A., Shanks, A., et al. (2020). Sugammadex versus neostigmine for reversal of neuromuscular blockade and postoperative pulmonary complications (STRONGER). *Anesthesiology, 132*, 1371–1381. https://doi.org/10.1097/aln.0000000000003256 (accessed on 28th June 2025).

22. Kim, H., Ahn, E., Oh, E. J., & Bang, S. R. (2025). Perioperative coronavirus disease 2019 infection and its impact on postoperative outcomes: Pulmonary complications and mortality based on Korean National Health Insurance Data. *Journal of Personalized Medicine, 15.* https://www.semanticscholar.org/paper/f6d7312a4cce907b0853550d33a2763d805a246c (accessed on 28th June 2025).

23. Kına, S. F., Türkmen, O., Özkan, R., Avcı, G., Sezgi, A., Tönge, A. E., & Erten, E. (2025). Hyperbaric oxygen therapy in emergencies: Approaches to mechanical ventilation and anesthesia. *Eurasian*

Journal of Anesthesiology and Intensive Care. https://www.semanticscholar.org/paper/938caffc214017c45f450aa36c6290e0dd585ce2 (accessed on 28th June 2025).

24. Lapisatepun, W., & Arkarattanakul, S. (2020). Early recognition and treatment of malignant hyperthermia in pediatric patient during bronchoscopy. *Case Reports in Anesthesiology, 2020*, 1–3. https://doi.org/10.1155/2020/6562896 (accessed on 28th June 2025).
25. Laurenza, C., Ansart, L., & Portier, K. (2020). Risk factors of anesthesia-related mortality and morbidity in one equine hospital: A retrospective study on 1,161 cases undergoing elective or emergency surgeries. *Frontiers in Veterinary Science, 6.* https://doi.org/10.3389/fvets.2019.00514 (accessed on 28th June 2025).
26. Lee, O., Shin, Y. C., Ryu, Y., Yoon, S., Kim, H., Shin, S., Heo, J., et al. (2023). Comparison between percutaneous transhepatic gallbladder drainage and upfront laparoscopic cholecystectomy in patients with moderate-to-severe acute cholecystitis: A propensity score-matched analysis. *Annals of Surgical Treatment and Research, 105*, 310–318. https://www.semanticscholar.org/paper/5c6ba909525172baae4c63c31f9e693fd51cb051 (accessed on 28th June 2025).
27. Ljungqvist, O., Scott, M. J., & Fearon, K. C. H. (2017). Enhanced recovery after surgery. *JAMA Surgery, 152*, 292. https://doi.org/10.1001/jamasurg.2016.4952 (accessed on 28th June 2025).
28. Mahmood, F., Matyal, R., Skubas, N. J., Montealegre-Gallegos, M., Swaminathan, M., Denault, A., Sniecinski, R. M., et al. (2016). Perioperative ultrasound training in anesthesiology: A call to action. *Anesthesia & Analgesia, 122*, 1794–1804. https://doi.org/10.1213/ane.0000000000001134 (accessed on 28th June 2025).
29. Monnazzi, M., Santos, M., Gabrielli, M. A., Tsuha, G. F., Ribeiro Neto, C. A., & Carlos, E. (2024). Hematologic response to hypotensive anesthesia during orthognathic surgery. *Concilium.* https://www.semanticscholar.org/paper/7976eb490b3d9175dd37ad471a4bd4eaf38c270d (accessed on 28th June 2025).
30. Ndikontar, R., Etoundi, P. O., Tochie, J. N., Bengono Bengono, R. S., & Ze Minkandé, J. (2020). Malignant hyperthermia, a rare perioperative complication: Case series and literature review. *Oxford Medical Case Reports, 2020.* https://doi.org/10.1093/omcr/omaa101 (accessed on 28th June 2025).
31. Oumer, K. E., Ahmed, S. A., Tawuye, H. Y., & Ferede, Y. A. (2021). Outcomes and associated factors among patients undergone emergency laparotomy: A retrospective study. *International Journal of Surgery Open, 36*, 100413. https://doi.org/10.1016/j.ijso.2021.100413 (accessed on 28th June 2025).
32. Shaughnessy, J. J., & Zechmeister, E. B. (2016). *Research methods in psychology.* https://doi.org/10.24926/8668.2201 (accessed on 28th June 2025).
33. Subhani, A. Z., Subhani, A. A., Hasan, A., Mansoor, V. B., Abbas, H., & Rashid, H. (2025). Prevention of maternal hypotension following spinal anesthesia in emergency C-sections; prophylactic phenylephrine infusion versus colloid cooled–a randomized control trial. *Insights-Journal of Health and Rehabilitation.* https://www.semanticscholar.org/paper/7b48c270d58be130210e998f8ba58c737dd652c7 (accessed on 28th June 2025).
34. Sulton, C., McCracken, C., Simon, H. K., Hebbar, K., Reynolds, J., Cravero, J. P., Mallory, M. D., et al. (2016). Pediatric procedural sedation using dexmedetomidine: A report from the Pediatric Sedation Research Consortium. *Hospital Pediatrics, 6*, 536–544. https://doi.org/10.1542/hpeds.2015-0280 (accessed on 28th June 2025).

35. Tamire, T., Demelash, H., & Admasu, W. (2019). Predictive values of preoperative tests for difficult laryngoscopy and intubation in adult patients at Tikur Anbessa Specialized Hospital. *Anesthesiology Research and Practice, 2019*, 1–13. https://doi.org/10.1155/2019/1790413 (accessed on 28th June 2025).

36. Waljee, J. F., Li, L., Brummett, C. M., & Englesbe, M. J. (2016). Iatrogenic opioid dependence in the United States. *Annals of Surgery, 265*, 728–730. https://doi.org/10.1097/sla.0000000000001904 (accessed on 28th June 2025).

37. Wax, R. S., & Sandrock, C. (2020). Practical recommendations for critical care and anesthesiology teams caring for novel coronavirus (2019-nCoV) patients. *Canadian Journal of Anesthesia/Journal Canadine Anesthesia, 67*, 568–576. https://doi.org/10.1007/s12630-020-01591-x (accessed on 28th June 2025).

38. Wilnerzon Thörn, R. M., Forsberg, A., Stepniewski, J., Hjelmqvist, H., Magnuson, A., Ahlstrand, R., & Ljungqvist, O. (2024). Immediate mobilization in post-anesthesia care unit does not increase overall postoperative physical activity after elective colorectal surgery: A randomized, double-blinded controlled trial within an enhanced recovery protocol. *World Journal of Surgery.* https://www.semanticscholar.org/paper/709537adfcc1fbfdfa123df7fee163d806a025a1 (accessed on 28th June 2025).

39. Ziganshin, M., Marakanov, R. M., Mulyukov, A. R., Baboyan, D. O., Nadyrgulov, R. B., & Gilyazitdinov, N. M. (2024). Epidemiology of complications in anesthesiology and possible ways of their prevention. *Acta Biomedica Scientific.* https://www.semanticscholar.org/paper/f3bc2792df83ba0c81b3f94da3c35739a021d0d0 (accessed on 28th June 2025).

40. Żyluk, A. (2024). Wide awake local anesthesia no tourniquet in hand surgery: An analysis of adverse events and complications. *Pomeranian Journal of Life Sciences, 70*, 15–17. https://www.semanticscholar.org/paper/da64c065e13089dc90d3aa7338f4d88ed9d118b7 (accessed on 28th June 2025).

41. Сметанин, В. Н. (2024). Some aspects of HCAI prevention in medical organizations. https://doi.org/10.34660/inf.2020.81.58.013 (accessed on 28th June 2025).

PRINCIPLES OF POST-ANESTHESIA CARE

12

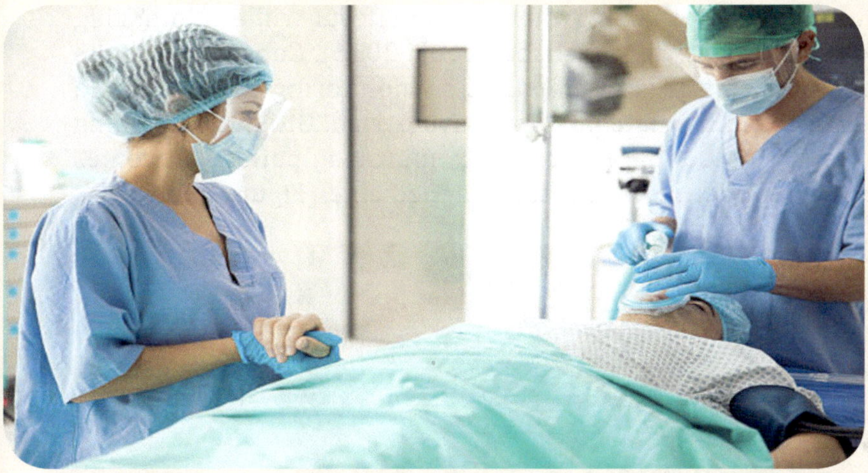

LEARNING OBJECTIVES

After studying this chapter, you will be able to:

1. Understand the anesthesia
2. Discuss the post-anesthesia care unit (PACU)
3. Explain the Patient assessment in PACU
4. Focus on the recovery process following anesthesia
5. Understand Complications and interventions
6. know Patient education and support

Introduction

Post-anesthesia care cannot be overemphasized, as it is an important part of patient recovery following surgical procedures. The introduction of innovations in anesthesia practice, such as the ideal anesthetic, is a milestone in perioperative medicine. This new approach, focusing on the application of a receptor-based magnetic resonance model of anesthesia, has the potential to alter anesthesia delivery, potentially removing systemic side effects associated with anesthetic drugs in the past (Golyanishchev et al., 2016). An appreciation for the principles of post-anesthesia care consists not only of complete knowledge of such advances but also awareness of the implications for patient safety and recovery outcomes. The addition of leading-edge technology and a sound nursing practice foundation serves as the foundation of an effective post-anesthesia care unit. With surgery evolving, so must the nursing practice and educational bases of caregivers. The growing number of day surgery units in the United Kingdom is one example of the need for increased nursing education that takes into account the evolving surgical demand. A study found that the education of new graduate staff nurses did not adequately cover contemporary operating room procedures, leaving the workforce insufficiently trained to manage the nuances of post-anesthesia care (Mitchell et al., 2005). The lack of this knowledge compromises the potential for optimal patient recovery and necessitates the redesign of nursing school curricula. With a focus on post-anesthesia principles, nurse education can prepare future professionals not only to understand anesthesia technologies but also to apply evidence-based practices in the postoperative setting. In addition, greater focus on patient-centered care underscores the importance of individualized post-anesthesia strategies aligned with technological innovation. The post-anesthesia care of the future is likely to rely on interdisciplinary teamwork, in which anesthesiologists, nurses, and allied health professionals collaborate to design tailored recovery pathways. With the integration of electromagnetic models of pharmacodynamics into anesthesia administration, as proposed by current studies, optimizing therapeutic effects while minimizing adverse interactions takes on a tangible dimension (Golyanishchev et al., 2016). Consequently, the role of healthcare professionals will shift to placing greater emphasis on monitoring, assessing, and responding to patients' individual needs in the immediate postoperative period. Ultimately, gaining knowledge of post-anesthesia care concepts is essential not only for improving patient outcomes but also for shaping the future of anesthesia practice within today's medicine (Figure 12.1).

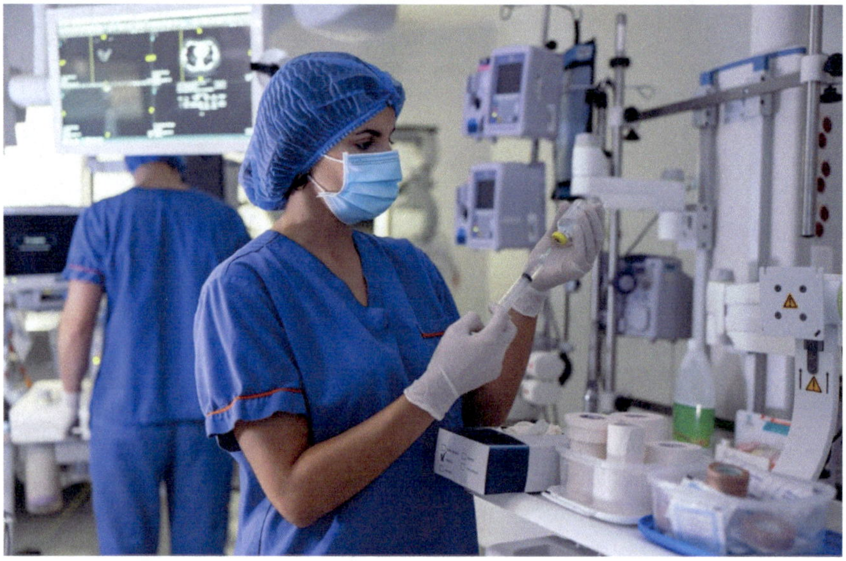

Figure 12.1. The significance of post-anesthesia care.

Source: https://cdn.prod.website-files.com/5babc11099f97ea5dbcf24d5/65b829131c46647c8f3729de_pacu-nurse.jpg.

Definition of Post-Anesthesia Care

Post-anesthesia care is a significant phase in the sequence of patient care that immediately follows surgical procedures involving the application of an anesthetic at the conclusion. It is intended to enable safe recovery from the effects of anesthesia, potentially varied in terms of duration and intensity depending on the character of the anesthetic applied. Such post-anesthesia recovery is typically performed in a dedicated unit known as the post-anesthesia care unit (PACU) where patients are constantly observed and monitored under close supervision for potential anesthetic complications. The objectives of post-anesthesia care include management of pain, observation of vital signs, and identification of any abnormal physiological response that arises as a result of the anesthetic wearing off. Successful post-anesthesia care places not only patient safety first but also overall outcomes at risk through immediate detection and adjustment of any emergent issues. Post-anesthesia care is defined to encompass many practices and protocols aimed at preserving physiological stability and facilitating recovery. This involves vigilant monitoring of the patient's vital signs, such as oxygen saturation, heart rate, and blood pressure, to detect early signs of complications, such as hypoxia or cardiopulmonary instability. The application of advanced monitoring devices, such as bioimpedance machines, also helps determine patients' responses to treatment and the severity of postoperative pain, underscoring the critical role of technology in patient evaluation in the PACU environment. For instance, the ANSPEC-PRO system is being piloted as a pain-level monitor in post-anesthesia recovery, both showcasing its potential to improve patient outcomes and demonstrating the need for continued innovation in postoperative care technology (Copot et al., 2020). Thus, post-anesthesia care is necessarily an ongoing multi-faceted process with close monitoring, assessment, and intervention. The complications that arise in post-anesthesia care underscore the importance of a comprehensive understanding and strategy in this regard. Tissue edema, particularly pulmonary edema, may be an important complication at this time, thereby affecting patients' outcomes. Modern strategies suggest careful fluid management, moderation of the inflammatory response, and monitoring equipment to minimize complications such as pulmonary edema (Assaad et al., 2017). Use of transpulmonary thermodilution as a monitor for the accumulation of water in the lung is an example of the efforts being made to enhance postoperative care by providing feedback of real-time data to assist therapeutic decision-making. Such technology not only helps in improving the management of complications but also enables a better understanding of the physiology of the patients as they emerge from the anesthetized state. Lastly, the post-anesthesia care definition reflects a commitment to patient safety, optimal recovery, and application of new technologies in the continuum of surgery (Figure 12.2).

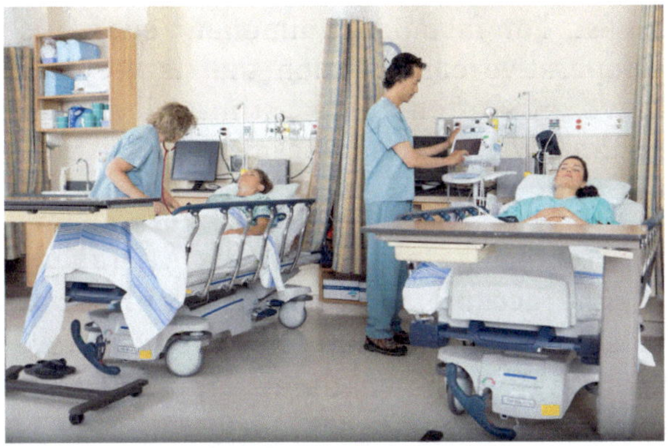

Figure 12.2. Post-anesthesia care.

Source: https://images.ctfassets.net/5ghoewqh73wu/3PzAbJEkC7LjaqaUG23itV/6c287af9cf12e11461569c89d5e10005/PACU_Nurse.jpg?w=1000&h=667&fl=progressive&q=50&fm=jpg.

Importance of Post-Anesthesia Monitoring

Effective post-anesthesia care is vital to ensuring patient safety and optimal recovery following surgical procedures. Post-anesthetic patients often exhibit differential physiologic responses that require close monitoring. Such stringent monitoring allows caregivers to detect any unusual complications early, such as respiratory depression, hypotension, or mental status change. For example, advances such as the development of the ANSPEC-PRO model enable real-time monitoring of pain levels and other critical parameters, thus providing greater insight into patient comfort and response during recovery. These technologies are only part of a broader movement to leverage monitoring technologies for enhanced patient care, as shown by evidence of the statistically significant, positive correlation between new monitors and traditional pain-measuring techniques. Thus, post-anesthesia monitoring represents a critical lifeline to ensure patient safety and satisfaction throughout recovery. Also, post-anesthesia monitoring is not merely for observation; it plays a vital role in the early recognition of complications, allowing intervention at the earliest. For instance, pulmonary edema is a perioperative complication that is very well-known but often underestimated and will presumably have a significant influence on the patient's outcome.

Monitoring strategies that have parameters for fluid accumulation can help differentiate the etiology and initiate treatment protocols accordingly. The bedside application of transpulmonary thermodilution (TPTD) illustrates how emerging monitoring techniques enhance patient care by identifying fluid overload early, before symptoms become evident. Its applicability is invaluable for risk stratification of high-risk individuals, enabling clinicians to optimally individualize interventions and reduce the risk of adverse events. Therefore, the introduction of new monitoring modalities in post-anesthesia care is required to enhance patient safety and improve the overall quality of care. In summary, the function of post-anesthesia monitoring is enhanced by its multi-angled implications to patient safety, complication prevention, and evidence-based decision-making in practice. Continued monitoring is necessary to provide healthcare providers with crucial information regarding a patient's hemodynamic stability and general recovery status. It also shows an evolving sensitivity to the nuances of post-anesthesia care, in which individualized strategies based on each patient's circumstances are paramount. As awareness of the implications of interventions such as minimizing fluid overload and optimizing pain control with newer technology increases, the principles of post-anesthesia care evolve to more fully embrace a holistic approach. By actively seeking strict monitoring procedures, as evidenced by the use of equipment such as ANSPEC-PRO and TPTD, practitioners can achieve significant improvements in patient outcomes and enhance the recovery process after surgical procedures (Figure 12.3).

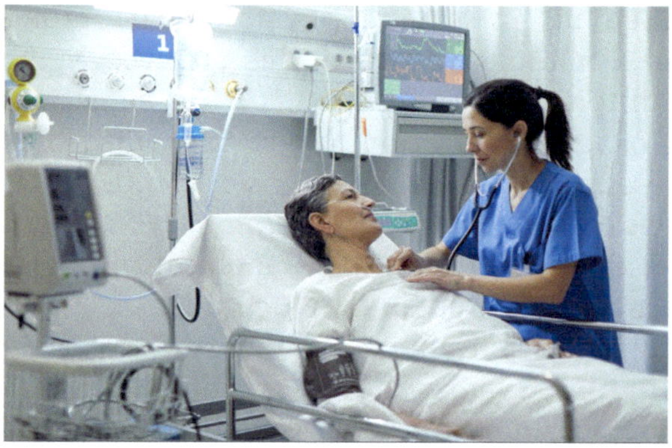

Figure 12.3. Importance of post-anesthesia monitoring.

Source: https://radiusky.com/wp-content/uploads/2020/12/postanesthesiamonitoring.jpg.

12.1. Understanding Anesthesia

Learning Outcome

1. Types of anesthesia
2. Mechanisms of action
3. Risks associated with anesthesia

Anesthesia is an important component of modern surgical procedures, providing patients with pain relief and comfort during invasive procedures. An understanding of its basics, including the drug properties of anesthetic agents, is compulsory for both patients and clinicians. Anesthetics are typically classified as general and local, with distinct mechanisms. General anesthesia permits temporary loss of consciousness. It facilitates extensive surgical manipulation, while local anesthesia is applied for pain relief at a defined location without altering the patient's overall level of consciousness. This dichotomy necessitates understanding the varying dosing regimens and the physiological consequences that may follow anesthesia, and prepares the ground for effective post-anesthesia care to achieve optimal patient outcomes. By assessing the safety and efficacy of anesthetic methods, health care professionals can better prepare for potential complications during recovery, thereby enhancing patient safety and satisfaction. Furthermore, the post-anesthesia care unit (PACU) is a key component of the continuum of care following anesthesia administration. Within it, patients are strictly observed for any type of undesirable response, especially respiratory or cardiovascular morbidity resulting from the anesthesia endured during surgery. The effectiveness of PACU care can typically be proved by adhering to established protocols and inter-professional relationships among healthcare professionals. Post-anesthesia innovation, as demonstrated in several case studies, has shown that standardized recovery pathways can significantly improve patient safety outcomes. The case studies reveal concrete actions hospitals implemented to enhance their anesthesia protocols, demonstrating the benefits of continuous learning and adaptation in clinical practice. These practices provide invaluable insights to healthcare systems aiming to create a culture of safety and enhance procedural effectiveness in the PACU, which is indispensable for integrated patient recovery processes (Blumenthal et al., 2006). Finally, the educational aspect in the context of understanding anesthesia is most significant, primarily since it encompasses interdisciplinary practice. Medical education is increasingly recognizing the importance of interprofessional collaboration among health professionals such as anesthesiologists, nurse anesthetists, and operating room staff. Face-to-face interaction across discrete health roles, particularly in educational settings, promotes a better understanding and respect for each profession's unique contribution to patient care. Evidence indicates that third-year medical students exposed to certified nurse-midwives, for example, graduate with a better appreciation of collaborative practice arrangements and develop a greater interest in working alongside such professionals in the future. Interdisciplinary training emphasizes the value of learning from one another's expertise, ultimately resulting in better outcomes in post-anesthesia care settings. Enhancing understanding and knowledge among future healthcare professionals can lead to a better consistency in patient safety and quality care in anesthesia practice (Hanson et al., 2005) (Figure 12.4).

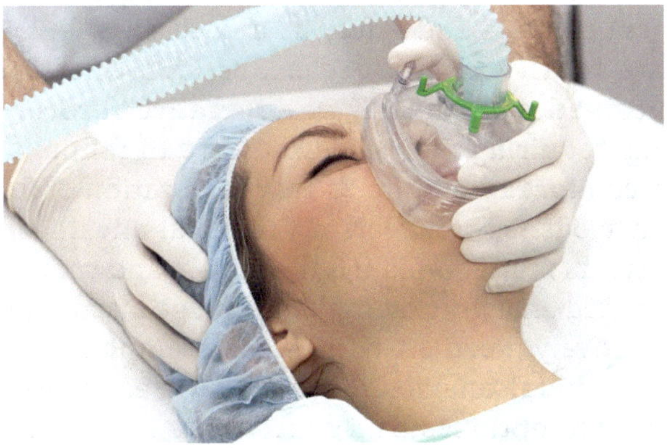

Figure 12.4. Anesthesia is a pivotal component of modern surgical procedures.

Source: https://cdn.britannica.com/41/183141-050-BD55C5AB/patient-anesthesia.jpg.

12.1.1. Types of Anesthesia

Anesthesia is one of the most important aspects of modern medicine, enabling surgical procedures and operations to be performed with very little pain for the patient. The primary types of anesthesia are general, regional, and local, each serving a distinct role depending on the type of surgery. General anesthesia induces unconsciousness and insensibility to pain all over the body and allows for massive surgery with complete immobilization and lack of awareness. Regional anesthesia, on the other hand, is the injection of anesthetic agents near nerves to inhibit sensation in a specific segment, which is best suited for surgery in limbs or lower regions. Finally, local anesthesia is applied for minor procedures, numbing a small area to prevent pain, but with the patient being consciously awake. It is imperative to know these differences in order to produce post-anesthesia care plans that meet specific patient needs effectively. In the practice of post-anesthesia care, the type of anesthesia is important in determining recovery procedures and pain control protocols. General anesthesia recoveries are usually followed by a broad range of pain, sedation, and nausea in patients, hence the need for strict monitoring to offer them comfort and safety as a necessity. This is particularly essential because residual effects of anesthetics can impair postoperative recovery, thus requiring individualized care to minimize discomfort and facilitate easy restoration of full consciousness. Conversely, regional anesthesia patients may complain of local pain and require directed analgesic therapy to manage discomfort effectively. Further, with greater emphasis on multimodal analgesia, which utilizes various drugs to optimize pain relief while minimizing opioid use, anesthesiologists also play a central role in orchestrating postoperative care that not only manages acute pain but also lays the foundation for long-term outcomes (Pozek et al., 2018). The connection between anesthetics and postoperative convalescence is once more emphasized in recent studies, which note the importance of a tailored approach to combating postoperative complications of chronic pain. A substantial minority of patients experience postsurgical pain that persists over a prolonged duration, emphasizing the importance of preoperative assessment and postoperative management to achieve pain control. Risk factors such as preoperative use of opioids, anxiety, and drug addiction can potentially enhance the risk for chronic postoperative pain. With greater collaboration between anesthesiologists and surgical teams, enhanced recovery pathways, and new anesthesia techniques, such as those provided by the latest monitoring platforms, such as ANSPEC-PRO, can be applied to achieve the best possible patient outcomes (Copot et al., 2020). These recommendations address not only short-term operative pain but also minimize long-term opioid dependency, thus serving the overall goals of patient care in an age of modern anesthesiology.

12.1.2. Mechanisms of Action

In post-anesthetic care, it is important to be aware of the mechanisms of action of anesthetic medications to achieve the best patient outcomes. Anesthetics possess various mechanisms of action, with central and peripheral nervous system effects. Intravenous agents propofol and ketamine, for instance, have different effects on GABA receptors as well as NMDA receptors that influence neurotransmitter discharge and the general excitability of the brain. This subtle interaction not only produces sedation but also influences patients' recovery patterns as they return from unconsciousness to consciousness. Hence, knowledge of these mechanisms assists clinicians in developing appropriate monitoring strategies and anticipating issues during the recovery phase, ultimately maximizing post-anesthesia care. Furthermore, the heterogeneity of anesthetic agents underscores the significance of individualized approaches to post-anesthesia monitoring. Electroencephalographic (EEG) signs are essential for assessing the depth of anesthesia by reflecting the brain states induced by different agents. The significance of monitoring stems from the fact that, for instance, sevoflurane can induce typical EEG patterns reflecting a particular level of unconsciousness distinct from its counterparts, such as isoflurane or nitrous oxide. These discoveries of the differential anesthetic effects not only facilitate good decision-making by anesthesiologists but also maximize post-anesthesia patient safety. Therefore, the application of EEG signatures represents a valid approach to ensuring a successful recovery shift. Besides pharmacologic considerations, the response to critical incidents during anesthesia underscores the importance of integrated post-anesthesia care. A thorough grasp of the mechanisms of response to critical incidents is a prerequisite to building facilitation models for anesthesia health professionals. As reported by many studies, formalized critical incident stress management programs significantly reduce psychological effects on anesthetists and enhance their capacity to provide quality care. For example, initiatives to empower certified registered nurse anesthetists (CRNAs) following critical incident work aim to address the need to address both emotional and cognitive responses likely to present in crisis situations. At the end of the day, establishing an environment where clinical staff are free to work through critical incidents appropriately enhances the overall post-anesthesia care experience for patients and medical practitioners (Hickey et al., 2019) (Figure 12.5).

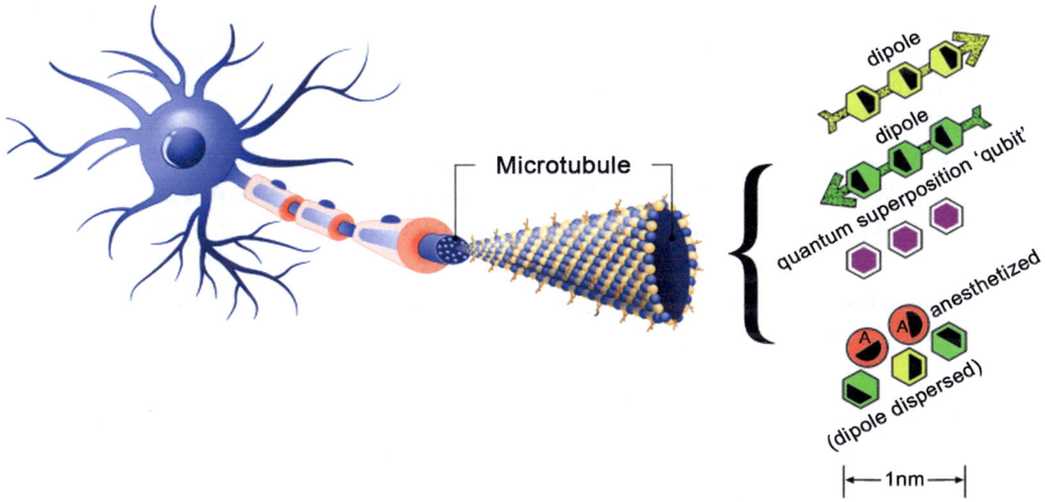

Figure 12.5. The mechanisms of action of various anesthetic agents.

Source: https://media.springernature.com/lw685/springer-static/image/chp%3A10.1007%2F978-1-4939-9891-3_6/MediaObjects/439706_1_En_6_Fig2_HTML.png.

12.1.3. Risks Associated with Anesthesia

Anesthesia administration is a vital component of surgery, but it involves inherent risks that must be addressed cautiously during post-anesthesia care. One such relevant issue is the risk of chronic postoperative pain, which affects a significant minority of patients. The problem often leads to excessive opioid use, further increasing opioid dependence as well as its complications. Patient characteristics such as preoperative opioid use, anxiety, and substance abuse may predispose patients to this issue. As a countermeasure, anesthesiologists are uniquely positioned to implement multimodal analgesia regimens that can effectively reduce opioid usage. With the utilization of personalized intraoperative medications and the creation of effective analgesic strategies for discharge, prolonged opioid exposure can be prevented. The cooperative behavior of anesthesiologists and surgeons in such instances is critical to successfully addressing and managing these risks, thereby enhancing patient outcomes in post-anesthesia care (Pozek et al., 2018). Another major risk with the administration of anesthesia is developing perioperative complications, a good example of which includes pulmonary edema. The fluid management strategy employed during the perioperative time is critical in avoiding this risk. Fluid overload can lead to increased capillary permeability and inflammatory responses, threatening patient recovery. In response, treatment guidelines authorizing monitoring of precautionary fluid use are essential. Use of transpulmonary thermodilution (TPTD) as an in-bed device is a recent technique for quantitative assessment of lung water content. It allows one to identify fluid overload in patients early on, before the overt presentation of pulmonary edema occurs. Through the integration of TPTD data, clinicians can make appropriate therapeutic choices, thereby maximizing patient safety and optimizing outcomes in high-risk postoperative patients (Assaad et al., 2017). The psychological dimensions of anesthesia also deserve consideration, as they may manifest in several postoperative complications. Preoperative anxiety and distress about surgery may increase a patient's perception of pain, making recovery after anesthesia more complicated. In addition, the administration of certain anesthetic drugs can interfere with mental functions and lead to postoperative cognitive dysfunction (POCD) in elderly patients. POCD poses a considerable challenge both to patients and health care personnel during recovery. Application of complete postoperative monitoring programs that observe mental status and deal with psychological consequences can be beneficial under such circumstances. Additionally, creating reassurance and calm conditions can decrease anxiety, improving overall recovery scores. Understanding the interaction between psychology, anesthesia, and recovery emphasizes the necessity for advanced and interprofessional care strategies in post-anesthesia settings.

Test Your Knowledge

1. What are the common risks associated with anesthesia, and how can they be minimized through proper assessment and monitoring?
2. How do patient-specific factors and the type of anesthesia influence the likelihood of anesthetic risks and complications?

12.2. Post-Anesthesia Care Unit (PACU)

Learning Outcome

1. Purpose and function of the PACU
2. Staffing and training requirements
3. Equipment and technology used in the PACU

The PACU is a key part of the recovery process following surgical procedures, serving as the most important bridge between the operating room and the final transfer to a ward or discharge. Such an area is designed to monitor and regulate patients as they recover from anesthesia, stabilizing vital signs and making certain complications are addressed promptly. Historically, the PACU has played not just a role in physiological monitoring, but also in pain management and emotional support of families and patients. This holistic approach is necessary to ensure a sense of security during a potentially disorienting recovery. Furthermore, increased emphasis on patient-centered care has amplified the PACU's role, positioning it at the center of quality improvement efforts to enhance patient outcomes and satisfaction. Emphasis on communication and workflow productivity within the PACU has become more important as census and surgical caseloads expand. The challenges faced in a high-demanding PACU environment can lead to frequent work disruptions, potentially compromising the quality of patients' care. As determined by existing studies, such disruptions can encroach on nurses' ability to perform at their best, leading to decreased job satisfaction and, consequently, potential delays in patient recovery (Martin et al., 2015). Implementation of change-oriented strategies, for example, enhancing communication among the multidisciplinary team, is intended to reduce such oversights.

For example, the adoption of contemporary communication technology would streamline operations and enhance coordination among health providers, thereby reducing oversight in patient care. Moreover, the invention of new monitoring devices, such as the ANSPEC-PRO prototype, is an example of how practices continue to improve within the PACU in a bid to improve the assessment and management of pain. Recent observational trials validated the device's efficacy in the evaluation of bioimpedance and pain intensity measurements compared during postoperative recovery (Copot et al., 2020). This technology innovation not only improves the precision of pain management but also enhances the nurse's ability to provide personalized care by monitoring immediate patient responses. This integration of technology and traditional care practices reflects the need for continuous improvements within the PACU environment, ultimately leading to better patient outcomes and experiences post-surgery. Thus, the PACU is more than a recovery room; it is an integral component of the healthcare delivery system that balances patient safety and satisfaction with the demands of modern surgical procedures (Figure 12.6).

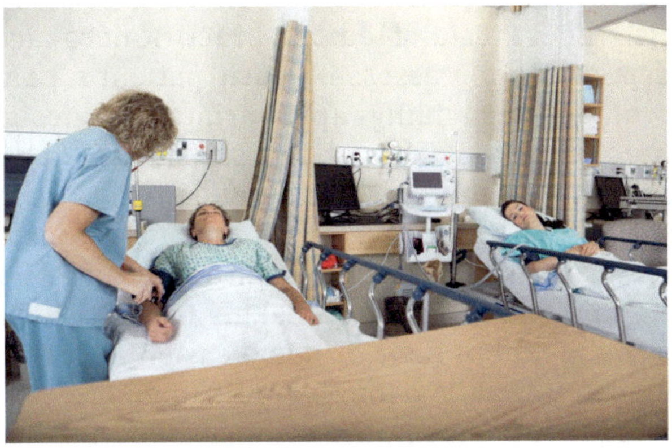

Figure 12.6. The post-anesthesia care unit (PACU) plays a critical role in the recovery process.

Source: https://images.ctfassets.net/5ghoewqh73wu/5rHwZUpXjzbel8Lb295UH/90d716b65ea90c899f1cacdd26ee711f/PACU_Nurse.jpg?w=1000&h=667&fl=progressive&q=50&fm=jpg.

12.2.1. Purpose and Function of the PACU

The PACU has an important role in the continuum of patient care following anesthesia procedures. As a transitional area, the PACU provides time and space for health professionals to monitor and take charge of patients after the dissipation of the effects of anesthesia. One of the primary purposes of the PACU is to maintain patients' safety by monitoring their vital signs closely through heart rate and blood pressure and detecting any complication that may arise during the initial recovery period. This monitoring is important, as it aligns with the goals of key healthcare campaigns, such as the Triple Aim Campaign, which aims to enhance patient experience and outcomes while lowering healthcare delivery costs (Cadwalader et al., 2015). This focused care environment seeks to minimize error and enable patients to safely emerge from anesthesia before they are transferred to other wards for further recuperation. Apart from observation, the PACU has vital functions in pain management and the management of side effects associated with anesthesia. Medical practitioners are responsible for assessing each patient's pain level and providing appropriate analgesia, thereby improving patient satisfaction and facilitating a quicker recovery. Effective pain control not only provides comfort for patients but also plays a critical role in reducing PACU length of stay, ultimately making the transition to the inpatient floor or home easier. Research indicates that maximizing pain management can reduce postoperative complications, further highlighting the PACU's role in recovery (Baek et al., 2010).

When patients recover and come around from the anesthetic, the staff of the PACU uses numerous interventions to avoid complications, such as nausea or respiratory depression, which are common after the administration of certain anesthetic drugs. Finally, the PACU is also an educational environment for patients and their relatives, providing vital information on postoperative care and recovery expectations. Educating patients on signs of complications, pain management measures, and activity restrictions creates an active role in their recovery and overall quality of care. This education is important because it enables patients to take charge of their health as they transition from PACU to the next phases of care. Ideal PACU communication also facilitates collaboration among healthcare providers, ultimately promoting strategies to improve patient outcomes and reduce medication administration or care delivery errors (Cadwalader et al., 2015). Thus, the PACU is not only interested in immediate recovery but also lays the groundwork for continued care, enabling enhanced long-term health outcomes among patients.

12.2.2. Staffing and Training Requirements

A good staffing model is central to the practice of post-anesthesia care, both safeguarding patient safety and quality of care. PACU requires a highly skilled workforce of nurses and practitioners who understand how to observe patients' recovery from anesthesia. Personnel should be educated in identifying manifestations of complications such as respiratory distress or altered consciousness, which are crucial in the early postoperative period. A good staffing ratio can truly impact patient outcomes; therefore, healthcare facilities must adhere to evidence-based best practices in determining the number of nurses to staff the PACU at any given time. A systematic resource capacity planning and control is crucial in this achievement, putting the healthcare managers in a position to make adequate decisions on staff levels and skill mix to enhance patient safety within the PACU (Boucherie et al., 2011). Training and education are significant components in establishing an effective workforce in the PACU environment. Nurses and other healthcare professionals require extensive training encompassing both theoretical proficiency and practical skills in post-anesthesia care. Such training is typically conducted through simulation exercises and on-site practice in identifying and managing potential complications. Additionally, ongoing professional development is necessary to update the employees on the latest advances in anesthesia technology and postoperative care. Enhancing staff knowledge and confidence through regular training sessions ultimately leads to improved patient outcomes. Evidence supports that well-trained staff can implement protocols that ensure patient comfort and safety during the recovery stage, underscoring the need for investments in high-quality training programs (Balatero et al., 2018). Moreover, the inclusion of interdisciplinary teamwork within the PACU significantly influences staffing effectiveness and the general healthcare delivery model. Cooperation among anesthesiologists, nurses, respiratory therapists, and other health professionals is required for the coordinated care of anesthesia-recovery patients. Interdisciplinary education enhances shared role and responsibility, understanding, communication, and workflow in the PACU. Teamwork enhances the effectiveness of interventions and the timely delivery of care. By placing a strong emphasis on a collaborative culture, hospitals can optimize staff resources while enhancing teams' capacity to manage the evolving needs of patients. Patient safety and satisfaction are further enhanced, establishing a leading standard of care in line with post-anesthesia care principles (Boucherie et al., 2011) (Figure 12.7).

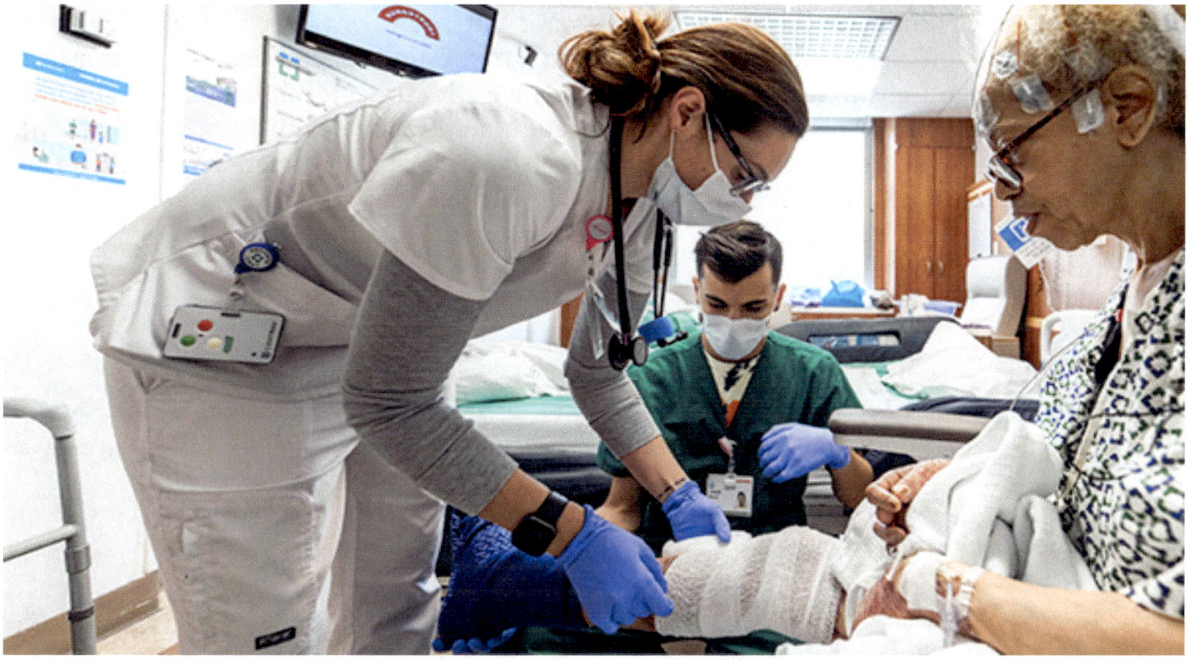

Figure 12.7. A robust staffing model is fundamental to the principles of post-anesthesia care.

Source: https://cdn-static.findly.com/wp-content/uploads/sites/2113/2022/12/06133737/HC15452-clvcln-cws-jobdescriptions-mobileheader-600x335-nursepatientsup.jpg.

12.2.3. Equipment and Technology Used in the PACU

The PACU has advanced technology and equipment designed to ease the monitoring and recovery of surgical patients. Central to such an environment are monitoring devices that provide immediate feedback on the patient's vital signs, such as heart rate, blood pressure, and oxygen saturation. This technology is critical for the immediate detection of postoperative complications, enabling prompt interventions. Apart from that, infusion pumps are used to administer medications and fluids intravenously, managing pain and hydration with high accuracy. Utilization of these machines not only ensures patient safety but also optimizes nursing workflow, allowing nurses to concentrate on critical elements of patient care throughout the recovery process. In recent years, technological advancements have also improved PACUs' operational effectiveness. The application of communication technologies has been observed to affect disturbances at work and international nurses' satisfaction in stressful environments such as the PACU. One study observed that improving the communication process through technology would lead to more interaction among perioperative teams, which in turn would produce better patient outcomes and efficiency in nursing (Martin et al., 2015). Yet, as with the initial findings indicating potential for improvement, the real impact on nursing performance was not extensive, suggesting that technological means alone cannot address the complex problems in such dynamic environments. Hence, a total approach, integrating efficient technology with qualified staff, must be given top priority to achieve the sought-after improvements in both patient care and employee satisfaction. Further exploration of equipment used in the PACU reveals specialized patient beds and safety and comfort equipment. Patient beds can be pre-mounted with electronic position control to enable patient evaluation and convalescence without placing undue stress on nursing staff. Further, the addition of suction equipment, oxygen therapy systems, and emergency equipment prepares the PACU for contingencies. Recent publications have called for ongoing evaluation of such equipment, specifically in its effectiveness at improving operational processes and patient care (Belien et al., 2025). As the future of post-anesthesia care continues to evolve, the strategic implementation of advanced equipment and technology will be essential to the success of safe, effective recovery processes for surgical patients.

Test Your Knowledge

1. What are the primary goals and functions of the Post-Anesthesia Care Unit in ensuring safe patient recovery after anesthesia?
2. Which vital parameters and clinical signs must be closely monitored in the PACU to detect early postoperative complications?

12.3. Patient Assessment in PACU

Learning Outcome

1. Vital signs monitoring
2. Pain assessment and management
3. Identification of complications

The PACU is a serious environment where patients are guaranteed safety and recovery during the postoperative period. Evaluation of the patient here is very important, as the nursing staff must evaluate a myriad of physiological parameters, from vital signs, consciousness level, to the severity of pain. To this effect, appropriate monitoring can prevent possible anesthesia complications, including respiratory depression or hemodynamic instability. Nurses use a variety of tools and measures, such as the numeric rating scale (NRS) for pain, to quantify and control patient pain effectively. Furthermore, this measurement process takes place in a high-stress, dynamic environment, necessitating rapid decision-making and effective communication among healthcare providers and family members, highlighting team-based care delivery in the PACU. To enhance the accuracy and efficacy of patient assessment in the PACU, emerging technologies are under consideration for their ability. One excellent example of advances in monitoring technology is the ANSPEC-PRO system, which uses bioimpedance analysis to more accurately measure nociceptive responses. The groundbreaking technique allows for continuous measurement of patient pain levels in real time, so interventions can be taken in a timely manner based on evolving patient needs. These innovations provide critical information that may supplement traditional evaluation methods, leading to better pain management therapies. The ANSPEC-PRO was recently validated in a trial of 26 patients in an observational setting, demonstrating its potential utility over traditional pain-monitoring instruments such as MEDSTORM. The encouraging findings of this trial highlight the importance of integrating advanced technology into post-anesthesia care practices, as it may significantly enhance the efficiency of patient assessment (Copot et al., 2020). In addition, the frequency of nurses' interruptions in the PACU is a problem that directly affects patient assessment and the quality of care.

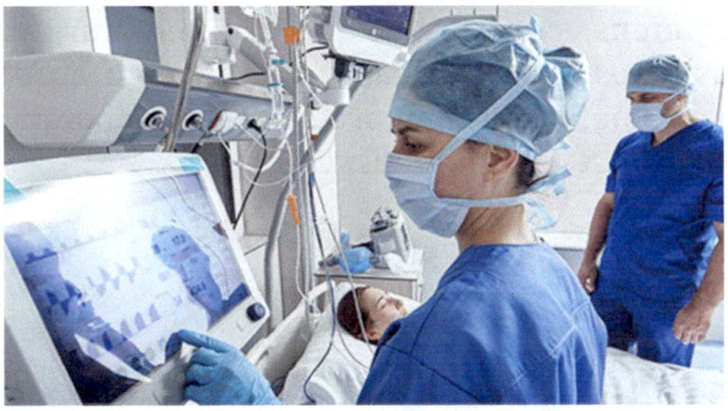

Figure 12.8. The post-anesthesia care unit (PACU) plays a critical role in ensuring patient safety and promoting recovery.

Source: https://members.acn.edu.au/images/acn/cpdlibrary/comprehensive-patient-assessment-and-management-in-the-pacu-500x280.jpg.

A more recent attempt to improve efficiency and nurse satisfaction in such a high-speed environment underscores the challenges faced in this setting. Even though the use of communication technology was intended to reduce such distractions, it did not have a significant impact on nursing efficiency. This points towards an engaging need for organizational improvements in the PACU, such as the incorporation of a clinical nurse leader (CNL) role to serve as a surgical nurse liaison. This initiative aims to foster communication and collaboration among the perioperative team to guarantee that evaluation of patients is conducted extensively and the center is always providing high-quality care. Introduction of a CNL with quality improvement skills later can ultimately reduce work interruptions and improve patient outcomes in the PACU (Martin et al., 2015) (Figure 12.8).

12.3.1. Vital Signs Monitoring

The value of monitoring vital signs following anesthesia cannot be overstated, as it is a central component of patient safety and recovery. The vital signs include heart rate, respiratory rate, blood pressure, and temperature, and as a group, they provide vital information about the physiological stability of the patient during the immediate postoperative period. Varying values from what is considered normal can yield clues to complications such as hypovolemia, respiratory distress, or inadequate analgesia. For instance, monitoring blood pressure and heart rate can detect premonitory signs of cardiopulmonary complications, prompting early intervention. In a case report of a 6-year-old skunk who was under anesthesia for a surgical procedure, hypoxemia was detected with vigilant monitoring of vital signs, emphasizing the importance of vigilant monitoring to prevent post-surgical complications (Marcilla et al., 2010). In addition, integration of new technologies into vital signs monitoring enhances the accuracy and reliability of data obtained. Monitoring equipment that continuously sends data provides real-time feedback on vital signs, allowing clinicians to respond quickly to any deviation from normal values. This capability is particularly vital in managing the variable physiologic responses during anesthesia recovery, when patients are exposed to variability in vital signs due to residual anesthetic effects or pain. Introduction of model-based control methods, which use feedback signals from monitoring devices, can make it possible to have more personalized interventions in managing a patient's analgesic needs (Chevalier et al., 2013). Therefore, such a development not only increases the practitioner's ability to maintain homeostasis but also minimizes risks encountered during recovery from anesthesia. Ultimately, careful monitoring of vital signs is paramount to enhancing a patient's well-being and ensuring an uneventful recovery from anesthesia. Use of standardized protocols for monitoring and assessing vital signs in a clinical setting is important to minimizing risks and maximizing patient care. In the post-anesthetic care period, careful assessment encompassing not only vital signs but also pain, consciousness, and general physical status is needed to identify potential complications early. As experience has demonstrated, early intervention, such as vigorous monitoring, can significantly reduce morbidity rates. Thus, with advancements in anesthesiology, vigilance is at the center of post-anesthesia care guidelines, ensuring patient safety in both routine and complex surgical procedures.

12.3.2. Pain Assessment and Management

Effective pain assessment and management are integral parts of post-anesthesia care, not just to patient comfort but also to the rate of recovery. Pain is a subjective experience; therefore, it requires an assessment approach that includes a range of self-report, observational, and clinical assessment tools. Clinicians must be skilled in applying a variety of pain scales appropriate to the patient's age and cognitive ability, especially in pediatric patients. Understanding pain during postoperative recovery enables clinicians to devise tailored management strategies that address patients' unique needs. Secondly, a thorough assessment allows the identification of chronic pain risk factors, thereby facilitating preventive interventions that healthcare providers can implement during the postoperative period. Use of multimodal analgesia is crucial in the prevention of opioid use and the reduction of risks associated with long-term use. Through the inclusion of various pharmacological as well as non-pharmacological methods, physicians can create a sound pain relief regimen that addresses numerous mechanisms of pain. For instance, application of regional anesthesia techniques may significantly lower systemic opioid demands while enhancing patient satisfaction. With the evolving pain management paradigm, collaboration between anesthesiologists and surgeons is critical; shared efforts in intraoperative medication plans and postoperative pain control strategies can significantly impact patient outcomes. Additionally, the use of advanced recovery pathways that incorporate customized pain regimens contributes to optimal surgical outcomes, thereby enabling patients to have a more comfortable and productive postoperative experience (Pozek et al., 2018).

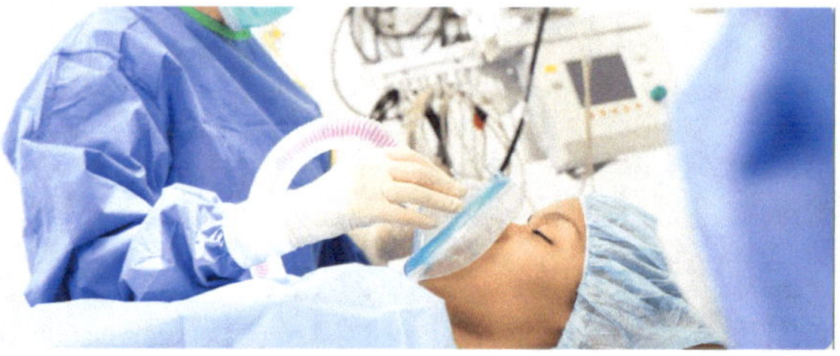

Figure 12.9. The pain assessment and management are critical components of post-anesthesia care.

Source: https://gargashhospital.com/uploads/blogs/24.png.

Second, and more particularly, there is a special challenge in managing pain in cases of pediatric cancers, where procedure pain comes to dominate the disease itself. The patient with cancer has a sequence of painful procedures, from diagnostic to therapeutic procedures, which are painful even though malignancy should not be painful usually. Adequate pain management in the population in question should address not only pharmacological but also psychological interventions. Cognitive-behavioral therapy, relaxation training, and preparation are among the techniques that can effectively alleviate distress and enhance coping abilities among adolescent patients. By placing both the physical and psychological aspects of pain control in pediatric oncology at the forefront, clinicians can significantly improve both the quality of care and the patient's experience during a challenging time (Liossi et al., 1999) (Figure 12.9).

12.3.3. Identification of Complications

In post-anesthetic care, recognition of complications is the most critical aspect of patient safety and recovery. Anesthetics are very safe, but, if anything, they may produce a variety of complications in the immediate postoperative period. Recognition of early warning signs of harmful events, such as respiratory depression, cardiovascular instability, or over-sedation, can make a massive difference in outcomes. Respiratory complications are damaging to oxygenation and require immediate correction to prevent hypoxia. Health care providers attention to monitoring the vital signs and patient response is critical, as these results not only enable timely intervention but also enable an adequate assessment of the patient's post-anesthesia status. For this reason, the inclusion of standard operating procedures for early detection of complications is significant, particularly in high-surgical-complexity institutions. Patient care with the more advanced forms of surgery, such as microvascular reconstructive surgeries, suggests the significance of recognizing complications. Anesthetic management becomes a significant consideration in patient outcomes in these situations, particularly as far as the probability of serious complications, such as hypoperfusion of flaps, is concerned. Present evidence indicates that careful monitoring and appropriate anesthetic management are effective in preventing this risk. A systematic review has established that awareness of hemodynamic changes and the use of special indicators, such as the hypotension probability indicator (HPI), can improve postoperative care by proactively managing variations in mean arterial pressure. The benefit of employing enhanced recovery protocols also underscores the importance of multidisciplinary collaboration in recognizing and addressing potential complications on the fly, while ensuring patient care is holistic and sensitive to dynamic clinical situations (GM et al., 2018). Moreover, effective communication within the healthcare team is critical for recognizing and managing complications in the post-anesthesia care setting. During recovery from anesthesia, the patient's status may change rapidly due to a variety of factors, including fluid balance, pain management, and the body's response to surgery. Joint discussions among surgeons, anesthetists, and nurses would improve the understanding of the patient's status and allow early intervention programs in the event of complications. For example, when a patient is hemodynamically unstable, immediate communication provides for collective action to enhance patient safety. Furthermore, continuous education and training of professionals on possible complications and early detection establishes a culture that prioritizes vigilance over everything else, ultimately leading to improved patient outcomes during the critical recovery phase (Blugerman et al., 2011).

Test Your Knowledge

1. What key parameters should be assessed in patients in the PACU to ensure safe recovery and effective pain control?
2. How do standardized pain assessment tools and multimodal analgesia strategies improve postoperative pain management in the PACU?

12.4. Recovery Process

Learning Outcome

1. Phases of recovery from anesthesia
2. Criteria for discharge from PACU
3. Role of the anesthesiologist in recovery

The post-anesthesia recovery process is a critical period that significantly influences patient outcomes. Adequate monitoring and observation during the period are important to prevent complications and ensure a smooth recovery in the operating room. Control of pain, level of sedation, and hemodynamic stability are among the factors that affect recovery. Adequate control of pain not only enhances patient comfort but also facilitates early mobilization, which is critical for overall recovery. Following findings from recent comparative studies, the use of tools such as the ANSPEC-PRO provides a quantitative method for measuring pain intensity, yielding data that can guide clinical interventions during the recovery process (Copot et al., 2020). Monitoring of patient's acute pain response guides the administration of analgesics, and responses can change accordingly, which enables the quality of care being delivered to be optimal within the immediate postoperative period. Together with pain relief, recovery involves evaluating the patient's return to baseline physiological function, including vigilance and the ability to perform daily activities. Clinical examination typically involves observing vital signs such as blood pressure, pulse, and oxygen saturation, as well as evaluating the patient's level of consciousness and responsiveness. Research indicates that recovery time should not only focus on physical recovery measures but also on patient-oriented outcomes like satisfaction and emotional well-being (Holmes et al., 2011). Tracking these facets is particularly important in modern healthcare as they play a pivotal role in determining overall patient experience. Key recovery pathways aim to maximize such assessments in order to provide patients with immediate attention based on their unique needs following anesthesia. Last but not least, the outcome of the recovery process is incorporated into post-anesthesia care ideas that aim to prevent complications and enhance overall recovery. Multidisciplinary cooperation among health professionals, including anesthesiologists, nurses, and pain management specialists, plays a crucial role in achieving successful patient outcomes. A smooth recovery plan with the inclusion of evidence-based practices, coupled with real-time monitoring of recovery parameters, aids in the identification of any deviation patterns from normal recovery at an early stage. Such proactive management is imperative, as it not only guarantees patient safety but also maximizes the utilization of healthcare resources. By ensuring a comprehensive strategy towards care and observation, the recovery process can maximize patient satisfaction and maximize long-term postoperative results, thereby upholding the principles of optimal post-anesthesia care (Figure 12.10).

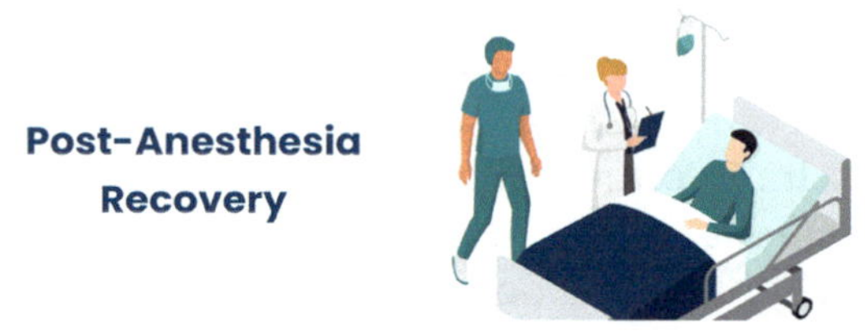

Figure 12.10. The recovery process following anesthesia is a critical phase that significantly influences patient outcomes.

Source: https://www.medicoverhospitals.in/images/articles/post-anesthesia-recovery-begumpet.webp.

12.4.1. Phases of Recovery from Anesthesia

The emergence from anesthesia to consciousness is a multifaceted process that can be divided into distinct phases, each of which is critical to the patient's safety and comfort. In the first phase, known as the emergence phase, the patients transition from unconsciousness to a state of wakefulness. Strict monitoring is needed during this time as the patients exhibit differential states of responsiveness depending on the anesthetic drugs given. This phase is characterized by the recovery of patients' airway reflexes, spontaneous breathing, and responsiveness to simple commands. Anesthesiologists must remain vigilant during this time, as airway obstruction can arise. A calm, soothing environment needs to be established to facilitate an easy transition, as this first stage lays the foundation for subsequent recovery milestones that dictate overall patient satisfaction and outcomes. Then there is the recovery phase, in which patients regain their faculties and start to reorient themselves after surgery. This is an essential phase for assessing pain control and for concluding that patients are stable enough to be moved to a less intensive recovery area. Multimodal analgesia techniques are of most value at this point, as they tend to counteract pain while lowering opioid consumption, minimizing the potential for complications and side effects that can occur in long-term opioid use. Collaboration between anesthesiologists and surgical teams can help integrate pain management techniques more closely in this phase of care, ultimately resulting in a faster and more effective recovery process. These protocols can be adjusted based on the individual needs of patients to minimize the causative factors of prolonged distress, such as anxiety or underlying medical conditions, as illustrated by Pozek et al. (2018). Recovery to homeostasis is the final phase of anesthesia recovery that sees patients regain normal physiological functions and are prepared for discharge. At this stage, frequent monitoring is crucial in order to identify any potential complications or lingering symptoms. The application of advanced monitoring technology, such as the ANSPEC-PRO device, can enable more effective objective quantification of patient pain intensity over time, as outlined in Copot et al. (2020). Use of such high-tech devices enables healthcare providers to tailor post-discharge plans to the individual patient's course of recovery, with unbroken, effective pain control extended even beyond the clinic setting. Understanding the importance of these stages, healthcare professionals can use evidence-based post-anesthesia care principles to optimize patient outcomes and enhance overall satisfaction during the recovery process.

12.4.2. Criteria for Discharge from PACU

In PACU, discharge criteria are vital for patient safety and satisfaction. The discharge criteria typically include stable vital signs, satisfactory respiratory status, and absence of unresolved pain or adverse effects of anesthesia. The patient should exhibit an improvement in level of consciousness to baseline or higher, reflecting the safe resolution of the anesthetic effect. In addition, the effectiveness of pain-control interventions is assessed to ensure patients can smoothly transition to the next phase of recovery without discomfort. Through these standards, not only is patient safety guaranteed, but complications are also minimized in the event of sending a patient home prematurely, emphasizing the critical role of PACU in the post-anesthetic care process. In addition to physiological evaluations, patients' psychological readiness is also a vital component of discharge criteria from PACU. Measures such as the readiness for hospital discharge scale (RHDS) can assist healthcare providers in evaluating patients' attitudes toward readiness, including knowledge of discharge instructions and perceived capacity to manage postoperative care at home. The instrument has been found to have good psychometric properties and hence enables practitioners to make decisions regarding patient readiness for discharge. When patients have clarity on their recovery plan, with or without follow-up care as may be required, it not only facilitates easier transition but also encourages active involvement in the recovery process, reiterating the holistic nature of discharge criteria. Last but not least is the critical role of good communication in the PACU as it has a direct impact on the discharge process. Inefficiencies and added stress to the nursing staff can result from communication breakdowns in the PACU, ultimately affecting patient outcomes. The use of communication technologies has been explored as a potential solution to enhancing workflow and minimizing disruptions in this frantic setting. The integration of these types of strategies, along with improved discharge criteria, could lead to increased patient and nurse satisfaction. For instance, the establishment of a surgical nurse liaison role could help bridge communication gaps, thereby allowing nurses to focus on direct patient care and making the discharge process more efficient, as noted in relevant research studies (Figure 12.11).

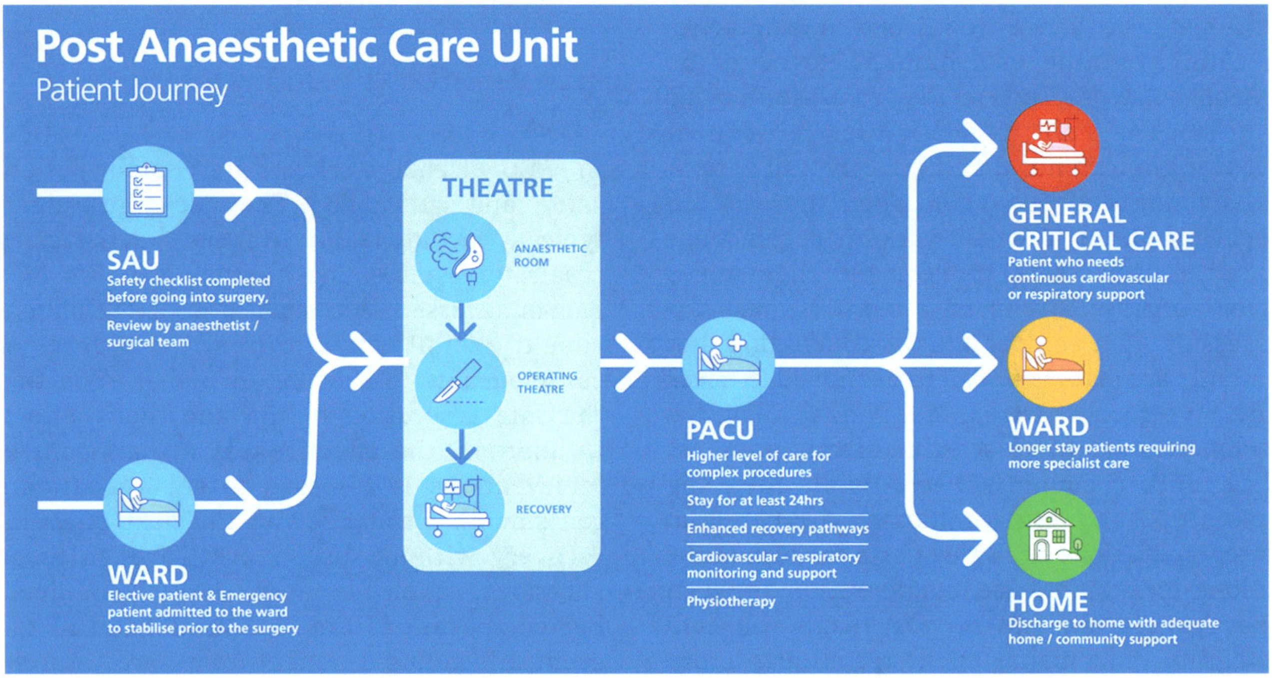

Figure 12.11. The criteria for discharge from the post-anesthesia care unit (PACU).

Source: https://www.southtees.nhs.uk/wp-content/uploads/2024/07/PACU-patietn-journey-800x400.jpg.

12.4.3. Role of the Anesthesiologist in Recovery

The anesthesiologist's function in post-anesthesia recovery is crucial in ensuring patient safety and comfort. Anesthesiologists must continue to monitor vital signs and neurological status as patients recover from anesthesia to an alert state. Monitoring of patients' pain and any complications due to anesthesia or surgery also falls within their functions. By using advanced monitoring devices, such as the ANSPEC-PRO tool, anesthesiologists can evaluate nociceptive responses in real time. This new technique provides comprehensive pain assessments and enables timely interventions to enhance recovery outcomes. Here, the anesthesiologist's skill not only allows easy recovery from anesthesia but also conditions for effective pain management techniques necessary for postoperative well-being (Copot et al., 2020). In this context, anesthesiologists have a leading role to play in the implementation of multimodal analgesia strategies designed to reduce opioid consumption during recovery. The impact of opioid abuse is severe, from chronic pain to addiction issues. Given that some of these patients are at risk for the development of chronic postsurgical pain, it then becomes incumbent upon anesthesiologists to implement varied modes of analgesia to address different patient profiles. For instance, regional anesthesia decreases the need for systemic opioids appreciably, allowing smoother recovery and reduction of side effects. Additionally, collaboration with surgical groups enhances the efficiency of postoperative pain management, upholding an integrative model of patient care that is essential in enhanced recovery pathways (Pozek et al., 2018). Last but not least, anesthesiologists' contribution to postoperative recovery goes beyond simple observation of the patient during the immediate postoperative time to encompass long-term outcomes. By meticulous assessment and titration of analgesic regimens based on the unique needs of each patient, anesthesiologists effectively prevent complications from ineffective pain control. The provision of care for pre-existing risk factors for long-term opioid use, such as a history of drug abuse or anxiety, highlights the role of the anesthesiologist during preoperative preparation and counseling of patients. Through continued engagement with patients throughout the perioperative process, anesthesiologists not only enhance recovery outcomes but also advocate for practices that improve the general well-being and safety of surgical patients in the postoperative period. Such efforts are thus core to providing the best possible surgical results consistent with post-anesthesia care principles.

Test Your Knowledge

1. What are the different phases of recovery from anesthesia, and what physiological changes occur in each phase?
2. What is the role of the anesthesiologist in monitoring, managing complications, and ensuring safe recovery during the postoperative period?

12.5. Complications and Interventions

Learning Outcome

1. Common complications post-anesthesia
2. Immediate interventions for complications
3. Long-term monitoring and follow-up care

Post-anesthesia recovery is a critical stage where anesthesia and surgical complications must be meticulously watched and addressed. One such concern is the risk of chronic postsurgical pain, which can complicate a patient's recuperation and lead to long-term opioid use. Such variables impacting this complication are preoperative opioid use, anxiety states, and substance abuse history. Managing such risks requires cooperation between the surgeon and anesthesiologist. Integrating multimodal analgesia protocols can prove beneficial in the sense of minimizing the need for opioids and creating a positive environment conducive to effective pain management. As the anesthesiologist customizes intraoperative drug regimes, he or she can reduce the risk of complications, ultimately contributing to better patient outcomes in the post-anesthesia care period (Pozek et al., 2018). Apart from pain management, the threat of pulmonary edema is another complication of post-anesthesia care.

Fluid overload administered during and after surgery results in pulmonary edema, which affects lung function and halts patient recovery. Successful treatment involves careful monitoring of fluid administration and implementing protocols that curb inflammatory processes and capillary permeability. Techniques like transpulmonary thermodilution (TPTD) have also been valuable tools in the healthcare provider's toolbox, yielding quantitative data on lung water deposition. Early diagnosis of fluid alterations can help prevent complications from overt pulmonary edema through intervention guidance. Not only do the technologies contribute to monitoring capability, but also to risk stratification, thus enabling individualized therapeutic interventions for critically ill patients in the perioperative setting (Assaad et al., 2017).

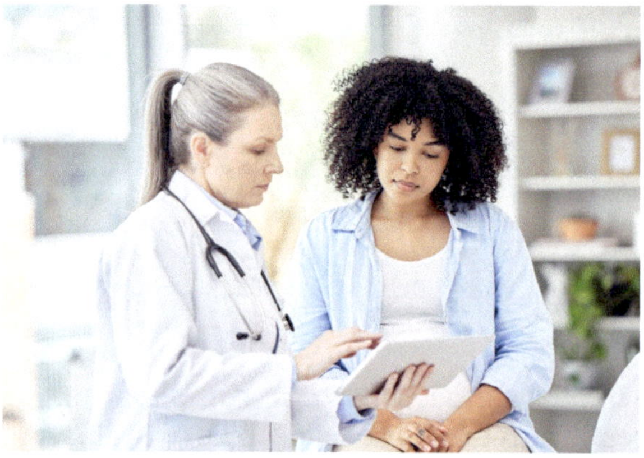

Figure 12.12. Post-anesthesia care encompasses a critical phase in which complications stemming from anesthesia.

Source: https://rivannamedical.com/wp-content/uploads/2024/10/shutterstock_2311883377.jpg.

The implementation of enhanced recovery pathways is further evidence of a proactive approach to managing post-anesthesia complications. Pathways make the continuum of care easier to navigate, as clinicians can optimize outcomes through systematic approaches. By facilitating early mobilization, nutritional supplementation, and adequate pain management, the recovery pathway prevents both surgical and anesthetic complications. They are typically discharged sooner, with higher overall satisfaction and lower complications. The organization of multidisciplinary teams also ensures that every stage of a patient's recovery process is considered, addressing both physical and mental problems. Ongoing evaluation and adaptation of these pathways will be necessary to accommodate evolving practice and emerging evidence, in order to deliver the highest quality care to the patient recovering from anesthesia (Assaad et al., 2017; Pozek et al., 2018) (Figure 12.12).

12.5.1. Common Complications Post-Anesthesia

Post-anesthetic care is a critical part of patient recovery, but various complications are expected following surgical procedures. Nausea, vomiting, and slow emergence from anesthesia are some of the predominant complications that usually take up clinical discussion space. These complications are most frequent during the first few hours postoperatively, when the patients' reaction to anesthesia can lead to pain and complications that could prolong the recovery time. Adequate management of such symptoms is crucial; it involves early assessment and intervention by the PACU nursing staff. Taking proactive actions, such as administering antiemetic drugs and strict monitoring, can go a long way to minimize the occurrence of such commonplace complications and hence enhance patient outcomes in the postoperative period. Treatment of such issues at an early point not only alleviates patient distress but may also assist in speeding up the return to the next phases of recovery. In addition, patients can experience respiratory complications after anesthesia. Postoperative respiratory depression is an important issue, particularly in individuals receiving opioids for pain management. The presence of residual anesthetic agents in the system can compromise airway reflexes and respiratory drive, resulting in hypoxemia or even respiratory arrest. Close monitoring of respiratory status is essential in identifying at-risk patients, particularly those with existing respiratory disease or postoperative patients following general anesthesia. By employing multimodal analgesia protocols, such as the use of non-opioid analgesics and regional anesthesia techniques, opioid use can be minimized and thereby the possibility of such respiratory complications (Pozek et al., 2018). Proper care strategies in post-anesthesia care will ensure patient safety and recovery. Furthermore, chronic postoperative pain is also a common complication that must be given due attention. Though most patients have tolerable pain after surgery, a proportion have chronic pain that hinders their recovery. The causes of this complication can be pain tolerance differences among patients, the type of surgery, and prior psychological states. Preoperative anxiety having a relation to persistent pain means that psychological interventions are also powerful for pain management (Pozek et al., 2018). develop personalized pain treatment plans that incorporate pharmacologic and non-pharmacologic interventions, encouraging a multidisciplinary approach to pain management. Postoperative education can also enable patients to actively engage in their own care postoperatively, reducing the risk of complications and overall increased satisfaction with the surgical experience (Figure 12.13).

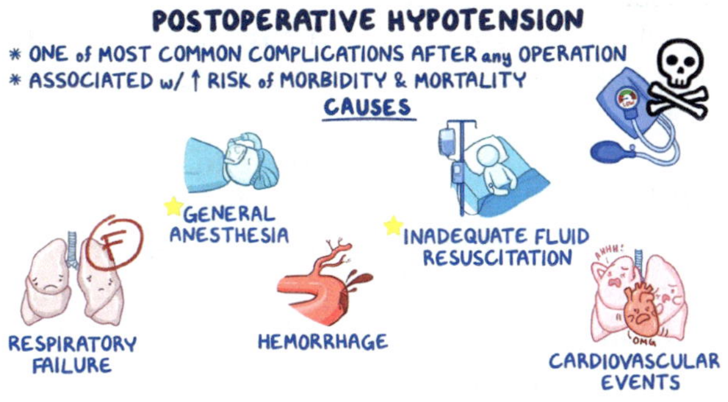

Figure 12.13. Common complications post-anesthesia.

Source: https://www.osmosis.org/_next/image?url=https%3A%2F%2Fd16qt3wv6xm098.cloudfront.net%2FUmX8Av1lSwefKUVNj-nCUE9XR-iCz_8W%2F_.jpg&w=3840&q=75.

12.5.2. Immediate Interventions for Complications

Early intervention is key in post-anesthesia care to manage potential complications that arise after surgery. A key area of concern here is the risk of opioid overdose leading to chronic postsurgical pain. The condition tends to become apparent in a limited period after surgery, and early intervention is therefore critical. The collaborative effort between surgeons and anesthesiologists is essential to managing the condition. By developing tailored intraoperative medication regimens and postoperative pain management strategies, clinicians can potentially reduce opioid use by a significant margin. Implementation of multimodal analgesia guidelines not only reduces opioid use but also enhances patient outcomes overall, with evidence to support being an aggressive approach towards pain management. These interventions ultimately aim to counter the risk of chronic opioid use and improve patients' recovery patterns, which is paramount in post-anesthesia care guidelines (Pozek et al., 2018). The most common complication requiring immediate adjustment is tissue edema, particularly pulmonary edema. Fluid management in post-anesthesia care practices is a fundamental component, where over-resuscitation has detrimental effects. Effective management techniques that all clinicians should adopt include monitoring and restricting fluid intake, thereby reducing inflammatory processes and capillary permeability. Advances in recent monitoring technologies, such as transpulmonary thermodilution (TPTD), provide informative information about lung water overload and other hemodynamic parameters, enabling more accurate fluid therapy. Clinicians can detect early signs of fluid imbalance before overt pulmonary edema using TPTD. This active monitoring not only enhances patient safety but also facilitates timely decision-making in high-risk surgical patients, which is essential in the practice of post-anesthesia care principles (Assaad et al., 2017).

Furthermore, the identification and management of emergent post-anesthesia complications require acute awareness of patient-specific factors influencing recovery. Complications may manifest as shifts in vital signs, altered mentation, or unexpected behavioral responses that require immediate clinical interventions. The use of systematic evaluation protocols ensures that abnormal recovery patterns are identified and addressed in a timely manner. interventions such as supplemental oxygen for hypoxia or intravenous fluid replacement for dehydration can have a striking effect on patient outcome. Additionally, comprehensive education of nursing staff and caregivers on the identification of post-anesthesia complications ensures an immediate and effective response. This proactive approach espouses a safe recovery environment, reflective of the principles of post-anesthesia care, and stresses the needs and well-being of patients during this acute phase of recovery. Such actions demonstrate a commitment to vigilant monitoring and intervention in the postoperative phase, as critical to preserving positive surgical outcomes.

12.5.3. Long-Term Monitoring and Follow-Up Care

Long-term follow-up and observation are integral components of post-anesthesia care, in which patients receive complete treatment following recovery from anesthesia. This is a very crucial period for the identification of any post-operative pains that may arise in a subset of patients after surgical treatment, like chronic pain or opioid use for an extended duration. Follow-up can prevent these complications if done appropriately, as pain management modalities are readjusted and medications are titrated. For instance, anesthesiologists can implement multimodal analgesia strategies that not only reduce the use of opioids but also enhance overall recovery, thus satisfying today's standards for postoperative care. The role of healthcare professionals in keeping patients active and aware of potential drug side effects cannot be overstated (Pozek et al., 2018). Furthermore, individualized postoperative follow-up allows it to be treated early in patients who are likely to have chronic postoperative pain or complications. Risk factors for prolonged opioid use, such as preoperative exposure to opioids and a history of substance abuse, highlight the need for close postoperative follow-up. Regular follow-up visits allow health care providers to monitor these risk factors and offer individualized care plans that include both pain management and psychosocial support. This aggressive approach is especially relevant in the setting of enhanced recovery pathways, whose aim is to optimize surgical success with the fewest complications. Multidisciplinary collaboration among various health care professionals, such as pain management specialists and anesthesiologists, enhances the likelihood of successful long-term outcomes for patients who are likely to face difficulty with recovery (Pozek et al., 2018). Lastly, it is important to note that long-term follow-up and monitoring must be patient-oriented and tailored to individual needs. The use of electronic health records can also significantly facilitate efficient communication between patients and their clinical care teams, enabling better monitoring of recovery and timely interventions. Those patients who are engaged in active participation in their follow-up treatment are likely to be more satisfied and have better results. Patient education on postoperative expectations enhances a supportive environment for recovery. Ultimately, post-anesthesia care standards must be directed towards long-term follow-up as an integral part of patient safety and health, thereby reinforcing the emphasis on continuous evaluation and revision of care algorithms in cooperation with patient-directed goals (Bonica et al., 2017) (Figure 12.14).

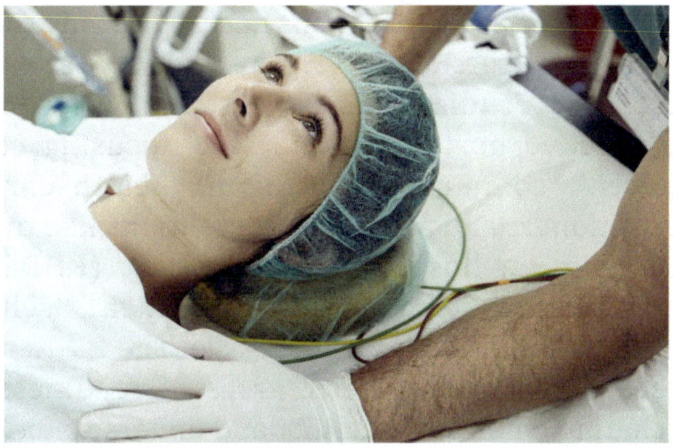

Figure 12.14. Long-term monitoring and follow-up care are integral components of post-anesthesia care.

Source: https://www.verywellhealth.com/thmb/w-cV8ALONTgbp1rMdot1cKmRRjU=/1500x0/filters:no_upscale():max_bytes(150000):strip_icc()/operating-nurse-soothing-patient-on-table-in-operating-room-596435375-57ab2f223df78cf4597c4dc7.jpg.

Test Your Knowledge

1. What are the common complications observed during the post-anesthesia period, and what immediate interventions are required to manage them?
2. How does early detection and timely intervention in the PACU help prevent serious postoperative outcomes?

12.6. Patient Education and Support

Learning Outcome

1. Importance of patient education post-surgery
2. Resources for patients and families
3. Strategies for effective communication

Effective patient education and support are critical components of post-anesthesia care, with direct consequences for patient outcomes and recovery experience. Anesthesia-treated patients can be in a state of vulnerability, expressed as confusion and altered sensory perceptions. Thus, the delivery of brief, clear, and individualized educational information about post-anesthesia expectations is critical to enhancing patients' knowledge retention and alleviating anxiety. Apparently, keeping patients well-informed about their immediate postoperative care, such as signs of potential complications and pain-relief techniques, allows them to assume responsibility for their own care. Evidence has shown that a well-organized educational process is related to greater patient satisfaction and lower hospital readmissions. By empowering patients with relevant information, health care practitioners foster a therapeutic relationship focused on self-care and adherence to postoperative instructions, thereby setting the stage for successful recovery. In addition, patient discharge readiness is an essential element of effective post-anesthesia care, focusing on effective communication among health care practitioners and patients. Interventions like the readiness for hospital discharge scale (RHDS) have been developed to quantify patients' self-reports of readiness for discharge. The 23-item measure assesses several areas of readiness, including emotional stability and understanding of follow-up care (Piacentine et al., 2006).

Utilizing such tools not only aids in assessing patient readiness but also aids in identifying those in need of further education or intervention before discharge. Hence, addressing these needs enhances the overall quality of care in the post-anesthesia period. With a focus on the patient's individual experience and perception, the healthcare team can better facilitate discharge procedures that align with patient expectations and needs. Finally, it is noteworthy that educational programs must adapt to evolving surgical practice to remain practical and relevant. The reported lack of attention to current surgical practice in nursing schools highlights a gap that should be addressed to enhance post-anesthesia care (Mitchell et al., 2005). By integrating current surgical methods and their implications into nursing programs, future nurses will be better able to provide targeted and evidence-based patient education. This alignment not only benefits nurses' professional development but also directly advances the provision of accurate and relevant information to patients. In conclusion, fostering a culture of ongoing education and support within nursing can significantly improve patient outcomes in post-anesthesia care, underscoring the pivotal role of patient education in the broader pursuit of healthcare excellence.

12.6.1. Importance of Patient Education Post-Surgery

Effective postoperative patient education is key to furthering healing and avoiding complications. Because of the consequences of anesthesia, patients are often disoriented, uncomfortable, and mentally slowed, sometimes keeping them from properly comprehending postoperative care instructions. Therefore, patient-specific education initiatives can enhance patient comprehension, ultimately resulting in enhanced compliance with recovery protocols. Evidence indicates that accurate, brief information on medication management, activity restrictions, and warning signs following surgery is crucial for preventing readmission and ensuring optimal outcomes. Postoperative time is a critical influence on the recovery course; as such, nursing professionals must place education at the top to empower patients and instill confidence in their ability to take care of themselves. These anticipatory measures not only aid recovery but also enhance patient autonomy by putting individuals in the driver's seat of their own recovery processes. Moreover, the effectiveness of educational interventions is boosted through personalized teaching methods that consider an individual's unique context, e.g., his/her prevailing knowledge, cultural background, and individual preferences. The application of a variety of learning aids—e.g., visual aids, written data, and oral advice—may meet various learning needs and enhance information retention. One study conducted in Day Surgery Units suggested that pre-registration training for nurses does not fully cover modern surgical practice, indicating a need for continuing education for healthcare professionals to remain up to date with current standards. Through expanded communication and ensuring that patient education methods are part of healthcare professionals' toolkits, the quality of care is significantly improved. The blended process maximizes the overall effectiveness of post-anesthesia care and minimizes the risk of complications, leading to an unproblematic transition from surgery to rehabilitation. Last but not least, feedback in the education process is very important in confirming knowledge retention and measuring the effectiveness of patient education programs. Regular follow-up, whether over the phone, via telehealth, or at a scheduled in-person visit, allows healthcare providers to address any areas of uncertainty that arise as patients progress through recovery. It is also an opportunity to remind patients of the key takeaways on medication adherence, activity levels, and side-effect monitoring. Active communication encourages patients to get clarification sooner, reducing the likelihood of complications. Besides, this supports the assertion that patient education is not an isolated event but a constant dialogue between patients and providers. As explicated through the review of pre-registration nurse training, the future of nursing encompasses embracing a culture of ongoing learning, enabling health professionals to educate patients appropriately in an evolving surgical landscape (Mitchell et al., 2005; Bonica et al., 2017) (Figure 12.15).

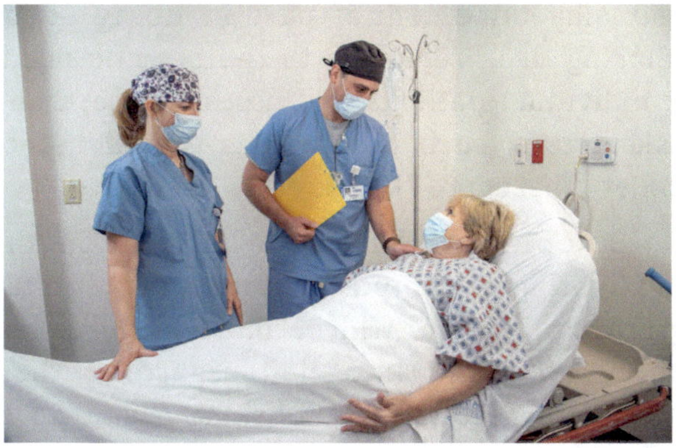

Figure 12.15. Importance of patient education post-surgery.

Source: https://www.matherhospital.org/wp-content/uploads/2021/06/Holding-Room-7-scaled.jpg.

12.6.2. Resources for Patients and Families

From a post-anesthesia care perspective, patient and family resources are paramount to ensuring a smooth transition from surgery to recovery. Anesthesia patients may experience different physical and emotional reactions afterwards, which is why it is important to provide sufficient support. Instructional materials that provide information on likely recovery processes, side effects, and self-care directions enable families to be actively engaged in the recovery process. Availability of such information promotes a sense of empowerment among relatives and patients, reducing fear and enhancing satisfaction with the treatment received. Moreover, resources such as helplines or support groups may offer an open line for the alleviation of concerns arising post-op. These resources help patients and family members bridge the gap between medical personnel and relatives, ensuring they do not feel abandoned as they navigate the complexities of recovery. Provider participation is essential in order to utilize resources effectively. Communication between patients, their families, and providers can have a profound impact on recovery outcomes. For instance, families with knowledge of the post-anesthesia care plan are better positioned to assess patients' status and provide early intervention when complications arise. In circumstances when such critical events do occur, as documented in the medical literature, access to supporting resources will buffer the experience of stress and develop resilience among caregivers and family members. Application of programs that support not just the recovering patient but also their relatives has been shown to enhance overall satisfaction with care experience, leading to improved health outcomes during the post-operative period. This combined view focuses on the inclusion of family involvement in post-anesthesia recovery plans. Ensuring that the needs of all concerned are addressed within the post-anesthesia program must be a collaborative effort among the healthcare teams. Healthcare institution leaders must prioritize creating and sharing policies that involve patients and families. For example, during crises like the COVID-19 pandemic, ethical dilemmas regarding resource allocation and prioritization of patient care have implications for both healthcare professionals and the families they serve. In addition to being diverted to clinical management, the resources also need to be directed towards managing open communication and providing emotional support for all concerned. Using models such as those outlined in attempts to improve healthcare, as currently established in the literature, organizations are more likely to navigate such issues. Upholding a commitment to patient and family resource enhancement is crucial to maintaining trust and enabling healthy care experiences across the care continuum (Hickey et al., 2019; Iserson et al., 2020) (Figure 12.16).

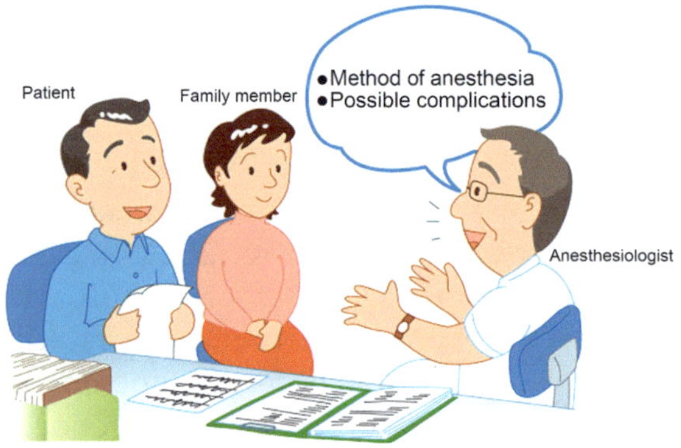

Figure 12.16. Resources for patients and families.

Source: https://anesth.or.jp/img/users/patient_guide_image_4_20200925.jpg?1604287835.

12.6.3. Strategies for Effective Communication

Effective communication in post-anesthesia care is crucial for achieving appropriate patient outcomes and satisfaction. Communicating effectively with patients regarding their surgical experience and expected recovery can indeed reduce anxiety and enhance trust. Medical professionals need to actively participate in dialogue involving the specifics of the anesthesia provided, possible side effects, and pain management techniques. This must be supported by written information that patients can refer to after discharge.

Because patients only retain part of what they are verbally communicated, supporting papers reinforce crucial information, enabling them to cope with recovery more effectively. Concentrating on an open-ended conversation among medical professionals and patients enhances comprehension and encourages patients to raise any concerns they may have during the recovery phase. The use of multimodal analgesia protocols is a communication strategy that directly impacts patient care in the post-anesthesia care unit. These protocols, which incorporate multiple modes of pain control, can be explained in detail to patients preoperatively so that informed decisions about pain control and opioid use can be made. Anesthesiologists also play an essential part in doing so by tailoring drug regimens to the specific needs of individual patients and assessing pertinent risk factors, such as previous opioid use or anxiety disorders (Pozek et al., 2018).

By openly sharing such information and highlighting the importance of an integrated approach, patients will be more likely to feel empowered and informed regarding their treatment. Secondly, establishing a culture of support encourages patients to ask questions, which in turn promotes better adherence to postoperative care and ultimately improved recovery outcomes. Finally, constant liaison amongst multidisciplinary teams is important for ensuring seamless post-anesthesia care. Effective teamwork entails regular briefings among surgeons, anesthesiologists, nurses, and pain specialists to review individual patients' cases and assess the effectiveness of administered analgesia. This integrative approach enables timely adaptations to pain management interventions and ongoing monitoring following recovery (Bonica et al., 2017). Applying standardized communication practices, such as checklists or electronic files, helps address gaps in patient information that affect continuity of care. In general, the synergy of precise guidelines and team collaboration in post-anesthesia care creates an environment that maximizes recovery while ensuring patients are cared for and informed along the way.

Test Your Knowledge

1. How does effective patient and family education improve recovery, compliance, and overall outcomes after anesthesia and surgery?
2. What types of educational resources and support services should be provided to patients and families to help them manage postoperative care at home?

SUMMARY

The post-anesthesia care guidelines are a fundamental protocol for enhancing patient safety and comfort following surgery. This period of care is critical, as it entails monitoring and management of potential anesthesia complications. Through systematic adherence to procedures, strict evaluation, and immediate intervention, healthcare providers can reduce risks to recovery during the postoperative period. A clear understanding of these principles benefits patients and reassures medical providers as they do the important work of sustaining health and wellness. Effective post-anesthesia care is more than a regulatory mandate; it reflects a dedication to delivering quality care with attention to patient safety and experience. The integration of extensive education and training for post-anesthesia practice is at the core of successful outcomes in this specialty of critical care. In educational settings, as explained in course material such as HMP 721.01 at the University of New Hampshire, post-anesthesia care principles reflect broader health practice management approaches centered on patient-oriented strategies (Bonica et al., 2017). Healthcare professionals must be trained in the physiological effects of anesthesia, potential complications, and proper postoperative care. Evidence-based practice-focused care providers are in a position to enhance their expert-level skills in monitoring patients and assisting in recovery from anesthesia to full awareness. Such training enhances patient care and harmonizes the interdisciplinary care necessary for optimal health outcomes. Finally, the evolving climate of anesthesiology and post-anesthesia care continually shapes and redefines best practice in the discipline. Evolving technology in monitoring and drugs supports the resilience of healthcare providers. As this analysis shows, the evolution of anesthesia and its utilization across various branches of medicine have underscored the importance of patient care as the hallmark of successful practice (Rang et al., 2015). Lastly, post-anesthesia care standards are based on a deep understanding of the ever-evolving science of anesthesia—and an ongoing commitment to further improvement in healthcare delivery. Embracing the complexities of patient recovery with dedication and expertise ensures not only the successful completion of surgery but also lays the groundwork for future growth in the science of anesthesiology.

In the post-anesthesia care environment, it is of primary importance to maintain patient safety and communication among healthcare providers. Effective communication is of primary importance in the post-anesthesia care unit (PACU), where nurses must work with patients, families, and a diverse group of surgical staff. High patient turnover rates can lead to frequent interruptions in nursing staff work, affecting the quality of care in this high-pressure environment. Integration of quality improvement initiatives, such as streamlining communication among members, is essential to reducing such disruptions, thereby improving nurse satisfaction and patient care. Prioritizing such adaptation highlights the complexity of care provided post-anesthesia and underscores the need to maintain interest in communication and workflow control in the PACU (Martin et al., 2015). The other important principle of post-anesthesia care is ensuring that a culture of safety exists within healthcare settings. Studies have shown that an environment in which medical team training is used to enable communication among staff is an important factor in reducing surgical mortality rates and improving overall quality of care. The implementation of standard communication practices, akin to those used in effective medical settings, can improve the timeliness and efficiency of postoperative patient management. Also, fostering organizational support, such as the VA's National Center for Patient Safety, promotes the certainty that healthcare practitioners are enabled to address safety concerns and conduct root-cause analyses once harm has ensued. Fostering a culture of safety and ongoing quality improvement advantages not only patients within the PACU but also staff morale and satisfaction (Chase et al., 2011). Lastly, effective post-anesthesia care is centered on thorough monitoring and assessment to detect complications as soon as possible. PACU nurses are tasked with constant observation of patients' vital signs, alertness levels, and pain control, all of which are significant to a successful recovery. Constant assessment enables detection of immediate post-operative and longer-term recovery complications. Besides, patient activation and education on postoperative care plans are effective ways to enhance compliance and satisfaction, resulting in improved health outcomes. Given the complexity of post-anesthesia recovery, nurses' roles in this environment are critical to addressing patient care complexities, ensuring responsiveness, and advocating for patients throughout the recovery process. By upholding these guidelines, health teams can administer high-quality and broad care during the crucial hours just after anesthesia (Martin et al., 2015).

KEY TERMS FROM THIS CHAPTER

Anesthesia
Anxiety
Electroencephalographic (EEG)
Holistic patient recovery
Patient education
Post-anesthesia care unit (PACU)
Anesthesiologists
Certified registered nurse anesthetists (CRNAs)
Healthcare
Patient assessment
Pharmacodynamics
Postoperative cognitive dysfunction (POCD)

CRITICAL THINKING QUESTIONS

1. **Which of the following is the most commonly used scoring system to assess readiness for discharge from the PACU?**
   a. Glasgow Coma Scale
   b. Aldrete Score
   c. ASA Physical Status
   d. Apgar Score
2. **What is the most common cause of airway obstruction in the immediate postoperative period?**
   a. Bronchospasm
   b. Laryngospasm
   c. Residual neuromuscular blockade
   d. Tongue falling back
3. **Which of the following is not a criterion in the Modified Aldrete Scoring System?**
   a. Activity
   b. Respiration
   c. Urine output
   d. Oxygen saturation
4. **The most appropriate initial management for hypoventilation in the PACU is:**
   a. Administer diuretics
   b. Increase IV fluids
   c. Provide ventilatory support and assess airway
   d. Give antiemetics
5. **Which of the following drugs is commonly used to treat postoperative shivering?**
   a. Ondansetron
   b. Ketorolac
   c. Meperidine
   d. Lidocaine

Short Answer Questions

1. Describe the key objectives of post-anesthesia care and the role of the Post-Anesthesia Care Unit (PACU).
2. Explain the criteria used to assess readiness for discharge from the PACU.
3. Outline the common respiratory complications in the immediate postoperative period and their management.
4. Discuss the causes and management of postoperative nausea and vomiting (PONV).
5. Describe the management of acute postoperative pain in the PACU.
6. Explain the causes, recognition, and treatment of postoperative hypotension in the PACU.

Answer to Critical Thinking Questions

1. (b); 2. (d); 3. (c); 4. (c); 5. (c)

REFERENCES

1. Assaad, S., Shelley, B., & Perrino, A. (2017). Transpulmonary thermodilution: Its role in assessment of lung water and pulmonary edema. *Journal of Cardiothoracic and Vascular Anesthesia, 31*(4), 1471–1480. https://doi.org/10.1053/j.jvca.2017.02.018Baek, C. W., Cha, S. M., Jung, Y. H., Kang, H., et al. (2010). The effects of changing from isoflurane to desflurane on the recovery profile during the latter part of anesthesia. https://core.ac.uk/download/12541579.pdf (accessed on 28th June 2025).
2. Balatero, J. S. (2018). Obstetric nurses' perceived barriers to immediate skin to skin contact after cesarean birth. https://core.ac.uk/download/159401074.pdf (accessed on 28th June 2025).
3. Belien, J., Cardoen, B., & Demeulemeester, E. (2025). Operating room planning and scheduling: A literature review. https://core.ac.uk/download/pdf/6347245.pdf (accessed on 28th June 2025).
4. Blugerman, G., D'Angelo, J. A., Habbema, L., Lisborg, R., et al. (2011). Application of the liposuction techniques and principles in specific body areas and pathologies. https://core.ac.uk/download/17179833.pdf (accessed on 28th June 2025).
5. Blumenthal, D., & McCarthy, D. (2006). *Committed to Safety: Ten Case Studies on Reducing Harm to Patients.* https://core.ac.uk/download/71350251.pdf (accessed on 28th June 2025).
6. Bonica, M., Students of Health Management 721.01, & University of New Hampshire. (2017). *Healthcare Management Primer*. https://core.ac.uk/download/215509297.pdf (accessed on 28th June 2025).
7. Boucherie, R. J., Hans, E. W., Hulshof, P. J. H., Kortbeek, N., et al. (2011). Taxonomic classification of planning decisions in health care: A review of the state of the art in OR/MS. https://core.ac.uk/download/pdf/11480704.pdf (accessed on 28th June 2025).
8. Brown, E. N., Pavone, K. J., Purdon, P. L., Sampson, A., et al. (2017). Clinical electroencephalography for anesthesiologists. https://core.ac.uk/download/127609503.pdf (accessed on 28th June 2025).
9. Cadwalader, J. (2015). Recreating the wheel: Redeploying pharmacy services to improve efficiency and patient safety. https://core.ac.uk/download/33562519.pdf (accessed on 28th June 2025).
10. Chase, D., & McCarthy, D. (2011). Advancing patient safety in the U.S. Department of Veterans Affairs. https://core.ac.uk/download/75777631.pdf (accessed on 28th June 2025).
11. Chevalier, A., Copot, D., De Keyser, R., Ionescu, C., et al. (2013). Fractional order impedance models as rising tools for quantification of unconscious analgesia. https://core.ac.uk/download/55782527.pdf (accessed on 28th June 2025).
12. Copot, D., Ghita, M., Ghita, M., Ionescu, C., et al. (2020). Pain detection with bioimpedance methodology from 3-dimensional exploration of nociception in a postoperative observational trial. https://core.ac.uk/download/322827629.pdf (accessed on 28th June 2025).
13. Golyanishchev, M. (2016). Hypothesis of Rfmra development–the receptor-focused magnetic and resonant anesthesia. https://core.ac.uk/download/301580510.pdf (accessed on 28th June 2025).

14. Gozalo Marcilla, M., Bosmans, T., Hellebuyck, T., De Decker, S., et al. (2010). Anesthetic and analgesic management of a skunk (*Mephitis mephitis*) undergoing a laminectomy for cauda equina compression. https://core.ac.uk/download/55759861.pdf (accessed on 28th June 2025).
15. Hanson, L., Kirby, R. S., & Tillett, J. (2005). Medical students' knowledge of midwifery practice after didactic and clinical exposure. https://core.ac.uk/download/213085474.pdf (accessed on 28th June 2025).
16. Hickey, J. V., & Slivinski, P. C. (2019). Implementation of a critical incident stress management program for nurse anesthetists. https://core.ac.uk/download/212903988.pdf (accessed on 28th June 2025).
17. Holmes, K. A., & Sneyd, J. R. (2011). Inhalational or total intravenous anesthesia: Is total intravenous anesthesia useful and are there economic benefits? https://core.ac.uk/download/29817529.pdf (accessed on 28th June 2025).
18. Iserson, K. V. (2020). Healthcare ethics during a pandemic. https://core.ac.uk/download/305124104.pdf (accessed on 28th June 2025).
19. Mitchell, M. J. (2005). Nursing knowledge and the expansion of day surgery in the United Kingdom. https://core.ac.uk/download/104292.pdf (accessed on 28th June 2025).
20. Piacentine, L., & Weiss, M. (2006). Psychometric properties of the Readiness for Hospital Discharge Scale. https://core.ac.uk/download/213077027.pdf (accessed on 28th June 2025).
21. Pozek, J. P. J., Schwenk, E. S., & Viscusi, E. R. (2018). Managing prolonged pain after surgery: Examining the role of opioids. https://core.ac.uk/download/213444274.pdf (accessed on 28th June 2025).
22. Prucher, G. M., Caporali, L., Lauretta, M. P., et al. (2018). Anesthetic challenging in microsurgical flap reconstruction: A systematic review. https://core.ac.uk/download/188826841.pdf (accessed on 28th June 2025).
23. Rang, A. (2015). Animal anesthesia: The race to recovery. https://core.ac.uk/download/41980349.pdf (accessed on 28th June 2025).
24. St. Martin, A. (2015). Inefficiency in the post anesthesia care unit: A quality improvement initiative. https://core.ac.uk/download/72052385.pdf (accessed on 28th June 2025).

INDEX

B

C